ESSENTIAL
HEALTH
ASSESSMENT

Janice Thompson, PhD, APRN, NP-C
Professor of Nursing
Quinnipiac University
Hamden, Connecticut

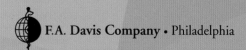

F.A. Davis Company • Philadelphia

F. A. Davis Company
1915 Arch Street
Philadelphia, PA 19103
www.fadavis.com

Printed in China

Last digit indicates print number: 10 9 8 7 6 5

Publisher, Nursing: Lisa B. Houck
Senior Content Project Manager: Elizabeth Hart
Electronic Project Manager: Sandra Glennie
Design and Illustration Manager: Carolyn O'Brien

As new scientific information becomes available through basic and clinical research, recommended treatments and drug therapies undergo changes. The author(s) and publisher have done everything possible to make this book accurate, up to date, and in accord with accepted standards at the time of publication. The author(s), editors, and publisher are not responsible for errors or omissions or for consequences from application of the book, and make no warranty, expressed or implied, in regard to the contents of the book. Any practice described in this book should be applied by the reader in accordance with professional standards of care used in regard to the unique circumstances that may apply in each situation. The reader is advised always to check product information (package inserts) for changes and new information regarding dose and contraindications before administering any drug. Caution is especially urged when using new or infrequently ordered drugs.

Library of Congress Cataloging-in-Publication Data

Names: Thompson, Janice (Professor of nursing), author.
Title: Essential health assessment / Janice Thompson.
Description: Philadelphia : F.A. Davis Company, [2017] | Includes bibliographical references.
Identifiers: LCCN 2016024586| ISBN 9780803627888 | ISBN 0803627882
Subjects: | MESH: Nursing Assessment–methods
Classification: LCC RT48 | NLM WY 100.4 | DDC 616.07/5–dc23 LC record available at https://lccn.loc.gov/2016024586

To all the nursing students around the world who will someday make a difference in patients' lives and all the practicing nurses who have already made a difference in patients' lives. I hope this text will provide you with the tools to safely and accurately assess your patients.

To my husband, Ken, and our four sons, as well as family and friends, who have stood by me trying to understand my drive to pursue this professional goal. Thank you for all your help, love, caring, and support to make this goal become a reality.

PREFACE

Health assessment is the foundation of safely caring for patients across the life span. Nurses need a concise, easy-to-follow guide that provides essential coverage of a routine head-to-toe focused or comprehensive health assessment. *Essential Health Assessment* is a new-generation core textbook for the undergraduate student nurse or a reference guide for the practicing nurse. Nurses must identify normal from abnormal findings and recognize when a finding is outside the spectrum of "normal." This book concentrates on essential, need-to-know information and techniques and excludes the nonessential information that does not need to be emphasized for health assessment. The focus is on typical findings, and abnormal findings are limited to those most commonly seen in clinical practice. A comprehensive review of systems and assessment techniques are in the print book, as well as documentation information on *DavisPlus* are provided to demonstrate how the nurse is to pull the assessment together. To cover health assessment across the life span, this book includes specialty chapters focusing on the newborn, pediatric, pregnant woman, and older adult populations.

Essential Health Assessment presents clear, sequential techniques with full-color step-by-step illustrations and photos. The size of this book makes it easy for students to carry to class or laboratory.

Chapter Organization and Standard Features

Each chapter is organized as follows:
Introduction
Review of Anatomy and Physiology
   Diagnostics
Health History
   Review of Systems
Preparation for Assessment
   Equipment Needed
   Sequence of Assessment
   Preliminary Steps
Focused Assessment
   Techniques, which include Normal and Abnormal Findings
Advanced Assessments
Patient Education

Within each chapter are the following standard features:

- **Review of Anatomy and Physiology** is a brief overview of basic anatomy and physiology of each body system as a refresher prior to assessment.
- **Diagnostics,** a section that appears immediately following the Review of Anatomy and Physiology, includes tests commonly used to assess and evaluate each body system.
- **Health History** covers the **Review of Systems,** which focuses on specific questions to identify present and past health patterns and history, health promotion practices, and cultural health beliefs. Risk factors are identified to alert the nurse to modifiable and nonmodifiable factors that can increase the likelihood of illness or disease. Examples guide students to gather subjective data about the patient's health status.
- **OLDCARTS Mnemonic** (Onset, Location, Duration, Characteristics, Aggravating/Alleviating factors, Relieving factors, Treatment, Severity) or the **OPQRST Mnemonic** (Onset, Provocation, Quality, Region or Radiation, Severity, Timing or Temporal): students are cued to use the mnemonics to identify attributes of a symptom.
- **Cultural Considerations** alert the reader to cultural variations influencing health beliefs and practices. Nurses provide culturally competent care by understanding and respecting a patient's health-care beliefs.

- **Preparation for Assessment** includes equipment, sequence, and any preliminary steps.
  - □ **Equipment** needed for each assessment is listed to help the nurse collect supplies prior to beginning the assessment.
  - □ **Sequence** and **Preliminary Steps** for the assessment offer guidance about organizing and preparing the patient and environment prior to performing the assessment.
  - □ **Techniques** are organized in a step-by-step sequence to guide the nurse to perform each assessment technique.
- **Advanced Techniques** are focused techniques that may be needed to further assess a specific system. The more common advanced techniques are at the end of each chapter, and the less commonly practiced assessments are documented online at *DavisPlus*.
- ***Healthy People 2020*** objectives and *United States Preventative Services Task Force* (USPSTF) recommendations have been integrated throughout chapters to alert students to current health promotion recommendations. Recommendations from other national specialty organizations provide the reader with references for patient education.
- **Patient Education** guides the nurse to health promotion topics that should be discussed with the patient for overall health and well-being.

Special Features

Special features are interspersed throughout each chapter to alert the reader to special considerations.

- **Tips** provide informative clinical information to help the student better understand the rationale for assessing an area or to alert students to a specific assessment finding.
- **Safe Effective Nursing Care (SENC)** is a key issue in nurses training and practice and is addressed in the following features:
  - □ **Patient-Centered Care** focuses on assessing the patient holistically as a full partner in care, keeping the patient informed and respecting the patient's values and needs. Holistic care reminds students that health assessment is more than techniques of the physical examination. Interviewing, actively listening, and teaching are critical components when providing individualized care.
  - □ **Safety Alerts** appear throughout the text. These alerts are intended to minimize risk for harm to the patient during assessment techniques and increase a nurse's awareness of assessment findings that need to be reported to the healthcare provider.
  - □ **Evidence-Based Practice** integrates best practices and new evidence in performing specific assessment techniques.
- **Cultural Considerations** boxes provide biocultural statistics, risks factors, or normal variants commonly seen in different cultures.

Student Resources

A wealth of resources on *DavisPlus* give students opportunities to reinforce and supplement their learning. Included in this toolbox are the following:

- **Advanced Assessment Techniques** are focused techniques that may be needed to further assess a specific system. All advanced techniques (print and online only) are compiled into one document for each relevant chapter for ease of use.
- **Audio Library** provides sample auscultation and percussion sounds.
- **Case Studies** are an exercise in critical thinking and documentation. Each case study provides a potential real-life clinical scenario with the scenarios taking place in a variety of healthcare settings. The case study will present normal and some of the more common abnormal variants. Students work through the three sections: Interview, Review of Systems, and Physical Assessment Finding, and practice documenting their findings.
- **Performance Checklists** are laboratory check-off sheets to document the steps of each technique and facilitate health assessment laboratory objectives.

Instructor Resources

- **Electronic Test Bank** has over 750 NCLEX-style questions, rationales, NCLEX descriptors, and page references for correct answers.
- **PowerPoint** presentations for each chapter augment instructor lectures, and interspersed **Clicker Questions** help evaluate student understanding.
- **Case Studies** are supplemental learning activities to reinforce critical thinking, documentation, and foundational health assessment knowledge. An answer key is provided to the instructor for each case study. Students are able to print out each case study and complete the documentation for in-class discussion or instructor review.
- The **Essential Health Assessment Practicum** is a comprehensive health assessment rubric for a 25-minute timed head-to-toe assessment. I have used this abbreviated assessment as a graded exercise at the end of the semester.

Health assessment is one of the core courses and skills that nurses will need throughout their nursing career. I hope that nursing students and practicing nurses develop and maintain the essential techniques to safely assess and care for patients. These health assessment techniques are foundational to nursing practice.

Janice Thompson, PhD, APRN, NP-C

ACKNOWLEDGMENTS

Coming together is a beginning: keeping together is progress; working together is success.

—Henry Ford

Writing a textbook is one of life's journeys that requires time, hard work, and perseverance to complete the project. This textbook would not have been published without the help and support of many individuals at F. A. Davis Company.

This text is a result of Lisa Houck, Publisher at F. A. Davis Company, having a vision that a new-generation textbook was needed for nursing students. Thank you, Lisa, for recognizing the need to publish innovative books that will enhance student learning.

I have had the privilege of working with Elizabeth Hart, Senior Content Project Manager, and Robin Richmond, Freelance Developmental Editor, who have been instrumental in giving me the strength and guidance needed to become an author. The expertise of both Liz and Robin helped me to achieve my goal. Thank you for your countless hours of outstanding support, guidance, and communication during this experience. I could not have done it without both of you.

Quinnipiac University (Hamden, Connecticut) has been my home away from home for many years. It is here that I have shared my knowledge of nursing and life with my students. I want to acknowledge and thank Quinnipiac University for the use of the health assessment labs during the photoshoot for this book. Also, I want to thank my colleagues for their encouragement and support throughout this scholarly endeavor.

Nursing is a helping profession. I would be remiss if I did not recognize the contributors, reviewers, and item writers who have helped me throughout many phases of this publication. I am very appreciative of your time and dedication to contribute to this textbook. By working together, you have all helped me to publish the first edition of *Essential Health Assessment*. Thank you!

CONTRIBUTORS

Cory Ann Boyd, EdD, RN
Associate Professor of Nursing
Quinnipiac University
Hamden, Connecticut
Chapter 22: Assessing the Child and Adolescent (co-author)

Jane Brophy, RN, MSN, CNM
Assistant Professor of Nursing
Trinity Washington University
Washington, DC
Chapter 21: Assessing the Newborn (co-author)

Kimberly Foisy, RN, MSN, CSMRN
Assistant Professor
Northern Essex Community College
Lawrence, Massachusetts
Chapter 17: Assessing the Neurological System (co-author)

Karen L. Gorton, PhD, RN, MS, ATC Ret.
Assistant Professor, Assistant Dean of Undergraduate Programs
University of Colorado College of Nursing—Anschutz Medical Campus
Aurora, Colorado
Chapter 16: Assessing the Musculoskeletal System (co-author)

Meredith J. Scannell, RN, CNM, MSN, MPH, PhD(c)
Clinical Instructor
Northeastern University
Research Nurse
Center for Clinical Investigation
Brigham and Women's Hospital
Boston, Massachusetts
Chapter 18: Assessing the Female Breasts, Axillae, and Reproductive System (co-author)

Leslie White, MSN, FNP-BC, APRN
Adjunct Faculty
Nurse Practitioner
Yale University; Quinnipiac University
New Haven, Connecticut
Chapter 23: Assessment of the Pregnant Woman

REVIEWERS

Sue Abuleal, MA, BSCN, RN
Nursing Educator
Camosun College
Victoria, British Columbia,
    Canada

**Carol Agana, MNSc, CNP,
    APRN**
Faculty
University of Arkansas
Eleanor Mann School of Nursing
Fayetteville, Arkansas

**Kathleen R. Albert, RN, MSN,
    CEN, CPEN**
Clinical Educator Emergency
    Department
Lowell General Hospital
Lowell, Massachusetts
Adjunct Faculty—RN-BSN
    Program
Emmanuel College
Boston, Massachusetts

**Ramona C. Anest, MSN,
    RNC-TNP, CNE**
Associate Professor
Bob Jones University
Greenville, South Carolina

**Linda Baumann, PhD, RN,
    APRN-C**
Professor Emerita
University of Wisconsin–Madison
Madison, Wisconsin

Julie A. Beck, RN, DEd, CNE
Associate Professor
York College of Pennsylvania
York, Pennsylvania

**Judith Belanger, RN, BSN,
    MSN/Ed, CNE**
Associate Professor of Nursing
University of New England
Portland, Maine

Sarah Bergman, MSN, RN
Assistant Professor
Nebraska Methodist College
Omaha, Nebraska

**Billie E. Blake, EdD, MSN,
    BSN, RN, CNE**
Associate Dean of Nursing;
    Director of BSN
St. Johns River State College
Orange Park, Florida

Simone Bollaerts, BN, IIWCC
Professor of Nursing
Mohawk College of Applied Arts
    and Technology
Hamilton, Ontario, Canada

**Judy Bornais, RN, BA, BScN,
    MSc, CDE**
Experiential Learning Specialist
University of Windsor, Faculty of
    Nursing
Windsor, Ontario, Canada

Teresa S. Boyer, MSN, APN-BC
Associate Professor of Nursing
Motlow College
Lynchburg, Tennessee

Shirley K. Comer, RN, JD, DNP
University Lecturer
Governors State University
University Park, Illinois

**Kimberly Jones Cooper, MSN,
    BSN**
Arkansas State University–
    Jonesboro Beebe Campus
Assistant Professor Beebe Site
    Coordinator
Beebe, Arkansas

**Claire M. Creamer, PhD, RN,
    CPNP-PC**
Assistant Professor Nursing
Rhode Island College
Providence, Rhode Island

**Margaret Davis, PhD, MSN,
    RN, CNE**
Associate Professor
Chamberlain College of Nursing
Atlanta, Georgia

Terry Delpier, DNP, RN, CPNP
Professor, Nursing
Northern Michigan University
Marquette, Michigan

**Jackie Sayre Dorsey, RN, MS,
    ANP**
Assistant Professor
Monroe Community College
Rochester, New York

Annemarie Dowling-Castronovo, AAS, BS, MA, PhD, RN, GNP-BC
Associate Professor, Interim Director of Undergraduate Nursing Studies
The Evelyn L. Spiro School of Nursing, Wagner College
Staten Island, New York

Mary Ann Dugan, DNP, CRNP, FNP-BC
Assistant Professor and Nurse Practitioner
La Salle University
Philadelphia, Pennsylvania

Tonya Eddy, MS(N), RN
Assistant Professor
Missouri Valley College
Marshall, Missouri

Janice Eilerman, MSN, RN
Assistant Professor–Nursing Faculty
Rhodes State College
Lima, Ohio

Sonya Franklin, EdD/CI, MHA, MSN, RN
Associate Professor of Nursing
Cleveland State Community College
Cleveland, Tennessee

Ronald C. Gonzalez, RN, MSN, MHA
Professor
College of Southern Nevada
Las Vegas, Nevada

Kelly Holder, MSN, RN, FNP
Dean, Health Sciences and Human Services
Piedmont Community College
Roxboro, North Carolina

Paul Jeffrey, RN(EC), BScN, MN, ACNP
Program Coordinator/Professor
Sheridan College
Brampton, Ontario, Canada

Patricia Kaufman, MSN, RN
Assistant Professor of Nursing
Cardinal Stritch University
Milwaukee, Wisconsin

Cathy R. Kessenich, DSN, ARNP
Professor of Nursing and MSN Program Director
University of Tampa
Tampa, Florida

Mary Knowlton, DNP, RN, CNE
Accelerated BSN Program Director
Western Carolina University
Asheville, North Carolina

Robin Eades Koch, RN, MSN, NNP-BC
Assistant Director/Program Director, Practical Nursing
Riverside College of Health Careers
Newport News, Virginia

Ramona B. Lazenby, EdD, RN, FNP-BC, CNE
Associate Dean and Professor of Nursing
Auburn Montgomery School of Nursing
Montgomery, Alabama

Jane Leach, PhD, RNC, IBCLC
Coordinator of Nurse Educator Program
Midwestern State University
Wichita Falls, Texas

G. Lindsay McCrea, PhD, RN, FNP-BC, CWOCN
Professor, Department of Nursing and Health Science
Associate Director, Semester Conversion Initiative
California State University, East Bay
Hayward Campus
Hayward, California

Jane M. Parks, RN, MSN
Assistant Professor
Creighton University School of Nursing
Hastings, Nebraska

Sharon L. Phelps, RN, MS, CNE
Curriculum Manager
Chamberlain College of Nursing
Downers Grove, Illinois

Kimberly B. Porter, MNSc, RN
Assistant Professor
University of Arkansas Little
 Rock
Little Rock, Arkansas

**Valeria Ramdin, PhD (c),
 APRN-BC, MS, CNE**
Faculty/Clinical Instructor
Northeastern University
Boston, Massachusetts

Sherry Ray, MSN, RN
Nursing Faculty
Arizona State University
Phoenix, Arizona

**Paula Reams, PhD, RN, CNE,
 LMT**
Professor, Chair Health Sciences
Kettering College
Kettering, Ohio

**Kathryn Reveles, PhD(c), DNP,
 APRN, CNS, CPNP-PC**
Associate Professor
Houston Baptist University
Houston, Texas

Catherine Rice, RN, EdD
Professor/Faculty in the
 Department of Nursing
Western Connecticut State
 University
Danbury, Connecticut

Debra L. Servello, DNP, ACNP
Assistant Professor of Nursing;
 ACNP Coordinator
Rhode Island College
Providence, Rhode Island

Joyce A. Shanty, PhD, RN
Associate Professor
Indiana University of
 Pennsylvania
Indiana, Pennsylvania

**Denise Schentrup, DNP,
 ARNP-BC**
Clinical Assistant Professor
University of Florida
Gainesville, Florida

**Mendy Stanford, BSN, MSN/
 Ed, CNE**
Executive Director of Nursing
 and Allied Health
Treasure Valley Community
 College
Ontario, Oregon

**Rebecca Sutter, MSN, APRN,
 BC, FNP**
Associate Professor, Nursing
Northern Virginia Community
 College
Medical Education Campus
Springfield, Virginia

Kathy Taydus
Assistant Professor
Jamestown Community College
Jamestown, New York

**Elaine Della Vecchio, PhD, RN,
 CCRN**
Assistant Professor
New York Institute of Technology
Old Westbury, New York

Judy Vansteenbergen RN, MSN
Adjunct Faculty
Quinnipiac University
Hamden, Connecticut
Southern Connecticut State
 University
New Haven, Connecticut

**Amber Williams, DNP, APRN,
 FNP-BC, RNC-MNN**
Director of RN-BSN and
 MSN-OL Programs
University of South Carolina
Columbia, South Carolina

Erica Yu, PhD, RN, ANP
Assistant Dean for Undergraduate
 Programs
University of Texas Health
 Science Center at Houston
 School of Nursing
Houston, Texas

**Tamara Zurakowski, PhD,
 GNP-BD**
Adjunct Associate Professor
University of Pennsylvania
Philadelphia, Pennsylvania

Tammy Zybell, MSN, MBA, RN
Faculty Manager/Instructor
Chamberlain College of Nursing
Homosassa, Florida

CONTENTS

1 Understanding Health Assessment

INTRODUCTION

The foundation of the healthcare delivery system is the interdisciplinary team that cares for the patients. Currently, there are about 3.6 million registered nurses (RNs) who provide care and assess patients in many different settings (American Nurses Association, Inc., 2017). Health assessment is a priority nursing skill that is the cornerstone of nursing care (Fawcett & Rhynas, 2012).

The Robert Wood Johnson Foundation Initiative on the Future of Nursing (2010) at the Institute of Medicine sought to build a blueprint for the future of nursing as part of larger efforts to reform the healthcare system (Institute of Medicine, 2010). The U.S. healthcare system is evolving, and care is becoming more focused on wellness, disease prevention, health promotion, and chronic illness management. In addition, healthcare reform provides many people with access to health care that they did not have previously. As a result, there continues to be an increased demand for everyday care through community health centers, professional home healthcare services, long-term care facilities, primary care providers' offices, and nonemergency settings that are close to home.

In 1981, the World Health Organization (WHO) adopted a program called Global Strategy for Health for All by the Year 2000. "Health for All" does not mean an end to disease and disability or that physicians and nurses will care for everyone. It means that resources for health are evenly distributed and that essential health care is accessible to everyone (WHO, 2016). Health for All proposes that health begins at home, in schools, and in the workplace and that people use better approaches for preventing illness and alleviating unavoidable disease and disability. In all settings, nurses are essential to ensuring access to needed care, and their knowledge and skills directly affect the quality of care that patients receive. In these areas, all patients need to be assessed by nurses.

Nursing is a practice profession. Health assessment is an essential skill to nursing practice. Assessing patients and being able to identify normal from abnormal findings is an essential role of the RN. Nurses must be able to use learned skills to collect information about patients' health and physical well-being.

There are growing trends of changing demographics and increased diversity throughout the world. Nurses assess individuals of different cultures across the life span and in every practice setting from birth to the end of a patient's life. Every person is unique, and each culture has its own health beliefs and practices. Cultural practices influence an individual's behavior to promote, maintain, and restore health and how, when, and with whom they seek help or treatment (Dossey & Keegan, 2013). Cultural considerations are important when assessing patients.

Assessment requires each nurse to be like a detective, investigating everything about what the individual reports, observing their nonverbal body language, and looking for clues that may indicate something out of the ordinary. Assessment is a skill that uses most of our perceptual senses: hearing, seeing, smelling, and feeling. Assessment skills are learned and need to be practiced to master the techniques of assessing an individual.

The new movement in health care is person-centered care (PCC), which emphasizes the intrinsic value of treating all patients as persons (Entwistle & Watt, 2013). Nurses work with individuals as copartners in care. The holistic caring process is a relational process; the nurse collaborates with the individual to pursue goals for health and well-being (Dossey & Keegan, 2013). Every nurse uses interpersonal skills to communicate and facilitate interventions to meet the needs of patients.

Nursing practice covers a broad continuum of care. Active collaboration with the individual and family in decision making, promotion of health, and prevention of stress and illness is part of this relationship (Dossey & Keegan, 2013). These collaborative relationships require listening, communicating therapeutically, and together with the individual, planning common goals.

DEFINITION OF HEALTH

Health is a term that has different meanings for each individual, family, community, or population. An individual's quality of life and level of functioning are dependent on their level of health. Nurses should have an understanding of each patient's definition of health and know and understand when individuals feel healthy or unhealthy. There are many definitions for health, including:

- The WHO defines health as the state of complete physical, social, and mental well-being and not merely the absence of disease and infirmity (WHO, 1946).
- Health is a balance of body, mind, and spirit.
- Health is influenced by each individual's external environment and physiological-biological, behavioral, and economic-political factors (Jeanfreau, Porche, & Lee, 2010) (Fig. 1-1).

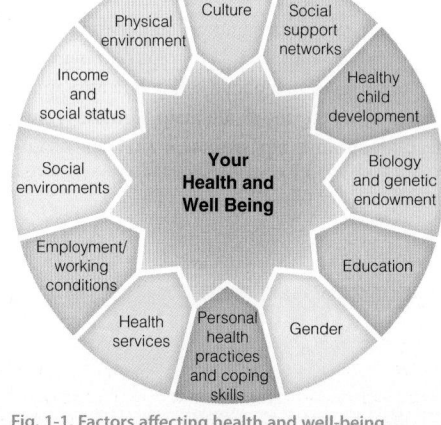

Fig. 1-1. Factors affecting health and well-being.

- The Centers for Disease Control and Prevention (CDC) identifies five determinants of health:
  1. genetics and biology (i.e., age and sex)
  2. individual behavior (i.e., alcohol use, unprotected sex, smoking)
  3. social environment (i.e., income and lifestyle)
  4. physical environment (i.e., where the individual lives)
  5. health services (i.e., insurance and access to health care) (CDC, 2014)

Healthy People 2020

The scope of health assessment encompasses many aspects of health that commensurate with the nation's federal initiative, *Healthy People* (Jeanfreau et al., 2010). *Healthy People* is a science-based framework updated every 10 years by the U.S. Department of Health and Human Services that identifies health and risk factors for diseases. The report stresses that individuals must take responsibility for their own health. *Healthy People 2020* has goals and objectives for health promotion and disease prevention. This framework establishes benchmarks and monitors progress over time to:

- encourage collaborations across the federal government, states, communities, and private and public sectors
- guide individuals toward making informed health decisions
- measure the impact of prevention activities.

Healthy People 2020 recognizes that specific disease outcomes, risk factors, and health determinants need to be addressed at various stages across the life span. Risk assessments are identified for particular age-groups, diseases, and health promotion (Box 1-1). Nurses should be familiar with the objectives and goals to integrate these into each patient's plan of care.

TIP A key role of nursing is to educate your patient and promote health and well-being; share your knowledge with your patient.

BOX 1-1 *Healthy People* Topical Areas

1. Access to health services
2. Adolescent health
3. Arthritis, osteoporosis, and chronic back conditions
4. Blood disorders and blood safety
5. Cancer
6. Chronic kidney disease
7. Dementias, including Alzheimer disease
8. Diabetes
9. Disability and health
10. Early and middle childhood
11. Education and community-based programs
12. Environmental health
13. Family planning
14. Food safety
15. Genomics
16. Global health
17. Health communications and health information technology
18. Health-related quality of life and well-being
19. Health-associated infections
20. Hearing and other sensory or communication disorders
21. Heart disease and stroke
22. Human immunodeficiency virus
23. Immunization and infectious diseases
24. Injury and violence prevention
25. Lesbian, gay, bisexual, and transgender health
26. Maternal, infant, and child health
27. Medical product safety
28. Mental health and mental disorders
29. Nutrition and weight status
30. Occupational safety and health
31. Older adults
32. Oral health
33. Physical activity
34. Preparedness
35. Public health infrastructure
36. Respiratory diseases
37. Sexually transmitted infections
38. Sleep health
39. Social determinants of health
40. Substance abuse
41. Tobacco use
42. Vision

(HHS, 2010)

U.S. PREVENTIVE SERVICES TASK FORCE

In 1984, the U.S. Preventive Services Task Force was initiated as an independent group of interprofessional national experts. The task force's goal is to use evidence-based medicine to improve the health of all Americans by making evidence-based recommendations about clinical preventive services such as screenings, counseling services, and preventive medications. The task force publishes "recommendation statements" for preventative services (USPSTF, 2013). Nurses should be aware of these recommendations for populations, specific genders, and age-groups.

LEVELS OF HEALTH PREVENTION

Preventative services include screening for disease, counseling, medications to prevent disease, and immunization recommendations. An individual's community can also enhance health promotion through social and environmental programs (Dunphy, Winland-Brown, Porter, & Thomas, 2013). There are three levels of prevention:

1. *Primary prevention* is the prevention of disease and disability and focuses on improving an individual's overall health and well-being (e.g., immunizations and health education).

2. *Secondary prevention* encompasses early screenings and detection of disease and treatment of diseases (e.g., colonoscopy to screen for colon cancer and medications to treat a curable illness).

3. *Tertiary prevention* encompasses the restoration of health after illness or disease has occurred (e.g., rehabilitation program for stroke patients).

TIP Health insurances and the individual's finances may influence the ability to have health promotion screenings.

HEALTH ASSESSMENT

Health assessment means assessing the whole patient. This includes:

- a method to establish a baseline health history by collecting pertinent patient health status data
- an organized, systematic, ongoing process of collecting, validating, and clustering data
- collecting different types of data about the individual's past and present health
- assessing factors influencing health and well-being, including (see Fig. 1-1)
  - ☐ physical health
  - ☐ behavioral aspects of health
  - ☐ spirituality
  - ☐ social factors
  - ☐ economic-political aspects of health
  - ☐ cultural variations
  - ☐ life span and developmental considerations
- Performing a physical examination.

THE NURSING PROCESS

The American Nurses' Association (ANA) has identified the nursing process to be the essential core of practice for the RN to deliver holistic, patient-focused care (ANA, 2017). The nursing process is a systematic, problem-solving process that assists the nurse in organizing the assessment to identify information about an individual's health and risk factors and develop a plan of care. This essential process collects information about the health status of the individual.

■ **TIP** Assessing a patient is always a priority role of the RN; this is a role that should never be delegated to the licensed practical nurse or unlicensed assistive personnel.

The five steps of the nursing process are as follows:

1. *Assessment* is the first, essential step requiring the nurse to collect and analyze information about the whole individual. This information includes physiological, psychological, psychosocial, spiritual, and cultural practices and beliefs.
2. *Diagnosis* involves analyzing a potential or actual health problem with a patient. Nursing diagnosis reflects the individual's actual or potential health risks or problems; the nurse uses clinical judgement and critical thinking to analyze all the information about the individual, synthesize and cluster the information, and hypothesize about the individual's health status (Wilkinson et al., 2015).
3. *Planning/Outcomes* involves working with the individual as a copartner in care to meet the needs or short- and long-term goals of the individual. The goals must be measurable and achievable.
4. *Implementation* of interventions includes the nursing and individual actions and plan of care to meet the individual's goals.
5. *Evaluation* is the ongoing process that assesses whether the short- and long-term goals have been met; this phase of the nursing process involves clinical judgment about whether the goals have been met or are unmet.

■ **TIP** The nursing process should include the individual, significant others, and the healthcare providers caring for the individual.

COGNITIVE SKILLS

Critical Thinking

Critical thinking is essential during the assessment process. Performing an assessment requires the nurse to be able to think, recall knowledge, and recognize the difference or deviations between normal and abnormal assessment findings. Critical thinking is an active, purposeful, and organized cognitive process involving creativity, reflection, problem solving, both rational and intuitive judgment, an attitude of inquiry, and a philosophical orientation toward thinking about how a nurse thinks (Dossey & Keegan, 2013). Critical thinking is a unique problem-solving, reflective process that uses (Fig. 1-2):

■ a combination of reasoned thinking, openness to alternatives, an ability to reflect, and a desire to seek truth (Wilkinson et al., 2015)
■ a process of purposeful and creative thinking about resolving problems
■ a multidimensional thinking process
■ reflective thinking
■ thinking "outside of the box"
■ questioning, interpreting information, and analyzing the situation and then synthesizing the information
■ development of alternative solutions to a problem.

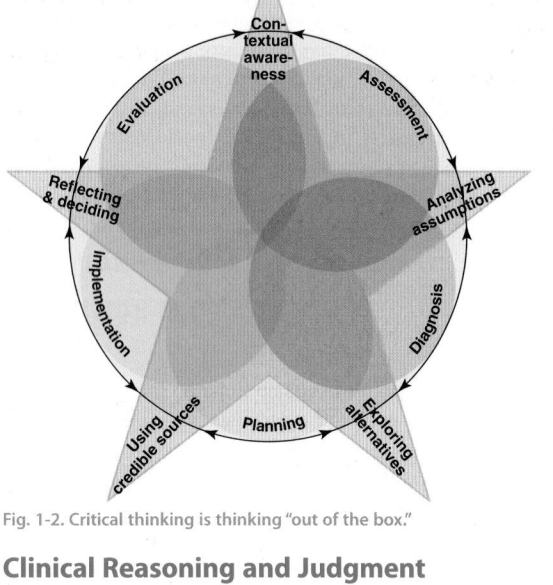

Fig. 1-2. Critical thinking is thinking "out of the box."

Clinical Reasoning and Judgment

Health assessment provides a surplus of data about the individual. Reviewing and analyzing normal and abnormal assessment findings is ongoing. Nurses must be able to collect, analyze, and interpret patient assessment findings to provide safe care for the patient.

PSYCHOMOTOR SKILLS

Assessment is a "doing" process. The four techniques of physical assessment are:

1. *Inspection,* looking
2. *Percussion,* tapping different areas of the body to assess underlying structures.

- *Clinical reasoning* uses an individual's history, physical signs, symptoms, laboratory data, and diagnostic imaging to arrive at a diagnosis and assess and formulate a treatment plan (Venes, 2013). Nurses collect these data to identify normal and abnormal findings, risk factors, health promotion, and prevention behaviors. Physical assessment findings are used to problem solve and develop the appropriate plan of care.
- *Clinical judgment* is defined as "an interpretation or conclusion about a patient's needs, concerns, or health problems and/or the decision to take action (or not), use or modify standard approaches, or improvise new ones as deemed appropriate by the patient's response" (Tanner, 2006).

Intuitive Thinking

Patient care assessment involves evaluation of data not only from a rational, analytic, and verbal mode but also from an intuitive, nonverbal mode. Dr. Patricia Benner, a nursing theorist, introduced the concept that expert nurses develop skills and understanding of patient care over time through a sound educational base as well as a multitude of experiences (Benner, 2011). Sometimes, the expert nurse has an intuitive inner sense (a feeling) about clinical situations and patients that is unsupported by observable facts. Intuitive thinking is a "gut feeling" that something may be wrong or that the nurse should do something, even if there is no real evidence to support that feeling. Intuitive patient encounters emerge as the nurse is open and receptive to the person's subtle cues (Dossey & Keegan, 2013). This is a skill that develops with experience.

3. *Palpation,* using your hands to feel surface characteristics
4. *Auscultation,* listening for sounds
These four techniques will be discussed thoroughly in Chapter 5.

COMMUNICATION SKILLS

- Health assessment requires essential therapeutic communication skills to obtain information about the individual.
- The purpose of communication is to exchange information about the patient's health and well-being (Fleischer et al., 2009).
- Communication facilitates a patient-centered relationship.
- Interpersonal communication skills and the ability of the nurse to communicate with patients, family members, and the interdisciplinary healthcare team are essential in health assessment.

Communication and interviewing techniques will be discussed more in Chapter 2.

FUTURE OF HEALTH CARE

On March 23, 2010, Congress passed and the President of the United States signed into law comprehensive healthcare legislation. The Patient Protection and Affordable Care Act (PPACA), also known as "Obamacare," provides higher-quality, safer, and more affordable and accessible care (Institute of Medicine, 2011). All individuals have the ability to buy health insurance through the health insurance marketplace. The PPACA's goal is to improve accessibility to health care, keep individuals healthy, help patients manage their chronic conditions better, and prevent illness. The healthcare system needs nurses to have strong assessment skills, educate patients, and advocate for patients.

Nurses have a leading role in being advocates for their patients and providing compassionate care. The new *Code of Ethics for Nurses with Interpretive Statements* (ANA, 2015) Provision 3 states the nurses promotes, advocates for, and protects the rights, health and safety of the patient. The ANA proclaims that every nurse is individually responsible and accountable for maintaining professional competence and must perform safe practice (ANA, 2015). Nurses need to listen carefully to each patient's self-report and be cognizant of the smallest details. Registered nurses are instrumental and have the knowledge and skills to thoroughly assess individuals in any practice setting.

Nurses need to maintain currency in their profession. Best practice assessments and instruments have been validated by research. Nursing research and evidence-based practice guide our assessments and clinical decisions to provide safe and effective care. Since the 1990s, there has been a paradigm shift to use evidence-based practice to guide nurses to make clinical judgements and use best practice protocols to provide optimum care to patients (Hoop & Rittenmeyer, 2012). The significance of evidence-based practice may be viewed in Box 1-2.

BOX 1-2 Significance of Evidence-Based Practice

- It has international importance.
- There are large, regional variations in use of evidence-based practices.
- There is rapid development of research but slow adoption of evidence-based practices.
- Only about half of all patients in the United States receive recommended care.
- There is a 28 percent improvement rate in patient outcomes when nurses use intervention based on research versus standard care.
- "Pay-for-performance" requires that evidence-based practices are used.

(Hopp & Rittenmeyer, 2012)

2 Interviewing the Patient for a Health History

INTRODUCTION

Interviewing and obtaining the health history are the key components to obtain baseline information about a patient. As early as 1953, Hildegard Peplau, a nursing theorist, emphasized the nurse-patient relationship as the foundation of nursing practice. Nurses interview patients in many different environments, including hospitals, long-term care settings, homes, clinics, and community centers. Communication and interviewing techniques are acquired skills (Varcarolis, 2011) and should be practiced. The process begins a therapeutic partnership between the nurse and the patient. During an interview, the nurse initiates the nurse-patient relationship and the patient relinquishes his or her independent role to that of a dependent role. The exchange of information, feelings, and concerns takes place during the assessment process. The nurse should be sensitive, nonjudgmental and genuine and demonstrate professionalism.

SENC Patient-Centered Care Privacy and confidentiality must be maintained and respected during the entire patient encounter. In April 2003, the Health Insurance Portability and Accountability Act (HIPAA) federally regulated and created a law to maintain confidentiality for all personal health information (U.S. Department of Health and Human Services, 2003).

THERAPEUTIC COMMUNICATION

Interviewing a patient requires therapeutic communication skills. Communication is a complex process that is influenced by a variety of personal, environmental, cultural, and social factors. It is the act of transmitting information effectively and a process of creating shared understanding (Barker, 2013). Nurses need to offer their presence, mutual respect, caring, and understanding during every patient encounter. As a healthcare provider, the nurse recognizes that each patient is unique and has feelings and beliefs.

Nurses are responsible for gathering vital health and personal information about the patient. During the patient encounter, the nurse needs to focus the direction of the interview to make sure all vital information is obtained and a clear understanding of the patient's concerns is acquired. Therapeutic communication encompasses the following dimensions for a patient-centered assessment:

- Empathy and compassion are a deep awareness of and insight into the feelings, emotions, and behavior of another person and their meaning and significance (Venes, 2013), and identifies a patient's feelings and concerns.
- Unconditional regard means respecting and accepting a patient as a unique individual.

- Genuineness is being honest with the patient. A nurse needs to be truthful and understanding with every patient encounter. Listen to the patient with an open heart and compassion.
- Respect is a moral value. It demonstrates that you have a positive feeling for every patient and accept each patient as a person who has unique qualities. As a nurse, you acknowledge that each patient is important and of value.

- Caring is the essence of nursing and connotes responsiveness between the nurse and the patient.

TIP During the interview, the focus of the patient encounter is to obtain truthful and reliable information about the patient. The pneumonic "CLEAR" in communication stands for Center, Listen, Empathy, Attention, and Respect (Box 2-1); these are foundational for successful interviewing.

BOX 2-1 Holistic Communication: Be CLEAR

Center yourself	• Pause for a moment. • Breathe deeply. • Connect with a feeling of love and compassion. • Create a silent intention that thoughts, words, and actions will be for the greater good.
Listen wholeheartedly	• Set aside your own thoughts, emotions, and feelings. • Focus on the person's agenda. • Do not judge or analyze. • Open your heart to what is being communicated.
Empathize	• Come from a place of genuine concern. • Have the ability to feel with a person, not be sorry for them. • Empathy involves an understanding that comes from sensing into the being of another.
Attention: be fully present	• Be aware of what you are feeling and sensing. Stay present with yourself. • Be the fullness of yourself to every moment—emotionally, mentally, physically, and spiritually.
Respect	• Respect all that is. • Respect yourself and set boundaries, if needed. • Respect the patient—honor cultural, social, ontological, and ideological differences. • Welcome diversity.

From L. Thornton, *Creating a Healing Environment. Course I: The Model of Whole-Person Caring* (Fresno, CA: self-published, 2010): 68, with permission.

PREPARATION

The nurse should prepare and plan for the interview. Preparation is key to being organized and ready to speak with the patient. Some pointers to prepare for the interview include the following:

- Reading the patient's record before seeing the patient will help you to prepare.
- The patient should stay dressed until you are ready to perform the actual physical assessment.
- Arrange for the interview to take place in a private environment that is free from distractions and noise, has good lighting, and has a comfortable temperature.
- Allow sufficient time to complete the interview and health history. Have a clock available to keep track of time but only glance occasionally at the clock.
- Never appear rushed during the interview. It is essential to allow sufficient time to interview, obtain a health history, and assess the patient.

- Sit or stand at the same level as the patient so the patient does not have to look up or down at you.
- Always introduce yourself to the patient and tell the patient approximately how long the interview should take.
- Reassure the patient that the health history is confidential.
- Encourage the patient to ask questions and to let you know if she or he ever feels uncomfortable.

SENC **Patient-Centered Care** Be sure to consider the developmental level of the patient. It is important to use words that the patient will understand and avoid medical terminology.

COMMUNICATION SKILLS

Effective and good communication skills are important in health assessment and essential to gathering information for a health history. Nurses must use professional etiquette during a nurse-patient interaction. Therapeutic communication is an active process that includes empathy and active listening while maintaining objectivity and professional boundaries (Patel & Jakopac, 2012). The purpose of communication is to:

- share content: the actual subject matter, words, gestures, and substance of the message (Wilkinson et al., 2015)
- share and exchange thoughts, perceptions, and feelings
- send, receive, and gather data

- share patient concerns
- exchange knowledge.

Nonverbal Communication

Nonverbal communication is communication without the use of spoken language. Nonverbal communication includes gestures, facial expressions, and body positions (known collectively as "body language") as well as unspoken understandings and presuppositions, and cultural and environmental conditions that may affect any encounter between people (American Heritage New Dictionary of Cultural Literacy, 2014). Patients communicate in different ways. While verbal and written communication skills are important, research has shown that nonverbal behaviors make up a large percentage of our daily interpersonal communication (Cherry, n.d.). Communication is said to be 10 percent to 20 percent verbal and 80 percent to 90 percent nonverbal (Varcarolis, 2011). The following are nonverbal visual cues to be aware of during an interview:

- physical appearance
- body language
- facial expression
- eye contact
- gestures
- facial grimacing
- tone of voice
- nonverbal sounds such as crying and moaning.

TIP Remember that both you and the patient convey nonverbal body language. During the interview, health history, and assessment be mindful of your body language.

CULTURAL CONSIDERATIONS Russians do not appreciate gestures such as standing with hands inserted in pockets, arms crossed over chest, or slouching postures when being interviewed. Until trust is established, many Russians are aloof when speaking with healthcare providers (Purnell, 2014).

COMMUNICATION TECHNIQUES

Effective Communication

Therapeutic communication will facilitate a therapeutic exchange between a patient and a nurse. Nurses must develop and refine communication skills to assess patients. While assessing patients, nurses need to be open to receive information in a nonjudgmental way. There are some helpful strategies that may be able to assist you to elicit or clarify information throughout the interview.

SENC Patient-Centered Care Some experiences may be difficult or painful for a patient to discuss. Ask permission to ask sensitive questions.

Effective communication includes the following:

- Be clear, concise, and honest in your communication.
- Be sure that you have a shared understanding of the patient's report, problems, and concerns.

- Avoid medical terminology that may not be understood.
- Keep your questions simple for clear understanding.
- Ask one question at a time, and wait for the patient to respond.
- Listen attentively and maintain eye contact (if culturally appropriate).
- Do not interrupt the patient while he or she is talking.
- Avoid taking excessive notes during the interview.
- Display nonverbal body language that says you are interested in hearing the patient's story (be cognizant of your posture, maintaining eye contact, and hand gestures).
- Always ask permission before touching a patient; take into account cultural considerations.

Some effective communication techniques include:

- **Active listening:** Pay close attention to the patient's report and nonverbal cues; maintain good eye contact and express a willingness to listen.
- **Active observing:** Concentrate on what you hear and see during the interview.

TIP Nurses should document what they see or observe during the interview such as the patient crying during the interview while discussing the recent loss of a spouse.

- **Broad opening questions:** Will allow the patient to report more spontaneous information and tell you their story. An example is, "What can I do for you today?"
- **Clarification:** Obtain clarification if the patient does not clearly express the problem or issue and you are confused about what the patient is saying to you. An example is, "I did not understand what you meant when you said the rash comes and goes. Can you explain what 'comes and goes' means?"
- **Confrontation:** Give the patient honest and respectful feedback about what you see or hear that is inconsistent with what the patient is telling you. An example of this is, "You told me that you do not have a drinking problem but you stated that you were arrested for drinking under the influence 3 months ago? Can we talk about how much alcohol you drink on a daily basis?"

SENC Patient-Centered Care Never sound angry or judgmental when confronting a patient; be cognizant of your tone of voice and nonverbal body language.

- **Empathy:** Identify, understand, share, and accept the patient's feelings. Empathy is caring about and for the patient as you are speaking together. An example of an empathetic response is, "I am sorry to hear that you have been in pain for this long. How has the pain affected your daily life?"
- **Respect:** Be respectful of what the patient is saying and feeling. An example of being respectful is, "This has been a difficult time for you

since your husband has been in jail. You are showing great strength in continuing to care for your children."

- **Exploring:** Encourage the patient to give you more details. An example is, "Tell me more about the pain in your back."
- **Facilitation:** Use simple verbal statements or words to encourage the patient to continue to tell the story. Use statements like "uh-huh," "Mm" or "And then?"
- **Focusing:** Ask specific questions to collect and clarify data that the patient may not be stating during the interview. An example of a focused question is, "How many stairs can you climb before you feel short of breath?"
- **Reflecting/Stating the Observed:** Repeat the patient's words specifically to encourage elaboration of the patient's self-report; this encourages more discussion. An example of reflection is
  Patient: "I cannot believe that I did not go for my mammogram and now I may have breast cancer."
  Nurse: "You sound upset. Are you angry that you did not go for your mammogram?"
- **Transitional statements:** Use transitional statements to help redirect the interview to another significant area. An example of a transitional statement is, "Now, I would like to discuss your family history."
- **Silence:** Refrain from speaking; planned absence of verbal remarks allows the patient and the nurse to think over or feel what is being discussed. If silence does not prompt a response within 5 to 10 seconds, the interviewer should try another skill as prolonged silence may make the patient feel uncomfortable (Fortin, Dwamena, & Smith, 2012). An example of a question you might ask is, "You appear to be quiet. Is there anything you would like to talk about?"
- **Summarizing:** State a brief summary at the end of the interview; this allows for clarification and accurate data of the patient's history or problem. An example of initiating a summary is "Let me summarize the important points."

Barriers to Therapeutic Communication

Communication is a reciprocal conversation. As healthcare providers, we must be aware of the barriers of communication. The following techniques should not be used during a patient-centered interview.

- **Leading the patient:** Do not lead the patient; patients tell you what they want you to hear and may not always be truthful in their self-report. For example, "Do you think that because your mother died of cancer you may also have cancer?"
- **Asking too many questions:** Only ask one question at a time for clarity and to disallow misunderstanding.
- **Not allowing enough response time:** Give the patient enough time to think through the answer.
- **Using medical jargon:** Use lay terms so the patient can understand you.
- **Assuming what the patient is saying:** Never assume what the patient is saying; this leads to misinterpretations. If you are unsure, ask the patient to clarify or give more information.
- **Taking the patient's responses personally:** Realize that the patient may be inappropriately displacing feelings or frustrations.
- **Using clichés:** Clichés (e.g., "you will feel better in the morning") show disregard for the patient's feelings. This is giving false reassurance. If you are unsure of an answer, tell the patient that you will try to find the answer.
- **Specifically asking "why" questions:** A patient may feel offended and feel like you are criticizing; a subtle approach is usually more comfortable (Wilkinson et al., 2015).
- **Offering false reassurance:** Never tell the patient that everything will be fine when it may not be.
- **Changing the subject inappropriately:** Sometimes nurses change the subject abruptly when the interview is uncomfortable; this is not helpful for the patient.

- **Giving opinions:** Do not give your own opinions. If the patient asks, "What should I do?" help to clarify the options, and provide information about the choices the patient has and refer the patient to talk with the healthcare provider.
- **Stereotyping:** Be objective during the assessment; every patient is unique and should be respected regardless of race, religion, gender, sexual preference, or age.
- **Using patronizing language:** Patronizing language communicates superiority or disproval. Statements such as, "you know better than that" is condescending. "Elder speak" such as "Dearie" or "Sweetie" describes ways that healthcare providers may unintentionally show disrespect to older adults (Wilkinson et al., 2015).

Special-Needs Patients

Communication depends on the ability to hear, speak, and understand. There are patients with sensory and neurological deficits who require special considerations.

Hearing-Impaired Patients

Hearing loss is a common human sensory deficit affecting the patient's ability to communicate.

- Make sure the patient's hearing aid(s) is turned on and the batteries are working.
- Reduce background noise in the room.
- Face the patient and speak slowly and clearly; use short and simple sentences.
- If the individual cannot hear, try to use written communication such as a whiteboard or paper and pencil if the patient can read and/or write.
- Confirm that the patient hears and understands.
- Allow for extra time and do not rush the assessment.
- Never shout at the patient.

Visually Impaired Patients

Patients who are visually impaired do not always tell the nurse. Visually impaired individuals can compensate for their loss of sight by developing stronger abilities in their remaining senses (Cohen et al., 2010).

■ Introduce yourself, and explain the purpose and sequence of the patient assessment.
■ Ask the patient:
  □ How much can you see?
■ Ask permission before you touch the patient; touching lets the patient know that you are listening and where you are sitting; allow the patient to touch you.
■ Be descriptive when giving directions; verbally give the person information that is visually obvious to individuals who can see. Describe the examination room.
■ If you are offering a seat or assisting the patient to the examination table, gently place the individual's hand on the back or top of the chair or examination table so the person can locate the seat or table. Offer assistance as needed.
■ Tell the patient if you are going to leave the examination room; ask if the patient needs assistance.

Aphasiac Patients

Aphasiac patients have an impairment of language or the inability to communicate through speech or writing because of brain dysfunction (Venes, 2013).

■ Make sure the environment is quiet and without distractions.
■ Allow extra time for the interview.
■ Communicate one question or sentence at a time.
■ Speak slowly and clearly.
■ Be honest; do not pretend if you do not understand what the patient is communicating to you.
■ Do not rush the patient as he or she is trying to communicate.

■ Write down questions or use pictures if the patient does not understand you; have the patient write or draw if the person cannot speak.

Cognitively Impaired Patients

Cognitively impaired patients have difficulty thinking with loss of short- or long-term memory. Assess the patient's orientation and ability to understand by:

■ Using simple focused questions.
■ Sitting in front and maintain eye contact.
■ Speaking slowly and clearly.
■ Communicating one question or sentence at a time.
■ Communicating with secondary sources if the patient is unreliable (i.e., aide or family member caring for the patient).

Aggressive or Challenging Patients

Aggressive or challenging patients may demonstrate increased agitation, restlessness, or irritability and may be uncooperative.

TIP A patient who is acting angry may simply be frightened, defensive, or resistant to the reason for seeking care. It is important for the nurse to take a step back from the patient who is angry and think about what is really going on (Lampert, 2014).

■ Be calm and reassuring; be empathetic.
■ Do not argue with the patient.
■ Speak softly and use simple questions.
■ Use reflective statements, such as, "I can understand why you feel this way."
■ Reassure confidentiality and safety.
■ Be alert and sensitive to nonverbal communication.
■ Keep out of striking distance.
■ Avoid cornering the patient; keep a clear pathway out of the room (Hogstel & Curry, 2001).

SENC Safety Alert If you ever feel unsafe, excuse yourself and leave the room.

Communicating With a Patient With a Language Barrier

A patient with a language barrier does not understand or speak English.

TIP If an interpreter is not available, the nurse should have a list of certified medical interpreters who can be available by phone.

- Ask the patient if he or she understands English; if the response is negative, ask the patient's preferred language.
- Use your resources to find a trained face-to-face interpreter; a professional interpreter will be able to convey objective information between you and the patient; ask the patient about any preference for a same-gender interpreter.
- Explain to the interpreter the purpose and goals of the assessment.
- The interpreter should explain the purpose and goals of the assessment to the patient.
- During the interview and assessment, look at the patient, not the interpreter.
- Ask simple and clear questions; provide time for the patient to ask questions.

TIP It is not recommended to use family members during an assessment to interpret for the patient for several reasons. A family member may

- Be subjective when giving information.
- Purposely omit information.
- Give his or her own opinion.
- Answer for the patient.
- The patient may not want the family member to know the truth.

Communicating With Patients With Low Health Literacy

Implementation of the Affordable Care Act (ACA) of 2010 has resulted in significant changes to the U.S. healthcare system. Among its many provisions, the ACA extends access to healthcare coverage to millions of Americans who have been previously uninsured. Many of the newly eligible health insurance consumers are individuals of low health literacy.

Patients with low health literacy may have difficulty understanding; many patients cannot read.

TIP Many patients are embarrassed to let you know that they cannot read. To assess whether a patient can read, give the patient a newspaper or a patient instruction sheet to read to you.

- Speak in very simple and clear language.
- Ask the patient if he or she understands your questions.
- Use pictures or diagrams, if necessary.

Cultural Considerations

A patient's culture can influence the interview process. A patient may have many different definitions and perceptions of health and illness. The patient's comfort level in regard to disclosing private issues with unfamiliar people, having physical closeness with unfamiliar people, involving significant other or family in the assessment process, and being addressed by first name varies among age, socioeconomic, and ethnic groups (O'Brien, Kennedy, & Ballard, 2008).

- Respect the patient's needs and preferences for modesty, uncovering only those parts of the body necessary for examination and treatment.
- Many cultures and religions have restrictions on touching, distance, and modesty, which may be affected by providers of the opposite sex or staff that are younger or older than the patient (The Joint Commission, 2010).

Some examples of cultural considerations are:

- American Indian/Alaskan Native Heritage: Same-gender healthcare providers are required for intimate care (Purcell, 2014).
- Asians: Avoiding eye contact shows respect (Varcarolis, 2010).
- Islamic culture and some religious Jews: Shaking hands with the opposite gender is viewed as culturally inappropriate (Fortin, Dwamena, Frankel, & Smith, 2012).

- People with French, British, and African backgrounds: Avoidance of eye contact by another person might be interpreted as disinterest (Varcarolis, 2010).
- American Eskimos: Silence is preferred and they may wait for several minutes before replying to a simple statement or greeting. If American Eskimos sense some intolerance from the nurse toward the use of silence, they may feel dominated and inferior, so the nurse should be cautious and not try to fill any silences (Dayer-Berenson, 2011).
- Cambodians: Be mindful of spacing and avoid prolonged eye contact; it is inappropriate to stare (Dayer-Berenson, 2011).
- Chinese: Most speak in a moderate to low voice tone and consider Americans to be loud. Be aware of your tone of voice when interacting with Chinese patients (Purcell, 2014).
- German Heritage: Feelings are considered private and difficult to share. Sharing one's feelings with others often creates a sense of vulnerability or is looked on as evidence of weakness (Purnell, 2014).
- Italian Americans: They tend to over-report symptoms or report their symptoms in a very dramatic manner (Dayer-Berenson, 2011). Language problems can face the nurse when the elderly or a new Italian immigrant seeks medical care. Cultural modesty may impact the ability to get adequate or complete answers to medical questions, even when an interpreter is used (Dayer-Berenson, 2011).

Types of Questions Used When Interviewing

Communication is an exchange of information. To gather information, there are two types of questions you can ask the patient during the interview.

- Open-ended questions allow the patient to express thoughts and encourage verbalization; this type of question allows the nurse to explore the focused topic more broadly. Patients are able to give you information in their own words. Some examples of open-ended questions and statements are:
  - ☐ "How do you remember to take all of your medications?"
  - ☐ "Tell me more about how you are feeling."
  - ☐ "What brings you to the clinic today?"

  TIP Information that the patient gives you is subjective data; use quotes if you are using the patient's exact words in your documentation. An example would be that the patient states: "I am so worried that I may have cancer."

- Closed-ended questions clarify and focus on specific problems, limit responses, and are usually answered with one-word responses such as "yes" or "no."
- During the health history, each inquiry should start with open-ended questions or statement to elicit patient information followed by closed-ended questions to gather specific details. An example would be, "Tell me about your daily eating patterns." Did you ever have to try to lose weight?"

THE INTERVIEW

The health history interview is a conversation with a purpose (Hogan-Quigley et al., 2012). It is a complex process that requires astute communication and observational skills. The nurse should prepare to interview the patient. Steps to prepare for the interview include the following:

- If available, review the patient's record.
- Organize your thoughts.
- Review how you will collect the data.
- Identify the goals for the interview.

- Assess your professional appearance and demeanor.
- Prepare the environment for comfort and privacy.

SENC Safety Alert Always wash your hands, preferably in front of the patient, before starting the interview, following standard precautions.

TIP If family members are present during the interview, the nurse should clarify who is present rather than assume wife, daughter, parent, or significant other. It is the nurse's responsibility to obtain permission from the patient for the family members to be present and participate in the interview process. Document who was present during the interview.

Three Phases of the Interview

- Phase One: Introductory Phase
  - ☐ Introduce yourself and explain your role.
  - ☐ Establish rapport and trust.
  - ☐ Explain the purpose or reason for the interview.
  - ☐ Tell your patient that you will be taking some notes.
  - ☐ State the approximate time frame for the interview.
  - ☐ Ask the patient if she or he is comfortable.

Example: "Hello Mrs. Mangos, my name is Trisha Feinstein and I am a registered nurse. I am here to interview you before Dr. Brown comes in to do your physical examination. The interview will take about 20 to 25 minutes, and I will be asking you questions about your health. I will be taking some notes on the computer for Dr. Brown to review. Are you comfortable?"

TIP Always introduce yourself and call the patient by the appropriate surname (Mr., Mrs., Ms., or Dr.), unless the patient tells you to call him or her by the first name.

- Phase Two: Working Phase
  - ☐ This is the longest phase of the interview.
  - ☐ Collect information about the patient.
  - ☐ Ask open- and closed-ended questions.
  - ☐ Have the patient self-report his or her history.
  - ☐ Be alert to nonverbal communication cues.
  - ☐ Identify patient problems and goals.
  - ☐ Ask the patient if he or she has any questions.
- Phase Three: Summarization Phase
  - ☐ Clarify the patient's report, needs, feelings, and concerns.
  - ☐ Summarize the patient's self-report by restating the findings and self-report to validate that both you and the patient perceive the health history the same way.
  - ☐ Confirm that the goals were validated by both you and the patient.

THE HEALTH HISTORY

The health history is one of the most important parts of the health assessment because it provides essential and critical information about the patient. This takes time. Each patient has personal beliefs about health and illness that are influenced by the patient's culture and perception of health.

TIP Remember that the patient is free to choose what to tell you and what to withhold from you (Wilkinson et al., 2015).

The health history contains the review of systems (ROS), a subjective report of all body systems by the patient. The patient will deny or report symptoms. The key is to make sure that you ask appropriate and specific questions to have a detailed description of the patient's health or problem.

TIP Patient reports specific symptoms are "pertinent positives." Patient denies specific symptoms are "pertinent negatives." These reported or denied symptoms are documented in the ROS. An example would be: "Reports nasal congestion, sneezing and watery eyes. Denies sinus headache/pressure, postnasal drip, and rhinorrhea."

Types of Health History and Sources

There are three types of health histories:

1. **Comprehensive health history:** A comprehensive health history looks at the whole patient and reviews all body systems; this health history takes time. For example, reviewing the patient systems from head to toe is routinely done during an annual examination.

2. **Focused or problem-based health history:** This type of health history focuses specifically on an acute problem or symptom that the patient is experiencing. Patients being seen in urgent care or the emergency room will have this type of health history. For example, if a patient is having difficulty breathing, the health history would focus on the respiratory and cardiac systems.

3. **Follow-up history:** This history occurs after a patient has been seen; it concentrates on new data since the last history. For example, a patient was originally treated and worked up for heart palpitations and is being seen two weeks later to evaluate the treatment.

Data are collected from two types of sources:

1. **Primary source** is the patient who is being interviewed and assessed.

2. **Secondary sources** are family members, significant others, or medical records of the patient.

   ☐ Secondary sources may be used if the patient has a sensory deficit or cannot communicate information due to a physical or psychological/cognitive disability.

Reliability of the source means the patient is communicating clear and accurate information and has the ability to recall past medical information. It is important to determine whether the patient is reliable. This may be done by asking patients questions that you can confirm the answers to, such as "What is your date of birth?"

Some patients may be unreliable because of decreased cognitive ability or mentation. Secondary sources will be needed to provide information for the health history. If this occurs, document "Patient is unreliable; report by patient's son." The information that the patient tells you during the health history will provide valuable information for the nurse when progressing to perform the health assessment. This interview process takes time and requires your full attention, good therapeutic communication skills, and building rapport and trust with the patient.

3 Taking the Health History

INTRODUCTION

The health history is an important part of the health assessment because it provides essential and critical sharing of information about the patient's past and present health. As a nurse, you will assess the patient using a holistic approach. Every patient is unique and has his or her own personal beliefs about health and illness that are influenced by their culture and their perception of health.

THE HEALTH HISTORY

The health history records subjective and essential data. Subjective data are pieces of information reported by the patient. Purposes of the health history include:

■ Document a database of past and present health including a medical history of medical problems, hospitalizations, and surgeries.
■ Document family history.
■ Identify psychosocial factors influencing health and well-being.
■ Identify self-care and health promotion practices.
■ Determine strengths and weaknesses of the patient.
■ Identify teaching needs.
■ Identify discharge needs or case management referrals.

SENC Patient-Centered Care During the health history, some of the questions may be uncomfortable for the patient to answer because the patient does not know how you will react or feels like you may judge them. Reassure the patient that you are here to help and the information will remain confidential.

Reason for Seeking Care

The reason for seeking care is synonymous with the chief complaint or the presenting problem. The reason for seeking care may focus on:

■ the history of present health (patient is here for an annual physical examination)
■ illness (e.g., general fatigue and weakness)
■ the presenting symptom(s) (e.g., cough and congestion).

Ask the patient:

■ What brings you here today?
  □ Specific details are required to attain necessary information about the patient and his or her health-related concerns. Open-ended questions will invite the patient's story. After the patient has finished speaking, you may have to explore the patient's self-report or ask more focusing questions.

History of Present Illness

You will be assessing patients who may or may not have a health problem. Some patients present for an annual physical assessment and do not have any health concerns or symptoms. If a patient does have a health concern or symptom, the history of the present illness documents the specific details of the symptom(s). Specific attributes of a symptom may be found using the subjective history-gathering mnemonic in Table 3-1 and the OLDCARTS mnemonic in Table 3-2.

TABLE 3-1 Mnemonic for Subjective History Gathering

Letter	Topic	Questions	Sample Responses
L	Location	Can you point to where the pain is?	Patient points to right lower quadrant.
M	Mechanism	What do you think is causing the pain?	"I don't know; maybe something I ate last night?"
N	New	Is this a new problem for you? Is this something that you have had before?	"I've never had a problem like this."
O	Onset	When did the pain start?	"Last night at 11 p.m."
P	Palliative	What makes your pain better?	"Nothing: I took some acetaminophen, and it didn't help."
	Provocative	What makes your pain worse?	"Bouncing in the car and lying flat seem to make it worse."
Q	Quality	Can you describe the pain?	"It's mostly achy, but it is sharp at times."
R	Radiation	Does your pain seem to go to other parts of your body?	"It hurts a little near my belly button."
S	Severity	On a scale of 1–10, what is your pain right now?	"It is about 7 out of 10."
	Setting	Does your pain seem to occur when you are in a specific place or doing something specific?	"It feels like a 9 sometimes." "No; it hurts all the time."
T	Timing	Has your pain changed over time? Are there certain times of the day that the pain is worse?	"It is a little worse in the last couple hours, but it is always there."
U	Unusual symptoms	Are you having any unusual symptoms? Do these seem related to your pain?	"I've been sick to my stomach and threw up once. I also feel warm. I think that I am nauseous because of the pain."
V	Valid	Do these symptoms seem real to you? (Try to determine if the complaint may be psychosomatic. Evaluate if dementia or delirium may be affecting subjective response.)	"Yes, I don't know what's going on."
W	Work	Have your symptoms prevented you from work, school, or activities of daily living (ADLs)?	"I stayed home from work today and don't feel like doing much."

Source: Campbell, Gilbert, & Lausten, 2010.

TABLE 3-2 OLDCARTS Mnemonic

Onset	When did the symptom begin?
	Identify date and time or time frame when the symptom started.
Location	Where specifically is the location?
	Is the symptom felt in another area of the body other than the specific location?
Duration	How long does it last?
	Does the symptom come and go (intermittent)?
	Is the symptom constant?
	Does the symptom occur during specific times?
Characteristics	What does it feel like?
	What does it look like?
Aggravating or alleviating factors	What makes the symptom worse?
	What makes the symptom better?
Related symptoms	Do you experience other symptoms?
	Concomitant symptoms occur at the same time such as nausea or headache.
Treatment	What have you taken or tried to alleviate the symptoms?
	This may include medications, treatments, or complementary or alternative treatments such as acupuncture.
Severity	How would you rate or describe the severity of the symptom?
	How does it affect your daily activities?

- Name
- Address
- Date of birth (DOB)
- Birthplace
- Age
- Gender
- Race
- Religion
- Primary language
  - Secondary language
- Marital status
- Occupation
- Health insurance
- Allergies (drug, environmental, food)
- Emergency contact

TIP Always document the type of reaction the patient has had to an allergen (e.g., pollen—watery eyes).

Military History

Nurses need to know how to interview and assess our veterans. In 2012, the American Academy of Nurses set forth a new initiative, "Have You Ever Served?" to increase awareness and improve the quality of veterans' health care. This one question is to identify and address healthcare issues rising from the veteran's military service. In 2015, the U.S. Census Bureau reported 21.8 million veterans in the United States with more than 1.3 million veterans serving during multiple wars (U.S. Census Bureau, 2015). Military experience varies based on the war or conflict, combat experience, and other variables (Johnson, 2013).

Biographical Data

Collecting general information about the patient gives the nurse the ability to identify any sensory and cognitive deficits. Nurses are also able to assess if the patient can understand the question, recall information, and is a reliable source.

General Questions About Military Experience

■ Would it be okay if I talked with you about your military experience?
■ When and where do you/did you serve?
■ What do you/did you do while in the service?
■ How has military service affected you?
　If your patient answers yes to any of the following questions, ask "Can you tell me more about that?"
■ Did you see combat, enemy fire, or casualties?
■ Were you or a buddy wounded, injured, or hospitalized?
■ Did you have a head injury with loss of consciousness, loss of memory, "seeing stars," or being temporarily disoriented?
■ Were you a prisoner of war?

Concerns About Military Exposure

■ Would it be okay if I asked about some things you may have been exposed to during your service?
　□ Veterans may have been exposed to many environments and chemical or biological agents and may have different health concerns depending on the war in which they served (Table 3-3).
■ What were you exposed to?
　□ Chemical (pollution, solvents, etc.)
　□ Biological (infectious disease)
　□ Physical (blast or explosion, bullet wound, heat, noise, radiation, shell fragment, vehicular crash, vibration, other injury)
■ What precautions were taken (avoidance, personal protective equipment, treatment)?
■ How long was the exposure?
■ How concerned are you about the exposure?
■ Where were you exposed?
■ Who else may have been affected (unit name, etc.)? (Veterans Health Administration, 2014)

Medications

Ask the patient:
■ What prescription and over-the-counter (OTC) medications do you take?
　□ Medications should include the name, dose, and how often it is taken.
　□ Patients should identify all types of medications that they are currently taking, including
　　• Prescription
　　• Vitamins
　　• Herbal and nonherbal supplements
　　• OTC medications
■ Have you ever had a blood transfusion? If so, when and why?

▮ **TIP** Ask the patient the reason for taking the medications. This will identify whether the patient is knowledgeable about the medications. Some patients do not know why they take their medications. Nurses should use this time to do patient teaching about medications and their actions.

Immunizations

Ask the patient:
■ What immunizations have you had?
　□ Vaccine-preventable diseases are near or at a record low (CDC, 2015). During this part of the history, patient education about recommended immunizations is encouraged. The immunization history should include all vaccinations the patient has received through life. Dates or years should be included. These may include the following:
　• hepatitis A
　• hepatitis B
　• herpes zoster (Zostavax)
　• influenza

TABLE 3-3 Veteran's Health Concerns

Environmental exposures	Asbestos Burn pit smoke Contaminated water (benzene, trichloroethylene, vinyl chloride) Endemic disease Hexavalent chromium Ionizing and non-ionizing radiation Jet fuel Lead Mustard gas Nerve agents Particulate matter Pesticides Tetrachlorodibenzo-p-dioxin (TCDD) and other dioxins	Gulf War (Operation Desert Shield/ Operation Desert Storm)	Chemical or biological agents Depleted uranium (DU) Dermatological issues Immunizations Infectious diseases (e.g., leishmaniasis) Oil well fires Reproductive health issues
		Vietnam, Korean DMZ, and Thailand	Agent Orange exposure Hepatitis C
		Cold War	Nuclear weapons testing (Atomic veterans)
Operation Enduring Freedom, Operation Iraqi Freedom, Operation New Dawn	Animal bites/rabies Combined penetrating Blunt trauma Burn injuries (blast injuries) Dermatologic issues Embedded fragments (shrapnel) Leishmaniasis Mental health issues Multi-drug-resistant *Acinetobacter* Reproductive health issues Spinal cord injury Traumatic amputation Traumatic brain injury Vision loss	WWII and Korean War	Cold injury Chemical warfare agent experiments Exposure to nuclear weapons (including testing or cleanup)

Veterans Health Administration, 2014.

- human papillomavirus (HPV)
- measles, mumps, rubella (MMR)
- meningococcal
- pneumococcal (polysaccharide)
- tetanus, diphtheria, pertussis (Td/Tdap)
- varicella

▇ **TIP** The most recent Centers for Disease Control and Prevention (CDC) immunization schedule can be found at http://www.cdc.gov/vaccines/schedules/.

Health Prevention and Promotion

Individuals should be maintaining their health and well-being. During the health history, it is good nursing practice to identify if the patient has been periodically having preventative checkups. These questions are integrated in the health history or review of systems.

Past History

Ask the patient about:
■ Past medical history related to
  □ childhood illnesses (measles, chicken pox, rheumatic fever)
  □ adult illness (i.e., diabetes, hypertension, cancer, sexually transmitted infections [STIs])
  □ accidents or injuries
  □ serious or chronic illnesses (cancer, arthritis, autoimmune diseases)
  □ hospitalizations (medical, surgical, obstetric, psychiatric, rehabilitative)
  □ surgeries (include year of surgery)
  □ mental or emotional illnesses.

▇ **TIP** Sometimes patients forget they had a specific type of surgery and you may see a scar when doing a physical assessment. For example, "I see that you have a scar on your shoulder. Did you have surgery?"

Family History

Gathering a complete and accurate family medical history is becoming more important as genetic medicine explains more diseases (American Medical Association, n.d.). The family history section reviews the health and illness history of family members.

■ The family history is helpful to determine whether there are any genetic or familial tendencies for a specific disease; it is valuable to identify family health patterns or tendencies.

■ A genogram (pedigree) is a pictorial diagram of a family tree; the diagram should include at least three or more generations (siblings, parents, grandparents); symbols identify the relationships, causes of deaths, and health and illness histories (Venes, 2013) (Fig. 3-1).

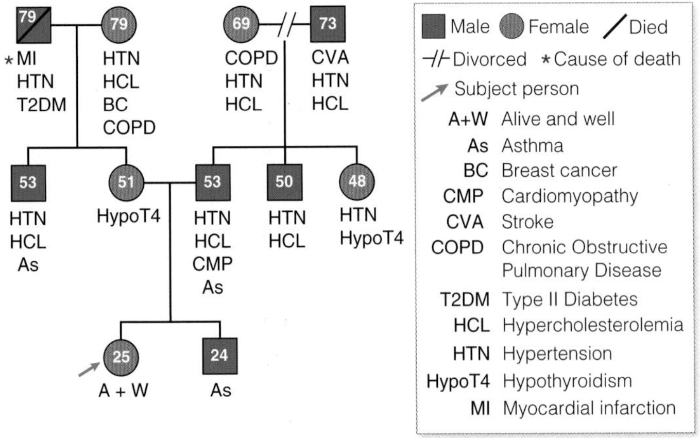

Fig. 3-1. Sample genogram.

PSYCHOSOCIAL ASSESSMENT

The psychosocial history collects information about many aspects of a patient's life; this reviews psychological or mental health and all aspects of the patient's social life.

The patient's lifestyle, relationships, employment, connections within the community, functional capacity, and environmental factors are reviewed to assess and obtain a clear picture of the whole patient. The following are fundamental topics included in the psychosocial assessment:

- **Behavioral:** daily habits, healthcare practices, and daily activities
- **Environmental:** physical and social environment (i.e., allergens, asbestos, housing, water)
- **Social:** human-to-human interaction, relationship to individuals, groups, institutions, organizational systems, culture, and spirituality
- **Financial and economic:** i.e., household management

The following are questions to ask the patient under each category.

Education

- Tell me about your education. Do you have a degree?
- What was your major in college or graduate school?

Occupation

- Are you employed outside of the home?
- What do you do for a living?
- Do you have medical benefits through work?
- Do you sit for long periods of time at work?
- What machinery do you use?
- Do you use safety precautions at work?
- Have you been exposed to fumes, loud noises, or environmental hazards?
- Do you think your job is affecting your symptoms?

Housing/Environment

- What type of house or apartment do you live in?
- Can you describe the neighborhood?
- What type of transportation is available to you?

Military Living Situation

- Would it be okay to talk about your living situation?
- Where do you live?
- Is your house safe?
- Are you in any danger of losing your housing?
- Do you need assistance in caring for dependents? (Veterans Health Administration, 2014)

Finances

- Are you able to financially support yourself?
- What is your economic situation?

Military Compensation and Benefits

- Do you have any service-connected condition?
- Would you like assistance in filing for compensation for injuries/ illnesses related to your service?

Exercise

- Do you regularly exercise? If so, what type of exercise? How long do you exercise?

Sleep/Rest

- How many hours per night do you sleep?
- Do you have difficulty falling asleep? Staying asleep?
- Do you have sleep apnea?

TIP The most common type of sleep apnea is obstructive sleep apnea. The airway collapses or becomes occluded during sleep and causes shallow breathing or breathing pauses for a couple of seconds or minutes. Sleep apnea is the leading cause of excessive daytime sleepiness (National Heart, Lung and Blood Institute, 2012).

Safety

- Do you wear seat belts?
- Do you use car seats?

- Do you wear a helmet when riding a bicycle or skiing?
- Do you have smoke or carbon monoxide detectors?
- How do you protect yourself when playing sports (such as, for males, a protective cup)?

Military Sexual Harassment, Assault Trauma

- Would it be all right to talk about sexual harassment or trauma that you might have experienced while serving in the military?
- Have you ever experienced physical, emotional, or sexual harassment or trauma?
- Is this past experience causing you problems now?
- Do you want a referral? (Veterans Health Administration, 2014)

Tobacco Use: Cigarettes or Cigars

- How many do you smoke daily? (Calculate the pack-years history.)

TIP The pack-years smoking history identifies the degree of tobacco exposure and a person's risk for developing disease such as emphysema or lung cancer.

  □ The pack-years history measures how many cigarettes the individual has smoked over a period of 1 year. There are 20 cigarettes in one pack.
  □ To calculate the pack-years history: Divide the number of cigarettes smoked daily by 20 and multiply this number by how many years the individual has smoked. For example, the individual has smoke 15 cigarettes daily for 21 years: $15/20 \times 21$ years = 16 pack-years.
- Do you chew tobacco?

Support Systems/Home Life

- Does anyone else live with you?
- Tell me about your family and friends.
- Who is your support system?

Stress/Coping Mechanisms

- Do you feel like you have any stress or stressors in your life?
- What do you do to relieve your stress?
  □ The BATHE assessment technique serves as a rough screening tool for anxiety, depression, and situational stress disorders. The BATHE technique consists of four specific questions about the patient's background, affect, troubles, and handling of the current situation; the assessment takes approximately 1 minute to complete (see Box 3-1).

Military Stress Reactions/Adjustment Problems

- Would it be okay to talk about stress?
- In your life, have you ever had an experience so horrible, frightening, or upsetting that, in the past month you:
  □ had nightmares about it or thought about it when you did not want to?
  □ tried hard not to think about it or went out of your way to avoid situations that reminded you of it?
  □ were constantly on guard, watchful, or easily startled?
  □ felt numb or detached from others, activities, or your surroundings? (Veterans Health Administration, 2014)

BOX 3-1 **The BATHE Technique**

B	Background: What is going on in your life?
A	Affect: How do you feel about that?
T	Trouble: What troubles you the most?
H	Handling: How are you handling that?
E	Empathy: That must be very difficult.

Lieberman III, JA and Stuart, MR. The BATHE Method: Incorporating Counseling and Psychotherapy Into the Everyday Management of Patients. Primary Care Companion *The Journal of Clinical Psychiatry*, 1999 Apr; 1(2): 35–38. Copyright 1999, Physicians Postgraduate Press. Adapted or Reprinted by permission.

Domestic Violence

During all assessments, the nurse must assess the patient's safety, any exposure to domestic violence, and interpersonal violence. The Affordable Care Act requires most health plans to provide annual screening and counseling for domestic and interpersonal violence. Domestic violence is a pattern of abusive behavior in any relationship that is used by one partner to gain or maintain power and control over another intimate partner. Domestic violence can be physical, sexual, emotional, economic, or psychological actions or threats of actions that influence another person. This includes any behaviors that intimidate, manipulate, humiliate, isolate, frighten, terrorize, coerce, threaten, blame, hurt, injure, or wound someone (U.S. Department of Justice, 2015).

The following questions should only be asked when the patient is alone. Ask the patient:

- Have you been hit, slapped, kicked, punched, forced to have sex, or otherwise hurt by someone within the past year?
- Do you feel safe in your current relationship?
- Do you feel threatened or controlled by a partner or ex-partner or anyone else in your life? (Feldhaus, Koziol-McLain, Amsbury, Lowenstein, & Abbott, 1997)

HITS is a domestic violence screening tool for use in the community (Box 3-2).

SENC: Evidence-Based Practice A new mobile app from Harbor House of Central Florida is working to turn smartphones and iPads in hospitals and doctors' offices into powerful screening tools that help identify victims of domestic abuse and direct them to the help they need. The R3 App, which stands for Recognize, Respond, and Refer, is the first mobile domestic violence screening tool in the United States and leverages the HITS process created 13 years ago by Dr. Kevin Sherin, Director of the Orange County (Florida) Health Department. This is an evidence-based screening tool that correctly identifies 91 percent of individuals in abusive relationships (http://www.harborhousefl.com/2012/01/r3-app-2/).

BOX 3-2 HITS: A Domestic Violence Screening Tool for Use in the Community

HITS Tool for Intimate Partner Violence Screenings

Please read each of the following activities and fill in circle that best indicates the frequency with which your partner acts in the way depicted.

How often does your partner?	Never	Rarely	Sometimes	Fairly Often	Frequently
1. Physically hurt you	○	○	○	○	○
2. Insult or talk down to you	○	○	○	○	○
3. Threaten you with harm	○	○	○	○	○
4. Scream or curse at you	○	○	○	○	○
	1	2	3	4	5

Each item is scored from 1 to 5. Thus, scores for this inventory range from 4 to 20. A score of greater than 10 is considered positive.

© 2003 Kevin Sherin MD, MPH. Used with permission.

Substance Abuse
■ Alcohol
- □ How often do you drink? If daily, how many drinks per day? What kind of alcohol?
- □ Have you been arrested for driving under the influence?

SENC: Safety Alert Moderate drinking has been defined as two standard drinks (e.g., 12 oz beer) per day for men and one drink per day for women and persons over age 65 years. Hazardous or "at-risk" drinking is defined as 14 drinks/week or more than four drinks/occasion for men and seven drinks/week or two drinks per occasion for women (Ferri, 2016).

■ Drugs
- □ Do you take or smoke any recreational drugs?
- □ Do you take any prescription pain medication on a regular basis?

SENC: Safety Alert Opioid abuse, especially heroin, is a growing public health problem. Ninety-one Americans die every day from an opioid overdose (CDC, 2016).

The CAGE-AID questionnaire is a substance abuse screening tool for alcohol and drug abuse and dependence in adults. The advantage of this screening tool is to assess for alcohol and drug problems conjointly rather than separately. When thinking of drug use, include illegal drug use and the use of prescription drug use other than prescribed. The questionnaire asks the following questions:
- Have you ever felt you needed to cut down on your drinking or drug use?
- Have people annoyed you by criticizing your drinking or drug use?
- Have you ever felt bad or guilty about drinking or drug use?
- Have you ever had a drink or used drugs first thing in the morning to steady your nerves or to get rid of a hangover?
  Scoring: Regard one or more positive responses as a positive screen.
  (Permission for use granted by Richard Brown, MD)

SENC: Evidence-Based Practice Brown and Rounds (1995) identified that the CAGE-AID exhibited 79 percent sensitivity and 77 percent sensitivity to one or more "yes" responses and 70 percent sensitivity and 85 percent specificity to two or more "yes" responses.

Another reliable questionnaire is a two-item conjoint screen (TICS) for alcohol and drug problems. This questionnaire is more sensitive to current drug and alcohol disorders rather than lifetime abuse. The questionnaire asks the following two questions:
- In the last year, have you ever drunk or used drugs more than you meant to?
- Have you felt you wanted or needed to cut down on your drinking or drug use in the last year?
  (Permission for use granted by Richard Brown, MD)

SENC: Evidence-Based Practice At least one positive result to the TICS detected current substance use disorders with nearly 80 percent sensitivity and specificity. The questionnaire performed particularly well with individuals who had disorders involving marijuana or cocaine. It is important to understand that the TICS can produce false positive results (Brown, Leonard, Saunders, & Papasouliotis, 2001).

Military Substance Abuse
- Have you ever used drugs such as heroin and cocaine?

Sexuality

Healthy People 2020 Goal
- Promote healthy sexual behaviors, strengthen community capacity, and increase access to quality services to prevent STIs and their complications.

A sexual history and risk assessment should be obtained to determine potential problems and identify areas that may require patient education (Williamson, 2010). Patients may be embarrassed to talk about their sexuality. This sensitive area requires the nurse to be compassionate and sensitive to the questions and answers.

■ **TIP** Nurses should know the difference between the terms "sex" and "gender." Sex commonly refers to physical characteristics; gender represents identity and self-image (Spack, 2013; Coleman et al, 2011).

■ Do not assume a patient's sexuality.

■ Gender-neutral language such as "partner or spouse" communicates to lesbian, gay, bisexual, and transgender patients that it is safe for them to be honest and open with the interviewer (Fortin, Dwamena, & Smith, 2012).

Patient-Centered Care

■ Some patients may not be comfortable talking about their sexual history, sex partners, or sexual practices. Try to put patients at ease and let them know that taking a sexual history is an important part of a health history and physical exam.

■ Sexual history may be assessed during a comprehensive or focused interview if the patient has signs or symptoms of STIs.

You might start the interview by saying:

■ "I am going to ask you a few questions about your sexual health and sexual practices. I understand that these questions are very personal, but they are important for your overall health."

■ "Just so you know, I ask these questions to all of my adult patients, regardless of age, gender, or marital status. These questions are as important as the questions about other areas of your physical and mental health. Like the rest of your visits, this information is kept in strict confidence. Do you have any questions before we get started?" (CDC, 2011)

Ask the patient:

■ Tell me about your sexual history.

■ Is there someone special in your life?

■ Are you sexually involved with another person?

■ Do you have sex with men, women, or both?

■ Are you practicing safe sex?

■ Are you or your partner having any sexual difficulties at this time? (Association of Reproductive Health Professionals, 2008)

■ **Female patient:** Do you have any pain during intercourse (dyspareunia)? Do you have any vaginal itching or drainage?

■ **Male patient:** Do you have any difficulty with ejaculating or having an erection? Do you have any colored drainage from your penis?

FUNCTIONAL ASSESSMENT

The functional assessment assesses a patient's ability to perform his or her activities of daily living (ADLs). During the assessment, you want to know if the patient is independent in performing ADLs or needs assistance. If the patient needs help, assess who helps and how much assistance is needed. This includes activities with:

■ bathing

■ dressing

■ eating

■ walking

■ housekeeping

■ meal preparation

■ shopping

■ driving

See Chapter 24, Assessing the Older Adult.

CULTURAL ASSESSMENT

Nurses care for patients from many different cultures. A cultural assessment identifies specific cultural factors that affect a patient's health (Box 3-3). Professional skill is needed to assess preferences of people of varying ethnicities or nationalities (Venes, 2013). The Institute of Medicine (IOM) (2011) report, "The Future of Nursing: Leading Change," noted that minority groups are expected to become a majority by 2042. Nurses continually need to develop cultural competence to develop increasing awareness about the similarities and differences of diverse cultures. Becoming culturally competent is a moral and ethical commitment to our patients, families, and communities (Hines, 2012). Each culture is unique, and nurses need the knowledge and skills to holistically consider the cultural considerations of each patient. During health assessment, observe and listen carefully to the patient's report. Display warmth, caring, and respect to encourage the patient to be open and share beliefs, concerns, and practices with you.

■ **TIP** Nurses should know where to access resources to assist them to provide cultural competent care. The National Center for Cultural Competence (2013) has many resources to guide nurses to provide and train to give culturally competent care. (https://nccc.georgetown.edu)

BOX 3-3 **Cultural Assessment Tool**

Client's Name _____

Ethnic Origin_____

Address_____ Birth Date_____

Name of Significant Other_____ Relationship_____

Primary Language Spoken_____

Second Language Spoken_____

How does client usually communicate with people who speak a different language?_____

Is an interpreter required?_____

BOX 3-3 Cultural Assessment Tool—cont'd

Available?_____

Highest level of education achieved?_____

Occupation_____

Presenting problem_____

Has this problem ever occurred before?_____

If so, in what manner was it handled previously?_____

What is the client's usual manner of coping with stress? _____

Who is (are) the client's main support system?_____

Describe the family living arrangements_____

Who is the major decision maker in the family?_____

Describe client's family members' roles within the family_____

Describe religious beliefs and practices_____

Are there any religious requirements or restrictions that place limitations on the client's care? _____

If so, describe_____

Who in the family takes responsibility for health concerns?_____

Describe any special health beliefs and practices that may vary from the conventional_____

From whom does family usually seek medical assistance in time of need?_____

Describe client's usual emotional/behavioral response to:

Anxiety_____

Anger_____

Continued

BOX 3-3 Cultural Assessment Tool—cont'd

Loss/change/failure_____

Pain_____

Fear_____

Describe any topics that are particularly sensitive or that the client is unwilling to discuss (because of cultural taboos)_____

_____

Describe any activities in which the client is unwilling to participate (because of cultural customs or taboos)_____

_____

What are the client's personal feelings regarding eye contact?_____

What is the client's personal orientation to time? (past, present, future)_____

Describe any particular illnesses to which the client may be bioculturally susceptible (e.g., hypertension and sickle cell anemia in Africans)

_____

Describe any nutritional deficiencies to which the client may be bioculturally susceptible (e.g., lactose intolerance in native and Asian Americans)

_____

Describe the client's favorite foods_____

Are there any foods the client requests or refuses because of cultural beliefs related to this illness? (e.g., "hot" and "cold" foods for Hispanic and Asian

Americans). If so, please describe_____

Describe client's perception of the problem and expectations of health care_____

From Townsend, M. (2010). *Nursing Diagnoses in Psychiatric Nursing Care Plans and Psychometric Medications*. Philadelphia, PA: F.A. Davis.

SPIRITUAL ASSESSMENT

Patients are bio-psycho-social-spiritual beings. Spirituality can have a positive influence on health and well-being. It can also play a vital role in illness and recovery.

There is a difference between religion and spirituality:

- Religion is an organized system of beliefs shared by a group of people; there are practices, behaviors, worship, and rituals associated with that system.
- Spirituality is multifaceted; it is a search for a meaningful and overall purpose of life and a sense of life's direction (Sheldrake, 2013).
- Spirituality is the essence of who we are and how we are in the world.
- The term is derived from the Latin *spiritus*, meaning breath and relates to the Greek *pneuma* or breath, which refers to the vital spirit or soul (Dossey & Keegan, 2013).
- Every culture has its own practices and beliefs. For example, Amish religious and cultural values include honesty, order, personal responsibility, community welfare, humility, nonresistance, nonviolence, and obedience to parents, church and God (Purnell, 2014).

A spiritual assessment is similar to the nursing process in that it is a process that begins when the patient is first assessed and continues throughout her or his care (Dunn, 2010). This assessment assists the nurse to get to know the whole patient, including her or his thoughts, beliefs, and way of life. A nurse is usually the healthcare provider who spends the time assessing and interviewing the patient and may offer his or her support by:

- praying with the patient
- offering the patient sacred space
- listening attentively and empathetically.

TIP Nurses should not be judgmental or biased when assessing the patient's spirituality or religion.

The FICA Spiritual History Tool was developed by Dr. Christina Puchalski and a group of primary care physicians to help physicians and other healthcare professionals address spiritual issues with patients (Table 3-4).

TABLE 3-4 **FICA Model for Spiritual Assessment Tool**		
F	*Faith and belief*	"Do you consider yourself spiritual or religious?" or "Do you have spiritual beliefs that help you cope with stress/difficult times?" If the patient responds, "No," the healthcare provider might ask, "What gives your life meaning?" Sometimes patients respond with answers such as family, career, or nature.
I	*Importance*	"What importance does your faith or belief have in our life?" "Have your beliefs influenced how you take care of yourself in this illness?" "What role do your beliefs play in regaining your health?"
C	*Community*	"Are you part of a spiritual or religious community?" "Is this of support to you and how?" "Is there a group of people you really love or who are important to you?" Communities such as churches, temples, and mosques, or a group of like-minded friends can serve as strong support systems for some patients.
A	*Address in care*	"How would you like me (your healthcare provider) to address these issues in your health care?"

Reprinted with permission from Christina Puchalski, M.D.

REVIEW OF SYSTEMS

The health history contains the review of systems (ROS), a subjective report of all body systems by the patient. This is a head-to-toe survey to uncover symptoms not elicited during the history of present illness; the patient reports his or her health status as it relates to each body system. During the ROS, the patient will either report and describe symptoms or deny symptoms. Be specific and document which symptoms were present or absent. Pertinent positive and negative responses should be documented for each system. Patients must understand your questions; do not use medical terminology. The key is to make sure that you ask appropriate and specific questions to have a detailed description of the patient's health or problem.

Each symptom should be fully described. Refer to the alphabetical Mnemonic for Subjective History Gathering (see Table 3-1) or the OLD-CARTS Mnemonic (see Table 3-2). Medications review and health promotion activities and screenings should be integrated throughout the ROS within pertinent body systems.

■ **TIP** If the patient is unreliable or unable to answer the questions, this must be documented. An example is, "Patient is unable to answer questions and is unreliable due to decreased cognition." The reason should be documented. If a secondary source answers the questions, the source should be identified, such as "Patient's husband is reporting the ROS on behalf of the patient."

The following section includes questions to ask the patient under each category.

General Status

- What is your perceived state of health? When was the last time you had a physical examination?
- Do you experience fever/chills, night sweats, weight changes, weakness, fatigue, general pain or discomfort, or mood changes (anhedonia *[the inability to feel pleasure from activities that were at one time pleasurable]*)?

Skin (See Chapter 8)

- Do you have any rashes/lesions, redness, itching/hives, easy or frequent bruising, change in moles, change in texture of skin, change in color of skin, wounds?
- Do you use sunscreen? If so, what strength? Do you go to tanning salons?
- Do you perform skin self-examination? If so, how often?
- Do you see a dermatologist? If so, who? When was the last time you saw a dermatologist for a skin check?

Hair on Body (See Chapter 8)

- Have you noticed any changes in hair distribution, brittle hair, hair falling out? If so, when did it start?
- Does your hair or scalp itch?

Nails (See Chapter 8)

- Have you noticed any change in the color or texture of your fingernails or toenails?
- Have your nails become thinner or thicker? Are your nails brittle?
- Do you bite your nails? Any recent nail infections?
- How do your care for your nails?

Head (See Chapter 9)

- Have you felt dizzy? Do you get headaches? If so, how often. Describe the type of headache.
- Do you have vertigo?
- Have you experienced trauma or an injury to your head?
- Do you see a neurologist? If so, who?

■ **TIP** Dizziness is feeling light-headed or unsteady. Vertigo is the sensation of moving around in space (subjective vertigo) or of having objects move about the person (objective vertigo). Vertigo is not a synonym for dizziness (Venes, 2013).

Eyes (See Chapter 11)

- Have you had your eyes examined by an optometrist or ophthalmologist? If so, when and by whom?
- Do you wear glasses? Any changes in vision, double vision (diplopia), eye pain, redness, discharge?
- Do you need to use safety glasses when working?

Ears (See Chapter 10)

- Have you had your hearing checked? If yes, when and by whom?
- Do you have any ringing in your ears (tinnitus), earwax, hearing loss, use of hearing aids, discharge, or ear pain?
- Do you need to wear ear protectors at work?
- Do you clean your ears? If so, how?

TIP An example of documentation for pertinent positives and negatives would be: Reports last ear exam by audiologist, Dr. _____, January 2016; reports constant tinnitus and hearing loss in both ears; wears hearing aids daily. Denies excessive earwax, discharge, pain, or use of Q-tips to clean ears.

SENC: Safety Alert Cotton-tip applicators are not recommended to clean the inner ear because when inserted into the ear canal, the cotton pushes the earwax farther into the inner canal.

Nose and Sinuses (See Chapter 9)

- Do you have nosebleeds, nasal drainage, any loss of smell, allergy symptoms?
- Do you get sinus infections or headaches?
- Do you have any difficulty with your sense of smell?
- Do you snore when you sleep?

Mouth and Throat (See Chapter 9)

- Have you been to the dentist? If yes, what is your dentist's name and how often do you get dental checkups?

- Do your gums bleed?
- Do you have pain on swallowing, difficulty swallowing (dysphagia), hoarseness, tongue burning, own teeth/dentures, mouth or tooth pain?

Neck (See Chapter 9)

- Have you felt any lumps on your neck?
- Do you have limited range of motion, or stiffness of your neck?
- Have you ever been in an accident and suffered whiplash?

Respiratory (See Chapter 12)

- Do you have a cough, chest pain, shortness of breath (SOB) (dyspnea), sputum production or blood in sputum (hemoptysis), or wheezing?
- Have you had a recent chest x-ray? If so, when?
- Have you been tested for tuberculosis?

Breasts (Male and Female) (See Chapters 18 and 19)

- Do you have any lumps, nipple discharge, breast pain, or prosthetics?
- Do you perform breast self-examination (BSE)? When? Tell me which method you use?
- Do you get mammograms? If so, how often? When was your last mammogram (if applicable)?

Cardiac (See Chapter 13)

- Do you have any chest pain, palpitations, dyspnea on exertion (DOE), SOB during sleep (paroxysmal nocturnal dyspnea)?
- Have you had an electrocardiogram? If so, when?
- Do you see a cardiologist? If yes, who is your cardiologist? When was your last visit (if applicable)?
- Do you have your cholesterol tested regularly?

TIP It is recommended to document the names of the healthcare providers that patients see on a regular basis.

Hematological
- Do you have any bleeding tendencies or bruising? Have you received any blood transfusions? If so, why did you need a blood transfusion?

Gastrointestinal (See Chapter 14)
- How would you describe your appetite?
- Do you get nauseous? Have you had problems with vomiting, vomiting blood (hematemesis), heartburn, or abdominal pain?
- Have you noticed any change in your bowel patterns such as constipation or diarrhea? Have you noticed any change in size (diameter) of the stool, blood in stool (melena), rectal bleeding?
- Do you have hemorrhoids?
- Have you had a colonoscopy? If so, when? By whom?
- Have you had an endoscopy? If so, when? By whom?

Urinary (See Chapter 14)
- Do you have frequency, urgency, or pain (dysuria) with urination?
- Have you noticed any increased urination at night (nocturia)?
- Have you noticed any blood in your urine (hematuria) or change in color?
- Do you have problems with urinary incontinence? Do you wear adult pads?
  For men, ask:
- Do you have difficulty or hesitancy starting a urine stream?
  For women, ask:
- Do you perform Kegel exercises?

TIP Kegel exercises strengthen pelvic floor muscles to prevent leakage of urine.

Musculoskeletal (See Chapter 16)
- Do you have any pain in your muscles, bones, or joints?
- Do you have any limitations with your range of motion of any extremities?

- Have you fallen? If so, when? Were you injured?
- Do you have muscle weakness or tremors?
- Do you use any assistive devices needed for ambulation?
- Do you have any swelling of joints, sciatica, or nerve pain?
- Do you get cortisone injections?
- Have you had physical therapy?

Peripheral Vascular (See Chapter 15)
- Do you have any tingling, burning sensations, or numbness of extremities?
- Do you have varicose veins?
- Have you noticed any change in the color of extremities?
- Do you have any pain in your legs with walking?
- Do you have any swelling or edema of the extremities?

TIP If a patient has pain with walking that goes away with rest, ask the patient how far he or she can walk without feeling pain (e.g., I can walk from my back door to my mailbox, which is about 100 feet).

Neurological (See Chapter 17)
- Have you ever had a seizure or fainting episode?
- Have you noticed any changes in your memory? When did this begin?
- Do you feel like you get confused at times?
- Do you have any changes in the five senses (seeing, hearing, smell, taste, touch)?
- Do you have any loss of coordination or a problem with balance?
- Have you noticed any tremors of your extremities?
- Do you have any muscle spasms?

Women's Health (See Chapter 18)
- Do you see a gynecologist? If so, how often? What is his or her name?
- **Women's health exams:** Have you had a mammogram? If so, when? Have you had a Papanicolaou test (Pap smear)? If so, when?

- When did you first start menstruating? How often do you menstruate? How long is your menstrual cycle? Any problems?
- **Menopause:** When did menopause start? Do you experience menopausal symptoms? If so, what type of symptoms?
- **STIs:** Have you noticed any perineal lesions or discharge, itching, or bleeding between periods?
- Has there been a change in your libido?
- What kind of birth control do you use?

Obstetrical History (See Chapter 23)

- How many, if any, pregnancies, deliveries (vaginal or cesarean section), miscarriages, abortions?
- Have you had any problems with infertility? If so, for how long?

Male Genital (See Chapter 19)

- Have you noticed any lesions, penile discharge, problems with erectile function, testis swelling or pain, change in libido, or hernias?
- Do you perform testicular self-examination? How often? Describe how you examine yourself.
- Have you had a prostate examination? If so, when? By whom?

MENTAL HEALTH ASSESSMENT

Healthy People 2020 Goal

Improve mental health through prevention and by ensuring access to appropriate, quality mental health services (HHS, 2010).

Patients can have changes in mental status for many reasons including disease, trauma, side effects of medications, and mental illness. Mental health assessment begins at the time that you meet and start interviewing the patient. Simply watch and listen to the patient carefully.

Mental health is a state of successful performance of mental function, resulting in productive activities, fulfilling relationships with other people, and the ability to adapt to change and to cope with challenges. Mental health is essential to personal well-being, family and interpersonal relationships, and the ability to contribute to community or society (HHS, 2010).

Mental illness affects women and men differently (HHS, 2010). Some disorders are more common in women, and some express themselves with different symptoms. Scientists are only now beginning to tease apart the contributions of various biological and psychosocial factors to mental health and mental illness in both women and men (National Institute of Mental Health, n.d.).

Mental health assessment is ongoing throughout the health assessment. Using open-ended questions encourages the patient to talk about issues of immediate concern and helps to establish rapport (Davis & Craig, 2009). During the assessment, you should be observing the following:

- **General appearance:** personal appearance, grooming, hygiene, whether the patient is dressed appropriately for the weather; posture during the assessment
- **Emotional reaction or affect can be of two types:**
  - ☐ Blunted affect is greatly diminished emotional response to a situation or condition.
  - ☐ Flat affect is virtual absence of emotional response to a situation or condition (Venes, 2013).
- **Speech pattern:** clarity, coherent, volume, articulation of words
- **Memory/cognition:** immediate, short term and long term
  - ☐ **Orientation to person, place, time, and situation:**
    - Person: What is your name?
    - Place: Where are you right now? What is your address?
    - Time: What is the today's date? What season are we in?
    - Situation: What are you doing right now?

- **Behavior and mood:** oppositional/resistant, submissive, defensive, open and friendly, candid and cooperative, shows subdued mistrust and hostility, excessive shyness, happy, sad, indifferent
  - □ Assessing for depression: a depressed mood or feelings of sadness on most days, decreased interest in social and daily activities, difficulty sleeping, chronic fatigue, and increased agitation, feelings of worthlessness, thoughts of death or suicide. Functional impairment is also a sign of depression.
  - □ Ask the patient:
    - Over the last 2 weeks, have you felt down, depressed, or hopeless?
    - Over the last 2 weeks, have you felt little interest or pleasure in doing things?

SENC: Evidence-Based Practice The U.S. Preventive Services Task Force recommends screening for depression in the general adult population, including pregnant and postpartum women. Screening should be implemented with adequate systems in place to ensure accurate diagnosis, effective treatment, and appropriate follow-up (U.S. Preventive Services Task Force, 2016).

According to the CDC (2015), suicide is the third-leading cause of death among individuals ages 10 to 14, the second for ages 15 to 34, the fourth in those ages 35 to 44, fifth for ages 45 to 54, and the eighth for ages 55 to 64. In 2013, suicide was the 10th-leading overall cause of death for all ages. There are nine simple questions to begin a suicide risk assessment:

1. How are you coping with what has been happening in your life?
2. Do you ever feel like just giving up?
3. Are you thinking about dying?
4. Are you thinking about hurting yourself?
5. Are you thinking about suicide?
6. Have you thought about how you would do it?
7. Do you know when you would do it?
8. Do you have the means to do it?
9. Have you ever attempted to harm yourself in the past? (Davis, Schuss, & Lockhart, 2014)

SENC: Safety Alert Never leave a patient alone if you suspect that he or she is having suicidal thoughts. Ask a healthcare provider to come assess the patient.

COGNITIVE ASSESSMENT

Mini-Mental State Examination

Cognitive impairment is no longer considered a normal and inevitable change of aging. Trauma, surgery, the aging process, and disease may affect or change a patient's cognitive level of functioning. Cognition involves:

- thinking skills
- language
- calculation
- perception
- memory
- reasoning
- judgment (Venes, 2013).

A cognitive assessment is performed to determine a patient's level of cognitive function. The Mini-Mental State Examination is a short assessment of 11 questions that test five areas of cognitive function: (1) orientation, (2) registration, (3) attention and calculation, (4) recall, and (5) language. The maximum score is 30. A score of 23 or lower is indicative of cognitive impairment. It takes only 5 to 10 minutes to administer, so it is practical to use repeatedly and routinely (Table 3-5).

TABLE 3-5 Sample Items From the Mini-Mental State Examination

Orientation to time	"What is the date?"
Registration	"Listen carefully, I am going to say three words. You say them back after I stop." Ready? Here they are… APPLE (pause) PENNY (pause) TABLE (pause) Now repeat those words back to me." (Repeat up to five times, but score only the first trial.)
Naming	"What is this?" (Point to a pencil or pen.)
Reading	"Please read this and do what it says." (Show examinee the stimulus form.) CLOSE YOUR EYES

Reproduced by special permission of the Publisher, Psychological Assessment Resources, Inc., 16204 North Florida Avenue, Lutz, Florida 33549, from the Mini-Mental State Examination, by Marshal Folsetin and Susan Folstein, Copyright 1975, 1998, 2001 by Mini Mental LLC, Inc. Published 2001 by the Psychological Assessment Resources, Inc. Further reproduction is prohibited without permission of PAR, Inc. The MMSE can be purchased from the PAR, Inc. by calling (813) 968-3003.

PATIENT EDUCATION

You will be learning all about the patient during the health history and ROS. The patient will be telling you whether he or she sees a physician regularly or is keeping up with recommended health screenings. Use this time as a teaching moment to share your knowledge. This is an optimal time for you to share recommended health screenings and discuss health promotion with the patient. Web sites to visit for recommended health screenings are as follows:

- American Cancer Society, http://www.cancer.org
- American Heart Association, http://www.heart.org/
- American Lung Association, http://www.lung.org
- CDC Eye Examinations, http://www.cdc.gov
- CDC Immunization Schedules, https://www.cdc.gov/vaccines/schedules/
- *Healthy People 2020*, http://www.healthypeople.gov
- U.S. Preventive Services Task Force, http://www.uspreventiveservicestaskforce.org/

DOCUMENTATION

The nursing history is documented per agency guidelines. There are many different types of forms and electronic health records used by institutions. Documentation should be clear, concise, and detailed. If written in the narrative form, subjective data should be documented using the patient's exact words using quotation marks. See Davis*Plus* for case studies with documentation exercises.

Assessing Nutrition and Anthropometric Measurements

INTRODUCTION

Good nutrition is important to maintain our overall well-being and to recover from illness. Nutritional intake affects overall growth and development. An old saying, "you are what you eat," is reflective of making the right choices for your everyday diet. Healthcare providers recognize the many benefits associated with a healthy eating plan, including:

■ decreased risk of chronic diseases, such as type 2 diabetes, hypertension, heart disease, and certain cancers
■ decreased risk of obesity
■ decreased risk of micronutrient deficiencies (CDC, 2014a).

Understanding the five basic food groups and how much we should eat of each category is a fundamental principle for healthy nutrition. The five basic food groups are (1) fruits, (2) vegetables, (3) grains, (4) protein, and (5) dairy. Simple screening and assessment of a patient's diet can identify whether healthy choices are being made and if the patient is at risk for nutritional imbalances.

A patient's state of health can be affected by too many or a deficiency of nutrients. Nearly 78 million adults in the United States deal with the health and emotional effects of obesity every day (American Heart Association, 2015). On June 17, 2013, the American Medical Association officially declared obesity as a disease that requires medical treatment and prevention (Pollack, 2013). Lack of attention to diet and nutrition may expose patients to the risk of developing malnutrition and its related complications, such as muscle wasting, poor wound healing, reduced immunity, longer hospital stays, and, ultimately, a reduced quality of life (Fletcher, 2009).

During the health assessment, nurses identify considerations that may influence an individual's diet. A patient's nutritional status can be influenced by many different factors including but not limited to:

■ cultural or ethnic influences on food choices and the meaning of food
■ economic considerations such as the cost of food
■ physical activity and expenditure of energy
■ physical condition of the patient and the patient's ability to eat food or go out and get food
■ psychosocial factors including mental health, religious beliefs, poverty, and lifestyle
■ available transportation to go out to purchase food
■ medications and their side effects that may cause anorexia
■ lack of knowledge about good nutrition, which may influence poor dietary intake.

Nurses need to be aware that assessing nutrition can be a sensitive topic to discuss with individuals. People do not always like to discuss what they eat, how much they eat, or foods they do not eat, even when they know that a particular food item is recommended. During this assessment, the nurse asks patients about eating habits, likes and dislikes, and special diets. Patients may not always be truthful in their report.

DEFINITION OF NUTRITION

Nutrition is the state of balance between nutrient intake and physiological requirements for growth and physical activity. Nutrition involves all the processes involved in the taking in and utilization of food by which growth, repair, and maintenance of activities in the body as a whole or in any of its parts are accomplished (Venes, 2013). Recent research shows that nutrition influences our genetic code. Nutrigenomics is a fast-moving field of research that combines molecular biology, genetics, and nutrition to regulate gene expression through specific nutrients (Kansas State University, 2010). Genetic variations influences an individual's metabolic rates, nutrient absorption, weight gain or loss, and how the individual responds to what they eat. The World Health Organization (WHO, 2016a) states that "nutritional disorders can be caused by an insufficient intake of food or of certain nutrients, by an inability of the body to absorb and use nutrients, or by overconsumption of certain foods."

Weight Loss

A person will lose weight by decreasing his or her caloric intake or burning more calories through physical activity. Losing weight can be a health benefit or a sign of underlying physical illness. Weight loss can be:

- **Planned:** Intentional, whereby the patient voluntarily loses weight:
  - ☐ A person who reduces his or her caloric intake by 500 calories or more per day than body requirements will lose 1 pound (0.45 kg) of body fat in 1 week.
- **Unplanned:** Unintentional, whereby the patient loses weight without trying to do so:
  - ☐ A 5 percent weight loss is an early indicator of increased risk of malnutrition (Fletcher, 2009).
  - ☐ A 10 to 20 percent weight loss indicates moderate protein-calorie malnutrition.
  - ☐ Weight loss of more than 20 percent indicates severe protein-calorie malnutrition (RX Kinetics, n.d.).

■ **TIP** Signs of unplanned weight loss are clothes and/or jewelry that have become loose fitting. Other signs are history of decreased food intake, reduced appetite, or swallowing problems over 3 to 6 months. Underlying disease or psychosocial/physical disabilities are also likely to cause weight loss (BAPEN, 2010).

Overnutrition

Modern society provides many opportunities for overeating and a sedentary lifestyle. Obesity is a national epidemic and a major contributor to some of the leading causes of death in the United States, including heart disease, stroke, diabetes, and some types of cancer (CDC, 2011). A person will gain weight when he or she consumes more calories than are burned through daily living:

- Overnutrition can be frequent or habitual overconsumption of nutrients by eating too much food in excess of body needs.
- The cause of overnutrition relates mostly to the excessive intake of carbohydrates and fats.

■ **TIP** One pound (0.45 kg) of fat = 3,500 calories.

- A person who eats 500 calories or more per day than body requirements will gain 1 pound (0.45 kg) of body fat in 1 week.

Malnutrition

Malnutrition is used to describe a deficiency, excess, or imbalance of a wide range of nutrients that can result in adverse effects on body composition and function. It can refer to individuals who are either overnourished or undernourished (Saunders, Smith, & Stroud, 2015). Individuals at risk for malnutrition may be seen in Box 4-1.

- Common causes of malnutrition include:
  - ☐ inadequate calorie consumption
  - ☐ inadequate intake of essential vitamins, minerals, or other micronutrients

- ☐ improper absorption and distribution of foods within the body (Venes, 2013).
- ■ Factors that may contribute to malnutrition include:
  - ☐ low income, which may influence the ability to buy food
  - ☐ chronic illnesses and illness causing decreased appetite, difficulty chewing and swallowing, side effects of medications, and a diminished sense of taste and smell, which may diminish appetite; lack of mobility, which may prevent the individual from buying or preparing food
  - ☐ dietary restrictions of salt, sugar, and fats, which may cause decreased appetite and food intake
  - ☐ mental health problems such as depression, loneliness, and drug and alcohol abuse which may contribute to anorexia and decreased food intake.

BOX 4-1

Individuals at Risk for Malnutrition
- Alcoholics
- Behavioral/mental health issues
- Children
- Chronically/acutely ill individuals
- Decreased cognitive function
- Elderly
- Illiterate individuals
- Individuals with disabilities
- Individuals who lack financial means
- Traumatic brain injury
- Substance abusers

DIAGNOSTICS

Blood work is an essential diagnostic tool to assess for anemia, lipid disorders, and nutritional status:

- ■ Complete blood count (CBC) is a basic test used for screening. The following parts of the CBC are important measures of red blood cell (RBC) indices to diagnose anemia:
  - ☐ RBC count checks for anemia and evaluates normal erythropoiesis (the production of RBCs).
  - ☐ Hemoglobin is the protein molecule in RBCs that carries oxygen from the lungs to the body's tissues and returns carbon dioxide from the tissues to the lungs. Hemoglobin levels will be lower in individuals with anemia and nutritional deficiencies.
  - ☐ The hematocrit is the proportion, by volume, of the blood that consists of RBCs; this indicates iron status. The hematocrit is expressed as a percentage. For example, a hematocrit of 25 percent means that there are 25 mL of RBCs in 100 mL of blood. Levels will decrease if the individual is anemic or has nutritional deficiencies.
  - ☐ Mean corpuscular volume (MCV) is the average size of RBCs; MCV increases or decreases along with an increase or decrease in mean cell hemoglobin; high or low levels identify iron, folic acid, or Vitamin B anemias.

- ☐ Mean cell hemoglobin is the average amount of hemoglobin in the average red cell. This test helps to identify the severity and type of anemia.
- ☐ Red cell distribution width is the measurement of the variability of RBC size; higher numbers indicate greater variation in size (Nabili & Shiel, 2008). This test helps identify the cause of the anemia.
- ☐ Platelet count is the calculated number of platelets in a volume of blood. Platelets are important for blood clotting and plugging damaged blood vessels.
- ■ Vitamin B_{12} deficiency level is a deficiency of this vitamin: this may be related to an insufficient dietary intake of foods containing vitamin B_{12} or to stomach or intestinal disease (Van Leeuwen, Poelhuis-Leth, & Vroomen-Durning, 2013).
- ■ Folate level measures the water-soluble vitamin that is absorbed through the intestinal mucosa and absorbed in the liver; folate is necessary for RBC and white blood cell function, DNA replication, and cell division.

- ■ Folic acid deficiency causes anemia; it is a B-complex vitamin needed by our body to manufacture RBCs.
- ■ Ferritin level measures the amount of iron in the blood; it is a protein found inside cells that stores iron so that your body can use it later (MedlinePlus, 2012).
- ■ Prealbumin is an important marker for assessing protein deficiency; it is a preferred marker for protein-calorie malnutrition.
- ■ Serum albumin level measures a protein found in blood; it decreases with poor nutrition and illness as it is the main transport of protein in our body (Van Leeuwen, Poelhuis-Leth, & Vroomen-Durning, 2013), measures visceral protein status, and serves as an indicator of long-term protein status.
- ■ Triglyceride level measures fats in the blood; it screens for high cholesterol.

CULTURAL CONSIDERATIONS

An essential component of providing culturally competent care is the recognition of differences among individuals. This includes diet and eating patterns. Nurses need to be alert to cultural preferences and dietary habits (Table 4-1).

TABLE 4-1 Cultural Considerations for Nutrition Assessments	
Culture	Nutritional Consideration
African American	The popular term for African-American cooking is "soul food." Traditional diets are high in fat, cholesterol, and sodium and low in fiber, fruits, and vegetables. A person with "high blood" (a term often used for high blood pressure) should avoid or reduce intake of salt, pork, red meats, and fried foods. A person with "low blood" (a term often used for low blood pressure) is encouraged to eat liver, greens, eggs, fruits, vegetables, and garlic. Dispel myths and teach factual information about recommendations to treat high and low blood pressure problems.

Continued

TABLE 4-1 Cultural Considerations for Nutrition Assessments—cont'd

Culture	Nutritional Consideration
Chinese	Believe nutrition is essential to health. Traditional Chinese medicine uses food and food derivatives to prevent and cure diseases and illnesses and increase strength in weak and older people. Foods are considered yin and yang to prevent sudden imbalances and indigestion. A balanced diet is considered essential for physical and emotional harmony.
Iranian heritage	Food is a symbol of hospitality. Food is classified into two categories, *garm* (hot) and *sard* (cold), that sometimes correspond to high-calorie and low-calorie foods. Hot tea is the most popular drink. Dairy products are dietary staples, particularly eggs, milk, yogurt, and feta cheese. Strict Muslims avoid pork and alcoholic beverages. Incorporate Iranian foods and dietary practices into health teaching to improve compliance with dietary restrictions.
Korean	Food is highly valued; the most distinguishing feature of Korean food is the spiciness. Breakfast is considered the most important meal. Most Koreans Americans are at high risk for calcium deficiencies due to lactose intolerance.
Mexican American	Food choices vary widely, depending on the region of Mexico from which the person comes. Rice, beans, and tortillas are primary foods. The noontime meal is the largest meal of the day; sweetened fruit drinks are popular; many individuals balance food choices according to the "hot and cold theory." Herbal teas are commonly used to maintain health and treat illnesses.
Germans	Infatuation with food can lead to overeating. Real cream and butter are used. Gravies, sauces, fried foods, rich pastries, and sausages are some of the favorite foods. Those who are ill receive egg custards, ginger ale, or tomato soup (without cream) to settle their stomach. Prune juice is given to relieve constipation. Soup from fresh tomato juice is used to treat migraine headaches. Encourage reducing portion size, overcoming harmful food rituals, and reducing fat intake.

From Purnell (2014).

RELIGIOUS CONSIDERATIONS

Since the beginning of time, dietary practices have been incorporated into the religious practices of people around the world. Some religious sects abstain, or are forbidden, from consuming certain foods and drinks; others restrict foods and drinks during their holy days; still others associate dietary and food preparation practices with rituals of the faith (FAQs.net, n.d.) (Table 4-2).

TABLE 4-2 Religious Dietary Restrictions

Religion	Dietary Restrictions
Buddhism	Restrictions vary but many Buddhists are vegetarians and refrain from the use of alcohol.
Catholicism	Meat on Ash Wednesday, Good Friday and all Fridays in Lent. Some Catholics do not eat meat on any Friday. Animal products such as fat, eggs, dairy, and broth are permissible, as is fish.
Hinduism	Meat, especially beef Alcohol
Islam	Alcohol, pork or pork products, birds of prey, carnivorous animals, blood, meat that is not slaughtered in the name of Allah, gelatin from non-Halal animals. Naturally grown food is ideal.
Orthodox Judaism	Pork and pork products, shellfish, and birds of prey; meat and dairy at the same meal. Fruits and vegetables must be washed to ensure a lack of insects. Three hours must be allowed between eating meat and dairy. Utensils, pots, and pans for dairy and meat must be kept separate, and those used for nonkosher food may not come into contact with kosher supplies. Grape products made by non-Jews may not be consumed.
Mormonism	Coffee, tea, alcohol, and large amounts of meat. Some Mormons avoid all hot drinks and some avoid all caffeinated beverages, such as soda.
Seventh Day Adventism	Alcohol Caffeine is to be avoided but is not strictly prohibited. Doctrine divides meat and fish into categories of "clean" and "unclean," sharing much in common with Jewish customs. Pork and shellfish are considered unclean while fish with fins and scales are clean.

From CNN (2010).

HEALTH HISTORY

A nutritional health history focuses on the clinical, physical, and psychosocial factors that may affect a patient's nutritional intake, or signs that the patient may already be experiencing difficulty eating a healthy diet (Fletcher, 2009). As part of this assessment, nurses must be alert to physical signs and symptoms of changes in nutritional intake. Ask the patient the following questions.

Food Preparation
- Who prepares your meals for you?
- With whom do you eat your meals?
  - □ Individuals who eat by themselves are less likely to prepare meals or eat regular meals; assess for weight loss.

- Do you have transportation to go the store to buy your food? If not, how do you get to the grocery store?
- Do you need any community resources to have meals on a regular basis?
  - □ Patients may have disabilities or financial difficulties preventing them from preparing, obtaining, or buying food; a referral to social services may be needed.
  - □ The Meals on Wheels Association of America is a program that delivers meals to people who are unable to purchase or prepare their own meals.

■ **TIP** Meals on Wheels has been guided by a single goal since the first known U.S. delivery by a small group of Philadelphia citizens in 1954—to support our senior neighbors to extend their independence and health as they age. What started as a compassionate idea has grown into one of the largest and most effective social movements in the United States, currently helping nearly 2.5 million seniors annually in virtually every community in the country (Meals on Wheels America, 2015).

Weight

- When was the last time you weighed yourself? How much did you weigh?
- Have you lost or gained weight? When did you start losing or gaining weight?
  - □ Weight changes are affected by an individual's:
    - changes in diet and eating patterns
    - resting metabolic rate (amount of energy to perform normal body functions)
    - metabolic/medical conditions such as diabetes, Cushing's syndrome, thyroid abnormalities
      - **Diabetes mellitus** is a metabolic disease producing high blood sugars; individuals with diabetes have a tendency to gain weight or be overweight.

- **Cushing's syndrome** is a hormonal disorder caused by high levels of cortisol; individuals with Cushing's syndrome have a tendency to gain weight.
- **Hyperthyroidism** is an overproduction of the thyroid hormones; basal metabolic rate increases causing weight loss.
- **Hypothyroidism** is decreased production of the thyroid hormones; basal metabolic rate decreases causing weight gain.
- psychosocial conditions such as stress, depression, sleep deprivation, and substance abuse

Dietary Preferences

- Do you follow a specific diet?
- Do you have any religious or cultural preferences influencing your diet?
  - □ Individuals may be following specific diets related to medical conditions such as heart disease, hypertension, diabetes, or gluten sensitivity.
  - □ Eating patterns between cultural and religious groups can be diverse.
  - □ Nutritional diversity is a result of culture, tradition, different lifestyles, and attitudes and beliefs toward food.

Dietary Supplements and Vitamins

SENC Safety Alert Excessive doses of vitamins can cause harm to the body.

- Do you take any dietary supplements? If so, how much? How often? Why do you take the supplement?
- Do you take any vitamins or herbal supplements? If so, what are they? Why do you take the vitamin or supplement?
  - □ A balanced diet should provide the necessary vitamins and minerals that we need. Individuals can take too many vitamins or herbal supplements and cause harm to their bodies. It is essential

that patients discuss with their healthcare provider any supplemental intake.

Appetite

- Tell me about your daily eating patterns.
- How would you describe your sense of taste or appetite?
  - □ Anorexia is a decreased appetite.
  - □ Ageusia is the absence of taste.
  - □ Dysgeusia refers to the presence of a metallic, rancid, or foul taste in the mouth.
  - □ Taking certain medications can cause a dry mouth or decrease the sense of taste and cause anorexia.
- Do you have difficulty swallowing or chewing your food?
  - □ Dysphagia is difficulty swallowing.
  - □ Individuals who have periodontal disease, few or no teeth, or poor fitting dentures have difficulty chewing food.
  - □ Patients who have been acutely or chronically ill may have difficulty eating or swallowing.

Food Intolerances/Allergies

- Are you allergic to any specific types of foods?
  - □ A food allergy is an immune system response. It occurs when the body mistakes an ingredient in food—usually a protein—as harmful and creates a defense system (antibodies) to fight it. The most common food allergies are nuts, fish, milk, eggs, soy products, and wheat.
- Do you have any diet intolerances?
  - □ Food intolerance is a digestive system response. It occurs when something in a food irritates a person's digestive system or when a person is unable to properly digest or breakdown the food. The most common food intolerance is to lactose, which is found in dairy products and milk. The most common symptom a patient experiences is diarrhea.
  - □ A gluten-free diet is a diet that eliminates the protein gluten; gluten is found in grains such as wheat, barley, or rye.

Water

- How much water or fluids do you take on a daily basis?
  - □ Water is your body's principal chemical component and makes up about 50 to 60 percent of your body weight. Water needs are dependent on the individual, his or her lifestyle, and climate and activity levels.
  - □ Dehydration is a condition that occurs when the loss of body fluids, mostly water, is greater than fluid intake. Vomiting, diarrhea, and excessive sweating may cause an individual to become dehydrated and cause electrolyte imbalances.

EQUIPMENT NEEDED

Paper measuring tape
Scale
Stadiometer

ASSESSING NUTRITION

The American Society for Parenteral and Enteral Nutrition (ASPEN) defines nutrition screening as "a process to identify an individual who is malnourished or who is at risk for malnutrition to determine if a detailed nutrition assessment is indicated" (Mueller, Compher, Druyen, & ASPEN, 2011). Registered nurses are often the first team members to interview a patient, and they communicate important nutritional information such as a client's response to food, including intake and tolerance to other team members (Lutz, Mazur, & Litch, 2015). Nurses are instrumental in screening, assessing, teaching, and referring patients to members of the interprofessional healthcare team. There are different ways to assess patients at nutritional risk:

1. The *nutritional screening tool* is brief enough that the information can be gathered in a short amount of time. If one factor is found, the screening is stopped, and the patient is declared at nutritional risk and referred to a dietician (Lutz & Przytulski, 2011) (Box 4-2).

▧ **TIP** The Joint Commission mandates that nutrition screening be done within 24 hours of admission to an acute care center when warranted by the patient's needs or condition (Joint Commission on Accreditation of Healthcare Organizations, 2008).

Nurses may collaborate with the interprofessional team (physician, dietician, social worker) to discuss nutritional concerns or assessment findings.

2. A *nutritional assessment* is an evaluation of a client's nutritional status (nutrient stores) based on a physical examination, anthropometric measurements, laboratory data, and food intake information (Lutz & Przytulski, 2011). It is a noninvasive assessment that will identify signs and symptoms of malnutrition.

FOCUSED ASSESSMENT

TECHNIQUE 4-1: **Inspecting General Appearance**

Purpose: To identify physical and psychological signs of malnutrition

ASSESSMENT STEPS

1. Inspect the general appearance of the patient, including:

- demeanor
- hair
- eyes
- lips
- tongue
- teeth
- gums
- skin
- nails
- mobility

2. Document your findings.
See Table 4-3 for normal and abnormal findings.

▧ **TIP** Patients who are healthy have good color and have an optimistic sense of well-being.

TABLE 4-3 Normal and Abnormal Findings of Nutritional Status

	Normal	Abnormal
Demeanor	Alert, responsive Positive outlook	Lethargic Negative attitude
Weight	Reasonable for build	Underweight Overweight, obese
Hair	Glossy, full, firmly rooted Uniform color	Dull, brittle, sparse; easily and painlessly plucked
Eyes	Bright, clear, shiny	Pale conjunctiva Redness, dryness Sunken
Lips	Smooth	Chapped, red, swollen
Tongue	Deep red Slightly rough One longitudinal furrow	Bright red, purple Swollen or shrunken Several longitudinal furrows
Teeth Dentures	Bright, painless Well-fitting dentures	Dental caries, painful or missing teeth Loose fitting dentures
Gums	Pink, firm	Spongy, bleeding, receding
Skin	Clear, smooth, firm, slightly moist	Rashes, swelling Light or dark spots Dry, cracked
Nails	Pink, firm	Spoon shaped or ridged Spongy bases Brittle
Mobility	Erect posture Good muscle tone Walks without pain or difficulty	Muscle wasting Skeletal deformities Loss of balance Muscle deconditioning

From Lutz et al. (2015).

BOX 4-2 Admission Nutrition Screening Tool

A. Diagnosis

If the patient has at least *one* of the following diagnoses, circle and proceed to section E to consider the patient at nutritional risk and stop here.

- Anorexia nervosa/bulimia nervosa
- Malabsorption (celiac disease, ulcerative colitis, Crohn's disease, short bowel syndrome)
- Multiple trauma (closed-head injury, penetrating trauma, multiple fractures)
- Pressure ulcers
- Major gastrointestinal surgery within the past year
- Cachexia (temporal wasting, muscle wasting, cancer, cardiac)
- Coma
- Diabetes
- End-stage liver disease
- End-stage renal disease
- Nonhealing wounds

B. Nutrition Intake History

If the patient has at least *one* of the following symptoms, circle and proceed to section E to consider the patient at nutritional risk and stop here.

- Diarrhea (>500 mL 2 days)
- Vomiting (>5 days)
- Reduced intake (<1/2 normal intake for >5 days)

C. Ideal Body Weight Standards

Compare the patient's current weight for height with the ideal body weight chart. If at less than 80 percent of ideal body weight, proceed to section E to consider the patient at nutritional risk and stop here.

D. Weight History

Any recent unplanned weight loss? No _____ Yes _____
Amount (lb. or kg) _____
If yes, within the past ____weeks or ____ months
Current weight (lb. or kg) _____
Usual weight (lb. or kg) _____
Height (ft., in., or cm) _____
Find percentage of weight lost:

$$\frac{\text{Usual weight} - \text{Current weight} \times 100}{\text{Usual Weight}} = \% \text{ Weight Loss}$$

Compare the percent weight loss with the chart values and circle the appropriate value.

Length of time	Significant (%)	Severe (%)
1 week	1–2	>2
2–3 weeks	2–3	>3
1 month	4–5	>5
3 months	7–8	>8
5+ months	10	>10

If the patient has experienced a significant or severe weight loss, proceed to Section E and consider the patient at nutritional risk.

E. Nursing Assessment

Using the above criteria, what is this patient's nutritional risk? (check one)

_____LOW NUTRITIONAL RISK
_____AT NUTRITIONAL RISK

From Kovacevich et al. (1997, p. 22).

Purpose: To identify baseline dietary patterns contributing to overnutrition or undernutrition:

ASSESSMENT STEPS

1. Ask the patient to tell you about his or her dietary patterns and factors influencing the patient's nutritional intake.
2. Ask the patient to identify what he or she has eaten or drank in the last 24 hours.

   ▐ **TIP** If the patient is asked to keep a 3-day diary, tell the patient to write down all the foods and beverage intake, immediately after eating. Behavioral eating patterns can be more adequately assessed.

3. Document the times and portion sizes or amounts of foods and beverages (Box 4-3).

   ▐ **TIP** During the diet recall, it is a good opportunity to discuss healthy portion sizes.

4. Review the data collected to identify overnutrition or malnutrition.
5. Document your findings.

   ▐ **TIP** The diet recall method may have recall bias; patients sometimes intentionally respond incorrectly to a question because they do not want you to know the truth about how much or how little they are eating.

BOX 4-3 **Example of Dietary Recall**

7:30 a.m.: Breakfast
2 scrambled eggs
4-oz glass of cranberry juice
Pieces of raisin cinnamon toast
1 cup of black coffee, 1 teaspoon (tsp) sugar

11 a.m.: Snack
1 large cinnamon Danish
1 cup of black coffee, 1 tsp of sugar

12:30 p.m.: Lunch
1 turkey sandwich, lettuce, salt, pepper, mayonnaise
1 small bag of salted potato chips
8-oz bottle of orange soda
2 chocolate chip cookies

4 p.m.: Snack
1 8-oz bottle of root beer soda

6 p.m.: Supper
4 pieces of cheese pizza
1 slice of Italian white bread with butter
1 8-oz glass of water
1 cup of black coffee with 1 tsp of sugar
1 slice of carrot cake

10 p.m.: Snack
½ cup of chocolate chip ice cream
4-oz glass of Sprite soda

Technique 4-2A: **Assessing Nutrition Through Direct Observation**

Purpose: To identify the amount of food a patient eats at mealtime

ASSESSMENT STEPS

1. Observe the patient eating during mealtime.

2. Note if the patient is having any difficulty swallowing or feeding himself or herself.

3. Document the percentage (0 through 100 percent) of the meal eaten.

> ■ **TIP** To calculate the percentage of intake, count the number of total food items for the meal. Condiments do not count. Each food item counts as 1 point. So, ¾ of the food item eaten = 1 point. Half of the food item eaten = ½ point. Less than or equal to ¼ eaten = 0 points. Divide the number of points by the total number of food items (e.g., 100% of meat eaten = 1 point), half-eaten vegetable = 0.5 point, no rice eaten = 0 points, half of dessert eaten = 0.5 point). Add total points/total food count = 2/4 = 50% of intake.

NORMAL FINDINGS

■ Meal eaten 75 to 100 percent

ABNORMAL FINDINGS

■ Meal eaten less than 75 percent on a regular basis

ANTHROPOMETRIC MEASUREMENTS

Anthropometric measurements are techniques to assess the physical dimensions and subcutaneous fat of an individual's body. These measurements assess the nutritional status of a patient and are compared to normative standards.

TECHNIQUE 4-3: **Assessing Height, Weight, and Body Mass Index**

Purpose: To estimate the amount of body fat

■ **TIP** Body mass index (BMI) is a screening tool that identifies the amount of body fat based on height and weight; it applies to adult men and women.

■ **TIP** A BMI is not diagnostic of the health of an individual; further assessments such as diet, physical activity, and family history are needed to determine if a BMI is a health risk (CDC, 2015). Nurses must remember that the BMI does not take into account muscle mass, bone density, body composition, and racial differences.

Equipment: Scale, stadiometer, BMI chart

ASSESSMENT STEPS

1. Ask the patient to remove shoes and place feet together before measuring height (Fig. 4-1).

2. Measure the patient's height by standing upright under a stadiometer.

3. Carefully lower the horizontal bar until it touches the top of the patient's head.

4. Record the measurement.

5. Weigh the patient on a scale; there are several different types of scales (Fig. 4-2).

■ **TIP** Scales need to be calibrated to zero prior to taking the patient's weight; when using a calibrated balance-beam scale, balance the scale by sliding both weight bars to zero.

6. Look at a BMI chart to identify where on the chart the height and weight intersect for the BMI (Fig. 4-3).

7. Record and interpret the BMI number.

8. Document height, weight, and BMI.

NORMAL FINDINGS

■ BMI is between 18.5 and 24.9.

ABNORMAL FINDINGS

■ BMI ≤ 18: Underweight

■ BMI ≥ 25 to 29.9: Overweight

■ BMI 30 to 39: Obese

■ BMI 40 or higher: Morbidly obese (CDC, 2015)

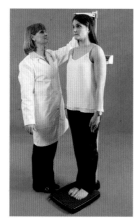

Fig. 4-1. Measuring height with stadiometer.

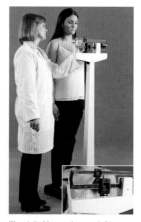

Fig. 4-2. Measuring weight using stand up scale.

Weight in pounds

Height	100	110	120	130	140	150	160	170	180	190	200	210	220	230	240	250	260	270	280	290	300
4'10"	21	23	25	27	29	32	34	36	38												
4'11"	20	22	24	26	28	30	32	34	36	38											
5'0"	20	21	23	25	27	29	31	33	35	37	39										
5'1"	19	21	23	25	27	28	30	32	34	36	38										
5'2"		20	22	24	26	27	29	31	33	35	37	38									
5'3"		19	21	23	25	27	28	30	32	34	36	37	39								
5'4"		19	21	22	24	26	28	29	31	33	34	36	38								
5'5"			20	22	23	25	27	28	30	32	33	35	37	38							
5'6"			19	21	23	24	26	27	29	31	32	34	36	37	38						
5'7"			19	20	22	24	25	27	28	30	31	33	35	36	38	39					
5'8"				20	21	23	24	26	27	29	30	32	34	35	37	38					
5'9"				19	21	22	24	25	27	28	30	31	33	34	36	37	38				
5'10"				19	20	21	22	24	25	27	28	30	31	33	34	36	37	39			
5'11"					20	21	22	24	25	27	28	29	31	32	34	35	36	38	39		
6'0"					29	20	22	23	24	26	27	29	30	31	33	34	35	37	38	39	
6'1"						20	21	23	22	24	25	26	27	29	30	32	33	34	36	37	38
6'2"					19	21	22	23	25	26	27	28	30	31	32	34	35	36	37	39	
6'3"						19	20	21	23	24	25	26	28	29	30	31	33	34	35	36	38
6'4"							20	21	22	23	24	26	27	28	29	31	32	33	34	35	37

Normal weight: 18.5-24.9
Overweight: 25-29.9
Obese: 30 and above

Extremely obese

Underweight

Fig. 4-3. Body Mass Index (BMI) chart.

SENC **Evidence-Based Practice** BMI provides the most useful population-level measure of overweight and obesity as it is the same for both sexes and for all ages of adults. However, it should be considered a rough guide because it may not correspond to the same degree of fatness in different populations and ethnic groups (WHO, 2016b).

TECHNIQUE 4-4: **Assessing Abdominal Circumference**

Abdominal circumference measures the distance around the abdomen.
Purpose: To measure abdominal fat
Equipment: Tape measure (cm)

SENC **Safety Alert** Centrally located abdominal fat deposition is considered to be an independent risk factor for cardiovascular disease in adults.

TIP Never take an abdominal measurement over clothing.

ASSESSMENT STEPS
1. Stand in front of the patient and palpate the right hip (right ilium) at the top of the right iliac crest to identify the greatest diameter of the abdomen.
2. Place the tape measure around the bare abdomen at the level of the iliac crest, which should also be close to the level of the navel (Fig. 4-4).
3. Pull the tape measure snugly around the abdomen.
4. Take the measurement after the patient breathes normally out (end of expiration).
5. Document the measurement.

TIP Measuring below the umbilicus, especially in obese patients, will be an inaccurate measurement.

NORMAL FINDINGS
- Males: ≤ 102 cm (40 inches)
- Females: ≤ 88 cm (35 inches)

ABNORMAL FINDINGS
- Males: > 102 cm (40 inches)
- Females: > 88 cm (35 inches) (CDC, 2014b)

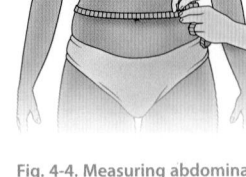

Fig. 4-4. Measuring abdominal circumference.

TECHNIQUE 4-5: Assessing Waist-to-Hip Ratio

Waist-to-hip ratio (WHR) is the ratio of the circumference of the waist to that of the hips.

Purpose: To assess body size and fat distribution

Equipment: Tape measure (inches or cm)

SENC Safety Alert Waist-to-hip ratio has been identified as a predictor of patients at risk for coronary heart disease.

ASSESSMENT STEPS

1. Place tape measure around the narrowest area of the waist between the hips and the 11th rib (Fig. 4-5).

2. Take measurement after a normal breath at the end of expiration.

3. Record the measurement in inches or centimeters.

4. Place the tape measure around the widest point of the hips (Fig. 4-5).

5. Record the measurement in inches or centimeters.

6. Calculate the waist-to-hip measurement by dividing the waist measurement by the hip measurement.

$$\text{waist-to-hip ratio} = \frac{\text{waist measurement (inches or cm)}}{\text{hip measurement (inches or cm)}}$$

7. Document your findings.

TIP Fat distribution can result in a pear-shaped figure (fat in the hip and thighs) or apple-shaped body (fat in the abdominal area) (Fig. 4-6).

NORMAL FINDINGS

- Men WHR < 0.95
- Women WHR < 0.80

ABNORMAL FINDINGS

- Indicates a health risk for heart disease and diabetes
- Men: WHR of 0.95 or higher
- Women: WHR of 0.80 or higher

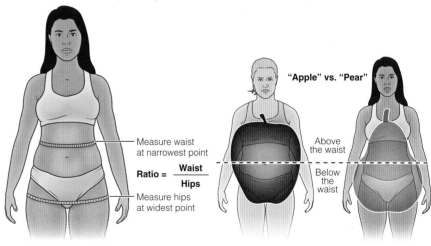

Fig. 4-5. Measuring waist-hip ratio.

Fig. 4-6. Fat distribution in adults.

ADVANCED ASSESSMENT

TECHNIQUE 4-6: Assessing the Mid-Upper Arm Circumference

Purpose: To assess body protein stores and skeletal muscle mass
Equipment: Tape measure (cm), marker

■ **TIP** Mid-upper arm circumference (MUAC) can be taken if patient is immobile or very ill. About 50 percent of the body's protein stores are located in muscle tissue (Lutz, Mazur, & Litch, 2015). It is an alternative indicator of nutritional status and allows an estimation of BMI to be made (Fletcher, 2009).

■ **TIP** There is evidence suggesting that a low mid-upper arm circumference is a more valid measure than a low BMI to define thinness in older persons (Wijnhoven et al., 2013).

ASSESSMENT STEPS

1. Place the patient in an upright sitting position.
2. Remove clothing from the nondominant arm.
3. Ask the patient to bend the nondominant arm.
4. Using the measuring tape, measure from the top of the shoulder (acromion process) to the tip of the elbow (olecranon process) (Fig. 4-7A).
5. Identify the mid-point of measurement and mark the arm at this point.
6. Ask the patient to allow his or her arm to hang by his or her side. Measure the arm at the mid-point mark making sure the tape measure is snug but not tight (Fig. 4-7B).
7. Document the measurement in centimeters (cm).

NORMAL FINDINGS

■ Male: ≥ 23 cm
■ Female: ≥ 22 cm

ABNORMAL FINDINGS

■ Decreasing measurements over time
■ Male: < 23 cm (malnourished); Female: < 22 cm (malnourished)

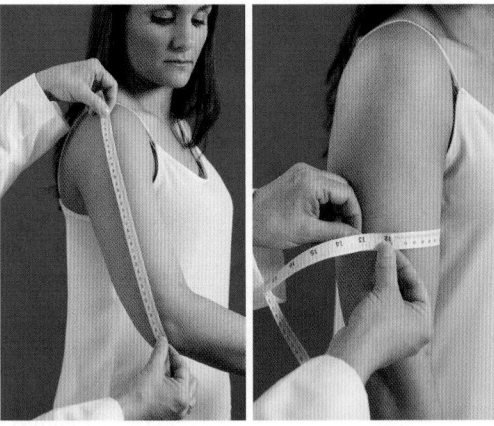
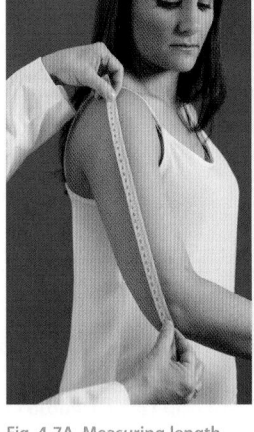

Fig. 4-7A. Measuring length.   Fig. 4-7B. Measuring circumference.

Healthy People 2020

Goals

- Promote health and reduce chronic disease risk through the consumption of healthful diets and achievement and maintenance of healthy body weights (HHS, 2010).
- Increase the proportion of primary care physicians who regularly measure the BMI of their patients.
- Increase the proportion of physician office visits that include counseling or education related to nutrition or weight.
- Increase the proportion of worksites that offer nutrition or weight management classes or counseling.
- Reduce the proportion of children and adults who are obese (HHS, 2010).

Nutrition is a key component of health and well-being. Patients need encouragement and guidance to develop and maintain good nutrition. The *2015–2020 Dietary Guidelines for Americans* focuses on balancing calories with physical activity, and encouraging Americans to consume more healthy foods like vegetables, fruits, whole grains, fat-free and low-fat dairy products, and seafood and to consume less sodium, saturated and *trans* fats, added sugars, and refined grains (Box 4-4) (HHS & USDA, 2015).

Teach patients to read labels on the backs of food boxes and cans. Recommended daily values are identified at the bottom of labels (see Fig. 4-8).

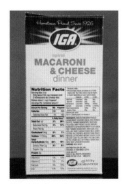

Fig. 4-8. Sample nutrition label.

MyPlate

MyPlate, the food guidance system from the U.S. Department of Agriculture (USDA), is based on the *Dietary Guidelines for Americans* and replaces the Food Pyramid. The new MyPlate provides a better visual of the five food groups and how they are recommended to balance one another in a meal

---

BOX 4-4 2015 Dietary Guidelines for Americans

Key Recommendations
Consume a healthy eating pattern that accounts for all foods and beverages within an appropriate calorie level.

A healthy eating pattern includes:
A variety of vegetables from all of the subgroups—dark green, red and orange, legumes (beans and peas), starchy, and other
Fruits, especially whole fruits
Grains, at least half of which are whole grains
Fat-free or low-fat dairy, including milk, yogurt, cheese, and/or fortified soy beverages
A variety of protein foods, including seafood, lean meats and poultry, eggs, legumes (beans and peas), and nuts, seeds, and soy products.
Oils

A healthy eating pattern limits:
Saturated fats and *trans* fats, added sugars, and sodium
Consume less than 10 percent of calories per day from added sugars
Consume less than 10 percent of calories per day from saturated fats
Consume less than 2,300 milligrams (mg) per day from sodium
If alcohol is consumed, it should be consumed in moderation-up to one drink per day for women and up to two drinks per day for men-and only by adults of legal drinking age.

From HHS & USDA (2015).

(Fig. 4-9). The purpose of MyPlate is to help consumers make better food choices at mealtimes and remind them to eat healthily. The program's website, ChooseMy-Plate.gov, provides all MyPlate information as well as additional nutrition resources to help consumers focus on key behaviors, such as balancing calories, foods to increase, and foods to decrease in one's diet.

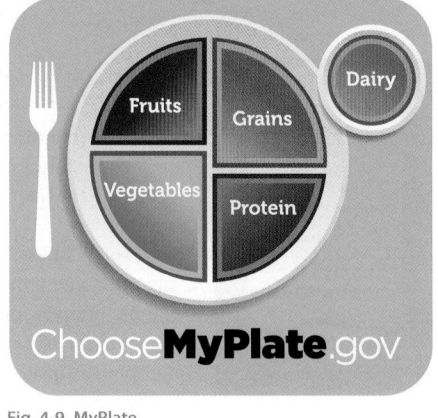

Fig. 4-9. MyPlate.

Healthy Eating Plate

■ The Healthy Eating Plate, a new visual guide for creating nutritious meals, was developed by Harvard School of Public Health (Fig. 4-10).

■ A representation of a plate is sectioned into colorful food portions and expands upon the USDA's recommendations.

■ The Healthy Eating Plate specifies that individuals should stick to whole grains instead of refined grains, eat healthy proteins such as fish or poultry rather than red or processed meats, and distinguish between healthy vegetables and potatoes.

■ The Healthy Eating Plate also includes a glass of water and healthy oils in its ideal meal, advising consumers to avoid butter and trans fat (Guzman, 2011).

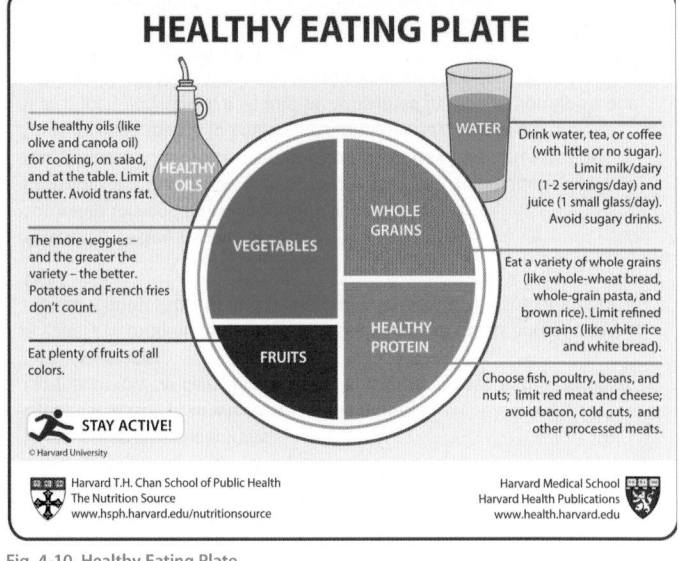

Fig. 4-10. Healthy Eating Plate.

SENC Evidence-Based Practice Siegrist and Dickinson Spillman (2010) surveyed a random population in a postal survey ($n = 1,043$) and developed a 13-question procedural nutrition questionnaire to identify patient knowledge related to a healthy diet. Results showed good procedural nutrition knowledge in consumers, yet substantial numbers of consumers hold misconceptions. Many consumers appear to be unfamiliar with the practical implications of the food pyramid, the concept of a balanced diet, and the importance of increasing fruit and vegetable consumption. Particularly older individuals and those following medically prescribed diets could benefit from more education on how to

Vitamin D

Vitamin D is obtained through our diet and by exposure to sunlight. It is needed to absorb calcium and promote bone growth.

- Natural foods have very little vitamin D. There are some vitamin-D fortified foods such as cereals, milk, yogurt, margarine, cheese, and orange juice.
- Vitamin D deficiency is diagnosed by a blood test, serum concentration of 25-hydroxyvitamin D.
- Research has shown that vitamin D decreases the risk of cancer, rickets (in children), osteomalacia or the weakening of bones (in older adults), and fractures.
- Patients should be tested for vitamin D deficiency.

SENC Evidence-Based Practice The Institute of Medicine (IOM, 2015) finds that the evidence "supports a role for vitamin D and calcium in bone health but not in other health conditions. The recommended dietary allowance for adults (ages 19 through 70 years) for Vitamin D is 600IU per day and calcium is 1,000–1,200 mg/day."

Water

Water is a major part of every tissue in the body; we can live only a few days without water (Grodner, Long Roth, & Walkingshaw, 2012).

The amount of water that is needed to keep our body healthy is influenced by our health, lifestyle, environment, and activity level.

- Individuals are recommended to have 9 to 13 cups (1 cup equals 8 ounces) of water a day from food and beverages.
- Lack of water causes dehydration; too much water causes overhydration.

SENC Safety Alert See Box 4-5 for signs of dehydration.

BOX 4-5 Signs of Dehydration

Dry mouth and mucous membranes
Irritability or confusion
Headache
Dizziness
Decreased urine output
Darker urine color
Fever

SENC Safety Alert Assess patient's intake and output closely when receiving intravenous fluids; too much fluid can cause fluid overload resulting in serious complications.

Weight Loss

Losing weight is never easy; weight loss takes time, hard work, and patience. Weight loss occurs with taking in fewer calories and burning more calories through activity. Some guidelines to lose weight are:

- Encourage reading nutrition labels.
- Promote new habits of purchasing food.
- Instruct on food preparation and avoiding high-calorie ingredients.
- Warn against overconsumption of high-calorie foods.
- Stress importance of water intake.
- Educate on reducing portion sizes.
- Encourage decreasing consumption of alcohol.
- Discuss energy value of protein, CHO, fats, and dietary fiber.
- Encourage exercise about 2.5 hours a week doing moderate-intensity aerobic and muscle-strengthening activities. Depending on the patient's schedule, he or she should exercise 30 minutes 5 days a week, or at least 150 minutes per week of moderate exercise, or 75 minutes per week of vigorous exercise (American Heart Association, 2014).

Assessment Techniques

INTRODUCTION

Health assessment requires essential data to accurately and safely care for every patient. Nurses need to be able to recognize the assessment findings that indicate serious problems and distinguish them from normal variants. The four assessment techniques that will provide objective assessment data are:

1. Inspection
2. Palpation
3. Percussion
4. Auscultation

Assessment techniques are learned; this takes time and practice.

PREPARATION FOR ASSESSMENT

Standard Precautions

Health assessment requires direct contact with the patient. Nurses must protect themselves from acquiring and transferring any infectious agents. The Centers for Disease Control and Prevention (CDC) and the Hospital Infection Control Practices Advisory Committee (HICPAC) reaffirm standard precautions as the foundation for preventing transmission of infectious agents during patient care in all healthcare settings (CDC, 2014). Standard precautions are the minimum infection prevention practices that apply to all patient care and include:

- Perform hand hygiene.
- Use personal protective equipment (e.g., gloves, gowns, masks) (Fig. 5-1).
  - □ Use gloves, mask, or gown to handle potentially contaminated equipment or if you come in contact with contaminated surfaces in the patient environment.
  - □ Use masks for respiratory precautions and encourage cough etiquette (CDC, 2014).

SENC Safety Alert
Healthcare–associated infections (HAIs) are major causes of morbidity and mortality in the United States. A growing proportion of these infections are due to resistant pathogens such as methicillin-resistant *Staphylococcus aureus* (MRSA) and multidrug-resistant Gram-negative bacilli (CDC, 2014).

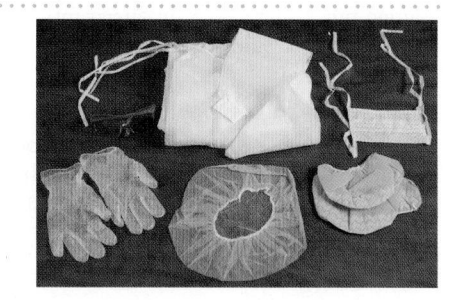

Fig. 5-1. Personal protective equipment.

TIP Healthcare–associated infections are a major concern to patients. Always try to wash your hands in front of the patient so the patient knows that you have performed hand hygiene.

SENC Evidence-Based Practice In a recent study, *Global implementation of WHO's Multimodal Strategy for Improvement of Hand Hygiene: A Quasi-Experimental Study,* an international team of researchers aimed to determine the effectiveness of WHO's Hand Hygiene Program, an education initiative that has been implemented in 168 countries and includes hand hygiene guidelines. Researchers analyzed hand hygiene across low, mixed, and high-resource hospital settings in five countries: Africa, Costa Rica, Italy, Pakistan, and Saudi Arabia. The researchers noted that nurses had the highest hand-washing compliance across all pilot sites before the intervention. Specifically, 71 percent of nurses complied with the guidelines, compared with 60 percent of doctors. Implementation of WHO's hand-hygiene strategy is feasible and sustainable across a range of settings in different countries and leads to significant compliance and knowledge improvement in healthcare workers, supporting recommendation for use worldwide (Allegranzi et al., 2013).

SENC Safety Alert A patient may have an allergy to latex. Symptoms of latex allergy include hives, rash, swelling, sneezing, headache, and a severe allergic reaction, anaphylaxis. Always ask your patient if he or she has a latex allergy; check to see whether you are wearing latex-free gloves and using latex-free equipment.

Patient's Rights

Patient-centered care is at the core of essential health assessment and performing health assessment techniques. Patients need to be respected and cared for without any type of discrimination. All patients have the right to be completely informed about the assessment and what to expect during the assessment. All patient findings must be confidential.

TIP A competent adult patient has the right to refuse being assessed. Nurses must document if a patient refuses an assessment and depending on the urgency of the assessment, the healthcare provider should be notified.

Patient Positions

Essential health assessment works best if you use an organized approach, working from noninvasive to invasive assessments. The nurse asks the patient to assume proper positions so that areas to be assessed are accessible. A patient's ability to assume different positions depends on his or her physical strength, limitations, and degree of wellness. Some patients may not be able to change positions independently. Be aware of your patient's ability to change positions and assist as necessary to ensure patient safety. During a complete head to toe assessment, minimal positional changes by the patient are advised for patient comfort. Try to cluster your assessments when the patient is sitting, standing, or lying down.

TIP The nurse should be standing on the right side of the patient when performing the exam because most examination techniques are performed with the nurse's right hand even if the nurse is left handed.

EQUIPMENT NEEDED

Gloves
Stethoscope
Tangential light

SEQUENCE OF ASSESSMENT

The sequence of assessment is dependent upon the specific body system or region being assessed.

1. Inspection
2. Palpation
3. Percussion
4. Auscultation

> **SENC Safety Alert** Always perform hand hygiene before and after the assessment.

TECHNIQUE 5-1: Inspection

Purpose: To look and assess the physical aspects of the body, posture, appearance, and behavior carefully

Equipment: Tangential lighting

Inspection should start when you first meet with the patient. There are two types of inspection:

■ **Direct inspection** is carefully observing and inspecting a specific area or the whole individual.
■ **Indirect inspection** is using specific equipment to improve your visualization of an area (i.e., ophthalmoscope to look at the internal structures of the eyes).

Inspection requires the use of three of your senses:

1. Seeing
2. Hearing
3. Smelling

Inspection requires:

■ Room temperature to be a comfortable level for the patient
■ Good lighting in the room
  □ Tangential lighting is a form of additional lighting placed at an angle in order to see more specific details for a specific assessment (i.e., tangential lighting, a penlight, is used to assess the characteristics of a skin lesion or mole) (Fig. 5-2).

    ▮ **TIP** Fluorescent lights can change the color of the skin. Natural lighting is the best lighting, if available.

■ Draping the patient appropriately and exposing only the body part being assessed
■ Always observing and comparing the symmetry of body parts from one side to the other side

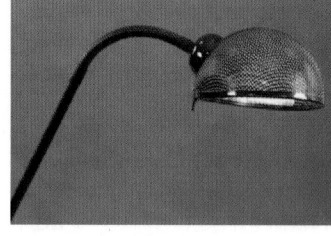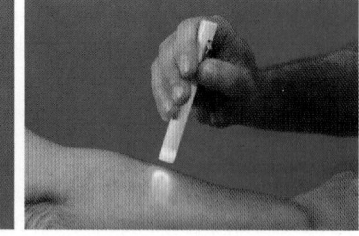

Fig. 5-2. Tangential lighting.

- Inspecting the following characteristics:
  - ☐ Location
  - ☐ Size
  - ☐ Color
  - ☐ Pattern
  - ☐ Shape
  - ☐ Odors
  - ☐ Symmetry
    - **TIP** Do not rush during inspection; inspection takes time and requires concentration.

TECHNIQUE 5-2: **Palpation**

Purpose: To touch and feel for surface characteristics
Equipment: Gloves (optional)

SENC Safety Alert Always wear gloves when palpating any part of the body with open areas, wounds, or internal structures of the body such as the tongue or mouth.

SENC Safety Alert Keep fingernails short. Long fingernails could cause discomfort or harm the patient while performing the assessment.

- There are two types of palpation: light palpation and deep palpation.
- There are three different parts of your hand that are more sensitive to assessing different surface characteristics (Fig. 5-3):
  - ☐ **Finger pads:** Assess fine discrimination and sensations on the surface areas such as texture, shape, consistency, pulses, and crepitus (popping sounds under the skin).
  - ☐ **Dorsal surface of the hand:** The back of the hand is used to assess temperature.
  - ☐ **Ulnar surface or ball of the hand:** Assess vibrations, fremitus (vibration on the body), and thrills (vibration over the chest wall).

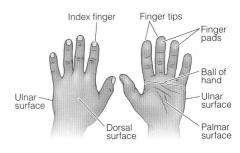

Fig. 5-3. Surfaces of hand used in palpation.

Technique 5-2A: **Light Palpation**

Purpose: To touch and feel for surface characteristics

Equipment: Gloves

1. Warm your hands.
2. Using the finger pads of your dominant hand, gently press down about 1 cm or ½ inch.
3. Gently press down or use light circular motions to palpate surface characteristics for:
   □ texture
   □ masses
   □ tenderness
4. Gently lift your fingers and move to the adjacent area; palpate the entire area that needs to be assessed (Fig. 5-4).

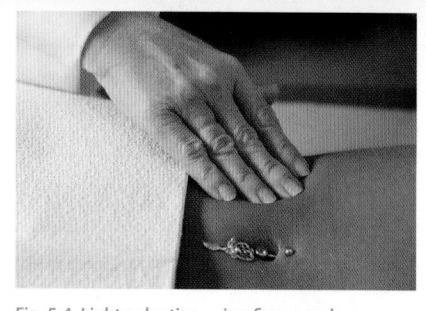

Fig. 5-4. Light palpation using finger pads.

Technique 5-2B: **Deep Palpation**

Purpose: To assess for location and size of internal organs, masses, and tenderness

Equipment: Gloves

■ Perform light palpation prior to deep palpation.

■ Light or deep palpation is determined by the depth of the structure being palpated and the thickness of the tissue overlying that structure.

> **SENC Safety Alert** If pain has been reported in an area, gently palpate this area last.

> **TIP** Deep palpation can be done using one or two hands (bimanual) (Fig. 5-5).

1. Warm your hands by rubbing them together.
2. Using the finger pads of your dominant hand or placing your dominant hand over your nondominant hand, gently press down 5 cm (about 2 inches or more) to assess:
   □ organ size and location
   □ masses
   □ tenderness
3. Gently lift your fingers to move to the adjacent area to assess.

> **TIP** Bimanual palpation can also be used to stabilize an internal organ.

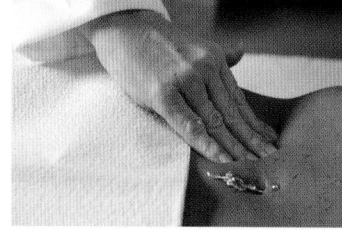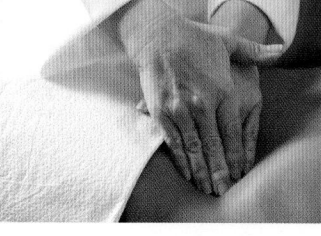

Fig. 5-5. Deep palpation using one hand, two hands, and bimanual technique assessing spleen.

TECHNIQUE 5-3: **Percussion**

Percussion creates a sound wave that vibrates; different tones are elicited depending on the underlying tissue density. There are three types of percussion: direct, indirect, and indirect fist (blunt).

Technique 5-3A: **Direct Percussion**

Purpose: To assess the size, consistency, and borders of body organs, and the presence or absence of fluid in body areas
1. Explain the technique to your patient.
2. Expose only the area that you will be percussing.
3. Using one or two fingertips, directly and lightly tap the area that needs to be assessed (Fig. 5-6A).
   ▊**TIP** Closing your eyes may help you to concentrate on the specific sounds you hear while percussing.
4. Listen carefully for the sound and identify the following characteristics:
   ☐ Pitch (frequency of the sound wave vibrations) is described as high, low, or dull.
   ☐ Intensity is described as:
     • soft tones are heard over solid tissue
     • moderate tones are heard over fluid-filled areas
     • loud tones are heard over air-filled spaces.
       ▊**TIP** As the density of the underlying structure increases, the percussion sounds become softer.
   ☐ Duration is the length of time the sound is heard.
   ☐ Quality of sound (what does it sound like?)
   ☐ There are five specific percussion sounds (Table 5-1):
     • Tympany is heard over abdominal areas that may be filled with abdominal gas or air-filled structures.
     • Dullness is heard over solid organs, fluid collection, or areas of consolidation (such as a tumor or mass).
     • Resonance is heard over normal lung fields.
     • Hyperresonance is heard over air-filled spaces such as lung fields in a patient with emphysema.
     • Flatness is heard over increased tissue density such as bones.

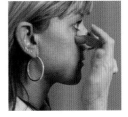

Fig. 5-6A. Direct percussion.

Technique 5-3B: **Indirect Percussion**

Purpose: To assess the size, consistency, and borders of body organs, and the presence or absence of fluid in body areas
1. Explain the technique to your patient.
2. Expose only the area to be percussed.
3. Lay your middle finger of your nondominant hand (the pleximeter) on the area to be assessed. The middle finger is the only finger that should be in contact with the skin while percussing.

TABLE 5-1 Percussion Sounds

Sound	Intensity	Pitch	Quality	Example of Structure
Tympany	Loud	High	Drum-like	Gastric air-filled structures in abdomen such as the intestines Heard over a chest indicates excessive air (i.e., pneumothorax)
Dull or thudlike	Soft to moderate	Medium	Thud-like	Liver Full bladder Solid organs or mass Fluid or solid tissue replaces air in the lung (i.e., pneumonia)
Resonance	Moderate to loud	Low	Hollow	Normal lung
Hyperresonance	Very loud	Low	Booming	Hyperinflated lungs (i.e., chronic obstructive lung disease or asthma)
Flatness	Soft	High	Dull	Muscle Bone Joints Solid mass

4. Flex your wrist of your dominant hand and tap your middle finger of this hand (the plexor) on the interphalangeal joint of the middle finger of your nondominant hand to elicit a sound (Fig. 5-6B).

▀ **TIP** Each tap should be short and sharp to produce a sound.

5. Listen carefully to the percussion sounds.

Technique 5-3C: **Indirect Fist Percussion (Blunt Percussion)**

Purpose: To assess organ tenderness

Equipment: Gloves

1. Explain the technique to your patient.

2. Expose only the area that you will be percussing.

3. Gently lay your nondominant hand over the area to be assessed.

4. Make a fist with your dominant hand.

5. Using the ulnar surface of your closed fist and using moderate intensity, hit the dorsum of the nondominant hand (Fig. 5-6C).

6. Ask the patient if he or she experiences any discomfort.

▀ **TIP** Indirect fist percussion is commonly done to assess for kidney inflammation.

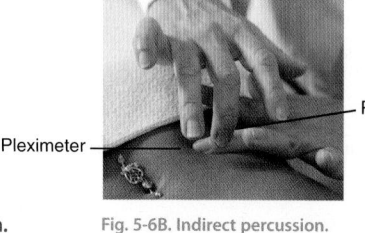

Fig. 5-6B. Indirect percussion.

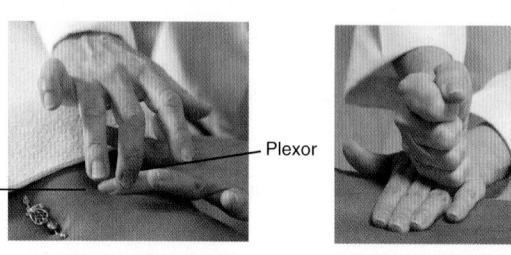

Fig. 5-6C. Indirect fist percussion.

TECHNIQUE 5-4: **Auscultation**

There are two types of auscultation: direct and indirect.

Purpose: To listen to cardiovascular, respiratory, gastrointestinal, and peripheral vascular sounds produced by the body

Equipment: Stethoscope (Fig. 5-7)

Doppler ultrasonic blood flow detector (Fig. 5-8)

Auscultation amplifies the following characteristics of sound:

- Duration (length of time)
- Intensity (loud or soft)
- Pitch (high or low)
- Quality (e.g., musical, blowing, bubbly)

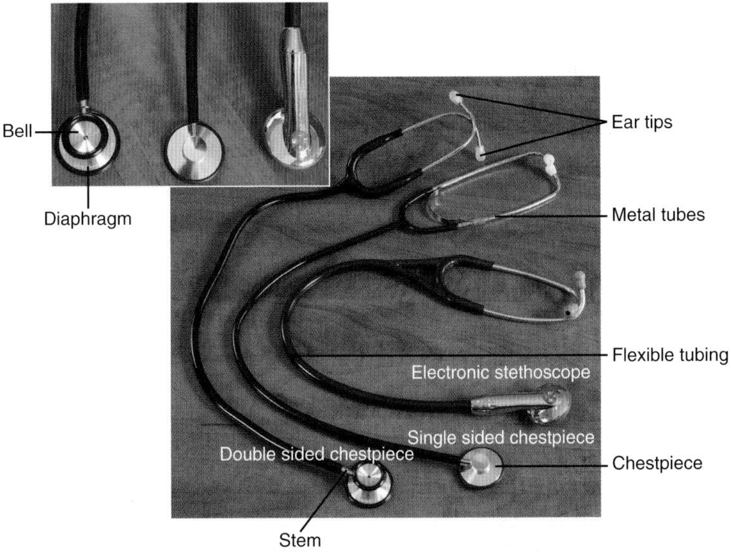

Technique 5-4A: **Direct Auscultation**

Purpose: To listen to sounds produced by the body:

1. Ensure there is a quiet environment.
2. Explain the technique to your patient.
3. Expose only the area that you will be directly auscultating.
4. Place your ear near the exposed area.
5. Listen for about a minute for sounds.

   ■ **TIP** Most common sounds that can be heard without equipment are respiratory and gastrointestinal sounds. Always confirm sounds with a stethoscope.

Technique 5-4B: **Indirect Auscultation**

Purpose: To listen to sounds produced by the body with an amplification device

Equipment: Stethoscope

1. Explain the technique to your patient.
2. Expose only the area to be auscultated.
3. Warm the stethoscope by gently rubbing your hand over the diaphragm or the bell of the stethoscope.

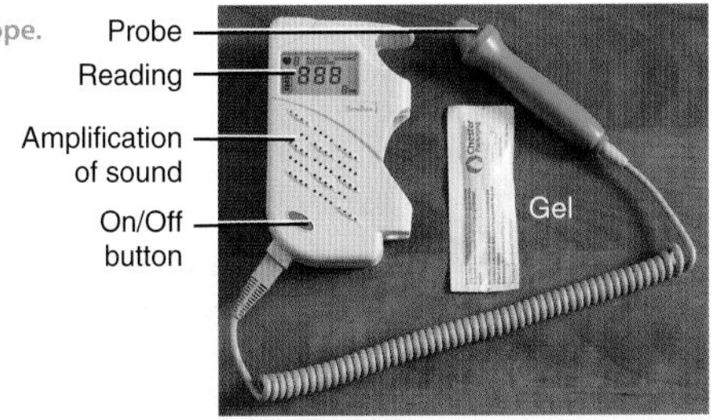

Fig. 5-7. Parts of the stethoscope.

Bell · Diaphragm · Ear tips · Metal tubes · Flexible tubing · Electronic stethoscope · Single sided chestpiece · Double sided chestpiece · Chestpiece · Stem

Probe · Reading · Amplification of sound · On/Off button · Gel

Fig. 5-8. Doppler ultrasonic blood flow detector.

TIP The bell of the stethoscope is used best to hear low-pitched sounds (e.g., vascular sounds and heart murmurs); the diaphragm of the stethoscope is best used to hear high-pitched sounds (e.g., respiratory sounds and bowel sounds).

4. Firmly place either the diaphragm or the bell of the stethoscope on the area to be assessed (Fig. 5-9).

TIP If the patient has much hair on the area to be auscultated, wet the hair with a warm washcloth to decrease the friction.

5. Concentrate and listen to the sounds.
6. When finished auscultating, clean off your stethoscope with an alcohol swab.

SENC Safety Alert Clean the stethoscope after each patient to prevent cross-contamination of bacteria and germs; a 70 percent alcohol solution is effective (Stem Cell Research.net, 2012). If you are unsure if the stethoscope is clean, always wipe off the diaphragm or bell with an alcohol solution prior to assessing the patient.

TIP The stethoscope and Doppler must be placed directly on the skin; never auscultate over clothing because artifact sounds may be heard.

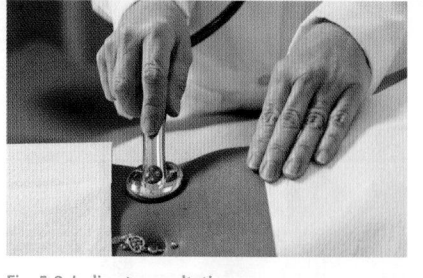

Fig. 5-9. Indirect auscultation.

General Survey and Assessing Vital Signs

INTRODUCTION

Patient care decisions and treatment depend on correct and essential assessment data (Tomlinson, 2010). There are many components to a health assessment that assess factors that influence a patient's health. As a healthcare provider, nurses are instrumental in collecting subjective and objective data during health assessment. The general survey and assessing vital signs are the first step in performing a physical assessment.

EQUIPMENT NEEDED

Thermometer
Sphygmomanometer

Stethoscope
Watch with a second hand

SEQUENCE OF ASSESSMENT

1. General survey
2. Temperature
3. Pulse

4. Respiratory rate
5. Blood pressure

TECHNIQUE 6-1: Surveying the Whole Person

Purpose: To assess the general well-being and behavior of the patient

The assessment begins with a general observation of the patient when you first meet and greet the patient and continues throughout the entire assessment. During the general survey, use your senses of sight, hearing, and smell. As you progress through the comprehensive, focused, or follow-up assessment, you will collect more specific subjective and objective data.

ASSESSMENT STEPS

1. Greet the patient and introduce yourself to the patient.

2. Explain your role and the purpose of the assessment.

3. As you begin interviewing the patient, make the following general observations about the patient:

☐ Physical appearance
  • Health: Does the patient look healthy, chronically ill, or ill?
  • Age: Does the patient look his or her stated age?
  • Patient hygiene, grooming, appropriate dress for climate or season; note body odors and breath
  • Body structure: tall, short, muscular, thin, or overweight; symmetry of body structures

☐ Behavior and mental status
  • Level of consciousness: alertness and orientation
  • Behavior: calm, restless, cooperative, eye contact, clarity of speech

CULTURAL CONSIDERATIONS Always take cultural considerations into account when performing the general survey. It is against some cultural norms to have direct eye contact with the healthcare provider. In the European American culture, eye contact is interpreted as attentiveness and honesty and people are taught to "look people in the eye" when talking. In many cultures, however, including Hispanic, Asian, Middle Eastern, and American Indian, eye contact is thought to be disrespectful or rude, and lack of eye contact does not mean that a person is not paying attention. Women may especially avoid eye contact with men because it can be taken as a sign of sexual interest. Do not force a patient to make eye contact with you. He or she may be treating you with greater respect by not making eye contact.

The Provider's Guide to Quality and Culture, *Non-Verbal Communication.* http://erc.msh.org/mainpage.cfm?file=4.6.0.htm&module=provider&language=.

☐ Facial expression: relaxed, stressed, frowning, facial grimacing, symmetrical
☐ Mood: happy, depressed, flat affect
  ■ **TIP** A depressed patient may have poor posture, hunched shoulders, avoid eye contact, appear sad, look and act tired, have dark circles around his or her eyes, and be overweight or underweight due to poor eating habits.
☐ Speech: clear, difficulty articulating words, slurring speech
  • Health literacy: patient's ability to understand health information

CULTURAL CONSIDERATIONS A nurse should assess the patient's fluency in English or understanding of the English language if the patient is communicating without an interpreter. Do not automatically assume that a patient with a heavy accent is not fluent or that just because it appears a patient is fluent that the patient comprehends the conversation. The easiest and quickest way to assess comprehension is to ask the patient to repeat back information or his or her understanding of the question (Dayer-Berenson, 2010).

- ☐ Mobility
  - Gait: steady and straight, difficulty walking, limping, or using an assistive device
  - Posture: stands or sits up straight; stooped posture, slumping in chair
  - Range of motion: ability or inability to move all joints and extremities; participate in the exam
- ☐ Signs of pain, respiratory, cardiac or gastrointestinal distress

SENC Safety Alert Always remember to look for signs of airway, breathing, or circulatory problems; these are areas of concern that require priority-focused assessments.

- Pain: facial grimacing, limited movement, guarding
- Respiratory distress: signs of difficulty breathing
- Cardiac distress: complaints of chest pain, skin color changes
- Gastrointestinal: holding or rubbing stomach, guarding abdomen
- General discomforts: fatigue, decreased endurance

NORMAL FINDINGS

- **Health:** appears healthy with no signs of illness or debilitation
- **Physical appearance:**
  - ☐ Age: patient looks stated age
  - ☐ Hygiene: well groomed, appropriately dressed for climate, no odors
  - ☐ Body structure: well built, symmetrical body structures
- **Level of consciousness:** alert and oriented × 4 (person, place, time, situation); calm and cooperative; may or may not have direct eye contact (depends on culture), speech clear, facial expression relaxed and symmetrical; mood calm; reports understanding reason for assessment
- **Mobility:**
  - ☐ Gait: steady and symmetrical, no difficulty walking
  - ☐ Posture: stands straight, sits up straight without support
  - ☐ Range of motion: ability to move all joints and extremities, actively participates in the exam
- **Distress:** No signs of general discomfort or pain, no signs of respiratory, cardiac, or gastrointestinal distress

ABNORMAL FINDINGS

- Physical appearance
  - ☐ Frailty, cachectic (wasting syndrome), fatigue may be a sign of acute or chronic illness
  - ☐ Age: patient looks much older than stated age; may indicate chronic stress or illness
  - ☐ Patient hygiene: unkempt grooming, inappropriate dress for climate, clothing that is too tight or too loose may indicate weight gain or weight loss; odors of the body or breath may indicate weight gain or weight loss, altered mental status, or cognitive dysfunction
    - **TIP** Poor hygiene and dress may be related to finances or lack of resources.

■ Behavior and mental status
  □ Level of consciousness: disoriented, decreased mentation (Chapter 3, Psychosocial Assessment; Chapter 17, Neurological Assessment)
  □ Behavior: inappropriate (Chapter 3, Mental Health Assessment; Chapter 17, Neurological Assessment)
  □ Mood: depressed, flat affect (Chapter 3, Mental Health Assessment)
  □ Speech: difficulty articulating words, slurring speech (Chapter 17, Neurological Assessment)
■ Mobility
  □ Gait and posture: unsteady difficulty walking, limping, poor posture (Chapter 16, Musculoskeletal Assessment)
  □ Range of motion: inability to move all joints and extremities; unable to participate in the exam (Chapter 16, Musculoskeletal Assessment)
■ **Distress:** signs of respiratory distress (Chapter 12, Respiratory Assessment); signs of cardiac distress (Chapter 13, Cardiovascular Assessment); signs of pain (Chapter 4, Pain Assessment); signs of gastrointestinal distress (Chapter 14, Abdominal Assessment)

VITAL SIGNS

Vital signs are an important measurement to determine overall health and the body's response to health and illness. Vital signs include measuring a patient's:

■ Temperature
  □ Body temperature is regulated by the thermoregulatory center in the hypothalamus that balances heat production and heat loss.
  □ Body temperature varies with the time of day and the site of measurement (Venes, 2013).
■ Pulse rate
  □ Pulse rate reflects heart rate; the number of times your heart beats per minute (bpm)
  □ The heart is a muscular organ that contracts and relaxes, forcing blood from the heart into the systemic arteries; the amount of blood that is forced out of the heart with each heartbeat is called stroke volume.
  □ Pulse is the force of blood against the walls of the arteries. This generates a rhythmic wave of pressure that is felt at various points in the body as a pulse.
■ Respiratory rate
  □ The respiratory center is located in the medulla oblongata and pons in the brain stem; this portion of the brain controls the rate and depth of respiration. The main organs of the respiratory system are the lungs (see Chapter 12).
  □ Breathing frequency; the number of breaths taken within 60 seconds
  □ Respiratory rate equals one inhalation and exhalation of breath

- Blood pressure
  - ☐ Blood pressure (BP) is the force of blood being exerted on the walls of the arteries as it is being pumped out of the heart. This pressure within the vascular system is influenced by:
    - Cardiac output is the volume of blood pumped out by the heart in 1 minute.
    - Stroke volume is the volume of blood pumped out by the heart during each contraction.

$$\text{Cardiac output} = \text{stroke volume} \times \text{heart rate}$$

    - The tension of the force of blood that is exerted on the walls of arteries by the strength of the contraction of the heart; reflects the elasticity of blood vessels (Venes, 2013). Elasticity of the blood vessels influences the BP; increased stiffness increases BP; increased dilation decreases BP.
    - Volume of circulating blood; the more volume creates increased pressure in the vessels
    - Viscosity: the thickness of the blood; increased viscosity causes increased peripheral resistance
    - Peripheral vascular resistance: the smaller the diameter of the blood vessels, the greater the peripheral vascular resistance
  - ☐ BP is recorded as two numbers—the systolic (pressure in arteries as the heart contracts) over diastolic (pressure in arteries as the heart relaxes between beats). The measurement is written one above or before the other, with the systolic number on top and the diastolic number on the bottom (National Heart Lung and Blood Institute, 2015).
- Pain assessment has been recognized as the fifth vital sign (see Chapter 4).

Normal vital signs change with age, sex, weight, exercise tolerance, and condition (Dugdale, 2011). Vital signs can change and be affected by our physical, psychological, and environmental conditions. An essential principle for assessing vital signs is always reviewing and comparing a patient's baseline or prior vital signs to the current readings.

PREPARATION FOR ASSESSMENT

During vital sign assessment, the environment should be at a comfortable temperature and quiet.

Neither the nurse nor the patient should be talking while the assessment is being performed. The following guidelines are used prior to taking specific vital signs.
- Temperature
  - ☐ The accuracy of a temperature measurement is influenced by how well the person uses the equipment, for example, how the probe is positioned and whether the probe is held steadily in place for the correct period of time (Davie & Amoore, 2010).
- Pulse rate
  - ☐ This is best assessed while the patient is resting.
- Respiratory rate
  - ☐ This is best assessed while the patient is resting.
- Blood pressure
  - ☐ The patient should not have caffeine or cigarettes in the preceding 30 minutes.
  - ☐ Patient should be sitting minimally 5 minutes in a chair with his or her back supported, feet flat on the floor, and legs uncrossed prior to taking the BP.

TIP If your back is not supported, your diastolic BP measurement may be increased by 6 mm Hg; crossing your legs has shown to raise your systolic BP 2 to 8 mm Hg (Monk, 2010).

TECHNIQUE 6-2: **Assessing Temperature**

Purpose: To assess the body's core temperature

Measuring patient body temperature is a part of routine and essential nursing care. Temperature can be taken several different ways. The site and measuring device chosen are based on a number of factors:

- Age of patient
- Mental status and cognition
- Physical condition
- Safety and nurse's technique with using the temperature device

Body temperature is measured in two different degrees:

- Celsius (C)
- Fahrenheit (F)

   TIP Conversions from Celsius to Fahrenheit (Table 6-1)

Factors that affect temperature measurement include:

- time of day and circadian rhythms: Body temperature can vary as much as 1°F to 2°F (0.5°C to 1°C) and is lowest in the morning (2 to 4 a.m.) while resting and is warmest in the afternoon (4 to 6 p.m.) while active
- age of the patient: older patients have decreased ability to control body temperature
- gender: hormonal fluctuations may increase or decrease temperature; when a woman ovulates, her temperature rises
- exercise increases the basal metabolic rate causing body temperature to rise
- environmental temperatures can increase or decrease body temperatures
- stress and emotions can trigger stimulation of the sympathetic nervous system causing body temperature to rise.

TABLE 6-1 **Conversion From Celsius to Fahrenheit**

Fahrenheit/Celsius	Conversion Calculation
°F to °C	Deduct 32, then multiply by 5, then divide by 9
°C to °F	Multiply by 9, then divide by 5, then add 32

SENC Safety Alert The U.S. Environmental Protection Agency (EPA) encourages consumers, businesses, and other organizations to use nonmercury thermometers whenever possible (EPA, 2012). Mercury thermometers are being banned from use in many healthcare organizations. Mercury thermometers contain a liquid inside that is harmful for both humans and the environment. Mercury is a toxic substance that can create health risks in very small amounts. Upon breaking a thermometer that contains 0.5 to 1.5 grams of mercury, a health risk can be created in a small room if the mercury is not cleaned up due to the evaporation of the mercury that would be present in the air. Health-wise, mercury can affect one's kidneys, brain, liver, and spinal cord. Mercury can also alter one's ability to taste, move, and see (Waxman, 2003).

Technique 6-2A: Assessing Oral Temperature

Purpose: To assess the core body temperature

The oral sublingual site has a rich blood supply from the carotid arteries that quickly responds to changes in inner core temperature.

▓ **TIP** The oral temperature should not be used on a patient who cannot follow directions, has decreased mentation, or breathes through his or her mouth.

Equipment: Electronic thermometer

▓ **TIP** Always make sure your thermometer is fully charged and calibrated.

ASSESSMENT STEPS

1. Take the thermometer off the charger prior to assessing the patient.
2. Explain the procedure to the patient.
3. Ask the patient if he or she has smoked or consumed any hot or cold foods or beverages in the last 30 minutes; if so, wait until 30 minutes has passed to maintain the accuracy of the reading.
4. Take the thermometer probe out of the holder and attach a plastic disposable probe cover.
5. Ask the patient to open his or her mouth and lift up his or her tongue.
6. Gently place the thermometer probe underneath the tongue (sublingually) (Fig. 6-1).
7. Ask the patient to gently but firmly close his or her mouth.
8. Observe the calculation of the thermometer. A sound or blinking will occur as the temperature reading registers.
9. Dispose of the dispensable thermometer probe cover.
10. Return the thermometer to the charger.
11. Document the site and temperature reading.

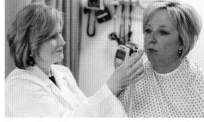

Fig. 6-1. Assessing temperature using an electric thermometer.

NORMAL FINDINGS

■ 97.5°F to 99.5°F or 36°C to 38°C
■ Daily fluctuations may be 1° F or 2° F

ABNORMAL FINDINGS

■ <97.7°F to >100°F or <36.5°C to >37.8°C
  □ Hypothermia is a core body temperature below 35°C (95°F) (Venes, 2013).

SENC Safety Alert Hypothermia should be confirmed by temperature readings at two different core locations (Venes, 2013).

SENC Safety Alert Hyperthermia (pyrexia) is an elevated body temperature greater than 37.8°C (>100°F).

Technique 6-2B: **Assessing Tympanic Temperature**

Purpose: To assess the core body temperature

Equipment: Tympanic thermometer

The eardrum is close to the hypothalamus in the brain that regulates the body's temperature.

A tympanic thermometer uses infrared radiation and a thermopile detector at the tip of the instrument to measure the infrared energy given off from the patient's eardrum in a calibrated length of time; temperature is assessed within 2 to 3 seconds.

SENC Safety Alert A tympanic thermometer should not be used on a patient who is experiencing ear pain, ear drainage, or has a large amount of wax in the ear.

ASSESSMENT STEPS

1. Explain the procedure to the patient.

2. Take the tympanic thermometer off the charging stand.

3. Attach a clear dispensable plastic ear probe.

4. Gently pull the upper earlobe up and back.

5. Insert the ear probe snugly pointing it toward the tympanic membrane (Fig. 6-2).

6. Push the button to register the temperature reading.

7. Once the temperature reading registers, dispose of the dispensable thermometer probe cover.

8. Return the thermometer to the charger.

9. Document the site and temperature reading.

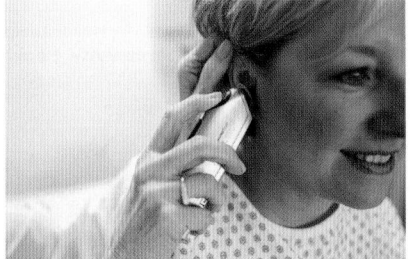

Fig. 6-2. Assessing temperature using a tympanic thermometer.

NORMAL FINDINGS

■ 98.2°F to 100°F or 36.8°C to 37.8°C

ABNORMAL FINDINGS

■ <98.2°F to >100°F or <36.8°C to >37.8°C

Technique 6-2C: **Assessing Temporal Temperature**

Purpose: To assess core body temperature

Equipment: Temporal artery thermometer

The thermometer reads the infrared heat waves released by the temporal artery, which runs across the forehead just below the skin.

TIP Each temporal artery thermometer may have different directions. Read the specific directions for correct application of the temporal artery thermometer.

ASSESSMENT STEPS

1. Explain the procedure to the patient.

2. Place the sensor head of the temporal artery thermometer at the center of the forehead midway between the eyebrow and the hairline.

3. Press the button down to start the scan.

4. Slowly slide the thermometer straight across the forehead toward the top of the ear maintaining direct contact with the skin (Fig. 6-3).

■ **TIP** Lifting the temporal artery thermometer off the skin will affect the reliability of the temperature.

5. Stop when you reach the hairline and release the button.

6. Lift up the thermometer from the skin and read the temperature on the display screen.

7. Dispose of the dispensable thermometer probe cover.

8. Return the thermometer back to the charger.

9. Document the site and temperature reading.

NORMAL FINDINGS

■ 98.7°F to 100.5°F or 37.1°C to 38.1°C

ABNORMAL FINDINGS

■ <98.7°F to >100.5°F or <37.1°C to >38.1°C

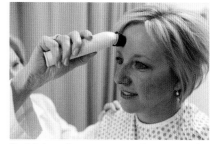

Fig. 6-3. Assessing temperature using a temporal artery thermometer.

Technique 6-2D: Assessing Rectal Temperature

Purpose: To assess core body temperature

Equipment: Electronic thermometer with rectal probe, gloves, lubricant

Rectal temperature is considered an accurate route for assessing body core temperature because it is an indication of deep visceral temperature.

SENC Safety Alert Rectal temperatures can stimulate the vagus nerve in the rectum. Rectal temperatures are contraindicated with the following patients:

■ Patients who had rectal surgery
■ Patients with disease of the rectum
■ Patients who have low white blood cell count
■ Patients who have blood clotting disorders
■ Patients with neurologic disorders
■ Patients with cardiac disease
■ Patients with diarrhea
■ Patient who has hemorrhoids

■ **TIP** In some institutions, rectal temperatures require a healthcare provider's order.

ASSESSMENT STEPS

1. If the patient is conscious, explain the procedure to the patient.

2. Put on clean gloves.

3. Position the patient on his or her side.
4. Remove the rectal temperature probe from the electronic thermometer base.
5. Insert probe into the disposable probe cover.
6. Lubricate the tip of the probe with lubricant.
7. Gently insert the tip of the thermometer into the rectum about 1 inch (Fig. 6-4).
8. Hold the probe in place until the temperature reading registers.
9. Slowly remove the probe from the rectum and discard the disposable plastic cover and gloves in the garbage.
10. Assist or place the patient in a comfortable position.
11. Return the thermometer back to the charger stand.
12. Document the site and temperature reading.

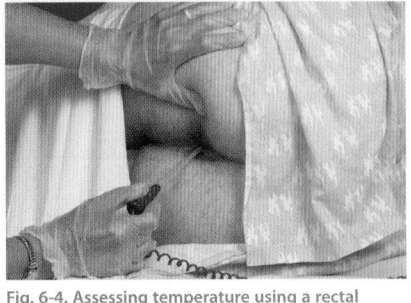

Fig. 6-4. Assessing temperature using a rectal thermometer.

NORMAL FINDINGS
■ 98.7°F to 100.5°F or 37.1°C to 38.1°C

ABNORMAL FINDINGS
■ <98.7°F to >100.5°F or <37.1°C to >38.1°C

SENC Evidence-Based Practice Sund-Lavender & Grodzinsky (2009) made the following suggestions to promote evidence-based practice when assessing temperature:
■ Evaluate body temperature in relation to the individual's baseline temperature.
■ Axillary body temperature measurement is not recommendable as an assessment of core body temperature in adults.
■ The same site of measurement should be used as much as possible.
■ Time, site of measurement, and administration of medication antipyretics should be noted in the patient record.

TECHNIQUE 6-3: Assessing the Pulse

Purpose: To assess the heart rate
Equipment: Watch with a second hand
A pulse can be felt as the heart pumps blood out to the aorta to the arterial system in the body. You will feel a pulsation in some of the blood vessels close to the skin's surface (see Chapter 15). The two key areas to check a pulse to assess the heart rate are:
1. Radial pulse is most commonly assessed if the patient has a regular heart rate.
2. Apical pulse is a more reliable and accurate location to assess the heart rate.

Technique 6-3A: **Palpating the Radial Pulse**

Purpose: To assess the heartbeat through the wall of the radial peripheral artery at the wrist:

ASSESSMENT STEPS

1. Explain the technique to the patient.

2. Gently place your second and third finger pads of your dominant hand on the radial artery at the flexor aspect of the wrist laterally along the radius bone (Fig. 6-5).

    ■ **TIP** Do not use your thumb because it has its own pulse that you may feel.

While palpating the pulsation, note the following characteristics of the pulse:

    ☐ Rhythm of the pulse: regular versus irregular; missed or paused beats; or an abnormal pattern of beats.

    ☐ Amplitude (strength) of the pulse is the force of the blood in the arterial system. This is measured on a scale of 0 to 3 (Table 6-2).

3. Holding your watch in the opposite hand, start counting the pulsations (heartbeats) for 60 seconds starting the count with number 1.

4. Document the site of the pulse, pulse rate, rhythm, and amplitude.

    ■ **TIP** It is good nursing practice to count the pulse for 60 seconds; this allows you to accurately assess the pulse for rate, rhythm, and amplitude.

    SENC Safety Alert If the pulse is irregular, always take an apical pulse for 60 seconds.

NORMAL FINDINGS

■ Rate: Resting pulse: 60 to 100 bpm; well-conditioned athletes 40 to 60 bpm.

■ Rhythm: regular

■ Amplitude: 2+

ABNORMAL FINDINGS

■ Pulse rate less than 60 and greater than 100

    ☐ Bradycardia is a heart rate less than 60 bpm

    ☐ Tachycardia is a heart rate greater than 100 bpm

■ Rhythm: irregular with pauses may be indicative of an irregular heart rate (arrhythmia)

■ Amplitude: absent (no heart rate), weak (decreased stroke volume), or bounding (increased stroke volume) may be indicative of changes in the circulatory system

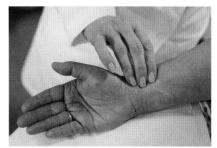

Fig. 6-5. Assessing a radial pulse.

Scale	Description
0	Absent: pulse cannot be felt
1	Weak or thready; pulse is barely felt and can be easily obliterated by pressing with the fingers
2	Normal quality: pulse is easily palpated, not weak or bounding
3	Bounding or full: pulse is easily felt with little pressure; not easily obliterated

TABLE 6-2 **Documentation for Amplitude of Pulse**

Wilkinson & Treas (2015).

TECHNIQUE 6-4: **Auscultating an Apical Pulse**

Purpose: To assess the heart rate
Equipment: Stethoscope, watch with a second hand
ASSESSMENT STEPS
1. Explain the technique to the patient.
2. Warm the stethoscope.
3. Uncover the left side of the patient's chest.
4. Gently place the diaphragm of the stethoscope directly over the left fifth intercostal space at the midclavicular line (apex of the heart) (Fig. 6-6).
5. Auscultate the heartbeat, assessing the rate and rhythm.
6. If heartbeat is regular, count the beats per minute for 30 seconds, then multiply by 2; if irregular, count the beats for 60 seconds.
7. Wipe off the stethoscope with an alcohol swab to clean the diaphragm.
8. Document the site and apical pulse rate.
NORMAL FINDINGS
■ Rate: resting pulse: 60 to 100 bpm; well-conditioned athletes 40 to 60 bpm
■ Rhythm: regular
ABNORMAL FINDINGS
■ Pulse rate less than 60 and greater than 100
■ Rhythm: irregular with pauses may be indicative of an irregular heart rate (arrhythmia)

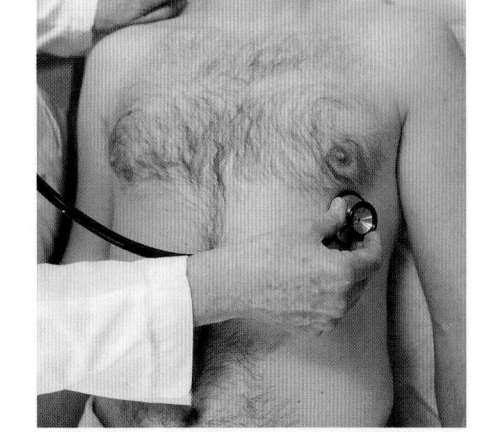

Fig. 6-6. Assessing the apical pulse at the left fifth intercostal space.

SENC **Safety Alert** If the pulse is irregular or weak, it may be related to the heart's inability to pump blood. Assess the radial pulse rate and the apical pulse rate. Determine if there is a pulse deficit, a difference between the apical and radial pulse rates. A pulse deficit is a difference in beats between the apical and radial pulse; this may be a sign of a cardiac arrhythmia.

TECHNIQUE 6-5: **Assessing the Respiratory Rate**

Purpose: To assess the pulmonary ventilation
Equipment: Watch with a second hand

TIP Changes in respiratory function are increasingly recognized as the most sensitive indicator of patient deterioration (Massey & Meredith, 2010).

■ Respiratory rate is the number of breaths a person takes in 1 minute. One breath constitutes an inspiration and expiration.
■ Respiratory rate is influenced by several factors:
 □ Exercise is a muscular activity and increases the respiratory rate.
 □ Pain causes an increase in respiratory rate and decreases the depth of respirations.
 □ Stress is the result of sympathetic stimulations and increases the respiratory rate.
 □ Fever increases the respiratory rate.
 □ Substance abuse can increase or decrease respiratory rate.

SENC Safety Alert Be alert to respiratory rate changes with temperature elevation. As the temperature rises 1°F (0.6°C), the respiratory rate may increase 4 breaths per minute.

 □ Illness and certain pathological conditions increase or decrease the respiratory rate.
 □ Medications can increase or decrease respirations (i.e., morphine sulfate has a side effect of respiratory depression).
 □ Position changes influence expansion of the lungs; sitting up (Fowler's or semi-Fowler's position) or standing is the best position for improving respiratory depth; lying down (prone position) reduces respiratory depth.
  TIP The best time to take a respiratory rate is after taking the pulse. Leave your fingers on the pulse, and assess the respiratory rate while the patient is resting. Sometimes, if the patient is aware that you are watching them breathe, the respiratory rate will change.

ASSESSMENT STEPS

1. Observe the patient's rise (inspiration) and fall (expiration) of the chest area.
2. Observe the following characteristics of the respirations:
■ Depth: even pattern, deep or shallow respirations
■ Rhythm: regular or irregular
■ Effort: amount of work required to take a breath
3. Count the number of respirations for 60 seconds.
4. Document the rate, depth, rhythm, and effort.
  TIP If you are having difficulty assessing respirations, place the diaphragm of the stethoscope over the trachea, and auscultate to the breath sounds.

SENC Safety Alert Assess patients for labored breathing or dyspnea (difficulty breathing) (see Chapter 12).

NORMAL FINDINGS

■ 12 to 20 breaths per minute; pattern is even; rhythm is regular.

ABNORMAL FINDINGS

■ Less than 12 breaths and more than 20 breaths per minute
■ Depth: deep or shallow respirations

- Rhythm: irregular
- Effort: using accessory muscles to breathe
- Specific abnormalities of respiratory rates (see Chapter 12)

TECHNIQUE 6-6: **Assessing Blood Pressure**

Purpose: To assess circulatory blood volume as the heart contracts and relaxes

BP measurement is done routinely and essentially to assess a patient's cardiovascular health. BP fluctuates throughout the day and night and is affected by many factors (Table 6-3). Three of the most common sites to take the BP are:

- Upper arm
- Forearms
- Thigh

TABLE 6-3 **Factors Affecting Blood Pressure**

Factor	Description
Gender	Men have slightly higher BP than women of comparable age.
	After menopause, women's BP increases possibly due to a decrease in estrogen.
Family history	Family history of hypertension increases the risk for developing hypertension.
Lifestyle	Diets high in sodium
	Alcohol consumption of three or more drinks per day
	Obesity increases risk for high BP
Diurnal variations	BP changes related to a person's schedules and routine
Exercise	Regular exercise decreases BP
Body position	BP higher with standing
	Readings are higher if arm is above the heart's level or unsupported at patient's side
	Higher if feet are dangling or legs are crossed.
Stress	Stressors increase BP
	"White coat hypertension" BP rises when being examined by a healthcare provider
Pain	Acute, short term pain increases BP
	Severe, prolonged pain can decrease BP

TABLE 6-3 Factors Affecting Blood Pressure—cont'd	
Factor	**Description**
Medications	Over-the-counter, herbs, illicit drugs, and medications can alter BP
Diseases	Diseases of the circulatory, renal, liver, and other major organs may affect BP.

Wilkinson & Treas (2015).

CULTURAL CONSIDERATIONS The age-adjusted prevalence of hypertension in non-Hispanic African Americans (32.4 percent) is substantially higher than that in non-Hispanic whites (23.3 percent) and Mexican Americans (20.6 percent) (Dreisbach, 2013).

Technique 6-6A: Assessing Blood Pressure in the Upper Arm

Purpose: To assess circulatory blood volume as the heart contracts and relaxes

Equipment: Manual sphygmomanometer, stethoscope, paper tape measure, electronic BP automated device (optional)

SENC Safety Alert The American Heart Association (2014) recommends an automatic, cuff-style, bicep (upper-arm) monitor. Wrist and finger monitors are not recommended because they yield less reliable readings.

■ **TIP** Always look in the patient's record to compare BP readings.

ASSESSMENT STEPS

1. Explain the technique to your patient.
2. Ask the patient if he or she has smoked or had any caffeine in the last 30 minutes; if no, proceed to take the patient's BP; if yes, wait until 30 minutes has lapsed.
3. If the patient is ambulatory, have the patient sit in a chair with his or her feet flat on the floor for 5 minutes.
4. Ask the patient not to move, talk, or cross his or her legs while taking the reading (Hyatt, 2011).

   ■ **TIP** The inflatable part (bladder) of the BP cuff should cover about 80 percent of the circumference of your upper arm. The cuff should cover two-thirds (40%) of the distance from your elbow to your shoulder (Sheps, 2010) (Fig. 6-7).

5. If sitting, seat the patient comfortably with back supported, legs uncrossed, and palm facing up, the arm resting at the level of the fourth intercostal space (heart level) and not tensed; if the patient is in supine position in the bed, place the arm flat with palm facing up on a pillow so that the arm is at heart's level.

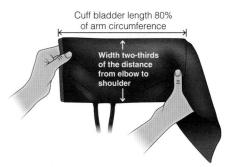

Cuff bladder length 80% of arm circumference

Width two-thirds of the distance from elbow to shoulder

Fig. 6-7. The "ideal" cuff with a length-to-width ratio of 2:1.

■ **TIP** A BP cuff should never be placed over any clothing, on an arm that has an intravenous or dialysis shunt, or the side of a recent mastectomy or surgical procedure.

6. Use a paper measuring tape, and measure the circumference of the midpoint of the upper arm between the shoulder and the elbow; choose the correct cuff size for your patient (see Table 6-4).

7. Wrap the deflated cuff around the patient's arm about 2.5 cm (1 inch) above the brachial artery and wrap evenly; make sure the artery marker is pointing to the brachial artery.

■ **TIP** If you could fit one finger under the BP cuff, it is not too tight.

8. Have the patient support the bare arm on the exam table or in your arm at the patient's heart level (Fig. 6-8).

■ **TIP** The manometer should be at your eye level.

9. Turn the manual valve clockwise on the BP cuff to close it.

10. Palpate the brachial artery at the antecubital fossa or the radial artery at the wrist, and continue to feel for the pulsation of the brachial or radial artery.

11. Start squeezing the bulb at the end of the rubber tube attached to the BP cuff. When you no longer feel the pulsation of the brachial artery, make note of this number on the sphygmomanometer. Slowly release the manual valve to deflate the BP cuff. This estimates the systolic pressure.

12. Place the bell or the diaphragm of the stethoscope on the brachial artery, and inflate the BP cuff 30 to 40 mm Hg above the palpable systolic BP number (Anderson, 2009). The numerical reading should be read to the nearest 2 mm Hg.

■ **TIP** If the palpable systolic value is unknown, you can inflate the cuff to 160 to 180 mm Hg. If pulse sounds are heard right away at these values, inflate to a higher pressure (Anderson, 2009). It is also good practice to review the patient's record for previous readings.

13. Slowly release the manual valve (2 to 3 mm/sec) to deflate the BP cuff, and listen for the first rhythmic Korotkoff sounds heard as blood begins to flow through the artery; this first sound is the systolic reading.

■ **TIP** Korotkoff sounds are the sounds heard in auscultation of blood pressure. These sounds arise from a combination of turbulent blood flow and oscillations of the arterial wall. They were first described by a Russian physician, Nikolai Korotkoff (1874–1920). There are five Korotkoff sounds (see Table 6-5) (Venes, 2013).

14. Listen carefully for an auscultatory gap; an auscultatory gap, also called a silent gap, is the interval of pressure where the Korotkoff sounds become diminished or absent. The presence of an auscultatory gap is frequently associated with increased vascular stiffness (Frech, Penrod, Battistone, Sawitzke, & Stults, 2012). The auscultatory gap happens when the first Korotkoff sound fades out for about 20 to 50 mm Hg only to return (Shrestha, 2011). Record the location in the reading where you hear an auscultatory gap (Fig. 6-9).

TABLE 6-4 Measuring Cuff Size

Arm Circumference	Cuff Size	Cuff Size
22 to 26 cm	Small adult size	12 × 22 cm
27 to 34 cm	Adult size	16 × 30 cm
35 to 44 cm	Large adult size	16 × 36 cm
45 to 52 cm	Adult thigh size	16 × 42 cm

Pickering et al. (2005).

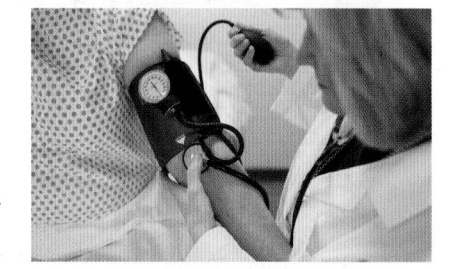

Fig. 6-8. Assessing BP with arm at heart level.

TABLE 6-5 Korotkoff Sounds

Korotkoff Sound	Description
First	As you deflate the BP cuff, you will initially hear a sound that occurs during systole. It is a tapping sound that corresponds to the pulse (systolic BP).
Second	Occurs as you further deflate the cuff. It is a soft, swishing sound caused by blood turbulence.
Third	Begins midway through the BP and is a sharp, rhythmic, tapping sound.
Fourth	Like the third sound, but softer and fading.
Fifth	Silence; it corresponds with diastole (diastolic BP).

Wilkinson & Treas (2015).

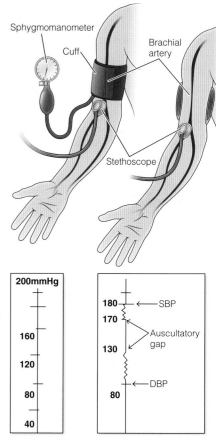

Fig. 6-9. Auscultatory gap.

15. Continue to listen as the BP cuff pressure is released, for the last Korotkoff sound that you are able to hear; this last sound is the diastolic reading.

16. Document the location and BP reading.

SENC Safety Alert If the BP reading is high, wait for about 2 minutes and retake the BP in the opposite arm. Document the higher of the two BP readings (systolic number/diastolic number) (Ferri & Alvero, 2016).

SENC Safety Alert Isolated systolic hypertension occurs if the systolic number is greater than 140 and the diastolic number is less than 90. This type of high blood pressure can lead to stroke, heart disease, or kidney disease (Sheps, 2014).

NORMAL FINDINGS
■ Normotensive (Normal BP); systolic reading is less than 120; diastolic reading is less than 80.

ABNORMAL FINDINGS (SEE TABLE 6-6)
■ Hypotension is blood pressure that is below normal limits.
■ Hypertension is blood pressure greater than or equal to 140 systolic or greater than or equal to 90 diastolic.

TABLE 6-6 Categories for Blood Pressure Levels in Adults Age 18 and Older*			
Category	**Systolic (Top Number)**		**Diastolic (Bottom Number)**
Normal	Less than 120	And	Less than 80
Prehypertension	120–139	Or	80–89
Hypertension Stage 1	140–159	Or	90–99
Hypertension Stage 2	160 or higher	Or	100 or higher
Hypertensive crisis (emergency care needed)	Higher than 180	Or	Higher than 110

Measure in millimeters of mercury, or mm Hg.
From American Heart Association (2016).

SENC Safety Alert Patients with chronic kidney disease or diabetes should maintain their blood pressure less than 130/80 mm/Hg.

Technique 6-6B: **Assessing Blood Pressure in the Forearm**

Purpose: To assess circulatory blood volume as the heart contracts and relaxes
Equipment: Manual sphygmomanometer, stethoscope, paper tape measure, electronic BP automated device (optional)
When patients' upper arms are not accessible and/or when cuffs do not fit large upper arms, the forearm site is often used for BP measurement (Schnell, Morse, & Waterhouse, 2010).

ASSESSMENT STEPS

1. Explain the technique to your patient.
2. Ask the patient if he or she has smoked or had any caffeine in the last 30 minutes; if no, proceed to take the patient's BP; if yes, wait until 30 minutes have elapsed.
3. If the patient is ambulatory, have the patient sit in a chair with his or her feet flat on the floor for 5 minutes.
4. Ask the patient not to move, talk, or cross his or her legs while taking the reading (Hyatt, 2011).
5. Using a measuring tape, measure the forearm in centimeters at the widest point closest to the elbow: choose a correctly sized BP cuff.
6. Wrap the deflated cuff around the patient's upper forearm about 2.5 cm (1 inch) below the brachial artery; make sure the artery marker is pointing down toward the radial artery.
7. Have the patient support the bare arm on the exam table or in your arm at the patient's heart level; patients in supine position should have their arm resting on a pillow at heart level.

8. Turn the manual valve clockwise on the BP cuff to close it.

9. Palpate the radial artery at the wrist, and continue to feel for the pulsation of the radial artery.

10. Start squeezing the bulb at the end of the rubber tube attached to the BP cuff. When you no longer feel the pulsation of the radial artery, make note of this number on the sphygmomanometer. Slowly release the manual valve to deflate the BP cuff.

11. Place the bell or the diaphragm of the stethoscope on the radial artery, and inflate the BP cuff 30 to 40 mm Hg above the palpable systolic BP number (Anderson, 2009).

12. Slowly release the manual valve to deflate the BP cuff, and listen for the first rhythmic, low-frequency Korotkoff sounds heard as blood begins to flow through the artery. This is the patient's systolic pressure; this first sound is the systolic reading.

13. Continue to listen as the BP cuff pressure is released, for the last Korotkoff sound that you are able to hear; this last sound is the diastolic reading.

14. Document location and BP reading.

Technique 6-6C: Assessing Blood Pressure in the Thigh

Purpose: To assess circulatory blood volume as the heart contracts and relaxes
Equipment: Manual sphygmomanometer, stethoscope, paper tape measure
This technique is only done if the BP cannot be taken in the arms.

ASSESSMENT STEPS

1. Explain the technique to the patient.
2. Place the patient preferably in the prone position; if patient cannot lie on his or her stomach, place the patient in the supine position with the knee slightly flexed.
3. Measure the thigh in centimeters between the knee and the hip; choose the correct size cuff.
4. Wrap the deflated cuff around the patient's thigh about 2.5 cm (1 inch) above the popliteal artery; making sure the artery marker is pointing down toward the popliteal artery (Fig. 6-10).
5. Turn the manual valve clockwise on the BP cuff to close it.
6. Palpate the popliteal artery and continue to feel for the pulsation of this artery.
7. Start squeezing the bulb at the end of the rubber tube attached to the BP cuff, inflating the BP cuff until you no longer feel the pulsation of the popliteal artery. (This is the palpable systolic BP.) Make note of this number on the sphygmomanometer. Release the manual valve to deflate the BP cuff.
8. Place the bell or the diaphragm of the stethoscope on the popliteal artery, and inflate the BP cuff 30 to 40 mm Hg above the palpable systolic BP number (Anderson, 2009).

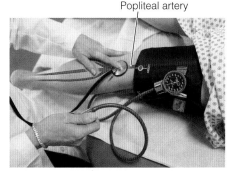

Popliteal artery

Fig. 6-10. Assessing BP using the thigh and popliteal artery.

9. Slowly release the manual valve to deflate the BP cuff, and listen for the first rhythmic low-frequency Korotkoff sounds heard as blood begins to flow through the artery. This is the patient's systolic pressure; this first sound is the systolic reading.
10. Continue to listen as the BP cuff pressure is released, for the last Korotkoff sound that you are able to hear; this last sound is the diastolic reading.
11. Document the location and BP reading.

   ▌ **TIP** Values obtained from thigh measurement may be higher than arm pressures due to increased hydrostatic pressure related to the lower position of the thigh (Jahangir, 2011).

ADVANCED ASSESSMENTS

TECHNIQUE 6-7: **Assessing Orthostatic Vital Signs**

Purpose: To assess blood volume with change of positions
Equipment: Manual sphygmomanometer, stethoscope, watch with second hand
Orthostatic hypotension (postural hypotension) is a form of low BP that occurs when you stand up from a sitting position or from lying down. Patients who have orthostatic hypotension complain of dizziness, or feeling lightheaded with change of position. A positive orthostatic pulse and BP may be a sign of decreased circulating volume (hypovolemia or dehydration), a side effect of medications, or a sign of a medical condition.

   SENC Safety Alert Closely monitor patients who may be at risk of falling because they feel dizzy or cannot stand up. Assess only the supine and sitting positions if the patient is unable to stand.

   SENC Evidence-Based Practice Orthostatic blood pressure position change from supine to standing has better diagnostic accuracy in volume-depleted adults compared to position changes from supine to sitting and then to standing. Orthostatic vital signs alone lack the sensitivity to reliably detect volume losses less than 1,000 mL. Symptoms such as dizziness and syncope, in combination with orthostatic vital signs, are more sensitive indicators of volume loss than vital sign changes alone. Therefore, symptoms and vital signs should be documented as the orthostatic variables (Witting & Hydorn, 2013).

ASSESSMENT STEPS
1. Explain the technique to the patient.
2. Place the patient in the supine position for 5 to 10 minutes prior to the first BP and pulse assessment.
3. Take the patient's pulse (see Technique 6-3) and BP (see Technique 6-4) in the left arm (Fig. 6-11A).
4. Do not remove the BP cuff.
5. Document the site, the pulse, and BP readings in the supine position.

6. Ask the patient to stand up.

7. Retake the patient's pulse and BP after 2 minutes while standing (Fig. 6-11B).

8. Document the site, the pulse, and BP readings in the standing position.

NORMAL FINDINGS
- No change in pulse rate or BP
- Pulse rate increases slightly (<20 bpm)
- BP drops slightly (<10 mm Hg)

ABNORMAL FINDINGS
- Pulse rate increases by 20 or more bpm
- Systolic BP decreases by 20 or more mm Hg
- Diastolic BP decreases by 10 or more mm Hg
- Patient becomes dizzy or loses consciousness (Witting & Hydorn, 2013)

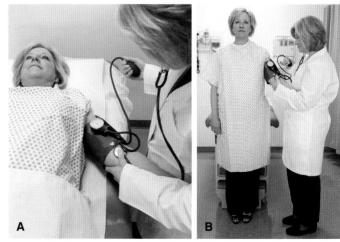

Fig. 6-11. Assessing orthostatic BP. (A) Laying supine. (B) Standing.

PATIENT EDUCATION

Healthy People 2020

Goal: **Improve cardiovascular health and quality of life through prevention, detection, and treatment of risk factors for heart attack and stroke; early identification and treatment of heart attacks and strokes; and prevention of repeat cardiovascular events (HHS, 2010).**

- Patients need to be taught the basics about taking their own temperature, pulse, and BP if needed and be aware of normal and abnormal findings. Knowing when to call the doctor should be discussed with all patients.

- About one in three adults in the United States has high BP. The condition itself usually has no symptoms. You can have it for years without knowing it. During this time, however, high BP can damage the heart, blood vessels, kidneys, and other parts of your body (National Heart Lung and Blood Institute, 2011).
- National Health and Nutrition Examination Survey predicts that by 2025 hypertension could affect more than 104 million people due to three main reasons:
  - ☐ Population growth in general
  - ☐ Aging population
  - ☐ Epidemic of obesity

- All patients should be taught about the risk factors of heart disease and high BP. High BP is a modifiable risk factor (one that can be modified through lifestyle changes) for heart disease and stroke. Lifestyle modifications for high BP include:
  - ☐ If overweight, lose weight:
    - Losing 10 pounds (4.5 Kg) of weight can lower the BP by 10 points
  - ☐ Limit alcohol:
    - Two drinks per day for men
    - One drink per day for women
    - One drink per day for older people (>65)
  - ☐ Exercise minimally 30 minutes preferably on all days.
  - ☐ Stop smoking.
  - ☐ Reduce sodium, saturated fats, and cholesterol.

Assessing Pain

INTRODUCTION

Pain is one of the most common and stressful symptoms encountered by patients (Kumar, 2011) and, in the United States, it is estimated that more than 76 million people suffer from pain (The Joint Commission, 2016). A subjective, universal experience, pain is undertreated, affects all aspects of daily living, and has an impact on a patient's quality of life. In 1995, Dr. James Campbell, in his Presidential Address to the American Pain Society (APS), presented the idea of evaluating pain as a vital sign (Campbell, 1995). In 1996, the APS introduced the phrase "pain as a 5th vital sign." This initiative emphasizes that assessing patients for pain is as important as taking vital signs. Considering the physical, psychological, social, economic, and spiritual effects of pain, it is possible to see how pain is multidimensional and can be challenging and difficult to assess objectively (Briggs, 2010). There are many factors that can affect the pain experience, including:

- age of the patient
- ethnicity, cultural, and religious background
- previous experience with pain
- nature of the injury or illness
- quality of life.

Patients react differently to pain and feel a variety of emotions such as fear, anger, helplessness, and depression during this experience. Nurses are instrumental in developing a trusting relationship with their patient, conduct a thorough pain assessment, and work with the patient to develop a plan of care for the most effective pain relief treatments (Briggs, 2010).

DEFINITION OF PAIN

Pain is a complex symptom that is difficult to define. Pain is a subjective experience that requires consciousness (Steeds, 2016). Some definitions include:

- An unpleasant sensory and emotional experience associated with actual or potential tissue damage, or described in terms of such damage (The International Association for the Study of Pain, 2011).
- Pain is a subjective, physical, and emotional experience shaped by cultural values and beliefs (Davidhizar & Giger, 2004).
- "Pain is whatever the experiencing person says it is, existing whenever he/she says it does" (McCaffery, 1968).

PHYSIOLOGY OF PAIN

The pain experience involves two processes: detection and interpretation.

Detection

Detection, or the transmission phase, is the generation and transmission of pain impulses from the site of injury (peripheral nervous system) to the central nervous system (CNS):

■ Pain impulses are initiated by activation of free nerve endings (pain receptors) called *nociceptors*. Pain receptors are everywhere in the body; these receptors are free nerve endings that are designed to detect tissue injury and are activated by three types of stimuli:
   □ Mechanical stimulus (e.g., pressure or stretching)
   □ Thermal stimulus (e.g., heat or cold)
   □ Chemical stimulus (e.g., bradykinins, serotonin, or histamine)
■ When tissue is injured and becomes inflamed, cells break down and release inflammation mediators such as prostaglandins, substance P, histamines, and cytokines. These substances cause an inflammatory reaction, thereby increasing sensitivity to pain.
■ During this phase, pain receptors release the pain stimulus; this stimulus is transmitted through peripheral nerves through the dorsal horn of the spinal cord and to the brain and back down the spinal cord. There are two main types of nerve fibers (nociceptors) that transport the pain signals to the CNS and submit these different sensations or qualities of pain: A-delta fibers and C fibers. Both these fibers terminate in the dorsal horn of the spinal cord (Fig. 7-1).
   □ A-delta fibers are the larger, thicker, nerve fibers that quickly travel through the nervous system; they are covered with myelin; pain will feel sharp, stinging, and acute; the patient is able to identify where the pain is; pain does not radiate.
   □ C fibers are smaller, thinner, unmyelinated nerve fibers that travel slowly through the nervous system; pain will feel diffuse, dull, burning, or achy; poorly localized; pain may radiate.

■ Ronald Melzack and Patrick Wall (1965) developed the gate control theory, which maintains that there is a transmission station, a gate, in the spinal cord that influences the flow of nerve impulses to the brain. Melzack and Wall theorized that pain impulses can be influenced by many factors, including a person's emotions and mind.

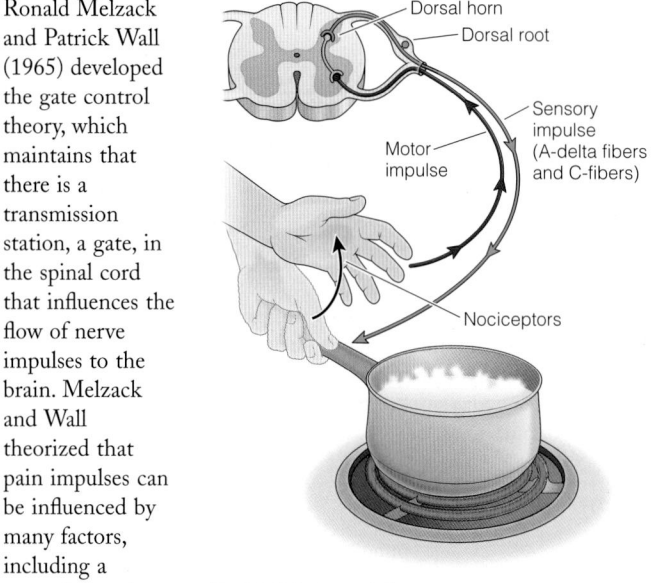

Fig. 7-1. Pain transmission.

   □ Certain nerve fibers traveling along the C fibers can be stopped before they ascend to the brain.
   □ Substantial gelatinosa cells in the dorsal horn of the spinal cord act as "gates" to regulate the flow of the impulses.
   □ The brain has a large influence on the gating mechanism; the sensation of pain can be blocked before the patient perceives the pain through alternative therapies such as massage, deep breathing, heat, and cold (Fig. 7-2).

Interpretation

Interpretation is the perception of pain.

- It is only when the noxious stimuli are actually interpreted in the higher cortical areas of the brain that we feel pain.
- Interpretation occurs once the impulses are in the CNS; incoming signals are modulated, this process is interpreted according to the individual's genetic make-up, sociocultural factors, beliefs, and expectations about pain, and cognitive experience (Casey, 2011).

TIP Modulation is a chemical system or third set of neurotransmitters that increases or decreases the transmission of pain impulses in the spinal cord.

- The thalamus is the part of the brain that receives the pain information from the spinal cord; the cortex of the brain interprets the sensation of pain.
- The limbic system accounts for an emotional response (e.g., crying) and conscious awareness.

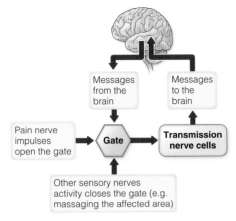

Fig. 7-2. Gate control theory of pain.

- Patient perceptions of pain include the following:
  - □ Pain threshold is the level at which the brain perceives a stimuli being painful (Guariglia, 2010).
  - □ Pain tolerance is how much pain and how long the patient is willing and able to endure the pain.

TIP Gender, stress level, and one's genetic make-up all contribute to sensitivity to pain.

SENC Evidence-Based Practice Research has investigated a wide variety of painful conditions that has suggested that there are gender differences in pain perception (Mogil & Bailey, 2010). Clinical findings have demonstrated that women are at increased risk for chronic pain and some data suggest that women may experience more severe clinical pain. Studies of experimentally induced pain have produced a very consistent pattern of results, with women exhibiting greater pain sensitivity and lower pain threshold compared with men (Ciaramella & Poli, 2015; Kvachadze, Tsagareli, & Dumbadze, 2015)

CULTURAL CONSIDERATIONS Culture is the framework that directs human behavior in a given situation. Not everyone in every culture conforms to a set of expected behaviors or beliefs, so cultural *stereotyping* (assuming a person will be stoic or very expressive about pain) can lead to inadequate assessment and treatment of pain (Weismann, Gordon, & Bidar-Sielaff, 2004). Nurses need to understand that different cultures react and treat pain differently (Table 7-1). Patients must be made to feel comfortable sharing their pain experience with the nurse.

TABLE 7-1 Pain Expression in Selected Ethnocultural Groups

Ethnic Group	Response to Pain
African Americans	Often viewed as a sign of illness or disease. Some believe that suffering and pain are inevitable and must be endured. Some believe that praying and laying on of hands may aid in freeing the person from pain and suffering; people who continue to have pain are considered to have little faith.
Amish Culture	Unlikely to display pain and physical discomfort.
Arab Americans	Often view pain as unpleasant and something that should be controlled. Tend to express pain openly with immediate family members but may act in a more restrained manner in the presence of healthcare providers. The nurse may assess pain relief as adequate; family members may demand additional analgesia.
Chinese Americans	Expressions of pain are described in terms of more diverse body symptoms. Often believe pain is related to the influence of imbalances of the *yin* and *yang*. Usually cope with pain by using externally applied oils and massage as well as warmth, sleeping on the area of pain, relaxation, and aspirin.
European Americans	Pain is the "fifth vital sign." Offer and encourage pain medications, and explain that it will help the healing process.
Jewish Culture	Verbalization of pain is acceptable; individuals want to know the cause of their pain. Relief of pain is important. In ultra-Orthodox denominations of Judaism, taking medication on the Sabbath that is not necessary to preserve life may be viewed as "work" and unacceptable. Teach patients about the potential life-threatening sequelae of their condition as well as the exceptions to Jewish laws that permits them to take medications.
Korean Culture	Some Korean Americans are stoic and are slow to express emotional distress from pain; others are expressive and discuss their smallest discomforts; monitor for nonverbal cues and facial expressions of pain.
Puerto Rican Culture	Individuals tend to be loud and outspoken in expressing pain. Herbal teas, heat, and prayer are often used to manage pain.

Adapted from Purnell, L. (2014). *Culturally competent health care*. Philadelphia, PA: F.A. Davis.

TYPES OF PAIN

There are many different causes and types of pain. Nurses need to assess the different factors influencing the pain experience.

Duration of Pain

Pain has different time frames. Pain can be **acute** (short term), **chronic** (long term), **intractable** (constant), or **intermittent** (comes and goes). The feeling of pain varies depending on where in the body the pain is felt. Pain can be identified as follows:

- **Acute pain** begins suddenly and is usually sharp in quality; results from nociceptor activation due to damage to tissues. Acute pain typically resolves once the tissue damage is repaired (Chekka, Benzon, & Jabri, 2011). An example of acute pain is pain related to an inflamed appendix (appendicitis). Acute pain may:
  - ☐ be associated with injury, trauma, or surgery
  - ☐ be of short duration and protective in nature.

- **Chronic or persistent pain** continue longer than three months or past the time of normal tissue healing. Patients describe this pain as debilitating, disabling, or intolerable (Venes, 2013). The most common sites of chronic pain are the back, head, and joints (Marcus, 2014). An example of chronic pain is arthritic pain, which causes pain and stiffness in the joints.
  - □ Pain signals remain active in the nervous system for weeks, months, or years.
  - □ Emotional effects include depression, fatigue, anger, anxiety, and fear of reinjury.
  - □ Functional effects include inability to work, disability, and inability to perform activities of daily living.
  - □ The cause may be unknown but is often associated with chronic illness.

SENC Evidence-Based Practice: Chronic Pain and the Military
Chronic pain is highly prevalent among U.S. military veterans treated in the Veterans Affairs (VA) system of care, with upward of 50 percent of VA medical patients reporting chronic pain. Stratton et al. (2015) conducted a study to examine the equivalence of three varying lengths of a cognitive behavioral therapy group protocol for the management of chronic pain in a clinical care setting. Across groups, veterans showed improvements in negative pain-related thinking and decreases in pain-related disability and distress. In general, patient outcomes regarding pain-related distress and disability for the 6-week group were equivalent or better than the 12- and 10-week groups. Preliminary results support the effectiveness of brief behavioral interventions for chronic pain. Research supports the use of cognitive behavioral therapy for the treatment of chronic pain.

There are physical changes in acute and chronic pain (Table 7-2).
- **Intractable pain** is constant pain that is resistant to treatment or incurable; it continues even with interventions that attempt to

TABLE 7-2 Physical Changes in Acute and Chronic Pain

Acute Pain	Chronic Pain
Sympathetic Nervous System	*Parasympathetic Nervous System*
↑Blood pressure, pulse, respiratory rate	Blood pressure, pulse, respiratory rate remain normal
Pupils become dilated	Pupils do not dilate
Skin becomes sweaty (diaphoretic)	Skin remains dry
↑Restlessness	No restlessness
↑Verbal responses (crying, moaning)	No verbal response
Nausea	No nausea
Tissue damage or injury	Decrease in functional capacity

alleviate the pain. An example of intractable pain is pain from advanced cancers.
- □ Very severe, unremitting pain
- □ Affects every aspect of the patient's life

Sources of Pain
- **Cutaneous pain** originates from the skin and subcutaneous tissue; it is superficial pain, described as sharp pain with short duration. An example is a skin laceration.
- **Colicky pain** fluctuates in intensity from severe to mild and most often occurs in waves (Venes, 2013); usually related to spasms in the intestines.
- **Nociceptive pain** results from damage or inflammation to the sensory nerves (nociceptors) in soft tissue; it may be described as dull, sharp, or achy pain. There are two types of nociceptive pain:
  - □ **Somatic pain** is diffuse, sharp, and well localized; it can often be reproduced by touching or moving the area or tissue involved;

arises from tissues such as skin, muscle, joints, bones, and ligaments; often known as musculoskeletal pain. An example of somatic pain is rheumatoid arthritis.

☐ **Visceral pain** is vague or poorly localized and usually originates from internal organs; feels achy and crampy; is caused by compression in and around the organs, ischemia, inflammation, or stretching of the abdominal cavity (Jacques, 2009). An example of visceral pain is the chest pain from a myocardial infarction.

■ **Neuropathic pain** is caused by injury or damage to nerves; this pain feels sharp, stings, burns, and the patient may experience numbness and tingling sensations. An example of neuropathic pain is leg and foot pain related to diabetes.

■ **Phantom limb syndrome** is a poorly understood type of neuropathic pain that is felt in a body part that has been removed. The brain still receives pain messages from the nerves that originally carried impulses from the missing limb (Flor, Diers, & Andof, 2013). Phantom limb pain (PLP) varies in character from neuropathic-type descriptors such as sharp, shooting, or electrical-like, to more nociceptive-specific adjectives such as dull, squeezing, and cramping. It can be localized to the entire limb or just one region of the missing limb (Hsu & Cohen, 2013).

SENC Evidence-Based Practice: Limb Loss and the Military The number of women veterans and service members with traumatic limb loss may be expected to grow, and little is known regarding their health and healthcare needs. Katon and Reiber (2013) found that, compared with men, women with traumatic limb loss had similarly high levels of persistent physical and mental health conditions. Both men and women with traumatic limb loss reported extremely high levels of migraine headaches, with women reporting an approximately threefold higher prevalence of migraine than men. Compared with men, women also had higher rates of prosthesis receipt and rejection, but lower rates of replacement.

These study findings highlight some potential issues specific to women veterans, which may require additional clinical attention.

■ **Psychogenic pain** has no organic or structural cause. The main mechanism proposed for the development of this condition is psychological trauma and suppression of the painful emotions (Atarodi, 2010).

Transmission of Pain

Pain can travel through nerve transmission to other parts of the body. Two types of transmitting pain are:

■ **Radiating pain** starts in one area and spreads out to another part of the body (e.g., toothache that radiates to the ear or head).

■ **Referred pain** is felt in an area away from the actual source of the pain (e.g., gallbladder pain may be felt in the shoulder or upper thoracic region of the back) (Fig. 7-3).

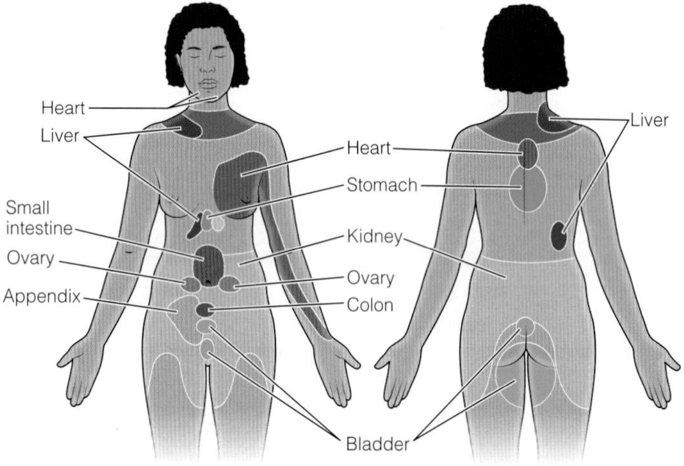

Fig. 7-3. Referred pain.

PAIN ASSESSMENT

Pain is a subjective report and is difficult to measure and validate. Accurately assessing pain refers specifically to the ability to correctly discriminate a patient's level of pain (Ruben et al., 2015). All patients should be asked whether they are experiencing pain. Inadequate pain assessment is one of the major factors of undertreatment of pain (Li, Herr, & Chen, 2009). The most reliable method for assessing pain is to have the patient describe the pain in his or her own words (Lehne, 2013). The "gold standard" for assessing pain is the patient's self-report of pain (Paulson-Conger, Leske, Maidl, Hanson, & Dziadulewicz, 2011). Start the assessment with an open question such as *"Can you describe your pain?"* Patients may start by describing the quality of pain as:

- aching
- dull
- knifelike
- sharp
- throbbing
- tingling.

■ **TIP** Have the patient point to the location of the pain and where the patient feels the pain.

Document the patient's own words when describing pain. An example is: *"I have a constant burning pain in my upper chest for the past week. I am nauseous and have no appetite. At night, I sit up because it is worse when I lay flat in bed."* Once the patient has completed the description, use focused questions to document the specific information necessary to assess pain. Specific information to assess pain should include:

- Duration of the pain: Is the pain constant? Does it come and go?
- Timing of the pain: Does it occur in the morning? After meals? Does it occur when walking?
- Quality of the pain: Does it feel sharp or dull?
- Aggravating factors: What makes the pain worse?
- Alleviating factors: What makes the pain better? What helps the pain go away?
- Concomitant symptoms: What other associated symptoms are occurring during the pain such as nausea, vomiting, headache?
- Treatment: Has the patient taken medication or treated the pain? Has the patient seen any other healthcare providers?
- Severity: How severe is the pain?

■ **TIP** Always ask what medications the patient is taking to try to alleviate the pain. Ask when the last dose was taken and whether the medication was effective.

CULTURAL CONSIDERATIONS Nurses should ask the patient whether he or she has any health or cultural beliefs related to the cause and treatment of pain. Nurses should have access to assessment tools that come in different languages for those patients that do not speak English.

During the pain assessment, be observant of nonverbal body language indicative of pain. This may include the following:

- Facial grimacing or tense or anxious facial appearance
- Tired look; moves slowly
- Posture: Fetal position or limping; tense muscles
- Verbal vocalization such as crying, moaning, sighing, or not articulating words
- Protective guarding, bracing, or rocking back and forth
- Rapid breathing

PAIN ASSESSMENT TOOLS

Accurately assessing pain refers specifically to the ability to correctly discriminate a patient's level of pain (Ruben, van Osch, & Blanch-Hartigan, 2015). A pain assessment tool should be used to assess severity of pain and the effectiveness of interventions.

- The assessment tool needs to be easy to understand by nurses, staff, and patients, and must be a valid and reliable measure of pain (Cox, 2010).
- When assessing pain, combining assessment validations is more reliable than just using one type of assessment. For instance, a patient's self-report and an assessment scale is better than self-report alone.

TIP Remember that not all patients are able to read and interpret the meaning of words or numbers. Make sure the patient understands the pain assessment questions and pain rating scales.

TIP Listen carefully during the patient's report; pay attention to the details of the description.

Mnemonics to Assess Pain

There are several memory aides to identify descriptors and attributes of pain. Because pain is a subjective experience, every individual feels pain differently.

OLDCARTS Pain Assessment

- Onset
  - □ When did the pain begin?
- Location/Radiation
  - □ Where do you feel the pain? Does the pain radiate?
- Duration
  - □ How long does the pain last? Is it constant or intermittent?
- Character
  - □ What does the pain feel like?
- Aggravating or alleviating factors
  - □ What makes the pain worse? What makes the pain better?
- Related symptoms
  - □ What symptoms do you have with the pain?
- Treatment
  - □ How do you relieve the pain? What medications do you take? Who has treated your pain?
- Severity
  - □ How would you rate or describe the severity of the symptom?
  - • Use a pain scale and the patient's own words
  - □ How does it affect your daily activity?

OPQRST Pain Assessment (Powell et al., 2010)

- O = Onset of pain
  - □ When did you first feel the pain?
- P = Provocation and palliates
  - □ What causes the pain?
  - □ What makes the pain better or worse?
- Q = Quality
  - □ What does the pain feel like?
- R = Radiation and region
  - □ Where is the pain located?
  - □ Is it confined to one place?
  - □ Does the pain radiate? If so, where to?
  - □ Did it start elsewhere, and is it now localized to one spot?
- S = Severity
  - □ How severe is the pain?
  - □ Rate the pain on a scale of 0 to 10 (with 0 being no pain and 10 being the worst pain possible).

- T = Timing or temporal
  - □ When did the pain start?
  - □ Is it present all the time?
  - □ Are you pain-free at night or during the day?
  - □ Are you pain-free on movement?
  - □ How long does the pain last?

Pain Assessment Scales

There are several different scales and descriptors used to assess pain. When considering which pain scale to use, consider the patient's age, level of education, language skills, eyesight, and lifespan variations (Wilkinson et al., 2015). Some examples of pain assessment scales are as follows:

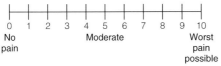

Fig. 7-4. Numeric rating scale.

- **Numeric Rating Scale:** This scale asks the patient to verbally estimate his or her pain on a scale of 0 to 10, with 0 representing no pain and 10 representing the worst possible pain (Fig. 7-4).

- **Wong-Baker Faces Pain Rating Scale:** This is administered by explaining to the patient that each face is for a person who feels happy because he or she has no pain (no hurt) or sad because he or she has some or a lot of pain. Face 0 is very happy because he or she does not hurt at all. Face 2 hurts just a little bit. Face 4 hurts a little more. Face 6 hurts even more. Face 8 hurts a whole lot. Face 10 hurts as much as you can imagine, although you do not have to be crying to feel this bad. Ask the patient to choose the face that best describes how he or she is feeling. This rating scale is recommended for people ages 3 years and older who are able to understand the instructions (Fig. 7-5).

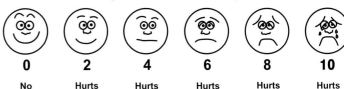

Wong-Baker FACES® Pain Rating Scale

0	2	4	6	8	10
No Hurt	Hurts Little Bit	Hurts Little More	Hurts Even More	Hurts Whole Lot	Hurts Worst

©1983 Wong-Baker FACES® Foundation. www.WongBakerFACES.org
Used with permission. Originally published in *Whaley & Wong's Nursing Care of Infants and Children*. ©Elsevier Inc.

Fig. 7-5. Wong-Baker FACES® Pain Rating Scale.

- **Verbal Descriptor Pain Scale (VRS):** This is for a patient who is able to describe pain using words such as mild, moderate, or severe (Fig. 7-6).

- **Iowa Pain Thermometer (IPT)** (Fig. 7-7): The IPT is a modified verbal descriptor scale made up of seven pain-describing words associated

---

Verbal Descriptor Scale

Patient's name:_____ Date:_____

Instructions: Please place a check mark next to the phrase that best describes the current level of your pain.

_____ The most intense pain imaginable

_____ Extreme pain

_____ Severe pain

_____ Moderate pain

_____ Mild pain

_____ Slight pain

_____ No pain

Fig. 7-6. Verbal descriptor rating scale.

---

with seven varying levels of pain intensity. Patients are asked to visualize a thermometer with the temperature rising and relate it to

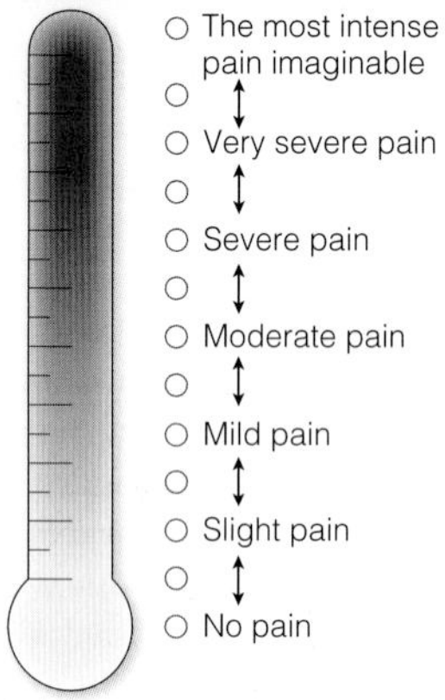

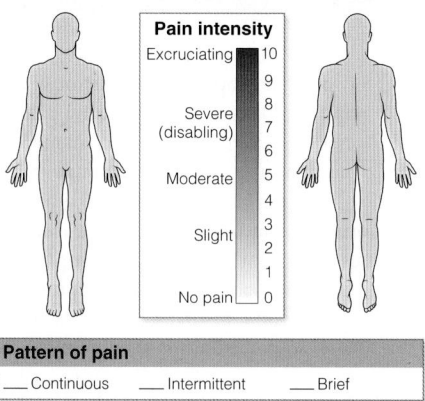

Fig. 7-7. Iowa pain thermometer. (With permission from Keela Herr.)

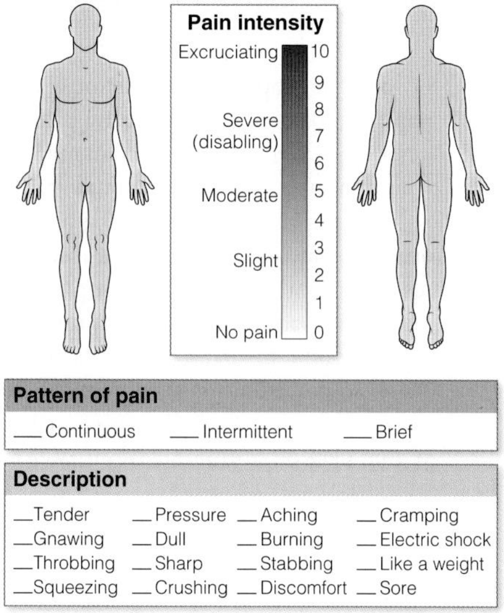

- ○ The most intense pain imaginable
- ○
- ○ Very severe pain
- ○
- ○ Severe pain
- ○
- ○ Moderate pain
- ○
- ○ Mild pain
- ○
- ○ Slight pain
- ○
- ○ No pain

Pain intensity

Excruciating	10
	9
	8
Severe (disabling)	7
	6
Moderate	5
	4
Slight	3
	2
	1
No pain	0

Pattern of pain

___ Continuous   ___ Intermittent   ___ Brief

Description

___Tender	___Pressure	___Aching	___Cramping
___Gnawing	___Dull	___Burning	___Electric shock
___Throbbing	___Sharp	___Stabbing	___Like a weight
___Squeezing	___Crushing	___Discomfort	___Sore

Fig. 7-8. Pain assessment tool. (With permission from Royal Brompton & Harefield NHS Foundation Trust.)

their feelings of pain. As the temperature rises, so does the feeling of pain intensity. The thermometer is used as a tool to measure current pain in patients who have difficulty communicating verbally or cognitive deficits.

■ **Pain Assessment Tool** (Fig. 7-8): The Pain Assessment tool offers a multidimensional approach to assessing pain. The nurse marks off on a body diagram the location of pain and circles the pain intensity on a 0 (no pain) to 10 (excruciating pain) scale. The pattern of pain and description of pain are checked off on the tool.

SENC Evidence-Based Practice The Iowa Pain Thermometer (IPT), Numerical Rating Scale (NRS), Verbal Rating Scale (VRS), and Faces

Pain Scale-Revised (FPS-R) are among the most common measures of pain intensity used by clinicians and researchers. Evidence supports the reliability and validity of each of these measures across many populations (Li, Herr, & Chen, 2009; Ware, Epps, Herr, & Packard, 2006).

■ **PainQuILT™** is a free, online evidence-based pain assessment and tracking tool for people with chronic pain and the healthcare professionals who care for them (Fig. 7-9):

　□ Consists of 16 icons to represent aching, burning, dull, electrical, freezing, heavy, pinching, pins and needles, pounding, shooting, sharp, stabbing, stiffness, squeezing, throbbing, and "other" pain.

　□ Patients use the mouse to "drag-and-drop" a miniature copy of their descriptive icon onto a virtual body-map to show the location, quality, and intensity of their pain.

　□ The PainQuILT™ may be viewed at https://app.painquilt.com

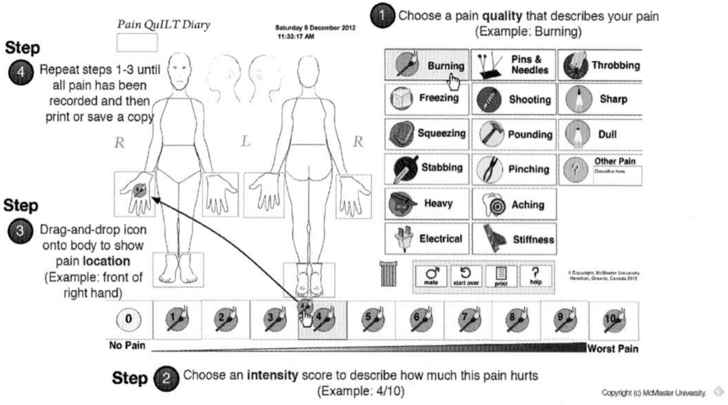

Fig. 7-9. PainQuILT™. (Copyright © McMaster University.)

ASSESSING THE COMMUNICATIVELY IMPAIRED PATIENT

Nurses must be aware that there are patients who cannot communicate how they are feeling because they cannot speak or may be cognitively impaired and cannot communicate effectively. The American Society for Pain Management Nursing addresses five populations of patients who may be unable to self-report:

- Older adults with advanced dementia
- Infants and preverbal toddlers
- Critically ill/unconscious patients
- Persons with intellectual disabilities
- Patients at the end of life (Herr et al., 2011).

A hierarchy of pain assessment techniques has been recommended as a guide to assess patients who are unable to self-report (Pasero & McCaffery, 2011):

- Self-report: This may include a simple yes/no answer; blinking of eyes (one blink means yes; two blinks means no).
- Search for potential causes for the pain.
- Observe patient behaviors for nonverbal cues.
- Proxy reporting: Credible information can be obtained from a family member or another person who knows the patient well.
- Utilize behavioral pain assessment tools, as appropriate (Herr et al., 2011):
  - □ **Critical Care Pain Observation Tool (CPOT).** You can assess nonverbal patient indicators of pain in four areas: facial expression, body movements, muscle tension, and ventilator compliance (Gélinas et al., 2008) (Table 7-3).

SENC Evidence-Based Practice The Critical-Care Pain Observation Tool is one of the few behavioral pain scales that have been developed and validated for the purpose of detecting pain in nonverbal critically ill adults (Gélinas et al., 2011).

  - □ **Pain Assessment in Advanced Dementia (PAINAD) Scale.** This can be used to assess pain in patients who are cognitively impaired, noncommunicative, or suffering from dementia and unable to use self-report methods to describe pain. The total score ranges from a minimum of 0 to a maximum of 10 (Table 7-4).

SENC Evidence-Based Practice Paulson-Conger, Leske, Maidl, Hanson, and Dziadulewicz (2011) compared two nonverbal assessment tools, the Pain Assessment in Advanced Dementia (PAIDAD) and the Critical-Care Pain Observation Tool (CPOT). A descriptive, comparative, prospective design ($n = 100$) was used; data were collected over a 6-month period in different critical care areas. Results indicated that there was no difference in PAINAD and CPOT scores for assessing pain in nonverbal patients in critical care. The results supported the reliability of these two pain tools to be used in nonverbal patients in critical care.

Nurses should be familiar with standard assessment tools used at their healthcare or community agencies. A structured assessment will facilitate a thorough pain assessment. Subjective and objective information along with data from the health history will help nurses and healthcare providers to alleviate pain through pharmacological and nonpharmacological treatment plans.

TABLE 7-3 The Critical Care Pain Observation Tool

Indicator	Description	Score
Facial Expression	No muscular tension observed	Relaxed, neutral 0
	Presence of frowning, brow lowering, orbit tightening, and levator contraction	Tense 1
	All of the above facial movements plus eyelid tightly closed	Grimacing 2
Body Movements	Does not move at all (does not necessarily mean absence of pain)	Absence of movements 0
	Slow, cautious movements, touching or rubbing the pain site, seeking attention through movements	Protection 1
	Pulling tube, attempting to sit up, moving limbs/thrashing, not following commands, striking at staff, trying to climb out of bed	Restlessness 2
Muscle Tension	No resistance to passive movements	Relaxed 0
Evaluation of passive flexion and extension of upper extremities	Resistance to passive movements	Tense, rigid 1
	Strong resistance to passive movements, inability to complete them	Very tense or rigid 2
Compliance with the ventilator (intubated patients)	Alarms not activated, easy ventilation	Tolerating ventilator movement 0
	Alarms stop spontaneously	Coughing but tolerating 1
OR	Asynchrony; blocking ventilation, alarms frequently activated	Fighting ventilator 2
Vocalization (extubated patients)	Talking in normal tone or no sound	Talking in normal tone or no sound 0
	Sighing, moaning	Sighing, moaning 1
	Crying out, sobbing	Crying out, sobbing 2
Total Range		0–8

Gélinas C, et al. *Am J Crit Care.* 2006; 15(4); 421.

TABLE 7-4 **Pain Assessment in Advanced Dementia (PAINAD) Scale**

Indicator	Score = 0	Score = 1	Score = 2	Total Score
Breathing (independent of vocalization)	Normal	Occasional labored breathing Short period of hyperventilation	Noisy labored breathing Long period of hyperventilation Cheyne-Stokes respiration	
Negative Vocalization	None	Occasional moan/groan Low level, speech with a negative or disapproving quality	Repeated troubled calling out Loud moaning or groaning Crying	
Facial Expression	Smiling or inexpressive	Sad, frightened, frown	Facial grimacing	
Body Language	Relaxed	Tense, distressed, pacing, fidgeting	Rigid, fists clenched Knees pulled up Striking out Pulling or pushing away	
Consolability	No need to console	Distracted or reassured by voice or touch	Unable to console, distract, or reassure	
				Total:

From Warden, V., Hurley, A., & Volicer, L. (2003). Development and psychometric evaluations of pain assessment in advanced dementia (PAINAD) scale. *American Medical Directors Association, 4*, 9–15.

CHAPTER

8 Assessing the Skin, Hair, and Nails

INTRODUCTION

The skin, hair, nails, glands, and mucous membranes compose the integumentary system and contribute to an individual's own unique appearance. An assessment of the skin, hair, and nails can reveal much information about the patient's overall health status, including the body's internal homeostasis, functioning, and hydration status, as well as skin disease, vitamin deficiencies, and effects of medications.

REVIEW OF ANATOMY AND PHYSIOLOGY

Skin

- One of the largest and heaviest organs of the body
- Self-generating
- Protects internal environment from the external environment
- Involved in several functions of the body, including (Fig. 8-1):
  - □ sensation and perception
  - □ thermoregulation
  - □ fluid balance
  - □ synthesis of vitamin D
  - □ excretion
  - □ immunity

Layers of the Skin
Epidermis

- This is the avascular, outer layer of the skin that is replaced every 3 to 4 weeks.

- It primarily consists of keratinocytes (cells containing protein) and melanocytes (cells producing a pigment melanin) that give the skin and hair color.
- Pigmentation is determined by the number, size, and distribution of melanosomes, membrane-limited vesicles found within melanocytes; genetics plays a key role.
- Stratum corneum is the thin layer of dead skin that changes in thickness depending on its location; it is thicker on the palms of the hands and thinner around the eyes.
- It depends on the underlying dermis for nutrition.

Dermis

- This contains connective tissue, sensory nerve fibers, capillaries, collagen, and elastin.
- It is the part of the skin that adds strength and elasticity to the skin and gives individuals the ability to feel.

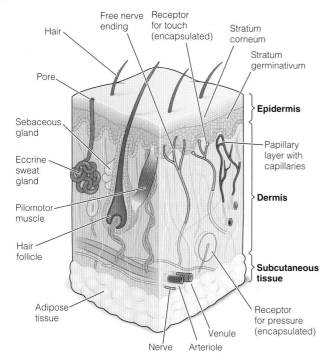

Fig. 8-1. Anatomy of the skin.

Hair

- Hair is made up of proteins and long chains of amino acids.
- Thin, flexible threads of keratin are found over much of the body, except the lips, nipples, soles of the feet, palms of the hands, labia minora, and penis.
- Hair grows from follicles (hair bulb and hair root) into the hair shaft.
- It is the visible projection from the epidermis.
- Growth is influenced by the production of hormones.
- There is a time frame for growth:
  - Eyebrow hair: lasts 3 to 5 months
  - Scalp hair: lasts 2 to 5 years
- Gray hair occurs due to a decrease in the number of functioning melanocytes.
- There are two types of hair:
  - Vellus: the fine, soft, nonpigmented hair over most of our body
  - Terminal: usually pigmented, dark, coarse, and thicker; develops during puberty; examples: pubic, axillary, and chest hair

Nails

- Nails are plates of keratin that start from the nail matrix in the epidermal layer and protect the fingernails and toenails (Fig. 8-2).
- The **cuticle** acts as a protective seal; if damaged, it can be an entryway for bacteria.

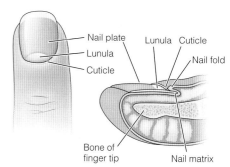

Fig. 8-2. Anatomy of the fingernails.

- This is where hair follicles and sebaceous, sweat, and apocrine glands originate.

Subcutaneous layer

- This is composed of adipose tissue and fat.
- It provides protection and insulation, and stores fat.
- Hair follicles have their roots in this layer.

- The **lunula** is a crescent-shaped white opaque area near the nail root.
- **Nailbeds** are pink due to highly vascular epithelial cells.
- **Growth:** Fingernail growth is approximately 1 mm per week. Growth is slower in toenails and slower in the summer than in the winter. Growth is affected by disease and hormone deficiency (Venes, 2013). Hair and nails are considered appendages of the skin.

Glands That Affect Skin, Hair, and Nails

Sebaceous Glands
- Located over the entire body except on the palms of the hands and soles of the feet
- Produce and secrete a protective oil through the hair follicles called *sebum*

Sweat Glands
There are two types of sweat glands:
- **Eccrine glands:** produce an odorless fluid to maintain body temperature and produce sweat; located in all skin especially the palms, soles of the feet, axilla region, and forehead.
- **Apocrine glands:** produce a body odor when reacting to bacterial decomposition and increases in response to emotional stress; located in the axillary and genital regions

DIAGNOSTICS
- **Skin biopsy** is a procedure to obtain a sample of tissue for examination under a microscope. This procedure diagnoses diseases, infections, and skin cancers.

HEALTH HISTORY

Review of Systems
The skin has many functions. It is important to remember that changes in skin could relate to a health problem that manifests as a skin problem. Assessment must start with a good history. Use focused, patient-centered interviewing to elicit specific information. Ask the patient about his or her daily routine of care for the skin, hair, and nails to assess baseline information. General topics for questions related to a skin problem are:
- onset or chronology of the skin problem
- quality or type
- quantity or severity
- timing
- location
- associated or alleviating factors
- associated symptoms or pertinent review of systems (ROS)
- treatment for any skin disorder.

TIP Use the OPQRST mnemonic (Onset, Provokes/Palliates, Quality, Radiates/Region, Severity, Time) to identify the attributes of a symptom. Ask the patient the following questions.

Medical and Family History
- Do you have a history or is there a family history of any skin problems or skin cancer (Box 8-1)?
- Do you have any systemic diseases that manifest through the skin?
- Do you take any medications for this skin problem?
- What are your symptoms?
- When did your symptoms occur?

Psychosocial History
- What are your skin care habits?
- What are your hair care habits?
- What are your nail care habits?

- Are you under any stress?
- Do you have any tattoos or body piercings? If so, have you had any reactions?

■ **TIP** Psychosocial habits can influence the skin, hair, and nails. Individuals under stress may bite their nails or have fine, brittle hair due to nutritional or vitamin deficiencies.

Allergies

- Do you have any environmental, medication (prescription, over the counter [OTC], herbal medicine), food, or other allergies?
  - ☐ Reactions to medications can cause skin rashes and hives.
  - ☐ If yes, have you developed any skin reactions? What was the specific reaction? How was it treated?

Skin Care

- Do you regularly examine your skin? If so, when?
  - ☐ Skin cancer is the most common and preventable cancer in the United States (American Cancer Society, 2017).

- Do you have yearly skin checks by a dermatologist? When was your last skin check? What is the name of the dermatologist?
  - ☐ The American Cancer Society recommends a yearly skin examination for individuals ages 20 and older and encourages individuals to know their pattern for moles, blemishes, freckles, and other marks on the skin.
- Do you wear sunblock when you are in the sun?
  - ☐ Sunblock with a sun protection factor (SPF) greater than 30 and water resistant is strongly recommended to prevent sun damage to the skin. It takes 15 minutes for your skin to absorb the sunscreen and protect you (American Academy of Dermatology, 2015a).
  - ☐ Sunblock should be reapplied after being in the water.
- Do you use indoor tanning?

SENC Evidence-Based Practice The American Academy of Dermatology (2014) found that increased numbers of teenage girls and young women are not being warned about the dangers of tanning beds by indoor tanning bed establishments. Studies have found that ultraviolet (UV) radiation from indoor tanning beds increases a person's risk of developing melanoma by 75 percent.

SENC Safety Alert The U.S. Food and Drug Administration (2015) has issued the following orders to address the risk to the public related to sunlamp products:

- Sunlamp products are to include a black box warning on the device that states that the sunlamp product should not be used on persons under the age of 18 years.
- Adult users over age 18 must sign a risk acknowledgement certification that states that they have been informed of the risks to health that may result from use of sunlamp products.

Skin Color
- Have you noticed any changes in the color of your skin (Box 8-2)?

CULTURAL CONSIDERATIONS African Americans encompass a gene pool of more than 100 racial strains; skin color among African Americans can vary from light to very dark. Lighter-skinned people appear more yellowish brown, whereas darker-skinned African Americans appear ashen (Purnell, 2014).

BOX 8-2 Changes in Skin Color

Changes in skin color could indicate systemic disease or problems with circulation.
- **Albinism**: Inherited disorder caused by the total or partial absence of an enzyme that produces melanin
- **Carotenemia**: A yellowing of the skin due to increased dietary intake of carotene in the diet, from foods such as carrots, sweet potatoes, pumpkin, corn, yams, spinach, and beans. The sclera of the eye does not become yellow.
- **Central cyanosis**: Bluish discoloration to the skin related to decreased circulating oxygen; best assessed in the oral mucosa, conjunctiva of the eyes, lips, and tongue.
- **Erythema**: Red, pink skin color; may indicate inflammation, fever, or increased blood flow. In carbon monoxide poisoning, the individual will have a bright red cherry face and upper trunk.

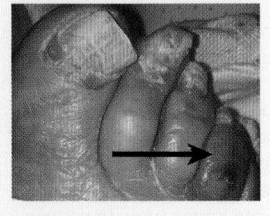
Erythema.

- **Hyperpigmentation:** Darker skin color
- **Hypopigmentation:** Lighter skin color
- **Jaundice**: Yellowing of the skin due to excessive levels of bilirubin in the blood

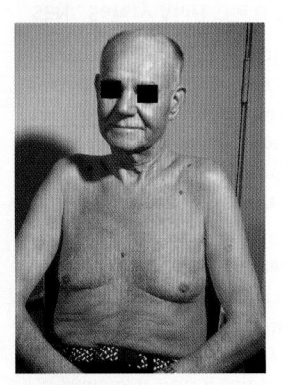
Jaundice.

- **Pallor/Pale**: Pale skin is seen in anemia, a decrease in circulating red blood cells or blood flow, or absence of oxygenated blood

BOX 8-2 **Changes in Skin Color—cont'd**

- **Peripheral cyanosis**: A blue, grey, slate, or dark purple discoloration of the skin or mucous membranes caused by deoxygenated or reduced hemoglobin in the blood; may occur with decreased cardiac output.

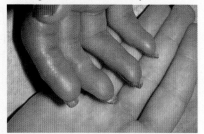

Peripheral cyanosis.

- **Vitiligo**: Autoimmune disorder that causes smooth, white patches of skin all over the body

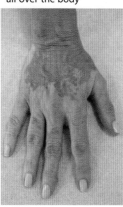

Vitiligo.

Skin Texture

- Have you noticed if your skin is soft, dry, scaly, swollen, flaky, or rough?
  - ☐ Skin conditions can affect the texture of skin (Box 8-3).

TIP Keloid formation is an overgrowth of connective tissue and commonly seen on dark skinned individuals (Purnell, 2014).

Moles or Lesions

- Have you noticed any new moles/lesions? If yes, have any of your moles/lesions changed in size, shape, or color (Box 8-4)?
- Have you noticed any changes in surface area, such as scaliness, oozing, or bleeding?

☐ Newly developed moles or changes in a mole could indicate skin cancer and should be checked by the patient's healthcare provider.

Rashes

Rashes can be chronic or acute and related to diet, stress, medications, allergies, hormone imbalance, autoimmune disease, kidney disease, toxic reactions, digestive problems, body imbalances, chemicals, and sun exposure. Ask the following:

- When did you first develop the skin rash?
- Is the rash constant or intermittent?
- Is this the first time? Where did the rash start?
- Did the rash spread?

BOX 8-3 **Conditions Affecting Skin Texture**

- **Autoimmune diseases**: can cause inflammation, redness, loss of hair, and changes in skin texture
- **Acne vulgaris**: a skin condition originating from sebaceous glands that can cause blemishes, cysts, bumps, pustules, and inflammation of the skin
- **Eczema**: causes chronic inflammation of the skin; itchy, dry, scaly patches of skin; this skin disorder has familial tendencies.

- **Hormonal conditions**: can change the texture of skin to be dry, oily, or moist; may change skin color.
- **Rosacea**: an inflammatory skin condition causing redness, swelling, and spider-like blood vessels to develop on the middle of the face

---

- Was the rash itchy, tender, or painful?
- Is there anything that makes the rash better or worse?
- Have you put any lotions or medications on the rash?

SENC Patient-Centered Care Patients with acute or chronic skin conditions or rashes may have changes in her or his body image, which affects self-esteem. Chronic aggravating symptoms can affect the patient's quality of life, level of functioning, and even activities of daily living (ADLs). Patients may have acute or chronic alterations in his or her skin that challenge the ability to cope with these changes. Being present with the patient and offering empathetic listening helps the patient feel comfortable during the self-report.

Hair

Hair changes can be related to diet, stress, genetics, infections, and endocrine disorders. Ask the following:
- Do you have a family history of hair loss?
- Have you noticed any changes in the texture of your hair?

- Is your hair dry or oily?
- Have you noticed any patchy or overall hair loss or hair breakage?

Nails

Nail changes can be related to nutrition, stress, systemic disease, vitamin or iron deficiency, infection, and nail biting or picking. Ask the following:
- Have you noticed any changes in your nails?
- Have you had previous nail problems?

SENC Patient-Centered Care The skin is a complex organ that can change acutely or chronically in response to different pathologies in the body. Skin assessment requires examination of the patient's most private and personal areas. Explaining to the patient what you are doing helps to inform and alleviate patient discomfort. Ask permission from the patient prior to examining these areas to ensure a trusting relationship. Maintain privacy and patient dignity throughout the assessment.

BOX 8-4 **Defining Primary and Secondary Lesions**

PRIMARY SKIN LESIONS

Primary skin lesions occur in reaction to the external or internal environment. They may be present at birth or develop during an individual's lifetime.

- **Macule:** A circular, small, flat spot less than 0.5 cm in diameter. Macules are red, brown, or white in color, and the color is not the same as that of nearby skin. They present in different shapes. Example: *freckle*

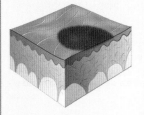

Macule.

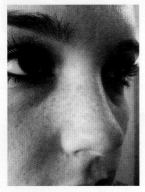

Freckle.

- **Patch**: irregular, flat, nonpalpable macule greater than 1 cm. Example: *Mongolian spots*
- **Papule**: A solid, elevated, spot that appears rough in texture and measures less than 0.5 cm in diameter. Papules are pink, red, or brown in color. Example: *mole*

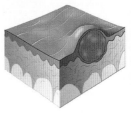

Papule.

- **Plaque**: A patch of closely grouped thickened papules measuring greater than 0.5 cm across. Plaque is red, brown, or pink in color with a rough texture. Example: *psoriasis*

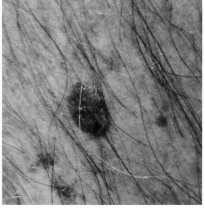

Mole.

Continued

BOX 8-4 Defining Primary and Secondary Lesions—cont'd

- **Vesicle:** Raised, round, or oval with serous blood or clear fluid measuring less than 0.5 cm in diameter. Example: *herpes simplex*

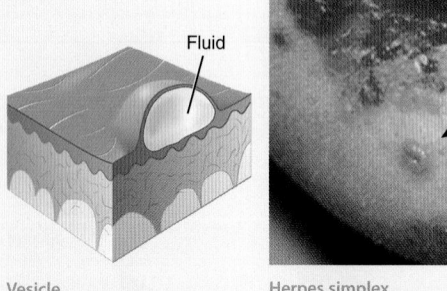

Fluid

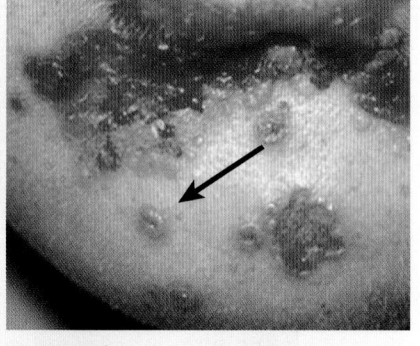

Vesicle.

Herpes simplex.

- A pustule is a raised vesicle filled with pus. Infection is the primary cause. Example: *acne*
- **Nodule** is solid, elevated, and palpable measuring less than 0.5 cm in diameter. Example: *fatty lipoma*

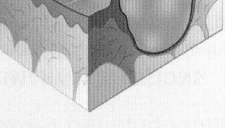

Solid

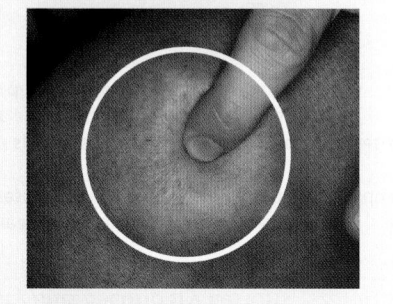

Nodule.

Benign fatty tumor (lipoma).

- **Tumor** is solid, elevated, and palpable measuring greater than 0.5 cm; may vary in shape and size.
- **Wheal** is defined by raised swelling, red bumps, or welts, and itchy skin. Wheals are red in color and are usually caused by an allergic reaction. Example: *hives*

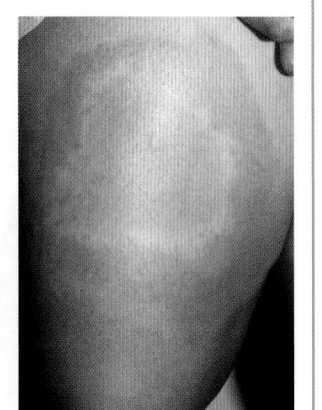

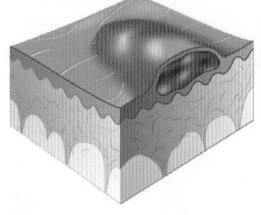

Wheal.

Hive.

- **Telangiectasia** are small, dilated blood vessels in the surface of the skin. Example: *rosacea*

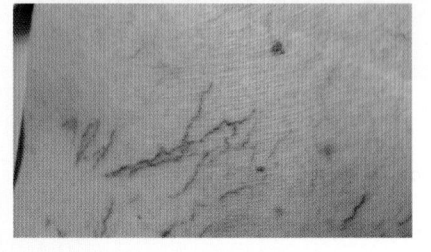

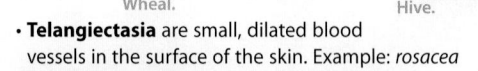

Telangiectasia.

BOX 8-4 **Defining Primary and Secondary Lesions**—cont'd

- **Cyst** is elevated, encapsulated, and filled with fluid measuring 1 cm or larger. Example: *sebaceous cyst*

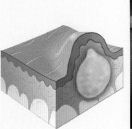

Sebaceous cyst.

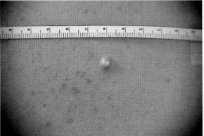

Keratogenous cyst.

SECONDARY SKIN LESIONS

Secondary skin lesions are progressive changes in primary lesions or trauma or injury to the primary lesion.
- **Scale** is a dry build-up of dead skin cells that usually flakes off the surface of the skin, such as in *psoriasis*.

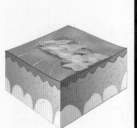

Scales.

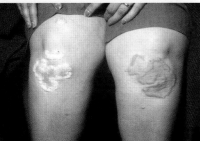

Psoriasis.

- **Crust** is a dried collection of blood, serum, or pus; part of the normal healing process, such as in *dried herpes simplex*.

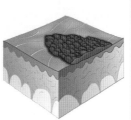

Crust.

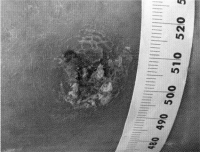

Dried herpes simplex.

- **Excoriation** is a hollow, crusted area with loss of the epidermis and an exposed dermis; may be caused by scratching the area, as in *chronic incontinence*.

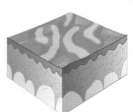

Excoriation.

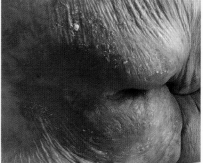

Buttock excoriation.

Continued

BOX 8-4 **Defining Primary and Secondary Lesions—cont'd**

- **Erosion** is a depressed area that is moist and shiny. There is a loss of superficial epidermis, such as in *candidiasis erosion*.

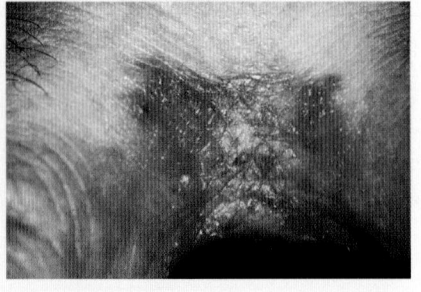

Erosion.

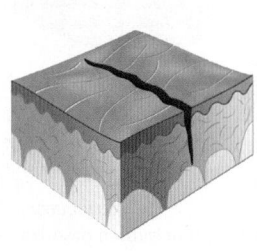

Candidiasis erosion.

- An **ulcer** is concave, exudative, and variable in size. Ulcers erode different layers of the skin, such as in a pressure ulcer. (See Box 8-5, p. 132.)

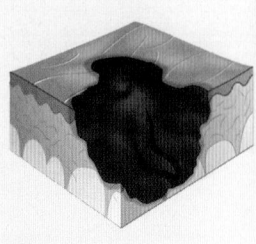

Ulcer.

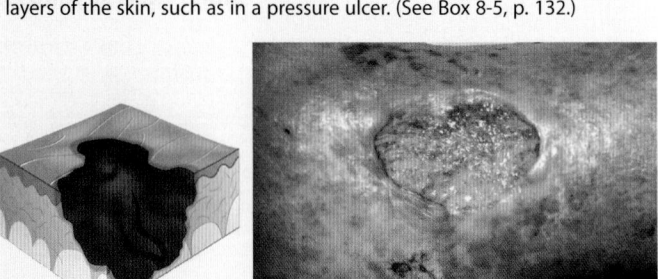

Stasis ulcer.

- A **fissure** is a linear break in the skin that involves the epidermal and dermal layers. They create small, deep, red fissures in the skin that is caused by a fungus.

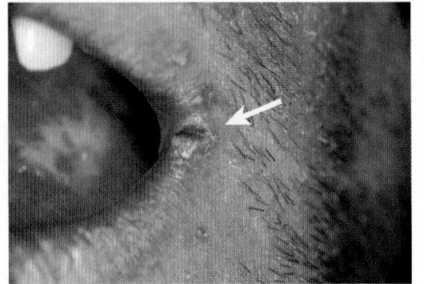

Fissure.

Cheilitis.

- A **scar** is discolored fibrous tissue that appears over healed surgical incisions and wounds. Scars can be red, blue, white, and silver in color.

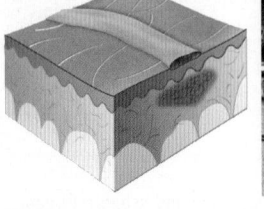

Scar.

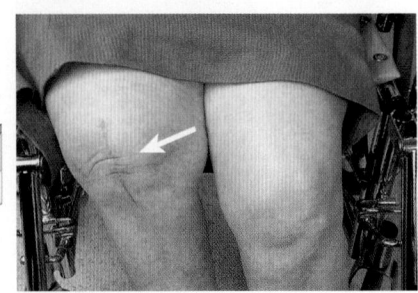

Surgical site.

BOX 8-4 **Defining Primary and Secondary Lesions—cont'd**

- A **keloid** is created by excessive collagen production extending beyond the original boundaries of a wound or incision. It is thick and raised.

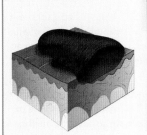

Keloid.

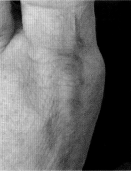

Keloids.

MOLES

A mole, which is a proliferation of melanocytes, is also called a nevus. Nevi is plural for nevus. Color is usually evenly pigmented in shades of brown with smooth borders. They measure less than 6 mm, and hair can grow out of them. Individuals average between 10 and 40 nevi.

- Atypical moles are called dysplastic nevi or **Clark's nevi**. They are larger with irregular, poorly defined borders. Color varies between shades of brown, tan, and pink. They have a greater potential for developing into melanoma.
- **Congenital nevi** are present at birth. They vary in size and can be greater than 10 cm. Color is usually tan, brown, red, or shades of black.

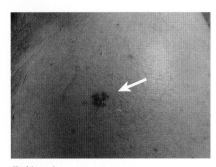

Clark's nevi.

PREPARATION FOR ASSESSMENT

Skin should be considered high priority in patient assessment because this organ can reveal significant information about the patient's health status. The skin assessment should be continuous throughout the entire assessment, and the two techniques, inspection and palpation, can be performed simultaneously. Always compare and contrast both sides of the body for symmetry, and assess starting with the head and ending with the feet.

■ **TIP** Lighting is critical during skin assessment. Fluorescent or artificial light may mask color and the presence of jaundice. It is best to assess skin in natural lighting, if available.

Preliminary Steps

1. Maintain privacy throughout the assessment.
2. Drape parts of the body for minimal exposure of the area you are examining.
3. Explain all steps of the assessment to the patient and ask permission to assess private areas.
4. Keep room warm and comfortable for the patient.
5. Perform hand hygiene.

SENC Safety Alert Intertriginous areas (under folds of skin) must be inspected; these areas trap moisture and can easily become infected. Intertriginous areas include:

- under the breasts
- under the stomach folds of an obese individuals (Fig. 8-3)
- groin areas
- under the arms

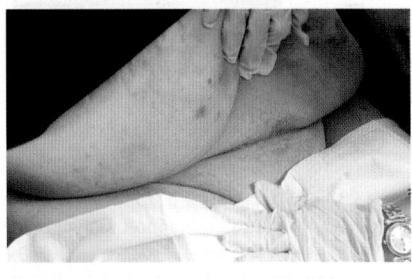

Fig. 8-3. Assessing intertriginous skin folds.

Equipment Needed

Personal protective equipment (gloves, gown, eye protection)
Paper tape measure
Penlight
Magnifying glass
Sterile cotton-tipped applicator

Sequence of Assessment

1. Inspection
2. Palpation

CULTURAL CONSIDERATIONS The U.S. Census Bureau reported in 2013 that Asians and Hispanics are the fastest growing ethnic groups, followed by Native Hawaiians, Pacific Islanders, American Indians, Alaska Natives, and African Americans. A large number of people in these ethnic groups have darkly pigmented skin and assessment may be challenging. Dark-skinned people typically have lighter tones of skin on their lips, nailbeds, and palms. Assess the conjunctiva, palm of the hand, and mucous membranes for color changes (Fig. 8-4).

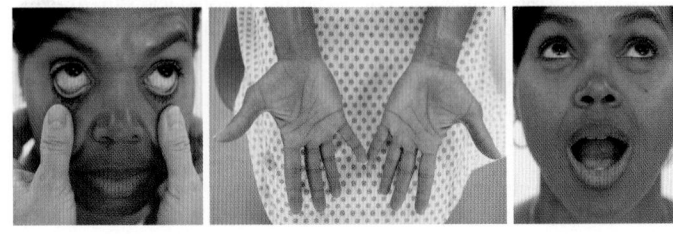

Fig. 8-4. Assessing dark-skinned individuals for color changes: conjunctiva, palms of hands, and oral mucosa.

TECHNIQUE 8-1: **Inspecting and Palpating the Skin**

Purpose: To identify changes in skin, including rashes, lesions, masses, and abnormal moles

SENC **Safety Alert** Always wear gloves if skin has an open area to protect yourself from bacteria or germs.

ASSESSMENT STEPS

1. Inspect the patient's hygiene, including odors of the body or breath.

2. Inspect the patient's color.

   a. Assess for cyanosis in the lips, oral mucosa, tongue, and extremities.

   b. Assess for pallor of skin in the lips, fingernails, and mucus membranes.

   c. Assess for jaundice of skin in the lips, sclera of the eyes, and across the rest of the body.

3. Palpate for temperature, comparing side to side using the dorsal surface of your hand (Fig. 8-5).

4. Palpate skin thickness. Remember that skin thickness varies. The thinnest skin is found on the eyelids, and the thickest areas of skin are found on the soles of the feet, palms of the hands, and elbows. Assess the hands and feet for calluses caused by pressure areas and rubbing (Fig. 8-6).

5. Palpate skin turgor. The best location to assess skin turgor is the clavicle area, but may also be done on the lower arm or abdomen. Pinch the skin between two fingers and let go. In a well-hydrated person, the skin returns to the flat position immediately. In the dehydrated person and someone who has lost a large amount of weight, the skin remains tented and slowly returns to the flat position (Fig. 8-7).

6. Palpate skin moisture.

   ▥ **TIP** Hyperhidrosis is excessive sweating of the body or hands, palms, armpits, feet, or face, due to an increased number of sweat glands. Excessive moisture or dryness of the skin may be indicative of an endocrine disorder.

7. Assess nevi, rashes, lesions, scars, and masses, making sure to identify location, distribution, pattern and configuration, color, and size, making sure to use a ruler to measure in centimeters (Table 8-1 and Table 8-2).

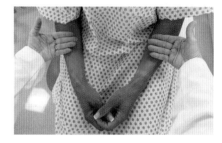

Fig. 8-5. Assessing skin temperature.

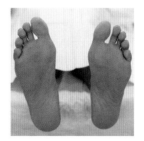

Fig. 8-6. Assessing calluses on feet.

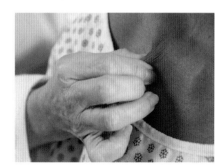

Fig. 8-7. Assessing skin turgor at clavicle.

TABLE 8-1 Distribution of Lesions

Area	Description	Area	Description
Diffuse/Generalized 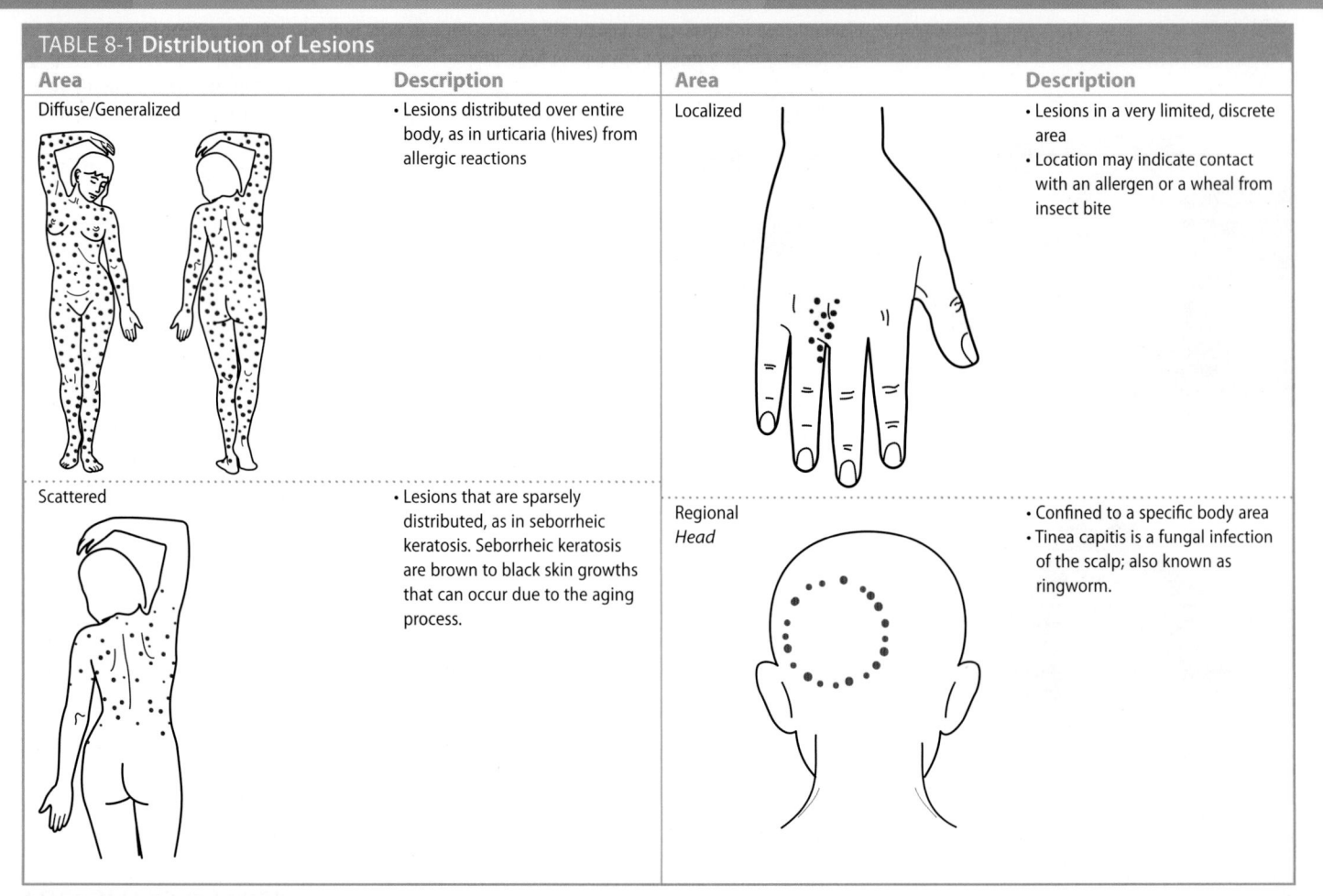	• Lesions distributed over entire body, as in urticaria (hives) from allergic reactions	Localized	• Lesions in a very limited, discrete area • Location may indicate contact with an allergen or a wheal from insect bite
Scattered	• Lesions that are sparsely distributed, as in seborrheic keratosis. Seborrheic keratosis are brown to black skin growths that can occur due to the aging process.	Regional *Head*	• Confined to a specific body area • Tinea capitis is a fungal infection of the scalp; also known as ringworm.

TABLE 8-1 **Distribution of Lesions—cont'd**

Area	Description	Area	Description
Regional *Torso* 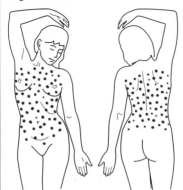	• Pityriasis rosea is a rash that starts usually on the torso as a large oval spot known as a herald patch or mother patch. Smaller patches will develop on the torso. Cause of the rash is still unknown.	Dermatome 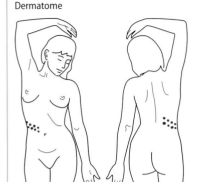	• Herpes zoster (shingles) is caused by the chicken pox virus; red, painful, vesicular rash occurring on a dermatone.
Extensor Surfaces 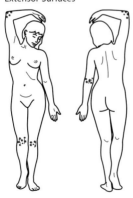	• Psoriasis is an autoimmune disease; red, rough scaly patches develop commonly on the extensor surfaces of the skin.	Hairy Areas 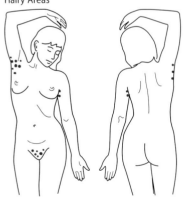	• Pediculosis, also known as body lice; infestation usually occurs in the hairy parts of the body causing itchiness and scratching in those areas.

Continued

TABLE 8-1 **Distribution of Lesions—cont'd**

Area	Description	Area	Description
Intertriginous Areas (Folds of Skin) 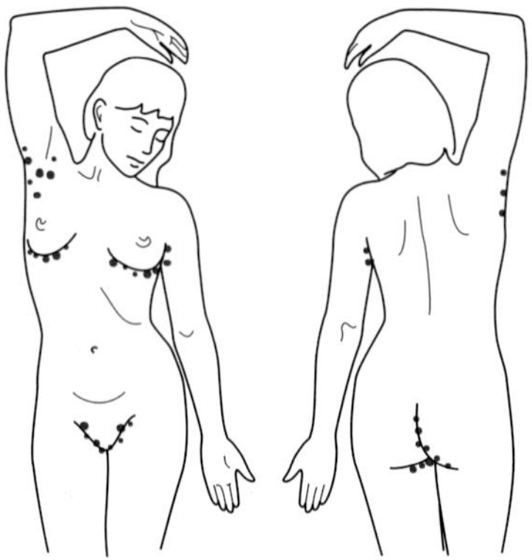 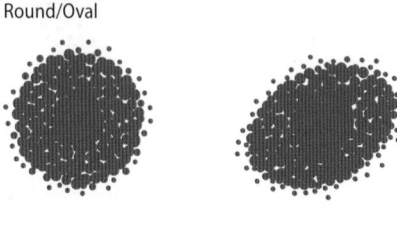	• Contact dermatitis, diaper rash, intertrigo (erythema and scaling of body folds)	Sun-Exposed Areas 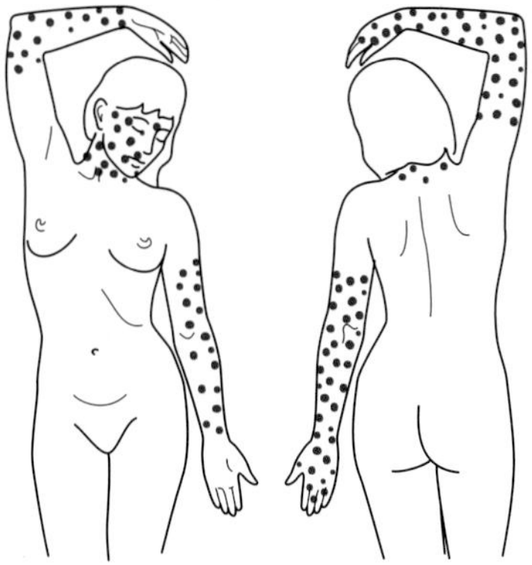 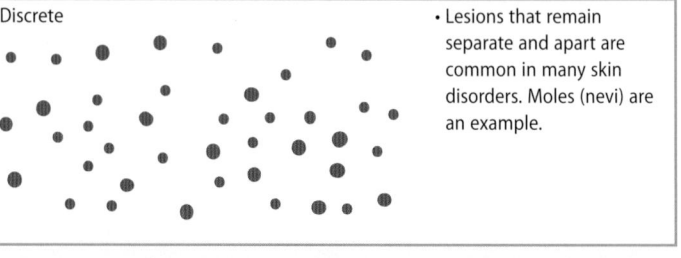	• Actinic keratosis (precancerous scaly skin lesion) and skin cancers (basal cell, squamous cell, and melanoma)

TABLE 8-2 **Pattern and Configuration of Lesions**

Pattern	Description	Pattern	Description
Round/Oval	• Coin or oval shaped, as in eczema. Eczema is an inflamed, irritated, itchy rash.	Discrete	• Lesions that remain separate and apart are common in many skin disorders. Moles (nevi) are an example.

TABLE 8-2 Pattern and Configuration of Lesions—cont'd

Pattern	Description	Pattern	Description
Grouped 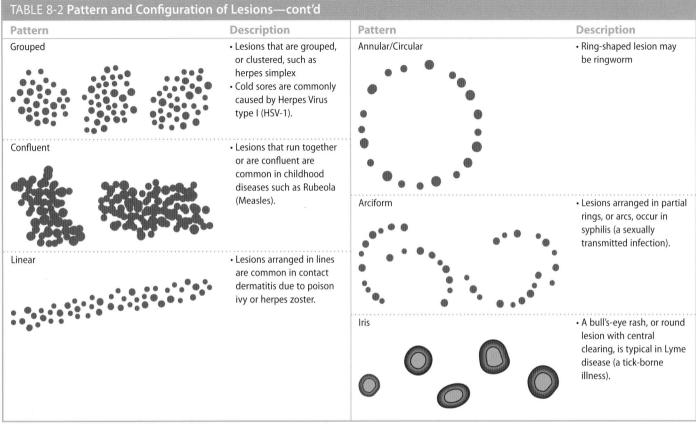	• Lesions that are grouped, or clustered, such as herpes simplex • Cold sores are commonly caused by Herpes Virus type I (HSV-1).	Annular/Circular	• Ring-shaped lesion may be ringworm
Confluent	• Lesions that run together or are confluent are common in childhood diseases such as Rubeola (Measles).	Arciform	• Lesions arranged in partial rings, or arcs, occur in syphilis (a sexually transmitted infection).
Linear	• Lesions arranged in lines are common in contact dermatitis due to poison ivy or herpes zoster.	Iris	• A bull's-eye rash, or round lesion with central clearing, is typical in Lyme disease (a tick-borne illness).

Continued

TABLE 8-2 Pattern and Configuration of Lesions—cont'd

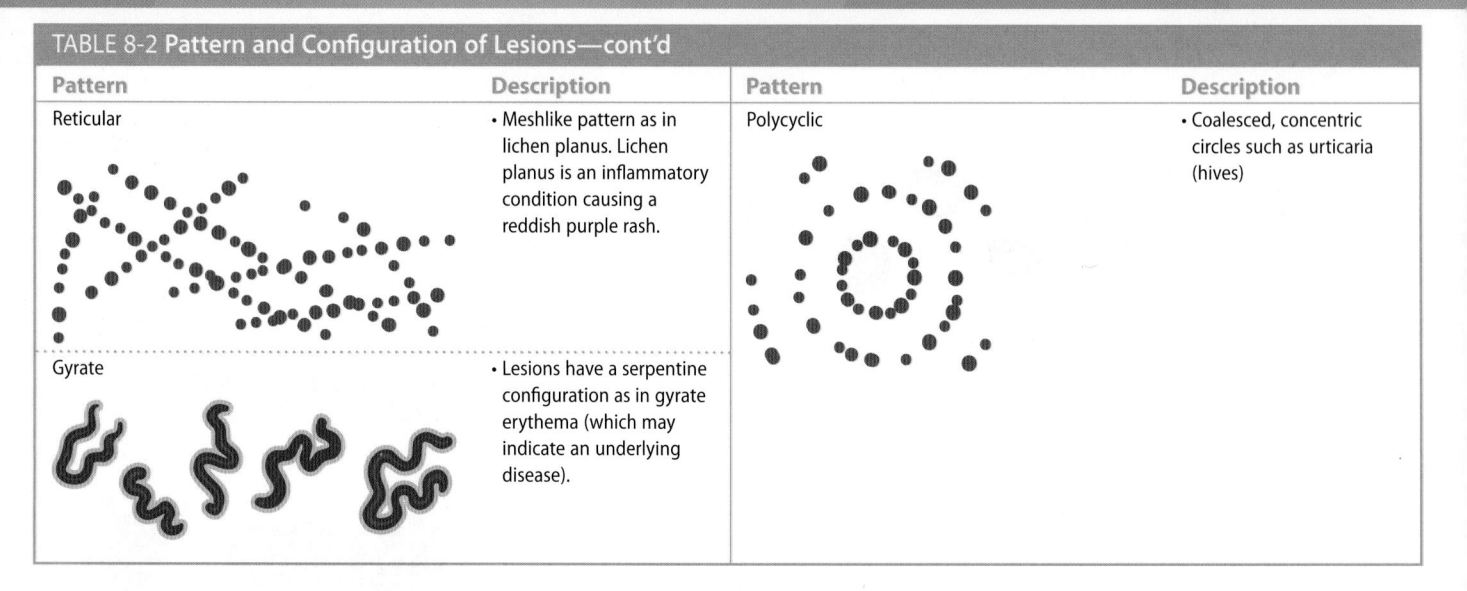

Pattern	Description	Pattern	Description
Reticular	• Meshlike pattern as in lichen planus. Lichen planus is an inflammatory condition causing a reddish purple rash.	Polycyclic	• Coalesced, concentric circles such as urticaria (hives)
Gyrate	• Lesions have a serpentine configuration as in gyrate erythema (which may indicate an underlying disease).		

☐ A magnifying glass may be necessary to enlarge and thoroughly assess a skin lesion. The Carter Skin Lesion Assessment Tree is an algorithm that can help you to assess types of primary and secondary lesions (Figs. 8-8, 8-9).

■ Assess all moles using the ABCDE mnemonic.

☐ **A** is for asymmetry—one half is unlike the other half.

☐ **B** is for border—an irregular, scalloped or poorly defined border.

☐ **C** is for color—is varied from one area to another; has shades of tan, brown or black, or is sometimes white, red, or blue.

☐ **D** is for diameter—usually greater than 6 mm (the size of a pencil eraser) but they can be smaller.

☐ **E** is for evolving—a mole or skin lesion that looks different from the rest or is changing in size, shape, or color. (American Academy of Dermatology, 2015b)

8. Assess tattoos and body piercings for signs of inflammation, infection or allergic reaction.

9. Document your findings.

The Carter Skin Lesion Assessment tree (primary lesion branch)

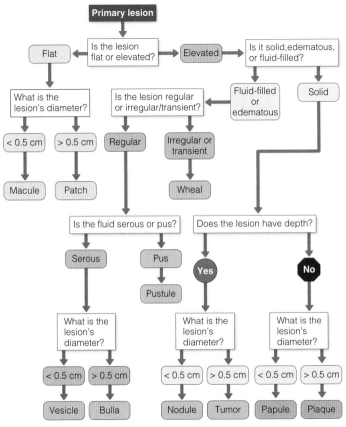

Fig. 8-8. Carter Skin Lesion Assessment tree for primary lesions. (Used with permission from Carter, K. F., Dufour, L. T., Ballard, C. N. Identifying Primary Skin Lesions, *Nursing* 2003: 33(12): 68-69.)

The Carter Skin Lesion Assessment tree (secondary lesion branch)

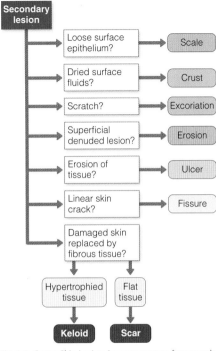

Fig. 8-9. Carter Skin Lesion Assessment tree for secondary lesions. (Used with permission from Carter, K. F., Dufour, L. T., Ballard, C. N. Identifying Secondary Skin Lesions, *Nursing* 2004: 34(1): 68.)

NORMAL FINDINGS
- Good hygiene, no odors
- Uniform color
- Skin warm, moist
- Skin turgor is less than 3 seconds
- No abnormal lesions (see Abnormal Findings)
- Nevi are uniform brown color, regular borders, less than 0.6 mm (Fig. 8-10).
- Tattoos and body piercings show no signs of redness, swelling, or inflammation.

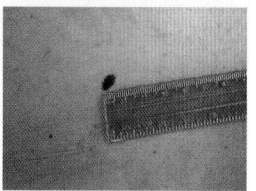

Fig. 8-10. Normal nevi (moles).

   TIP Cherry angioma is a benign, cherry red papule, of compressed blood vessels; commonly seen in individuals older than 30 years of age (Fig. 8-11).

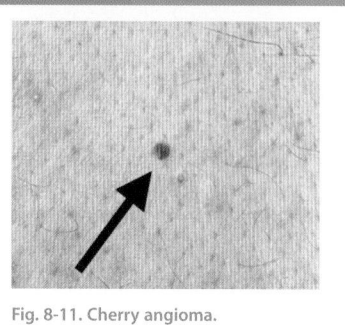

Fig. 8-11. Cherry angioma.

ABNORMAL FINDINGS
- Skin turgor is greater than 3 seconds, may be related to fluid loss.
- **Vascular Lesions**
  - ☐ **Ecchymosis** is a bruise caused by bleeding under the skin or mucous membranes; occurs as a result of local trauma.
  - ☐ **Hematoma** is an elevated collection of clotted blood within the tissue caused by a break in a blood vessel.
  - ☐ **Telangiectasia** is caused by vascular dilatation of a small group of blood vessels; occurs anywhere on the body but most often on the face and legs.
  - ☐ **Petechiae** are tiny, pinpoint hemorrhages caused by superficial bleeding from the capillaries of the skin; measure less than 3 mm; may be related to platelet deficiencies.
  - ☐ **Purpura** is a hemorrhagic red or purple spot or rash that is flat and does not blanch; measures 3 to 10 mm; may be associated with platelet disorders.
- **Skin Cancer Lesions**
  - ☐ **Basal cell carcinoma** presents as a pearl white, dome-shaped papule with overlying random telangiectasia; enlarges slowly and may ulcerate in the center; most common form of cutaneous malignancy (Fig. 8-12A).
  - ☐ **Squamous cell carcinoma** is a malignant cutaneous malignancy arising from keratinocytes of the skin or mucosal surfaces; thick, rough, scaly with a crusted surface and irregular borders; second most common type of skin cancer (Fig. 8-12B).
  - ☐ **Malignant melanoma** is a malignancy of the melanocytes arising in the skin; develops from a pre-existing lesion usually with an increase in size, change in color or appearance of a nevus; vary considerably in appearance; curable with early detection (Fig. 8-12C).

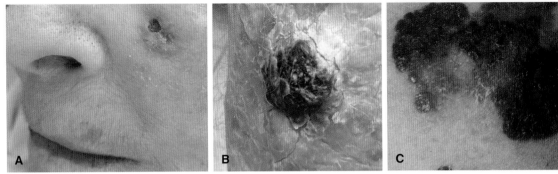

Fig. 8-12. Skin cancers. (A) Basal cell carcinoma. (B) Squamous cell carcinoma. (C) Malignant melanoma.

TECHNIQUE 8-2: Inspecting and Palpating the Hair and Scalp

Purpose: To assess for changes or abnormalities in the hair and scalp
Equipment: Gloves (optional)
Inspection of hair should include the body, hair, scalp, axillae, and pubic areas at 1 inch intervals

SENC Safety Alert Small white eggs found on the hairs of the scalp, axillae, beard or pubic area may indicate hair lice (singular called *louse*) (*Pediculus humanus*), parasitic insects. Head lice spread by direct contact with another infected person or through shared items such as a comb, hat or linens; lice crawl from one head to another or when a person comes in contact with an infected item. Lice cannot fly or jump. The key symptoms are scratching or itching at the infected site. The female lice lay eggs (nits) very close to the scalp area which can be confused with dandruff. Assess head lice using a fine-tooth comb, a magnifying glass, and a strong light. If nits or lice are found, use clear tape to pick them up (Rush, 2008). Topical treatment will be required.

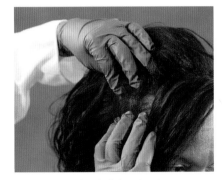

Fig. 8-13. Inspecting the hair and scalp.

ASSESSMENT STEPS
1. Put on gloves.
2. Assess general condition of the hair, including amount, distribution, and cleanliness.
3. Assess the condition of the scalp; inspect scalp skin and color, and inspect for lesions (Fig. 8-13).
4. Assess hair color.
5. Assess hair texture (thick, brittle, curly).

6. Palpate the scalp.

7. Discard gloves.

8. Document your findings.

NORMAL FINDINGS

- Hair clean, curly, or straight texture; uniform thickness and distribution
- Color brown, black, blonde, red, white, or gray
- Scalp clean and intact, no lesions
- Scalp nontender

ABNORMAL FINDINGS

- Brittle or thin hair
- Lesions on scalp; scalp red and tender
- **Alopecia**, defined as hair loss, may be due to nutritional deficiencies, medications, illness, endocrine disorders, radiation, or the physiological changes of aging.
- **Alopecia areata** of the scalp, or spot baldness, is a loss of hair in patches involving the scalp or beard; thought to be related to an autoimmune disorder.
- **Folliculitis** is inflammation of a hair follicle developing on the face, arms, legs, or buttocks; white pustules appear around the hair follicle; may be related to *Staphylococcus aureus* infection.
- **Hirsutism** is the excessive growth of thick, dark hair in women where normally the hair does not grow, including areas such as the face, chest, abdomen, arms, and legs; usually caused by abnormality of androgen production, metabolism, medications, or hormonal therapies.
- **Seborrhea dermatitis**, also called *cradle cap* in infants, is a chronic, greasy scale that accumulates and thickens on the scalp with or without redness; may extend to the forehead, eyebrows, and face.
- **Tinea capitis**, also called *scalp ringworm*, is a fungal infection of the scalp causing round, patchy hair loss, pustules, and scale on the skin.
- **Tinea versicolor**, also called *pityriasis versicolor*, is a fungal infection of the skin causing discolored patches or spots occurring anywhere on the body.

SENC Patient-Centered Care Male pattern baldness (androgenic alopecia) is more common than female pattern baldness; may start with a symmetrical receding hairline or vertex hair thinning. This may be a sensitive area of discussion.

TECHNIQUE 8-3: **Inspecting and Palpating the Fingernails and Toenails**

Purpose: To assess for healthy nails or presence of vitamin deficiency, malnutrition, disease, or infection.

ASSESSMENT STEPS

1. Inspect general condition of the nails, including cleanliness, thinness, and thickness (Fig. 8-14).

2. Inspect color and markings.

3. Inspect adherence to nailbed.

4. Inspect shape and contour.

5. Palpate the nailbeds.

6. Perform the capillary refill test. (See Chapter 15, page 274.)

7. Document your findings.

NORMAL FINDINGS

- Nails are smooth, short, of uniform thickness, and well groomed.
- Nail base angle is 160 degrees.
- Nails firmly adhere to the nailbed.
- Nailbeds are pink.
- Nails are nontender to palpation.
- Capillary refill is less than 3 seconds.
- No redness, exudates, or signs of infection or inflammation are found.
- Dark-skin individuals may have pigmented bands in their nails.
- Aging nails have longitudinal ridging of the nail (Fig. 8-15).
- White spots in the nail may result from forms of mild trauma (Fig. 8-16).

ABNORMAL FINDINGS

- Changes in color, shape, texture, or thickness indicate an abnormal finding.

    SENC Safety Alert Changes in the nail may also indicate a systemic disorder.

- **Beau's line** is a white, horizontal groove across the nailbed, usually caused by disease, toxic reaction, or trauma.
- **Onychomycosis** is thickening, yellow discoloration, and scaling of the nailbed due to a fungal infection; more common in diabetics and older individuals.
- **Paronychia** is a skin infection around the nail causing erythema, swelling, and tenderness at the nail fold.
- **Pitting** of nails is a sign of psoriasis; affects both fingernails and toenails; appears as indentations in different sizes, shapes, and depths; nails can disintegrate easily.
- **Splinter hemorrhages** appear as red streaks in the nails, caused by bleeding from capillaries under the nails.
- **Spoon nails** are flat or concave; outer edges flare out; dips or waves are visible on the surface of the nail; may be hereditary, related to a nutritional or systemic disease.

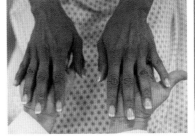

Fig. 8-14. Inspecting fingernails and toenails.

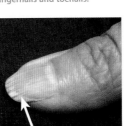

Fig. 8-15. Longitudinal ridging.

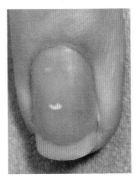

Fig. 8-16. White spots.

ADVANCED ASSESSMENTS

Wounds are assessed for healing or signs of infection. A wound is an alteration in the integrity of the skin. There are different types of wounds (Table 8-3).

TABLE 8-3 **Types of Wounds**

Type	Description
Abrasion	A scrape of superficial layers of the skin; usually unintentional but may be performed intentionally for cosmetic purposes to smooth skin surfaces
Abscess	A localized collection of pus resulting from invasion from a pyogenic bacterium or other pathogen; must be opened and drained to heal
Contusion	A closed wound caused by blunt trauma; may be referred to as a bruise or ecchymotic area
Crushing	A wound caused by force leading to compression or disruption of tissues; often associated with fracture; usually there is minimal or no break in the skin
Incision	An open, intentional wound cause by a sharp instrument
Laceration	The skin or mucous membranes are torn open, resulting in a wound with jagged margins
Penetrating	An open wound in which the agent causing the wound lodges in body tissue
Puncture	An open wound caused by a sharp object; often there is collapse of tissue around the entry point, making this wound prone to infection
Tunnel	A wound with an entrance and exit site

Source: Wilkinson, J. et al. (2015). *Fundamentals of nursing* (3rd ed., p. 902). Philadelphia, PA: F.A. Davis.

TECHNIQUE 8-4: **Assessing Wounds**

Purpose: To monitor for signs and symptoms of healing, inflammation, or infection
Equipment: Personal protective equipment, wound dressing supplies, paper tape measure, cotton-tipped applicator

> **SENC Safety Alert** Maintain standard precautions during all wound assessments; wear protective eyewear, gloves, or gowns as necessary to protect yourself.

ASSESSMENT STEPS
1. Collect wound dressing supplies.
2. Wash hands.
3. Check identification of patient and explain the technique to the patient.
4. Prepare and organize the area for assessing the wound and changing the wound dressing.
5. Identify the wound location and position patient.
6. Put on gloves, protective glasses, or gowns as needed.
7. Remove wound dressing using aseptic technique.
8. Assess wound for signs of inflammation, drainage, and healing.

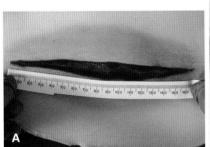
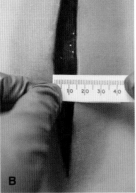
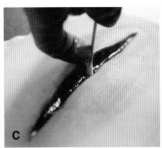
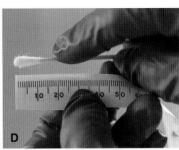

Fig. 8-17. Measuring (A) length, (B) width, (C) depth of a wound. (D) Measurement of depth.

9. Assess the approximation of the edges (wound edges come together).
10. **Measure the length:** Measure the longest axis of the wound with a tape measure; document in centimeters (Fig. 8-17A).
11. **Measure the width:** Measure the widest perpendicular axis of the wound with a tape measure; document in centimeters (Fig. 8-17B).
12. **Measure the depth:** Using a sterile cotton-tipped applicator, gently insert the applicator into the deepest area. Measure by placing your fingers on the applicator next to the wound edge. Position the applicator next to a tape measure (Fig. 8-17C). Measure in centimeters.
13. Perform wound care per healthcare provider's orders.
14. Discard dressing and supplies.
15. Remove personal protective equipment.
16. Reposition patient.
17. Wash hands.
18. Document your findings.

NORMAL FINDINGS
■ No signs of erythema, drainage, or inflammation
■ Wound size decreasing
■ Signs of healing.

ABNORMAL FINDINGS
- Prolonged healing
- Increased redness and inflammation
- Colored drainage (i.e., yellow or green)
- Wound dehiscence
  □ Occurs when the surgical incision opens up or fails to remain closed; usually a complication following surgery (Fig. 8-18A)
- Wound evisceration
  □ Protrusion of abdominal organs, usually the intestines, through a surgical incision site (Fig. 8-18B)

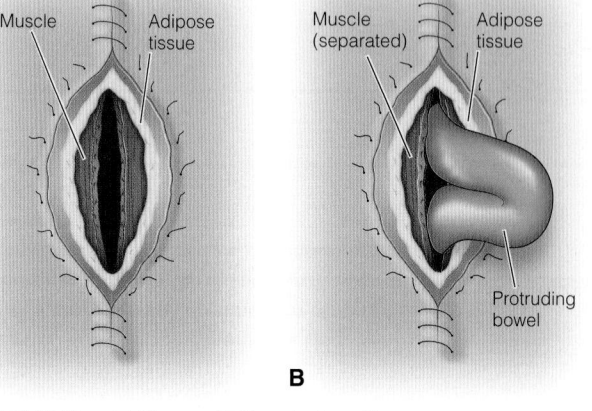

Fig. 8-18. (A) Wound dehiscence. (B) Wound evisceration.

TECHNIQUE 8-5: **Assessing Pressure Ulcers**

Purpose: To assess for signs of healing or inflammation (Box 8-5, Table 8-4)
Equipment: Personal protective equipment, wound dressing supplies, paper tape measure, cotton-tipped applicator

SENC Safety Alert Stage I pressure wound may be more difficult to see in African Americans and darker-skinned people. If you suspect the area is a pressure wound, assess skin temperature using the dorsal surface of your hand or a change in skin texture. Skin temperature will have increased warmth and skin texture may feel softer/harder or boggy. Dark-skinned patients rarely have a blanch response; irritation may cause hyperpigmentation (increased pigmentation) or hypopigmentation (reduced pigmentation), with no redness being visible (Sommers, 2011).

ASSESSMENT STEPS
1. Collect wound dressing supplies.
2. Check identification of patient and explain the technique to the patient.
3. Prepare and organize the area for change of dressing.
4. Identify the pressure wound location and position patient.

5. Put on gloves, protective glasses, or gowns as needed.

6. Remove wound dressing using aseptic technique.

7. Measure the length: Measure the longest axis using the clock face with a tape measure. Document in centimeters.

8. Measure the width: Measure perpendicular to the length using the widest perpendicular axis with a tape measure. Document in centimeters.

9. Measure the depth: Using a sterile, cotton-tipped applicator, gently insert the applicator into the deepest area. Measure by placing your gloved fingers on the applicator at the wound margins; place it against a ruler to measure.

10. Assess for undermining (a pocket under the edges of a wound) at each hour of the clock. Measure the deepest part of the undermining edge using a sterile, cotton-tipped applicator and measuring against a ruler (Fig. 8-19). Document the location of undermining using the numbers on a clock such as "undermining of 1.0 cm assessed from 9 to 11 o'clock."

   ■ TIP Linear measurement of a wound is known as the *clock method*. Use the body as the face of an imaginary clock. The head is always at 12 o'clock and the feet are always at 6 o'clock. On the feet, the heels are always at 12 o'clock and the toes are at 6 o'clock. Document the longest length using the face of the clock over the wound bed, then measure the greatest width (Morgan, 2012).

11. Assess for tunneling (a narrow passageway from the wound bed into adjacent tissues). Document the location of tunneling using the numbers on a clock. Assess the length of the tunneling using a cotton-tip applicator at the wound edge, similar to assessing the depth of a wound (Fig. 8-20).

12. Assess the wound perimeter.

13. Assess for redness and signs of inflammation.

14. Assess for exudate (drainage):
    ☐ Serous is fluid that is clear to straw colored.
    ☐ Serosanguineous is light red or pink in color.
    ☐ Sanguineous is red to dark red in color.
    ☐ Purulent is yellow or green in color, indicating infection.

15. Assess for presence of *slough*, which is yellow, moist, and stringy, indicating hydrated necrotic tissue (Fig. 8-21).

16. Assess for tenderness.

17. Assess for presence of *eschar*, which is dehydrated necrotic tissue causing a black discoloration. Eschar looks dry, leathery, and indurated (hard) (Fig. 8-22).

18. Perform wound care per healthcare provider's orders.

19. Discard dressing and supplies.

20. Remove and discard personal protective equipment.

21. Reposition patient.

22. Wash hands.

23. Document your findings.

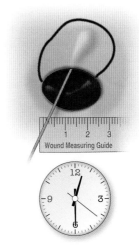

Fig. 8-19. Measuring undermining.

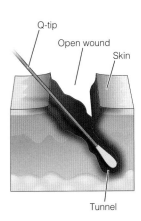

Fig. 8-20. Measuring tunneling.

■ **TIP** The Pressure Ulcer Scale for Healing (PUSH Tool) is a reliable tool to monitor the change in pressure ulcer status over time (Fig. 8-23, p. 136).

NORMAL FINDINGS

■ Pressure ulcer shows signs of healing.
■ Pressure ulcer has no signs of inflammation.
■ Wound base has pink, granulation, or epithelial tissue.
■ Weekly measurements are decreasing in size.

ABNORMAL FINDINGS

■ Presence of slough or eschar
■ Erythema
■ Inflammation
■ Increased drainage
■ Foul odor
■ Maceration around the perimeter

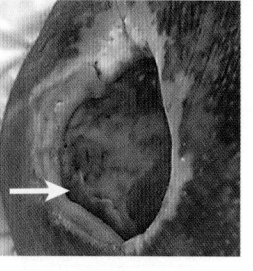
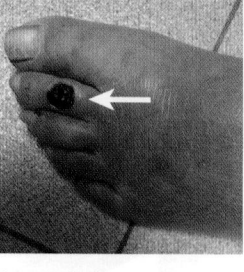

Fig. 8-21. Pressure wound slough.

Fig. 8-22. Eschar.

SENC Safety Alert Be aware that wound maceration is caused by excessive moisture from pooled drainage or a moist dressing that is inappropriately applied, left on too long, or overlaps healthy skin. The skin may appear pale or unhealthy or "pruned," which may peel or flake (Wilkinson et al., 2015). Teach patients, families, or healthcare providers about wound care and how to prevent maceration.

■ **TIP** The National Pressure Ulcer Advisory Panel has recently published "Prevention and Treatment of Pressure Ulcers: Quick Reference Guide" that can be found at http://www.npuap.org/wp-content/uploads/2014/08/Updated-10-16-14-Quick-Reference-Guide-DIGITAL-NPUAP-EPUAP-PPPIA-16Oct2014.pdf

---

BOX 8-5 **Pressure Ulcers**

Pressure ulcers are a type of lesion caused by unrelieved pressure; the most common sites for pressure ulcers are over bony prominences. They develop when the skin fails. The two most common causes of pressure ulcers are friction and shearing forces. Individuals most at risk for developing pressure ulcers include those who

• Are immobile or who have decreased mobility
• Have poor nutrition
• Are confined to a bed or wheelchair
There is also a risk of developing pressure ulcers secondary to decreased blood circulation. (See Table 8-4.)

BOX 8-5 **Pressure Ulcers—cont'd**

STAGING CRITERIA

There are four stages of pressure ulcers:

- **Stage 1**: Nonblanchable erythema of intact skin. Pain, increased warmth of skin, and edema may be present.

  TIP If the skin is blanchable (turns pale) when you press your finger on the erythema, this is not a pressure ulcer.

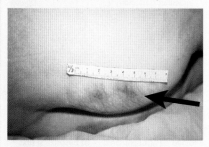

- **Stage 2:** Partial thickness tissue loss involving both epidermis and dermis. Ulcer is still superficial and appears as a blister, abrasion, or very shallow crater.

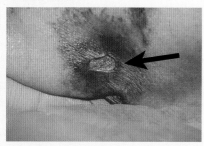

- **Stage 3**: Full thickness tissue loss involving subcutaneous tissue. Ulcer may extend to but not through fascia. A deep crater that may undermine or tunnel adjacent tissues.

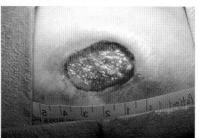

- **Stage 4:** Full thickness tissue loss with extensive involvement of muscle or bone, or supporting structures. This deep ulcer may involve undermining and sinus tracts of adjacent tissues. When eschar or slough covers an ulcer completely, the wound bed is obscured by eschar or slough and cannot be assessed; the ulcer is then documented as **unstageable**. Until the slough and eschar are removed, the wound will not heal. The slough and eschar will have to be removed for healing to take place and for the true depth of the wound to be measured.

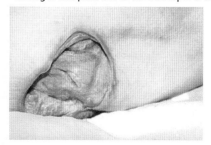

TABLE 8-4 The Braden Scale for Predicting Pressure Sore Risk

Note: Bed and chairbound individuals or those with impaired ability to reposition should be assessed upon admission for their risk of developing pressure ulcers. Patients with established pressure ulcers should be reassessed periodically.

Sensory Perception Ability to respond meaningfully to pressure-related discomfort	**1. Completely Limited** Unresponsive (does not moan, flinch, or grasp) to painful stimuli, due to diminished level of consciousness or sedation, *OR* Limited ability to feel pain over most of body surface.	**2. Very Limited** Responds only to painful stimuli. Cannot communicate discomfort except by moaning or restlessness. *OR* Has sensory impairment which limits the ability to feel pain or discomfort over 1/2 of the body.	**3. Slightly Limited** Responds to verbal commands but cannot always communicate discomfort or need to be turned, *OR* Has some sensory impairment, which limits ability to feel pain or discomfort in one or two extremities.	**4. No Impairment** Responds to verbal commands. Has no sensory deficit which would limit ability to feel or voice pain or discomfort.
Moisture Degree to which skin is exposed to moisture	**1. Constantly Moist** Skin is kept moist almost constantly by perspiration, urine, etc. Dampness is detected every time patient is moved or turned.	**2. Moist** Skin is often but not always moist. Linen must be changed at least once a shift.	**3. Occasionally Moist** Skin is occasionally moist, requiring an extra linen change approximately once a day.	**4. Rarely Moist** Skin is usually dry; linen requires changing only at routine intervals.
Activity Degree of physical activity	**1. Bedfast** Confined to bed.	**2. Chairfast** Ability to walk severely limited or nonexistent. Cannot bear own weight and/or must be assisted into chair or wheelchair.	**3. Walks Occasionally** Walks occasionally during day but for very short distances, with or without assistance. Spends majority or each shift in bed or chair.	**4. Walks Frequently** Walks outside the room at least twice a day and inside room at least once every 2 hours during waking hours.
Mobility Ability to change and control body position	**1. Completely Immobile** Does not make even slight changes in body or extremity position without assistance.	**2. Very Limited** Makes occasional slight changes in body or extremity position but unable to make frequent or significant changes independently.	**3. Slightly Limited** Makes frequent though slight changes in body or extremity position independently.	**4. No Limitations** Makes major and frequent changes in position without assistance.

TABLE 8-4 **The Braden Scale for Predicting Pressure Sore Risk—cont'd**

Nutrition	1. Very Poor	2. Probably Inadequate	3. Adequate	4. Excellent
Usual food intake pattern	Never eats a complete meal. Rarely eats more than one-third of any food offered. Eats two servings or less of protein (meat or dairy products) per day. Takes fluids poorly. Does not take a liquid dietary supplement, *OR* Is NPO and/or maintained on clear liquids or IV for more than 5 days.	Rarely eats a complete meal and generally eats only about one-half of any food offered. Protein intake includes only three servings of meat or dairy products per day. Occasionally will take a dietary supplement, *OR* Receives less than optimum amount of liquid diet or tube feeding.	Eats over half of most meals. Eats a total of four servings of protein (meat, dairy products) each day. Occasionally will refuse a meal, but will usually take a supplement if offered, *OR* Is on a tube feeding or TPN regimen, which probably meets most of nutritional needs.	Eats most of every meal. Never refuses a meal. Usually eats a total of four or more servings of meat and dairy products. Occasionally eats between meals. Does not require supplementation.
Friction and Shear	1. Problem	2. Potential Problem	3. No Apparent Problem	
	Requires moderate to maximum assistance in moving. Complete lifting without sliding against sheets is impossible. Frequently slides down in bed or chair, requiring frequent repositioning with maximum assistance. Spasticity, contractures, or agitation leads to almost constant friction.	Moves feebly or requires minimum assistance. During a move skin probably slides to some extent against sheets, chair, restraints, or other devices. Maintains relatively good position in chair or bed most of the time but occasionally slides down.	Moves in bed and in chair independently and has sufficient muscle strength to lift up completely during move. Maintains good position in bed or chair at all times.	
				TOTAL SCORE

Note: Patients with a total score of 16 or less are considered to be at risk of developing pressure ulcers. (15 or 16 = low risk; 13 or 14 = moderate risk; 12 or less = high risk)

NATIONAL
PRESSURE
ULCER
ADVISORY
PANEL

Pressure Ulcer Scale for Healing (PUSH)
PUSH Tool 3.0

Patient Name _____ Patient ID# _____

Ulcer Location _____ Date _____

Directions:

Observe and measure the pressure ulcer. Categorize the ulcer with respect to surface area, exudate, and type of wound tissue. Record a sub-score for each of these ulcer characteristics. Add the sub-scores to obtain the total score. A comparison of total scores measured over time provides an indication of the improvement or deterioration in pressure ulcer healing.

	0	1	2	3	4	5	Sub-score
LENGTH X WIDTH (in cm²)	0	< 0.3	0.3 – 0.6	0.7 – 1.0	1.1 – 2.0	2.1 – 3.0	
		6	**7**	**8**	**9**	**10**	
		3.1 – 4.0	4.1 – 8.0	8.1 – 12.0	12.1 – 24.0	> 24.0	
EXUDATE AMOUNT	0 None	1 Light	2 Moderate	3 Heavy			Sub-score
TISSUE TYPE	0 Closed	1 Epithelial Tissue	2 Granulation Tissue	3 Slough	4 Necrotic Tissue		Sub-score
						TOTAL SCORE	

Length x Width: Measure the greatest length (head to toe) and the greatest width (side to side) using a centimeter ruler. Multiply these two measurements (length x width) to obtain an estimate of surface area in square centimeters (cm²). Caveat: Do not guess! Always use a centimeter ruler and always use the same method each time the ulcer is measured.

Exudate Amount: Estimate the amount of exudate (drainage) present after removal of the dressing and before applying any topical agent to the ulcer. Estimate the exudate (drainage) as none, light, moderate, or heavy.

Tissue Type: This refers to the types of tissue that are present in the wound (ulcer) bed. Score as a "4" if there is any necrotic tissue present. Score as a "3" if there is any amount of slough present and necrotic tissue is absent. Score as a "2" if the wound is clean and contains granulation tissue. A superficial wound that is reepithelializing is scored as a "1". When the wound is closed, score as a "0".

4 – **Necrotic Tissue (Eschar):** black, brown, or tan tissue that adheres firmly to the wound bed or ulcer edges and may be either firmer or softer than surrounding skin.

3 – **Slough:** yellow or white tissue that adheres to the ulcer bed in strings or thick clumps, or is mucinous.

2 – **Granulation Tissue:** pink or beefy red tissue with a shiny, moist, granular appearance.

1 – **Epithelial Tissue:** for superficial ulcers, new pink or shiny tissue (skin) that grows in from the edges or as islands on the ulcer surface.

0 – **Closed/Resurfaced:** the wound is completely covered with epithelium (new skin).

PUSH Tool Version 3.0: 9/15/98
©National Pressure Ulcer Advisory Panel

www.npuap.org
11F

Fig. 8-23. PUSH Tool. (With permission from the National Pressure Ulcer Advisory Panel, 1998.)

Pressure Ulcer Healing Chart

To monitor trends in PUSH Scores over time
(Use a separate page for each pressure ulcer)

Patient Name _____ Patient ID# _____

Ulcer Location _____ Date _____

Directions:

Observe and measure pressure ulcers at regular intervals using the PUSH Tool.
Date and record PUSH Sub-scores and Total Scores on the Pressure Ulcer Healing Record below.

Pressure Ulcer Healing Record

Date					
Length x Width					
Exudate Amount					
Tissue Type					
PUSH Total Score					

Graph the PUSH Total Scores on the Pressure Ulcer Healing Graph below.

Pressure Ulcer Healing Graph

PUSH Total Score															
17															
16															
15															
14															
13															
12															
11															
10															
9															
8															
7															
6															
5															
4															
3															
2															
1															
Healed = 0															
Date															

NATIONAL PRESSURE ULCER ADVISORY PANEL

www.npuap.org
11F

PUSH Tool Version 3.0: 9/15/98
©National Pressure Ulcer Advisory Panel

Fig. 8-23, cont'd

PATIENT EDUCATION

The American Cancer Society recommends a yearly skin examination by a healthcare provider and encourages individuals to check their skin monthly after a bath or shower (Fig. 8-24). Individuals should know their pattern for moles, blemishes, freckles, and other marks on the skin (American Cancer Society, 2015c). A good time to have an annual skin exam is during your birthday month.

- Sun exposure is the most preventable risk factor for all skin cancers.
  - ☐ Protect your eyes by wearing sunglasses
  - ☐ Protect your head and face by wearing a hat
  - ☐ Protect your skin by wearing appropriate clothing and apply SPF of at least 30 or more to all exposed areas.
  - ☐ Remind patient to use plenty of sunscreen and reapply after being in the water.

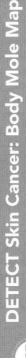

DETECT Skin Cancer: Body Mole Map

SPOT SKIN CANCER

Follow these instructions regularly for a thorough skin-exam: **1.** Learn what to look for **2.** Examine your skin **3.** Record your spots and remember: if you notice any change, contact your dermatologist to make an appointment. If you don't have one, visit **aad.org** to find one in your area.

1 The ABCDEs of Melanoma
What to Look for:

Melanoma is the deadliest form of skin cancer. However, when detected early, melanoma can be effectively treated. You can identify the warning signs of melanoma by looking for the following:

A ASYMMETRY — One half unlike the other half.

B BORDER — Irregular, scalloped or poorly defined border.

C COLOR — Varied from one area to another; shades of tan and brown, black, sometimes white, red or blue.

D DIAMETER — While melanomas are usually greater than 6mm (the size of a pencil eraser) when diagnosed, they can be smaller. See ruler below for a guide.

E EVOLVING — A mole or skin lesion that looks different from the rest or is changing in size, shape or color.

Examples:

2 Skin Cancer Self-Examination
How to Check Your Spots:

Checking your skin means taking note of all the spots on your body, from moles to freckles to age spots. Skin cancer can develop anywhere on the skin and is one of the few cancers you can usually see on your skin. Ask someone for help when checking your skin, especially in hard to see places.

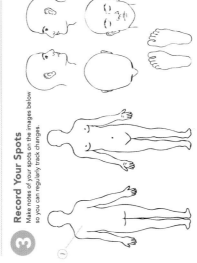

1. Examine body front and back in mirror, especially legs.

2. Bend elbows, look carefully at forearms, back of upper arms, and palms.

3. Look at feet, spaces between toes and soles.

4. Examine back of neck and scalp with a hand mirror. Part hair and lift.

5. Finally, check back and buttocks with a hand mirror.

3 Record Your Spots

Make notes of your spots on the images below so you can regularly track changes.

MOLE #	**A** Asymmetrical? Shape of Mole	**B** Type of Border?	**C** Color of mole	**D** Diameter/Size of Mole. Use ruler provided.	**E** How has mole changed?
1	OVAL, EVEN	JAGGED	PINK	1.5MM	YES, LARGER

Name: _____   Date: _____

© 2016 American Academy of Dermatology

Fig. 8-24. Body Mole Chart. (With permission from the American Dermatology Association.)

CHAPTER 9

Assessing the Head, Face, Mouth, and Neck

INTRODUCTION

The head, face, mouth, and neck is a complex region. The major senses of smell, taste, hearing, and vision originate in this region. The structures contained in the head affect almost every organ system controlling the body.

REVIEW OF ANATOMY AND PHYSIOLOGY

Head

The head is divided into two parts: the cranium and the face. There are 22 bones that make up the adult skull. Bones of the head and face are connected by connective tissue and immovable joints called sutures.

- Cranium (skull) is supported on the top of the vertebral column by the atlas, the first cervical vertebrae.
- There are eight cranial bones: frontal (1), parietal (2), temporal (2), occipital (1), ethmoid (1), sphenoid (1) (Fig. 9-1).

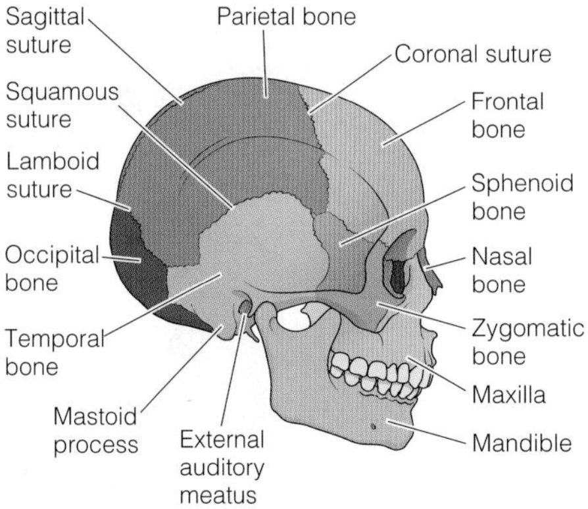

Fig. 9-1. Cranial bones and sutures.

- The frontal bone is the most important and forms the forehead above the eyeballs, gives each person's facial appearance.
- Cranial bones meet at meshed immovable joints called *sutures*; the major sutures are the sagittal, coronal, and lambdoidal.
- Cranial vault is the large part of the skull that protects the brain from injury. The cranium acts like a helmet to the brain.

DIAGNOSTICS

- **Computed tomography (CT scan)** is a noninvasive test that combines special x-ray equipment with sophisticated computers to produce multiple images or pictures of the inside of the body. CT scan of the head is ordered when a more detailed picture is needed for diagnosing and treating injuries, stroke, or pathology within the brain.
  - □ This scan can be done with or without contrast. The contrast material, an iodine dye, is used to make structures and organs easier to visualize.
- **Magnetic resonance imaging (MRI)** is a noninvasive test that uses a powerful magnetic field, radio frequency waves, and a computer to

produce detailed pictures of organs, soft tissues, bone, and virtually all other internal body structures.

- ☐ This is the most sensitive imaging diagnostic test that provides more detail to identify disease or abnormalities.
- ☐ This test provides even more detail than a CT scan and may be ordered if the information is not being seen using other diagnostic tests.

Face

The anterior region of the skull forms the face and contains 14 facial bones: zygomatic (2), vomer (1), palatine (2), nasal (2), maxillae (2), mandible (1), lacrimal (2) and inferior nasal conchae (2) (Fig. 9-2).

- ■ The **temporal artery** is a major artery of the head that branches from within the external carotid artery, has a palpable pulse superior to the zygomatic arch, is palpable in front of each ear.
- ■ **Temporomandibular joint** is a hinge joint connecting the upper temporal bone (part of the skull) and the mandible, the lower jawbone; allows the jaw to move forward, backward, and side to side; an articular disc made up of fibrocartilaginous tissue is positioned between the two bones.

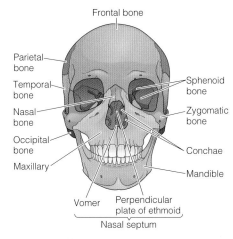

Fig. 9-2. Facial bones and structure.

- **Parotid glands** are the largest salivary glands that secrete saliva into the mouth through the Stensen's ducts. These glands are located superficial to and behind the mandible, and the ducts are on each side of the oral cavity.
- ■ The **submandibular gland** is located within the lower mandible; this gland drains saliva through the Wharton's ducts into the lower oral cavity.

Sinuses

Sinuses are air-filled spaces/hollow cavities that surround the nasal cavity and decrease the weight of the skull.

- ■ Sinuses give resonance to voice during speech.
- ■ There are four pairs of paranasal sinuses:
  - ☐ Frontal above the eyes; in the center of the forehead.
  - ☐ Ethmoid are between the eyes; deeper in the skull; not palpable for examination.
  - ☐ Sphenoids are behind the nasal cavity; deeper in the skull; not palpable for examination.
  - ☐ Maxillary sinuses are the largest; located in the cheekbones below the eyes.

DIAGNOSTICS

- ■ **Computed tomography (CT)** scan of the sinuses is an imaging test that uses x-rays with or without contrast dye to create detailed pictures of the air-filled spaces inside the face (sinuses). This scan may help to diagnose infection, nasal polyps, birth defects, or abnormalities of the sinuses.

SENC Safety Alert CT scans expose the patient to more radiation than an x-ray. The more CT scans that a patient has can increase the risk for cancer.

Nose

The nose is located centrally on the face; composed of bone (upper portion) and cartilage.

- Two **nostrils (nares)** are lined with mucous membranes.
- **Nasal septum** is midline; made up of cartilage and many blood vessels (Kiesselbach area); divides the nose into equal halves; receptors for cranial nerve I (olfactory) are located in the upper part of the septum and nasal cavity.
- **Turbinates** (superior, middle, inferior) are bony lobes on the lateral walls of the nasal cavity; compose most of the mucosal area and increase the surface area; enriched with airflow pressure and temperature-sensing nerve receptors.
- The nose warms, moistens, and filters air, inhaling and exhaling air, and smelling.
- **Adenoids** are clusters of lymphatic tissue behind the nose and are part of the immune system.

Mouth

Figure 9-3 shows the anatomy of the mouth and teeth.

- **Oral mucosa** is the mucous membrane epithelium lining inside the mouth. It is the first portion of the alimentary canal for ingestion and digestion of food.

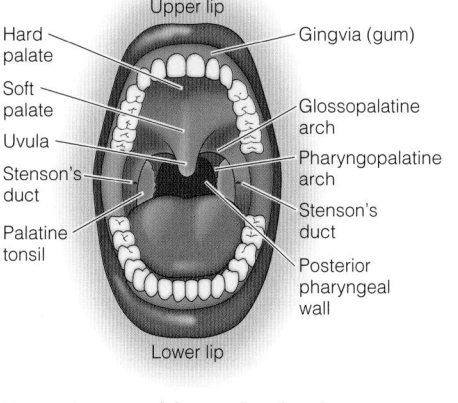

Fig. 9-3. Structure of the mouth and teeth.

Labels on figure: Upper lip; Hard palate; Soft palate; Uvula; Stenson's duct; Palatine tonsil; Gingvia (gum); Glossopalatine arch; Pharyngopalatine arch; Stenson's duct; Posterior pharyngeal wall; Lower lip

- **Lips** mark the transition of mucous membrane of the mouth to skin.
- **Cheeks** (buccal mucosa) are the lateral walls of the mouth.
- **Soft palate** is composed of muscle and connective tissue; responsible for closing off the nasal passages during the act of swallowing; uvula hangs midline from the soft palate.
- **Hard palate** is a thin, horizontal plate of the skull, located in the roof of the mouth; covered with stratified squamous epithelium.
- **Jaw bone (mandible)** is the largest and strongest bone of the face.
- Three **salivary glands** (parotid, submandibular, and sublingual) secrete saliva to start the process of digestion and moisten the mucosa. Salivary glands produce 0.5 to 1.5 liters of saliva per day (Braxton & Quinn, 2013).
- **Stensen's ducts (parotid duct)** are located in the upper buccal mucosa; this is the route saliva flows from the parotid gland into the mouth; ducts are pink; may be darker in dark-skin people.
- **Wharton's ducts** are located on each side of the lower oral cavity; drain saliva from the submandibular and sublingual glands.
- **Teeth** are rooted in the gums; 32 permanent teeth in an adult. Primary function is for chewing and breaking down food to initiate digestion of food.
- **Gingiva (gums)** are covered by mucous membranes; tough insoluble protein mucosa; area around the root of a tooth; attaches to the surface area of the tooth root (cementum) and the alveolar bone, thickened ridge of bone that contains the tooth socket.
- **Tongue** is a muscle located in the floor of the mouth; anchored to the hyoid bone and styloid process of the temporal bone; organ of taste; covered with moist mucosa; there are arteries, veins, and nerves in the tongue. It consists of symmetrical halves; separated by a fibrous septum, middle line; papillae, tiny bumps on the tongue, create a rough texture on about two-thirds of the top of the tongue; thousands of taste buds cover the surface of the papillae; aides in swallowing, and speech.

Throat (Pharynx)

Figure 9-4 shows the anatomy and structure of the throat.

- The anterior part of the neck in front of the vertebrae makes up the **nasopharynx** (upper part) and **oropharynx** (lower part), and consists of pharynx, larynx, trachea, and esophagus.
- **Trachea** (windpipe) is a cylindrical tube composed of cartilage and membranes; measures about four and a half inches in length; three quarters of an inch to an inch in diameter; always larger in males than females.
- **Epiglottis** is the flap that separates the trachea from the esophagus; prevents aspiration of food and fluids.
- **Tonsils** are soft masses of lymphoid tissue located in the back of the pharynx; part of the body's immune system.

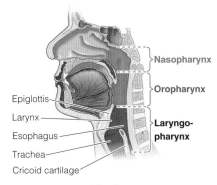

Epiglottis
Larynx
Esophagus
Trachea
Cricoid cartilage

Nasopharynx
Oropharynx
Laryngo-pharynx

Fig. 9-4. Structure of the pharynx.

DIAGNOSTICS

- **Swallowing evaluation** is usually initiated when difficulty swallowing foods or fluids (known as dysphagia) is observed or reported. A referral to a speech language pathologist is made. The speech pathologist will observe the patient closely while she or he eats and drinks to assess for dysphagia, difficulty swallowing.
- **Modified barium swallow study** is a radiologic procedure that assesses swallowing using a fluoroscope, an instrument used for viewing x-ray images on a screen. The patient is given barium, a white chalky mixture, to drink during the procedure. The mouth, throat, and esophagus are assessed.
- **Fiberoptic endoscopic evaluation of swallowing** requires a small, flexible endoscope to be passed through the nose into the pharynx. The physician is able to assess the structures of the throat and assess swallowing.
- **Throat culture** is commonly done to identify the organism causing a bacterial, viral, or fungal infection. A throat culture is completed by swabbing the back of the throat and placing in a culture medium; results take 1 to 2 days. Rapid strep test results are ready in 10 to 15 minutes.

Neck

The neck is formed by seven cervical vertebrae, muscles, and ligaments; supports the weight of the head.

- It protects the nerves that carry sensory and motor impulses from the brain to the body.
- The major muscles supporting the neck are the **sternocleidomastoid** and **trapezius muscles**; both these muscle groups form the anterior and posterior triangles of the neck (Fig. 9-5) and are used as landmarks when assessing the neck.
- The **hyoid bone** is a horseshoe-shaped bone between the chin and the thyroid cartilage, anchored only by muscles in the floor of the mouth. The base of the tongue rests on this bone and aids in tongue movement and swallowing; this is the only bone that is not attached to another bone in the body.
- **Thyroid cartilage** is the largest cartilage of the larynx (the voice box); formed by connecting two pieces of cartilage together; the fusion creates a prominence known as the *Adam's apple*. This cartilage protects the vocal folds.
- **Cricoid cartilage** is a ring of cartilage around the trachea; forms the lower and back part of the cavity of the larynx.

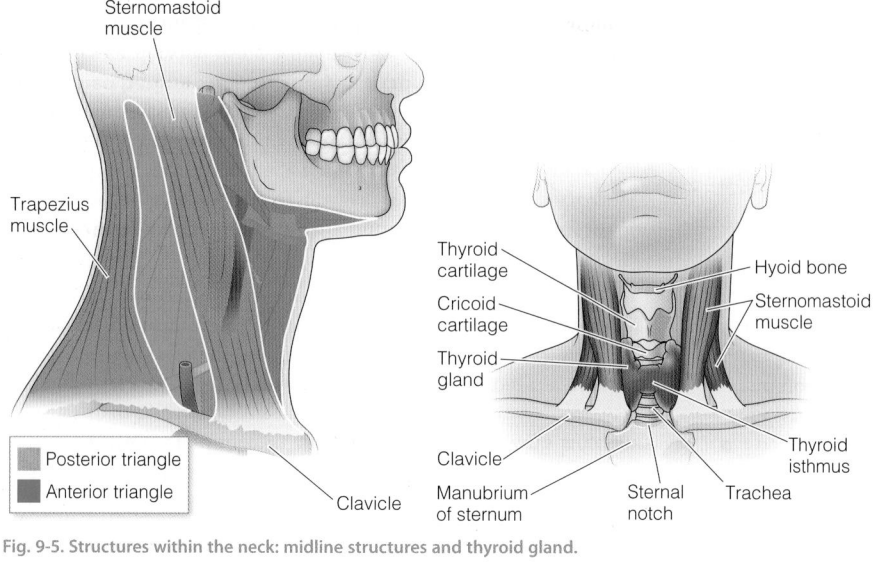

Fig. 9-5. Structures within the neck: midline structures and thyroid gland.

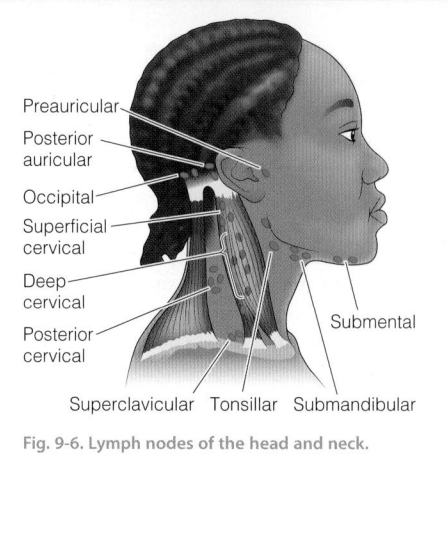

Fig. 9-6. Lymph nodes of the head and neck.

■ **Larynx** is located between the trachea and the base of the tongue; organ of voice.

■ **Trachea** (windpipe) is made up of cartilage and membranes; cylindrical tube extending from the larynx to the bronchi measuring approximately 4.5 inches in length; diameter is three quarters to one inch.

■ **Thyroid** is a butterfly-shaped gland in the anterior portion of the neck. It is the largest endocrine gland; has two lobes about 4 to 6 cm in length; isthmus connects the right and left lobes. This gland has a major role in metabolism and absorbs iodine and uses it to make hormones.

■ **Carotid arteries** are located on each side of the neck; transport oxygenated blood supply to the brain (see Chapter 15).

■ **Jugular veins** are located bilaterally on each side of the neck; these veins empty deoxygenated blood into the superior vena cava (see Chapter 15).

■ **Lymph nodes** are part of the lymphatic system (see Chapter 15); made up of reticular connective tissue filled with lymphocytes. Clusters of lymph nodes are found in the head and neck area and are named after their anatomical location (Fig. 9-6).

DIAGNOSTICS

■ **Thyroid-stimulating hormone (TSH)** is a blood test that evaluates thyroid gland functioning. Results can assess an overactive thyroid gland (hyperthyroidism) or underactive thyroid gland (hypothyroidism). An abnormal value indicates an excess (hyperthyroidism) or deficiency (hypothyroidism) of thyroid hormone available to the body.

■ **Triiodothyronine (T_3)** is a blood test that is used with the TSH and T_4 blood tests to diagnose an overactive thyroid gland. This hormone is converted from the T_4 hormone in the tissues. This test is commonly ordered if the TSH test is abnormal and the T4 levels are normal. The T3 test differentiates causes of thyroid malfunction and helps to diagnose hyperthyroidism.

- **Free thyroxine (Free T$_4$)** is a blood test to assess the functioning of the thyroid gland. T$_4$ is directly secreted by the thyroid gland. This test is commonly ordered with the TSH test to differentiate causes of thyroid dysfunction.

- **Thyroid scan** is a nuclear medicine test to assess the functioning of the thyroid gland, masses, or inflammation. Radioactive iodine in a pill form may also be given to the patient. The amount of radioactive iodine detected in your thyroid gland corresponds with the amount of hormone being produced in the thyroid gland (Topiwala, 2012).

HEALTH HISTORY

Review of Systems

The head is a complex region containing vital organs, cranial nerves, and four of our senses (hearing, seeing, smelling, and tasting). Reviewing past medical history (PMH), family history (FH), injuries, hospitalizations, and surgeries are important for any system. Focused questions are needed for a good history; use the OPQRST mnemonic (Box 9-1) for complaints of pain or a symptom. Psychosocial history needs to be carefully assessed. People who smoke and chew tobacco are at risk for cancer of the head, mouth, throat, and neck (Table 9-1).

BOX 9-1 **OPQRST Mnemonic**

O = Onset
P = Provokes or Palliates
Q = Quality of the pain
R = Region and Radiation
S = Severity
T = Timing

TABLE 9-1 **Risk Factors for Cancers of the Oral Cavity, Nasal/Paranasal Sinus, and Thyroid**

Oral cavity and oropharyngeal cancers	• Twice as common in men than women • Tobacco use including smoking or chewing tobacco • Smoking cigars or pipes • Alcohol • Sun increases risk of skin cancer of the lips • Weakened immune system • Human papilloma virus (CDC, 2016)
Nasopharyngeal cancers	• Twice as common in males than females • Most common in Chinese Americans, followed by other Asian-American groups, African Americans, Hispanics/Latinos, and whites • People who live in parts of Asia, northern Africa, and the Arctic region where nasopharyngeal cancer is common typically eat diets very high in salt-cured fish and meat • Epstein-Barr virus infection • Smoking (CDC, 2016b)
Thyroid cancer	• Family history of thyroid cancer • Occurs three times more often in women • Diets low in iodine • Exposure to radiation (ACS, 2017)

Head

SENC Evidence-Based Practice Head injuries are common, and there is a high risk of disability and death. People with head injuries are more likely to die up to 13 years after the event. Younger men are more likely to die after a blow to the skull. The increased risk of death years after the injury occurred might be explained by factors associated with the injury, rather than the actually injury itself (McMillan, Teasdale, Weir, & Stewart, 2011).

Ask the patient if she or he experiences the following:

- Dizziness or vertigo
- Fainting spells with loss of consciousness
- Seizures
  - ☐ A seizure is caused by abnormal electrical activity in the brain lasting seconds to minutes. Have the patient give a thorough history about the type of seizures, symptoms and medications taken for seizures.
- Headaches
  - ☐ Any unusually severe headaches? How frequent are your headaches? Do you have any other symptoms with headache such as nausea, vomiting, sensitivity to light (photophobia)?
    - • Communication of specific symptoms and location of pain is critical for describing the type of headache; also assess the patient's level of disability when experiencing the headache.
  - ☐ Types of headaches (Fig. 9-7)
    - • Tension or stress: feeling of pressure in the front of the head or both sides of the head or neck related to muscular contraction; feels like a band is tightening around the head; may be related to stress or poor posture.
    - • Cluster: a vascular headache; stabbing pain on one side of the face or behind one eye or at the temple near the forehead; pain is constant; occurs in "clusters" or periods of time.

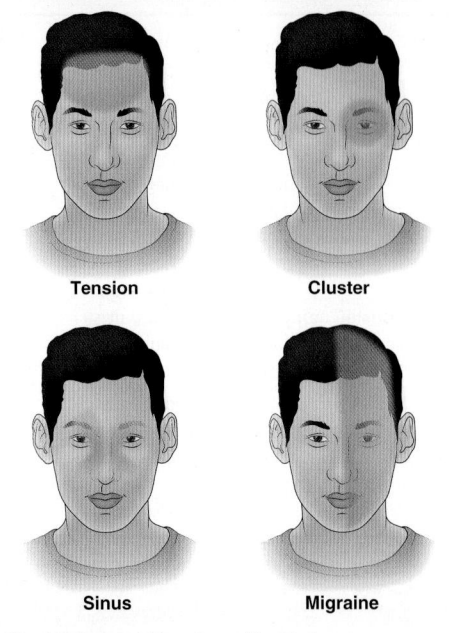

Tension   **Cluster**

Sinus   **Migraine**

Fig. 9-7. Types and locations of headaches.

TIP Cluster headaches occur at predictable times, most commonly in the very early morning between midnight and 3 a.m., and once again later in the day or early evening (Tepper, 2015).

- • Sinus: throbbing pain in front of the face; accompanied by upper respiratory symptoms.
- • Migraine headaches are vascular headaches; produce unilateral, pulsating, intense pain lasting from 4 hours to 3 days; cause nausea or vomiting, and are made worse with activity or precipitating factors; sensitivity to light, noise, and smells (Dunphy, Winland-Brown, Porter, & Thomas, 2015, p. 126).

Nose

- Do you have any problems with your nose?
- Do you have any problems breathing through your nose?
- Have you noticed any changes in your ability to smell?
- Do you have any of the following:
  - Nasal drainage
    - Rhinorrhea is a thin watery discharge from the nose (Venes, 2013); may have associated symptoms of nasal congestion or stuffiness.
  - Postnasal drip
    - Mucus drips from the back of the nose into the upper pharynx
    - Most common cause of a chronic cough especially at night
  - Sinus congestion
    - Sinus infection (sinusitis), occurs when the sinuses and nasal passages become inflamed; most sinus infections are viral infections and can last as long as 4 weeks; symptoms may include headache, nasal congestion, sinus pressure, fever, and cough that may be worse at night (American Family Physician, 2011).
  - Nosebleeds (epistaxis)
    - The nose has many tiny capillaries that are very close to the surface; nosebleeds can occur due to many reasons including picking the nose, dry nose, anticoagulants, bleeding disorders, and a foreign object in the nose.

TIP If a patient has a nosebleed on arrival, the patient should sit and lean forward to keep blood from running into the posterior pharynx. The patient should be instructed to continuously hold pressure on the nares by pinching the nostrils tightly, for 10 to 15 minutes (Morgan & Kellerman, 2014).

SENC Safety Alert Emergency medical attention is necessary if nosebleeds are severe, last longer than 30 minutes, interfere with breathing, or follow an injury (www.mayoclinic.com/health/nosebleeds/MY01201).

- Allergies
  - Common symptoms are sneezing, itchy eyes, and nasal congestion with watery nasal drainage.

Mouth

- Discuss daily hygiene for oral care. Do you experience dry mouth?
  - Xerostomia is a dry mouth; patient has decreased saliva. May be related to:
    - medications
      - People take medications on a daily basis that may cause side effects, the most common side effect related to the mouth is xerostomia (dry mouth) (Box 9-2).
    - systemic disease
    - radiation therapy
    - anxiety
    - dehydration

SENC Patient-Centered Care As people age, the mouth has a tendency to produce less saliva. A dry mouth can cause difficulty eating and talking and this may be embarrassing for the patient. Patients should be educated that there are oral rinses that could help with dry mouth.

BOX 9-2 **General Classification of Medications Causing Xerostomia**

DRUG CLASS
Anticholinergics
Anticonvulsants
Antidepressants
Antihistamines
Antihypertensives
Antineoplastics
Genitourinary smooth muscles relaxants and antispasmodics

SENC Safety Alert Decreased saliva in the mouth can cause dental decay and bad breath (halitosis); encourage dental hygiene and assessments.

☐ Excessive saliva
☐ Mouth pain
☐ Jaw pain may be related to:
  • temporomandibular joint (TMJ) disorder
  • teeth grinding (bruxism)
  • cardiac conditions such as heart attack
☐ Tooth pain
☐ Bleeding from the gums
  • Bleeding gums is a symptom of plaque buildup on the teeth; may also be related to systemic disease or clotting disorders.

■ **TIP** Oral health disparities are profound in the United States. Despite major improvements in oral health for the population as a whole, oral health disparities exist for many racial and ethnic groups, by socioeconomic status, gender, age, and geographic location. Some social factors that can contribute to these differences are lifestyle behaviors such as tobacco use, frequency of alcohol use, and poor dietary choices. Just like they affect general health, these behaviors can affect oral health. The economic factors that often relate to poor oral health include access to health services and a person's ability to get and keep dental insurance (CDC, 2015a).

Throat

■ Do you have any problems with swallowing (dysphagia), sore throat, pain, or hoarseness?
  ☐ Hoarseness means a change in the quality of voice; some causes are:
    • allergies
    • straining of the vocal cord
    • smoking
    • cancer
    • gastroesophageal reflux
    • neurological disorders.

Neck

■ Have you had any neck injuries?
■ Have you noticed any:
  ☐ stiffness
  ☐ pain
    • Patients may develop neck pain due to muscle strain or spasms; patients who do not use good ergonomics with repetitive motions are a great risk for neck complaints.
  ☐ swelling
    • Conditions of the thyroid gland may cause an enlargement of this gland.
    • Goiter is an enlargement of the thyroid gland; a goiter can occur if the thyroid gland is producing too much hormone (hyperthyroidism), too little hormone (hypothyroidism), or the correct amount of hormone (euthyroidism).
  ☐ lumps.
    • Lumps in the neck may be a sign of swollen glands, enlarged lymph nodes, infection, or a sign of an underlying medical condition.
■ Do you have any thyroid problems?

CULTURAL CONSIDERATIONS Cancers of the larynx and pharynx are more common among African Americans and Caucasians than among Asians and Latinos (American Cancer Society, 2016).

Equipment Needed

Gauze
Gloves
Penlight or otoscope
Stethoscope
Tongue blade
Cup of water

Sequence of Assessment

1. Inspection
2. Palpation
3. Auscultation

The entire head, nose, and throat region is assessed with the person in the sitting position. Explain the assessment as it moves forward. This assessment is noninvasive and should not cause any discomfort. Have the patient let you know about experiencing any discomfort or pain during the examination.

TECHNIQUE 9-1: Inspecting and Palpating the Head

Purpose: To assess for normal size and shape of the head
Equipment: Gloves (optional)
■ **TIP** Have the patient remove any hairpieces or accessories.
ASSESSMENT STEPS
Inspecting and palpating may be done simultaneously.
1. Put on gloves.
2. Inspect the patient's head for:
  □ size
  □ shape
  □ configuration
  □ movement.
3. Palpate the head (Fig. 9-8) and assess for tenderness, masses, or depressions.
4. Remove and discard gloves.
5. Document your findings.
NORMAL FINDINGS
■ Head is symmetric, midline, round.
■ Normocephalic; a person's head is normal shape and size for his or her age.

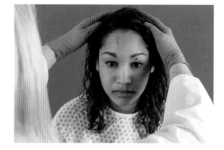
Fig. 9-8. Inspecting and palpating the head.

- Head erect and still; no involuntary movements.
- No pain, tenderness, masses, or depressions during palpation.

   ▆ **TIP** When documenting physical assessment findings, use the anatomical regions to specify the location of any abnormality on the head (see Fig. 9-1).

ABNORMAL FINDINGS

- Pain
- Tenderness
- A mass
- Involuntary movements
- Depression of the skull
- **Macrocephaly** is an abnormally large head size.
- Neurological disorders cause tremors, tics, or jerking movements of the head.

   ▆ **TIP** Tics are repeated, spasmodic contractions of the muscles, most commonly involving the head, face, neck, and shoulders.

TECHNIQUE 9-2: **Inspecting the Face**

Purpose: To assess facial appearance and symmetry

ASSESSMENT STEPS

1. Stand in front of the person and assess for appearance and shape of face:
   □ Round
   □ Square
   □ Oval
2. Assess for symmetry of the face (cranial nerve VII) (Fig. 9-9):
   □ Nasolabial folds (the distance from the corner of each nostril to the corner of the lip bilaterally; should be equal measurements.
   □ Palpebral fissures; inspect the distance between the upper and lower eyelids; should be equal distances.
3. Assess for facial expression:
   □ Does the patient make eye contact?
   □ Flat affect: showing no emotion of facial expressions
   □ Sad or happy affect
4. Assess for involuntary movements (muscles)
5. Assess the condition and texture of the skin

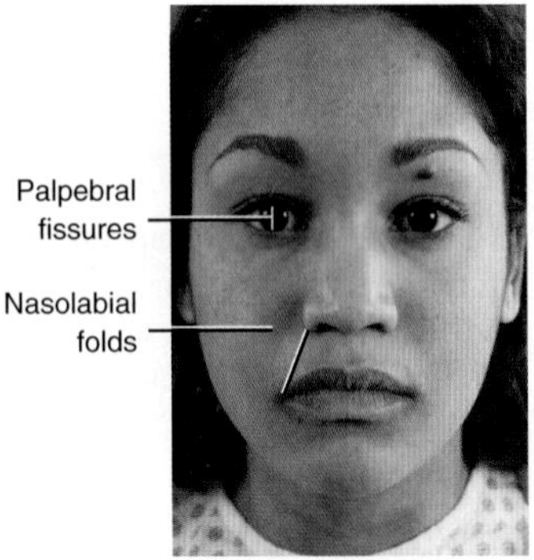

Fig. 9-9. Assessing nasolabial folds and palpebral fissures.

6. Assess for edema

7. Document your findings.

NORMAL FINDINGS

- Face (round, oval, or square)
- Bilaterally symmetrical facial structures
- Nasolabial folds and palpebral fissures equal
- Expression relaxed; makes eye contact
- No involuntary muscle movement; no visible pulsations
- Skin smooth and clear
- No edema

ABNORMAL FINDINGS

- Asymmetry of the face may be related to abscess, infection, enlargement of parotid gland, neurological disorders.
- Flat affect may indicate depression or chronic pain.
- **Acromegaly** is a syndrome of growth hormone excess by the pituitary gland; characterized by enlargement of the bones of the hands, feet, and face.
- Parkinson's disease causes a "masklike" facial appearance.
- Kidney diseases may cause swelling of the face or around the eyes (periorbital edema).
- Cardiac, respiratory, and autoimmune disorders may present with different facial changes (Table 9-2).

TABLE 9-2 Medical Conditions With Facial Identifiers

Medical Condition	Characteristic Name	Description of Facial Identifiers
Congenital aortic stenosis	Elfin face	• Prominent forehead • Short upturned nose • Widely spaced eyes • Full cheeks • Deep husky voice
Severe aortic insufficiency		• Head bobbing or head nodding with each heartbeat
Aortic regurgitation or heart failure	Corvisart facies	• Puffy cyanotic face • Swollen eyelids • Shiny eyes

TABLE 9-2 Medical Conditions With Facial Identifiers—cont'd

Medical Condition	Characteristic Name	Description of Facial Identifiers
Mitral stenosis		• Rosy cheeks or slightly cyanotic cheeks; dilated capillaries
Scleroderma		• Sharp nose • Shiny, tightly drawn skin on face
Systemic lupus erythematosus (SLE)		• Butterfly rash on face
Severe myxedema		• Dull, puffy face • Thickening of the tongue • Dry, rough skin • Pallor and lip pallor • Edema particularly pronounced around the eyes and does not pit with pressure
Myasthenia gravis		• Drooping eyelids (ptosis) • Weakness of the facial muscles; apathetic or depressed look
Graves' disease (hyperthyroidism)		• Lid lag: upper eyelid does not keep pace with the eyeball as it follows a moving object downward from above • Flushing of skin • Exophthalmos (protruding eyes) • Patient appears anxious
Trauma and basal skull fracture with bleeding into the middle fossa	Battle sign	• Discoloration behind the ear • Mastoid ecchymosis
Parkinson's disease		• Mask-like features • Lack of facial expression • Slowness to smile • Decreased blinking • Characteristic stare
Cushing's syndrome		• Face is round and puffy known as a moon face • Red cheeks • Excessive hair growth on face • Acne

Adapted from Massey, D. (2006). The value and role of skin and nail assessment in critically ill. *Nursing in Critical Care 11*(2), 80–85.

TECHNIQUE 9-3: **Palpating the Face**

Purpose: To assess tenderness, swelling, and inflammation
Equipment: Gloves (optional)

ASSESSMENT STEPS

Stand in front of the person and assess as follows:

1. Using the finger pads of both hands, gently palpate the face for tenderness and swelling.
2. Place your fingers in front of the earlobes and corner of the eyes and palpate the temporal arteries simultaneously in front of each ear to assess for tenderness or inflammation.
3. Place your fingertips in front of each ear at the zygomatic arch and ask the patient to open and close his or her mouth. Assess for any clicking sounds or decreased range of motion (ROM) of the jaw, including TMJ disorder (Fig. 9-10).
4. Document your findings.

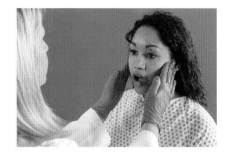

Fig. 9-10. Assessing the temporomandibular joint.

NORMAL FINDINGS

- No tenderness
- Temporal arteries nontender
- The TMJ has no clicking sounds or limited ROM. Mouth opens on the average 3 to 6 cm and moves laterally 1 to 2 cm.

ABNORMAL FINDINGS

- Temporal arteritis is an inflammation of the temporal arteries and blood vessels that supply blood to the head; cause is unknown; patients may complain of a throbbing headache on one side of the head, fever, jaw pain, and tenderness of the face and temporal area.
- TMJ disorder causes a clicking, popping, or grating sound; limited movement of the mouth; headaches, jaw, tooth, or ear pain.

TECHNIQUE 9-4: **Inspecting and Palpating the Nose**

Purpose: To assess for tenderness, inflammation, or deviation.

ASSESSMENT STEPS

1. Stand in front of the person and inspect the nose for the following:
   - ☐ Symmetry
   - ☐ Alignment of septum
   - ☐ Color
   - ☐ Swelling
   - ☐ Drainage

2. Gently palpate the nose for tenderness or swelling.

3. Document your findings.

NORMAL FINDINGS

- Nose symmetrical
- Septum straight and midline
- Skin color same as face
- No lesions, swelling, or deformity
- No drainage

ABNORMAL FINDINGS

- Asymmetry
- Deviated septum
- Swelling or inflammation
- Redness, bruising, lesions
- Tenderness or swelling while palpating
- Nasal drainage: amount (scant, moderate, copious), color (clear, yellow, green, bloody), consistency (thin, thick), with odor.

Technique 9-4A: **Assessing the Patency of the Nose**

Purpose: To assess for nasal passageway occlusion

ASSESSMENT STEPS

1. Ask the patient to press on the right naris to occlude the passageway.

2. Ask the person to inhale through the left naris with his or her mouth closed.

3. Ask the patient to press on the left naris to occlude the passageway (Fig. 9-11).

4. Ask the person to inhale through the right naris with his or her mouth closed.

5. Document your findings.

NORMAL FINDINGS

- Each nasal passageway is patent.

ABNORMAL FINDINGS

- Absence of sniff may be an indication of nasal congestion or obstruction; obstruction may be related to a foreign object.
- Rhinitis, an inflammation of the mucosa in the nose causing nasal congestion and sneezing, may be related to a viral or bacterial infection.
- Nasal polyp is a soft, painless, growth that protrudes into the nasal cavity; may block your nasal passages; can form as a result of allergic conditions or inflammation (Rogers, 2012, p. 142).

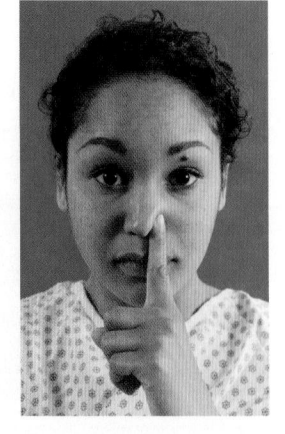

Fig. 9-11. Assessing for nasal patency.

TECHNIQUE 9-5: **Palpating the Maxillary and Frontal Sinuses**

■ **TIP** Percussion may be done instead of palpating the sinuses. Tap over the maxillary and frontal sinuses instead of palpating.

Purpose: To assess for tenderness or pain

ASSESSMENT STEPS

Stand in front of the person and assess the following:

1. Place your thumbs slightly below the eyebrows.

2. Press up and under the eyebrows, palpating the frontal sinuses (Fig. 9-12).

3. Assess for tenderness or pain.

4. Now, place your thumbs below the cheek bones, palpating the maxillary sinuses (Fig. 9-13).

5. Assess for tenderness or pain.

6. Document your findings.

NORMAL FINDINGS

■ No tenderness or pain is felt

ABNORMAL FINDINGS

■ Tenderness or pain that may indicate allergies or a sinus infection

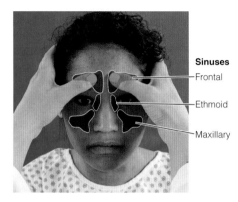

Fig. 9-12. Palpating the frontal sinuses.

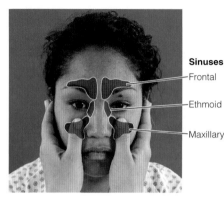

Fig. 9-13. Palpating the maxillary sinuses.

TECHNIQUE 9-6: **Inspecting and Palpating the Mouth**

Purpose: To assess the structures of the mouth for redness, tenderness, lesions, or abnormalities

■ **TIP** You need good lighting for visualization of all structures in the mouth and throat. Assess from the front of the mouth and work toward the back of the throat.

SENC Patient-Centered Care While assessing the mouth, the patient will have to keep his or her mouth wide open. This assessment may take some time. If you observe that the patient is having difficulty doing that, have him or her close the mouth for a rest period.

Equipment: Penlight, gloves, tongue blade, sterile gauze

SENC Safety Alert Always wear clean, nonsterile gloves during this part of the assessment because you will be coming in contact with the patient's saliva.

Technique 9-6A: **Inspecting the Lips**

■ **TIP** Female patients should remove lipstick prior to this assessment.

Purpose: To assess shape and integrity of the lips

ASSESSMENT STEPS

1. Stand in front of the person and inspect the lips for:
- ☐ symmetry
- ☐ color
- ☐ moisture
- ☐ lesions
- ☐ swelling.

NORMAL FINDINGS

- Lips are symmetric
- Upper lip is everted
- Pink, moist, no lesions, swelling, or cracking of skin

ABNORMAL FINDINGS

- Lips are inverted
- Swelling, erythema, lesions, cracking of skin

    ■ **TIP** A sore that does not heal in the mouth requires further evaluation.

    ☐ **Angular cheilitis** is inflammation at the corners of the mouth; sore, cracked corners of the lips; commonly caused by yeast infections, dry mouth, or vitamin deficiency.

    ☐ **Angioedema** is edema of the lips; usually related to an allergic reaction (Fig. 9-14).

    ☐ Pallor of lips may indicate decreased perfusion related to respiratory or cardiovascular problems.

    ☐ **Herpes simplex virus** manifests with cold sores or blisters on the lips.

        ■ **TIP** Preventing high-risk behaviors that include cigarette, cigar, or pipe smoking, use of smokeless tobacco, and excessive use of alcohol are critical in preventing oral cancers. Early detection is key to increasing the survival rate for these cancers (CDC, 2016b).

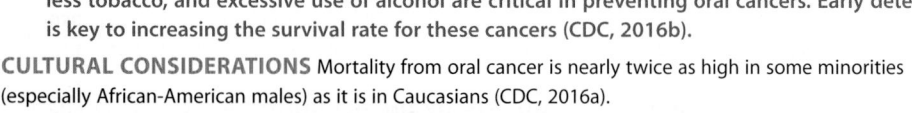

Fig. 9-14. Angioedema.

CULTURAL CONSIDERATIONS Mortality from oral cancer is nearly twice as high in some minorities (especially African-American males) as it is in Caucasians (CDC, 2016a).

Technique 9-6B: **Inspecting the Teeth**

Purpose: To assess for position, number, and integrity of teeth

■ **TIP Adults have between 28 and 32 teeth. Ask people if they have dentures or implants.**

ASSESSMENT STEPS

1. Inspect the teeth for:
- ☐ dentures, caps, or missing teeth
- ☐ color
- ☐ tooth decay.

2. Ask patient to clench teeth and assess for malocclusion, malposition of the teeth (Fig. 9-15).

NORMAL FINDINGS

■ Color of teeth white to an ivory color:
- ☐ Teeth may be stained yellow from smoking or brown from drinking tea or coffee.
- ☐ Age-related darkening (yellow or brown)

■ Clean, free of debris

■ Smooth edges

■ 32 teeth or 28 teeth if wisdom teeth have been removed
- ☐ The upper incisors should overlap the lower incisors; back teeth should meet

ABNORMAL FINDINGS

■ Loose, broken, painful teeth (Fig. 9-16)

■ Tooth decay

■ Malocclusion of the teeth:
- ☐ Protrusion of the upper and lower incisors
- ☐ Failure of the upper incisors to overlap the lower incisors
- ☐ Problems with the bite
- ☐ Back teeth do not meet

CULTURAL CONSIDERATIONS African Americans, non-Hispanics, and Mexican Americans aged 35 to 44 experience untreated tooth decay nearly twice as much as white, non-Hispanics (CDC 2015a).

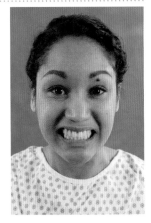

Fig. 9-15. Inspecting teeth while clenched.

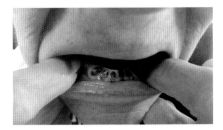

Fig. 9-16. Broken teeth.

Technique 9-6C: **Inspecting and Palpating the Buccal Mucosa**

Purpose: To assess for inflammation, lesions, or abnormalities

ASSESSMENT STEPS

1. If a patient has full or partial dentures, have her or him remove the dentures for inspection and palpation of gum area.

2. Inspect and palpate the buccal mucosa and gums.

3. Gently use a tongue blade to hold the tongue out of the way for full visualization of the gums and mucosa (Fig. 9-17).

NORMAL FINDINGS
■ Pink, smooth, moist, no lesions, swelling, or bleeding
■ Tight margin around each tooth
■ No tenderness with palpation

ABNORMAL FINDINGS
■ Red, inflamed, or bleeding mucosa; lesions
■ Tenderness with palpation:
  □ **Aphthous stomatitis** (canker sore) is the most common nontraumatic form of oral ulceration with 20% to 40% incidence in the population; ulcer formation is the main clinical presentation (Jefferson, 2011).
  □ **Gingivitis** is the mildest type of periodontal disease; red, swollen, bleeding gums.
  □ **Gingival hyperplasia** is an enlargement or overgrowth of the gum tissue; firm and nonpainful; may be related to systemic illness, side effects of medications such as phenytoin (Dilantin (used for seizure disorders)), and poor oral hygiene.
  □ **Periodontal disease** is a chronic infection of the gums. The gums pull away from the teeth and create open spaces that collect bacteria which causes chronic inflammation. The accumulation of bacteria damages and destroys the teeth, tissue, and underlying bone.
  □ **Thrush** is a candidiasis fungal infection that creates thick, white to yellow patches on the tongue or buccal mucosa; occurs frequently with a weakened immune system and antibiotic therapy.

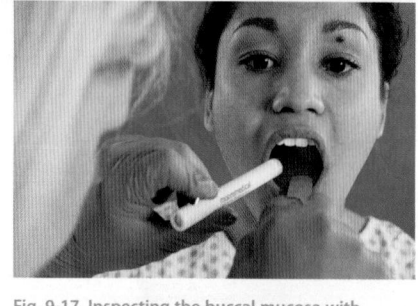

Fig. 9-17. Inspecting the buccal mucosa with tongue blade.

CULTURAL CONSIDERATIONS Some 47.2% of U.S. adults have some form of periodontal disease. In adults aged 65 and older, 70.1% have periodontal disease. Periodontal disease is higher in men than women, and greatest among Mexican Americans and non-Hispanic African Americans, and those with less than a high school education (CDC, 2015a).

Technique 9-6D: **Inspecting and Palpating Hard and Soft Palates**
Purpose: To assess for color, tenderness, or abnormal deviations
ASSESSMENT STEPS
1. Using a penlight, inspect the anterior hard and posterior soft palate (Fig. 9-18).
2. Inspect Stensen's ducts on each side of the soft palate.
  □ Stensen's ducts are the openings of the parotid glands on the buccal mucosa that allow saliva to flow from the parotid gland (see Fig. 9-2).
3. Using your index finger, gently palpate the following structures (Fig. 9-19):
  □ Hard palate
  □ Soft palate
NORMAL FINDINGS
■ Transverse rugae, irregular ridges are firm, pink to light red; moist
■ Stensen's ducts are draining

- No tenderness
- Soft palate is pink, moist; no lesions or ulcerations
- Integrity of hard and soft palate intact
- Nodular bony ridge down the middle of the posterior hard palate

ABNORMAL FINDINGS

- Deep red color, ulcerations, lesions, or growths
  - ☐ Hard palate is a shade of yellow if jaundice is present.
  - ☐ **Torus palatinus** is an abnormal growth that develops midline in the hard palate; surgically removed if the growth causes discomfort; may be hereditary.

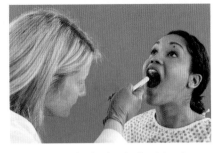

Fig. 9-18. Inspecting hard and soft palate using a penlight.

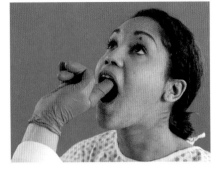

Fig. 9-19. Palpating hard and soft palate.

Technique 9-6E: **Inspecting and Palpating the Tongue**

Purpose: To assess color, movement, and abnormalities

ASSESSMENT STEPS

1. Inspect the dorsal surface of the tongue for color, lesions, or coating on the tongue (Fig. 9-20).
2. Ask the patient to stick out his or her tongue and assess the:
   - ☐ lateral edges of the tongue
   - ☐ voluntary movement of the tongue
   - ☐ fine tremors (fasciculations) of the tongue
   - ☐ position of tongue is midline (hypoglossal nerve, cranial nerve XII).
3. Ask the patient to touch the roof of the mouth with the tongue; inspect the:
   - ☐ floor of the mouth
   - ☐ frenulum, which is a small fold of mucous membrane dividing the tongue in half; secures the tongue
   - ☐ ventral surface of the tongue (Fig. 9-21)
   - ☐ Wharton's ducts:
     - • Wharton's ducts appear on each side of frenulum that drains saliva from the sublingual and submandibular glands into the lower part of the mouth.

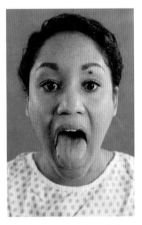

Fig. 9-20. Dorsal surface of the tongue.

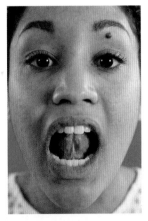

Fig. 9-21. Ventral surface of the tongue.

4. Using a sterile gauze, gently palpate the tongue for any lumps or nodules (Fig. 9-22).

5. Discard the gauze.

NORMAL FINDINGS

- Color pink and saliva present
- Papillae on dorsal surface
- Midline position
- Ventral surface smooth, pink, moist
- No lumps or nodules with palpation
- Wharton's and Stensen's ducts visible

   ■ **TIP** *Geographic tongue* is a harmless condition; the tongue is usually covered with tiny, pinkish-white bumps (papillae); patches on the tongue are missing papillae; tongue appears smooth, red "island," often with slightly raised borders (Fig. 9-23).

ABNORMAL FINDINGS

- Cracked, dry, red, presence of ulcers or lesions, bleeding, thick white or yellow coating on tongue.
   □ **Atrophic glossitis** is a smooth red or pink tongue; may indicate nutritional deficiencies.
   □ **Hairy tongue** is a white to dark overgrowth, hairy surface that may indicate systemic immune suppression or too much bacteria.
   □ **Leukoplakia** are patches on the tongue (usually white or gray); progresses to cancer 19% of the time (Jefferson, 2011).
   □ **Squamous cell carcinoma** of the tongue presents as a thickened white or red patch or plaque; may develop nodularity or ulceration; usually laterally on the tongue.
   □ Tongue lesions require a biopsy to determine if the lesion is cancerous.

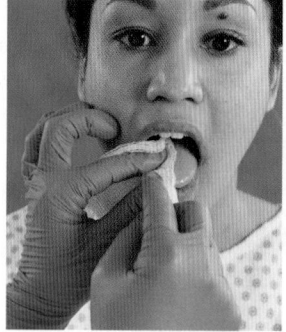

Fig. 9-22. Palpating the tongue using sterile gauze.

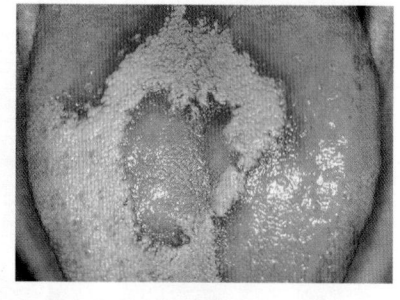

Fig. 9-23. Geographic tongue.

Technique 9-6F: **Inspecting the Pharynx and Tonsils**

Purpose: To assess for redness and inflammation

ASSESSMENT STEPS

1. Moisten a tongue blade with warm water.

   ■ **TIP** A moistened tongue blade may help to decrease the patient from gagging.

2. Ask the patient to open his or her mouth wide, tilt the head back, and say "aah." Using a penlight, inspect the rising of the soft palate and uvula (Fig. 9-24).

3. Using the tongue depressor to hold the tongue down, ask the patient to say "aah" again and assess the throat and tonsillar pillars.

   □ Note mouth odors.

      ■ **TIP** Halitosis is bad breath; may be related to problems with the teeth or periodontal disease.

4. Using the tongue depressor, gently touch the back of the pharynx to elicit a gag reflex.

5. Discard the tongue blade.

6. Remove and discard gloves.

7. Document your findings.

NORMAL FINDINGS

- Uvula rises midline symmetrically; glossopharyngeal (cranial nerve IX) and vagus (cranial nerve X) intact
- Throat pink
- Tonsils pink; may partially protrude or be absent
- Positive (presence of) gag reflex

ABNORMAL FINDINGS

- Asymmetrical rise of the uvula
- Throat deep red, inflamed, with drainage
- Throat pain
- Tonsils protruding with or without drainage
- **Tonsillitis** is a viral or bacterial infection of the tonsils; tonsils become enlarged, swollen, may have white or yellow drainage. Enlargement of tonsils is graded on a 1 to 4 scale (Fig. 9-25).
  +1 tonsils are visible and slightly protruding
  +2 tonsils are halfway between the tonsillar pillars and uvula
  +3 tonsils are almost touching the uvula
  +4 tonsils are touching each other
- **Pharyngitis** is a sore throat caused by inflammation of the mucous membranes of the back of the throat; may be related to viral or bacterial infection.

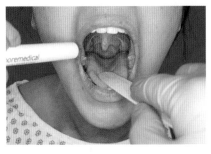

Fig. 9-24. Inspecting the uvula using a penlight.

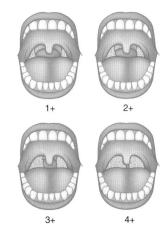

Fig. 9-25. Grading the tonsils.

TECHNIQUE 9-7: **Inspecting the Neck**

Purpose: To assess symmetry, movement, and swelling of the neck
Ask the patient to sit up straight with neck in the normal position and then slightly hyperextended.

ASSESSMENT STEPS
1. Assess the neck for symmetry and swelling.
2. Have the patient turn his or her head to assess range of motion (ROM) (Fig. 9-26):
☐ Turn neck side to side.
☐ Bend neck forward.
☐ Extend neck backward.
☐ Bend neck toward each shoulder.
▮ **TIP** Instruct the person to try to keep the shoulders down, not up, when bending the neck to the shoulder to increase the full visibility of the neck.

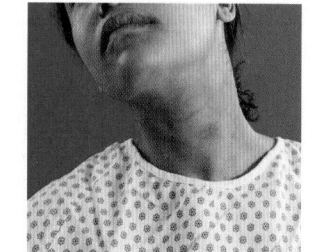

Fig. 9-26. Inspecting ROM of the neck.

NORMAL FINDINGS
▪ Neck is symmetrical; no swelling
▪ No pain with range of motion
▪ Full ROM of neck

ABNORMAL FINDINGS
▪ Asymmetrical
▪ Pain with movement
▪ Unable to turn neck
▪ **Torticollis** is a stiff neck with muscle spasm of the sternocleidomastoid muscle on one side of the body causing a lateral flexion contracture of the cervical spine musculature; may be congenital or acquired (Venes, 2013).

TECHNIQUE 9-8: **Inspecting and Palpating the Trachea**

Purpose: To assess for tracheal shift or deviation
▮ **TIP** A mass in the neck or pathology in the lung may cause the trachea to shift or deviate toward the affected or unaffected side.
Ask the patient to sit up straight and bend her or his head slightly forward to relax the sternomastoid muscles.

ASSESSMENT STEPS
1. Inspect the trachea below the thyroid isthmus.
2. Gently place your right index finger in the sternal notch (Fig. 9-27).

3. Slip your finger off to each side noting distance from the sternomastoid muscle.

4. Assess the symmetrical spacing on each side and note any deviation from midline.

5. Document your findings.

NORMAL FINDINGS
- Trachea is midline.
- Space is symmetric on each side.

ABNORMAL FINDINGS
- Trachea is deviated to the right or left side and away from the midline (Table 9-3).

    ▓ **TIP** Tracheal deviation may be related to masses, adhesions, and pathology affecting the trachea or the mediastinum in the center of the chest cavity.

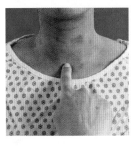

Fig. 9-27. Assessing the trachea at the sternal notch.

TABLE 9-3 Reasons for a Tracheal Shift

Trachea Deviates to Affected Side of Disease	Trachea Deviates to Unaffected Side
Pulmonary fibrosis	Tumor or aneurysm
Pleural adhesion	Thyroid lobe enlargement
Large pulmonary atelectasis (gas exchange impairment related to a partially or completely collapsed lung or buildup of fluid in the lung).	Pneumothorax (collapsed lung)

TECHNIQUE 9-9: **Inspecting the Thyroid**

Purpose: To assess size and mobility.

Equipment: Cup of water (optional)

Seat the patient with his or her head in a neutral or slightly extended position.

ASSESSMENT STEPS

1. Stand in front of the patient.

2. Inspect the neck for swelling or enlargement of the thyroid gland below the cricoid cartilage (Fig. 9-28A).

3. Have the patient take a sip of water (Fig. 9-28B) or swallow and observe the upward motion of the thyroid gland.

NORMAL FINDINGS
- Neck area at the site of the thyroid gland should have a smooth, straight appearance.
- Thyroid gland as well as cricoid and thyroid cartilage move up with swallowing.

ABNORMAL FINDINGS
- Neck is enlarged, asymmetrical.
- Gland does not move during swallowing.

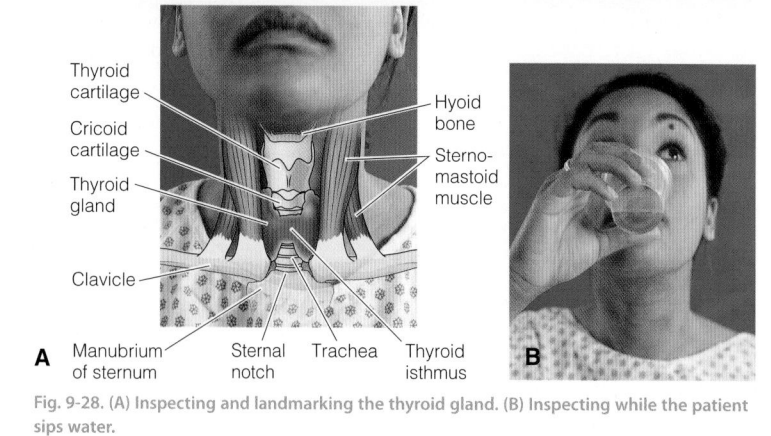

A Thyroid cartilage / Cricoid cartilage / Thyroid gland / Clavicle / Manubrium of sternum / Sternal notch / Trachea / Thyroid isthmus / Hyoid bone / Sterno-mastoid muscle

B

Fig. 9-28. (A) Inspecting and landmarking the thyroid gland. (B) Inspecting while the patient sips water.

Technique 9-9A: **Palpating the Thyroid**

Purpose: To assess the thyroid gland for smoothness, enlargement, nodules, or tenderness

Equipment: Cup of water (optional)

TIP The thyroid gland may be assessed using an anterior or posterior approach. Assessment is easier if you are able to find your landmarks first: cricoid cartilage, the isthmus of the thyroid gland, and suprasternal notch. It is important to remember the length of a thyroid lobe is only about 4 to 6 cm.

Posterior Approach

ASSESSMENT STEPS
1. Stand behind the patient.
2. Ask the patient to sit up straight with his or her neck slightly flexed to the right to relax the neck muscles.
3. Place your finger pads between the sternomastoid muscle and trachea on each side of the patient's neck slightly below the cricoid cartilage.
4. Have the patient take a sip of water or swallow and feel the rise of the thyroid gland.
5. Using your left hand finger pads, gently push the trachea to the right side (Fig. 9-29).

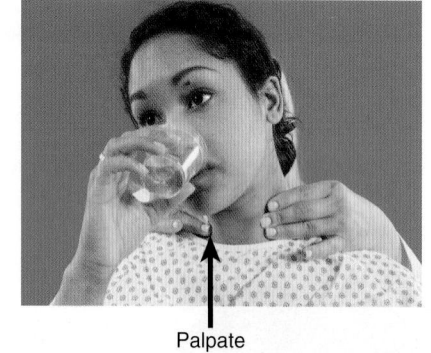

Palpate

Fig. 9-29. Palpating the thyroid gland: posterior approach.

6. Using your right hand finger pads, ask the patient to take a sip of water or swallow and gently palpate laterally the right lobe of the thyroid for smoothness, enlargement, nodules or tenderness.

7. Ask the patient to slightly flex his or her neck to the left to relax the neck muscles.

8. Using your right hand finger pads, gently push the trachea to the left side.

9. Using your left hand finger pads, ask the patient to take a sip of water or swallow and gently palpate laterally the left lobe of the thyroid for smoothness, enlargement, nodules or tenderness.

10. Document your findings. Specifically, document the size, shape, and location of any nodule.

NORMAL FINDINGS

- Lateral lobes may or may not be palpable.
- If palpable, the lobes are smooth, firm, and nontender.

ABNORMAL FINDINGS

- Enlargement of one or both lobes
- Tenderness, presence of lumps or nodules
- Texture has variations of firmness

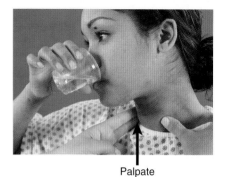

Palpate

Fig. 9-30. Assessing the thyroid gland: anterior approach.

Anterior Approach

ASSESSMENT STEPS

1. Stand in front of the patient.

2. Ask the patient to sit up straight with his or her neck slightly flexed to the right to relax the neck muscles.

3. Place your finger pads between the sternomastoid muscle and trachea on each side of the patient's neck slightly below the cricoid cartilage.

4. Have the patient take a sip of water or swallow and feel the rise of the thyroid gland.

5. Using your thumb of your right hand on the patient's neck slightly below the cricoid cartilage, gently push the trachea to the right (Fig. 9-30).

6. Position your finger pads of your left hand between the sternomastoid muscle and trachea, have the patient take a sip of water or swallow and gently palpate the right lobe of the thyroid for smoothness, enlargement, nodules or tenderness.

7. Ask the patient to slightly flex his or her neck to the left to relax the neck muscles.

8. Using your thumb of your left hand on the patient's neck slightly below the cricoid cartilage, gently push the trachea to the left.

9. Position your finger pads of your right hand between the sternomastoid muscle and trachea, have the patient take a sip of water or swallow and gently palpate the left lobe of the thyroid for smoothness, enlargement, nodules or tenderness.

10. Document your findings. Specifically, document the size, shape, and location of any nodule.

NORMAL FINDINGS

- Lateral lobes may or may not be palpable.
- If palpable, the lobes are smooth, firm, and nontender.

ABNORMAL FINDINGS

- Enlargement of one or both lobes
- Tenderness, presence of lumps or nodules
- Texture has variations of firmness.
- **Goiter** is an enlarged thyroid gland; may be related to hyperfunction or hypofunction of the thyroid gland.

Technique 9-9B: **Auscultating the Thyroid**

Purpose: Further assessment of an enlarged thyroid gland is necessary to check for presence of a bruit, increased, turbulent blood flow.

Equipment: Stethoscope

ASSESSMENT STEPS

Ask the patient to sit up straight with his or her neck slightly flexed.

1. Using the bell of the stethoscope, auscultate both lobes of the thyroid gland (Fig. 9-31).

2. Assess for a "whooshing" or abnormal sound.

3. Document your findings.

NORMAL FINDINGS

- No bruit is heard.

ABNORMAL FINDINGS

- A bruit, turbulent blood flow is heard related to increased blood flow.
  □ A bruit is a vascular sound usually heard with hyperthyroidism.

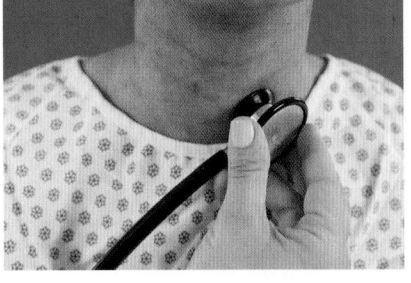

Fig. 9-31. Auscultating the thyroid gland.

PATIENT EDUCATION

Healthy People 2020

Goal: **Prevent and control oral and craniofacial disease, condition, and injuries, and improve access to preventive services and dental care (HHS, 2010).**

- Increase awareness of the importance of oral health to overall health and well-being.
- Increase acceptance and adoption of effective preventive interventions.
- Reduce disparities in access to effective preventive and dental treatment services.

Dental Health

The American Dental Association (2016) recommends:

- A dental exam twice per year.
- Brush all tooth surfaces for at least 90 seconds, twice daily using a soft toothbrush.
- Place your toothbrush at a 45-degree angle to the gums.
- All toothbrushes should be dry before storing, and toothbrushes should be replaced every 3 to 4 months or sooner if the bristles are frayed.
- Floss at least once a day, preferably more often.

- Brush your tongue to remove bacteria
- Avoid tobacco and alcohol.
- Use water-based moisturizers to protect lips.
- Maintain adequate hydration.

Head Safety

Traumatic Brain Injury (TBI)

TBI is an injury to the brain caused by an external force that can disrupt the normal brain cell functioning; symptoms include difficulty thinking, remembering, and concentrating. Prevention should include educating patients in the following areas:

- Fall Prevention
  - ☐ Reduce clutter and items you can trip over.
  - ☐ Securely fasten throw rugs to the floor.
  - ☐ Use cabinets for that which can be easily reached.
  - ☐ Wear shoes.
  - ☐ Become knowledgeable about the side effects of medications.

- Car Safety
  - ☐ Wear seat belts at all times.
  - ☐ Do not text or talk on the phone while driving.
- Recreational Safety
  - ☐ Wear a helmet. All recreational activities that involve wheels, asphalt, or concrete require the person to wear a properly fitting helmet to prevent brain injury (CDC, 2013a). For proper fitting of helmets, please see the Centers for Disease Control and Prevention website at http://www.cdc.gov/bam/safety/helmets.html.
  - ☐ Wear protective equipment (e.g., shin guards, eye and mouth guards)
  - ☐ Bicycle safety includes the following:
    - Riding on the right side of the road with traffic
    - Obeying traffic signs
    - Using hand signs
    - Stopping at intersections
    - Yielding right of way to pedestrians

CHAPTER
10 — Assessing the Ears

INTRODUCTION

The ears enhance quality of life. Hearing helps us to understand and function in the environment and assists us in communicating effectively. Hearing loss or impairment progresses slowly and is a sensitive topic for an individual. Hearing loss may be inherited, caused by maternal rubella or complications at birth, certain infectious diseases such as meningitis, chronic ear infections, use of ototoxic drugs, exposure to excessive noise, and aging (World Health Organization [WHO], 2016).

Routine health assessment is dependent on a person's ability to hear the questions that we ask. Assessing hearing starts with the first encounter noting whether "conversational hearing" is intact (Sanders & Gillig, 2010).

REVIEW OF ANATOMY AND PHYSIOLOGY

The ear is the sensory organ that identifies and interprets sounds (Fig. 10-1). It also has a role in maintaining equilibrium and body position. One ear is positioned at each side of the head at eye level. There are three parts to the ear: external ear (collects sound), middle ear (transmits sound), and inner ear (passes sound to the brain).

- The auricle (pinna) is the outer visible portion of the ear made up of flexible cartilage and skin; sebaceous glands are located on the surface; helps direct sound to the eardrum, the tympanic membrane. Anatomical structures of the auricle include the following:
  - □ Helix is the prominent outer rim of the auricle.
  - □ Tragus is the protuberance anterior to the auditory canal.
  - □ Lobule is the soft lobe on the bottom of the auricle.
- Ear canal is approximately 2.5 cm long and begins at the meatus of the auricle and ends at the tympanic membrane; hairs help to trap

debris; has small glands in the skin that produce ear wax (cerumen); cerumen cleans and lubricates the ear canal due to its slightly acidic nature and has bactericidal properties to protect the ear canal against foreign bodies (Harkin & Kelleher, 2011).
- The middle ear is an air-filled chamber behind the eardrum, which includes the three smallest bones (ossicles) in our body that transmit sound waves from the eardrum to the inner ear and the eustachian tube. The three ossicles are as follows:
  - □ Malleus has the manubrium, a long handle that attaches to the mobile portion of the tympanic membrane.
  - □ Incus acts like a bridge to connect the malleus and stapes.
  - □ Stapes is the smallest bone in the body.
- Eustachian tube connects the middle ear to the nasopharynx; equalizes ear pressure on each side of the tympanic membrane.

- Cranial nerve VIII brings sound and information about one's position and movement in space into the brain (Sanders & Gillig, 2010).
- Inner ear, or labyrinth, is responsible for transmitting sound waves through the auditory nerve (CN VIII) to the brain; it contains the following:
  □ Cochlea (organ of hearing) serves as the microphone in the ear, converting sound impulses and vibrations from the outer ear into electric impulses that are sent to the brain via the acoustic nerve (cranial nerve VIII); the organ of Corti is located in the cochlea and is the sensory organ of hearing.
  □ Three semicircular canals are located in the inner ear and assist in the perception of body position and maintenance of balance (Harkin & Kelleher, 2011).

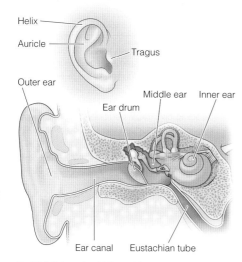

Fig. 10-1. External, middle, and inner ear.

Sound is described in terms of
- frequency: the pitch of sound, measured in Hertz (Hz)
- intensity: the loudness of sound, measured in decibels (dB).

DIAGNOSTICS

- **Audiometric testing** is a hearing evaluation to assess conductive and sensorineural hearing loss at different high and low frequencies:
  □ An audiologist has specialized training to perform hearing evaluations.
  □ The individual sits in a soundproof room or booth with a set of headphones that are connected to an audiometer, and is instructed to press a button every time she or he hears a tone at varied frequencies.
  □ The audiometer documents the results on a graph for interpretation (Sisson, 2010).

Tympanometry assesses the movement of the tympanic membrane and disorders of the middle ear. During this assessment, a soft ear bud is inserted into the ear canal, which changes the air pressure to move the tympanic membrane. The results of the changes in air pressure are recorded on a graph called a tympanogram. This graph identifies whether there is normal air pressure and normal mobility of the tympanic membrane. This assessment can identify problems leading to hearing loss, the presence of middle ear infections, fluid in the middle ear, and dysfunction of the Eustachian tube.

HEALTH HISTORY

Review of Systems

Hearing loss is usually gradual and occurs over time. Hearing assessment should start with some basic questions to determine if the individual reports being hard of hearing (HOH). Be alert to the patient's ability to hear your questions or if the patient asks you to repeat the question (Box 10-1).

■ **TIP** Observe the patient's nonverbal body language; leaning forward, tilting the head and ear toward you, and looking at your mouth are signs of hearing loss.

Medical History

■ Do you have difficulty hearing words when an individual is talking?
  □ Spoken words may sound mumbled, and the individual may have difficulty hearing above background noise.
■ Do you have difficulty communicating with others? Watching television?

□ Individuals with hearing loss have difficulty communicating with others on an equal basis.
■ Does background noise affect your ability to hear?
■ Do you have hearing loss? When did it start?
  □ Hearing loss can have a significant impact on everyday life, causing feelings of loneliness, isolation, and frustration.
  □ Hearing loss can have an economic impact; adults with hearing loss also have a much higher unemployment rate (WHO, 2014).
  □ Presbycusis is a natural process of hearing loss related to sensorineural hearing loss from death of cochlear hair cells. The most common pattern is symmetrical in which high frequencies are lost (Morrison, 2013).
  □ Hearing loss may be inherited
■ Have you had ear surgery or any injury to the ears?

BOX 10-1 **Do You Need a Hearing Test?**

If you are 18 to 64 years old, the following questions will help you determine if you need to have your hearing evaluated by a health professional. Answer YES or NO.

1. Do you have a problem with hearing over the telephone? ○Yes ○No
2. Do you have trouble following the conversation when two or more people are talking at the same time? ○Yes ○No
3. Do people complain that you turn the TV volume up too high? ○Yes ○No
4. Do you have to strain to understand conversation? ○Yes ○No
5. Do you have trouble hearing in a noisy background? ○Yes ○No
6. Do you find yourself asking people to repeat themselves? ○Yes ○No

7. Do many people you talk to seem to mumble (or not speak clearly)? ○Yes ○No
8. Do you misunderstand what others are saying and respond inappropriately? ○Yes ○No
9. Do you have trouble understanding the speech of women and children? ○Yes ○No
10. Do people get annoyed because you misunderstand what they say? ○Yes ○No

If you answered "yes" to three or more of these questions, you may want to see an otolaryngologist or an audiologist for a hearing evaluation.

Credit: "Do You Need a Hearing Test?," the National Institute on Deafness and Other Communication Disorders, National Institutes of Health, U.S. Department of Health and Human Services, adapted from Newman, C. W., Weinstein, B. E., Jacobson, G. P., & Hug, G. A. (1990). The Hearing Handicap Inventory for Adults [HHIA]: Psychometric adequacy and audiometric correlates. *Ear Hear, 11*, 430–433.

Environment

- Have you been exposed to loud noises (e.g., loud music, guns, machinery)?
  - Prolonged exposure to loud noise may cause wear and tear on the hairs or nerve cells in the cochlea that send sound signals to the brain. When these hairs or nerve cells are damaged or missing, electrical signals are not transmitted as efficiently, and hearing loss occurs (Harkin & Kelleher, 2011).

TIP Occupational hearing loss is one of the most common work-related illnesses in the United States. Four million workers go to work each day in damaging noise. Ten million people in the U.S. have a noise-related hearing loss (National Institute for Occupational Safety and Health, 2016).

Ears

- Do you wear hearing aid(s)? If so, for which ear?
  - A hearing aid is an electronic device that amplifies sound.
- Do you have a cochlear implant? If so, which ear? When did you have it implanted?
  - A cochlear implant bypasses damaged portions of the ear and directly stimulates the auditory nerve. Signals generated by the implant are sent by way of the auditory nerve to the brain, which recognizes the signals as sound (National Institute on Deafness and Other Communication Disorders, 2014).
- When was your last hearing test?

Do you have:
- Ear pain or earaches (use OPQRST or OLDCARTS mnemonic)?
- Ear discharge?
- Ringing or buzzing in your ears (tinnitus) (use OPQRST or OLDCARTS mnemonic)?
  - **Tinnitus** is the perception of sound when no actual external noise is present; it is commonly referred to as "ringing in the ears," and can manifest many different perceptions of sound, including buzzing, hissing, whistling, swooshing, and pulsing (American Tinnitus Association, n.d.). These can be symptomatic of an inner ear disorder.
- Dizziness is a feeling of lightheadedness; may lead to feeling faint and vertigo a feeling that the environment is moving; may feel like spinning, tilting, or falling. Both of these symptoms may be related to a dysfunction of the balance organs in the middle ear.

TIP Medications can damage the sensory nerves affecting hearing and balance; there are over 200 medications that are ototoxic. Tinnitus, ringing in the ears, may be the first sign of ototoxicity (Cone et al., 2013).

PREPARATION FOR ASSESSMENT

Equipment Needed
Otoscope
Tuning fork (412 Hz)

Sequence of Assessment
1. Inspecting the ear
2. Palpating the ear
3. Assessing hearing
4. Assessing the internal ear

Preliminary Steps
- Perform hand hygiene.
- Ears are assessed with the patient in the sitting position.
- The assessment is noninvasive and should not cause any discomfort.

■ Tell the patient to let you know if he or she is experiencing any discomfort or pain in the ears during the examination.

FOCUSED ASSESSMENT

TECHNIQUE 10-1: Inspecting the Ears

Purpose: To assess for ear deformities

ASSESSMENT STEPS

1. Stand in front of the patient and assess both ears for:
  □ size
  □ shape
  □ color
  □ symmetry
  □ landmarks
    • **Darwin's tubercle** is a congenital deviation that is a small cartilaginous protuberance on the helix of the ear (Fig. 10-2).

2. Assess the angle of attachment by doing the following:
  □ Draw an imaginary line from the external canthus of the eye to the top of the helix.
  □ Draw an imaginary line perpendicular to the ear (Fig. 10-3).
  □ Assess the angle of attachment.

3. Document your findings.

NORMAL FINDINGS

■ Equal size and shape bilaterally; normal size (4 to 10 cm)
■ Color same as facial skin
■ Symmetrical
■ Angle of attachment less than 10 degrees
■ No deformities, inflammation, nodules, or drainage

ABNORMAL FINDINGS

■ Asymmetrical
■ Lesions

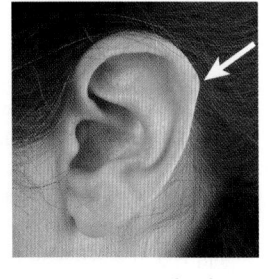

Fig. 10-2. Darwin's tubercle.

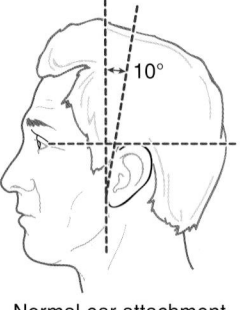

10°

Normal ear attachment

Fig. 10-3. Angle of attachment of the ears.

- Cysts
- Drainage
- Color is blue, red, white, or pale

SENC **Safety Alert** Bloody or clear drainage may be related to a perforated eardrum or head injury.

- **Cauliflower ear** occurs from repeated trauma or hitting the ear; a blood clot forms under the skin or there is damage to the cartilage causing a change in shape and structure of the ear; commonly seen in wrestlers or individuals who play contact sports.
- **Microtia** is a congenital deformity; the pinna is underdeveloped or incompletely formed; may involve one or both ears; less than 4 cm (approximately 1.5 inches) in vertical height in adults.
- **Macrotia** is abnormally large ears; greater than 10 cm (approximately 4 inches) vertical height in adults.
- **Tophi** are hard, whitish, or cream-colored, nontender deposits of uric acid crystals indicative of gout.

TECHNIQUE 10-2: **Palpating the Ears**

Purpose: To assess for tenderness

ASSESSMENT STEPS

1. Stand on the right side of the patient.
2. Gently palpate the right ear (Fig. 10-4).
  ☐ Auricles (Pinna)
  ☐ Tragus
  ☐ Earlobes
  ☐ Mastoid process
3. Stand on the left side of the patient and palpate the left ear.
4. Document your findings.

NORMAL FINDINGS

- No tenderness
- Firm consistency

ABNORMAL FINDINGS

- Tenderness may indicate inflammation.
- Swelling
- Hard lumps or nodules are present

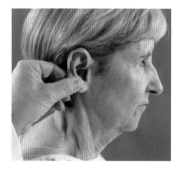

Fig. 10-4. Palpating the right ear.

TECHNIQUE 10-3: **Assessing Hearing (CN VIII)**

Purpose: To assess for impaired or loss of hearing

■ **TIP** Tests to assess hearing are subjective because you are relying on the individual's response to what he or she says is heard. The tests will only screen for hearing loss.

There are three types of hearing loss:

■ **Conductive hearing loss**, which is also considered middle ear hearing loss, is when sound is not conducted through the outer ear canal to the eardrum and the tiny bones (ossicles) of the middle ear; involves a reduction in sound level or the ability to hear faint sounds.

■ **TIP** Wax impaction is the most common cause of conductive hearing loss (Morrison, 2013).

■ **Sensorineural hearing loss**, which is considered inner ear hearing loss, occurs when there is damage to the inner ear (cochlea), or to the nerve pathways from the inner ear to the brain; speech may sound unclear or muffled; most common type of permanent hearing loss.

■ **Mixed hearing loss** includes both conductive and sensorineural hearing loss.

SENC Evidence-Based Practice The whispered voice test is an efficient method to assess hearing; it has 90 percent sensitivity and at least 80 percent specificity (Sanders & Gillig, 2010). Sensitivity indicates how likely the test is to be positive in a patient with a given disease entity. Specificity indicates how likely it is that someone without a given disease will have a negative test (Dunphy, Winland-Brown, Porter, & Thomas 2015).

TECHNIQUE 10-4: **Conducting the Whispered Voice Test**

Purpose: To assess for impaired or high-frequency hearing loss

ASSESSMENT STEPS

1. Explain the technique to the patient.

2. Place patient in the sitting position.

3. Stand behind the patient to his or her left side about 2 feet away so you cannot be seen (Fig. 10-5).

4. Ask the patient to cover the right ear that you are not testing.

5. Whisper six random letters/numbers toward the left ear. (i.e., k-g-t-2-2-0)

6. Have the patient repeat what you whispered.

7. If the patient responds incorrectly, repeat the test using a different number/letter combination.

8. Repeat steps 3, 4, 5, and 6 on the right side.

9. Document your findings.

NORMAL FINDINGS

■ Patient repeats at least three of the six letters/numbers correctly.

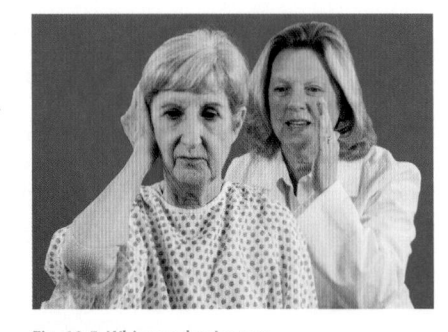

Fig. 10-5. Whispered voice test.

- Patient repeats fewer than three of the six letters/numbers correctly or did not hear what you whispered.
- Audiometric testing is in order when there are abnormal findings (Sanders & Gillig, 2010, p. 19).

TECHNIQUE 10-5: **Conducting the Weber Test**

Purpose: To assess unilateral hearing loss and functioning of the cochlear nerve (CNVIII).
Equipment: 512 Hz tuning fork
A tuning fork is a device that vibrates at a specific frequency when it is struck; it is used in simple tests for hearing and to assess vibration sense (Fig. 10-6).
ASSESSMENT STEPS

1. Place the patient in the sitting position.
2. Explain the technique to the patient.
3. Hold the base of a 512 Hz tuning fork with one hand without touching the tines.
4. Strike the tines on the back of your other hand to initiate the tines to vibrate.
5. Place the base of the tuning fork on the midline of the top of the patient's head (Fig. 10-7).
6. Ask the patient if she or he hears the sound equally on both sides or point to the ear in which the sound is heard louder.
7. To confirm results, strike the tines again on the back of your hand.
8. Ask the patient to hold a hand over the right ear, then after a couple of seconds have the person hold a hand over the left ear.
9. Ask the patient if he or she hears the sound louder in the left or right ear.
10. Document your findings.

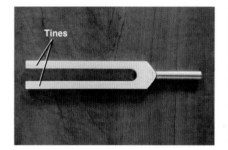
Fig. 10-6. Tuning fork.

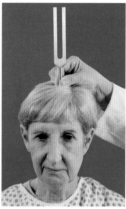
Fig. 10-7. Weber Test.

NORMAL FINDINGS
- Tuning fork sounds vibrate through the bones and the sound quality is heard equally in both ears.

ABNORMAL FINDINGS
- The bad ear seems to be softer; the damage is probably sensorineural hearing loss.
- The bad ear seems to be louder; the damage is probably conductive hearing loss.
- If the sound seems equally dull, the Weber test is inconclusive (Sanders & Gillig, 2010, p. 19).

TIP The Weber test should always be accompanied by the Rinne test to screen for hearing loss.

TECHNIQUE 10-6: **Conducting the Rinne Test**

Purpose: To assess hearing by bone conduction versus air conduction and middle ear disease
■ **TIP** The Rinne test is the more accurate test, if conductive hearing loss is suspected.
Equipment: 512 Hertz tuning fork, watch with a second hand

ASSESSMENT STEPS

1. Place patient in the sitting position.
2. Explain the technique to the patient.
3. Strike the tines on the back of your other hand to initiate the tines to vibrate.
4. Gently place the tuning fork on the mastoid bone (Fig. 10-8A), about 1 inch from the left ear; tell the patient to say "now" when he or she no longer hears the vibration sound. Time how many seconds the vibrations are heard by the patient.
5. Move the tuning fork tines perpendicular to the patient's left ear canal (Fig. 10-8B); tell the patient to say "now" when he or she no longer hears the vibrations. Time how many seconds the vibrations are heard by the patient.
6. Repeat steps 3, 4, and 5 on the right side.
7. Instruct the patient to tell you if she or he hears better with the tuning fork on the mastoid bone or next to the ear.
8. Document your findings.

NORMAL FINDINGS

■ **Positive Rinne:** Air conduction (AC) is heard twice as long as bone conduction (BC). (AC > BC)

ABNORMAL FINDINGS

■ **Negative Rinne:** Bone conduction is heard longer than air conduction (BC > AC) and is indicative of conductive hearing loss.

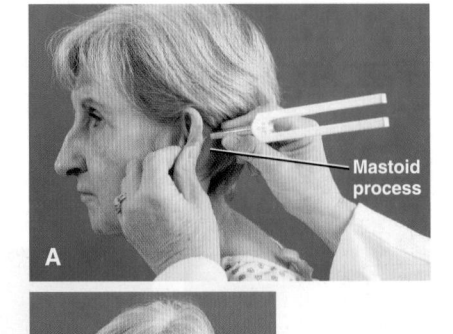

Mastoid process

A

B

Fig. 10-8. Rinne test.

SENC Evidence-Based Practice Edmiston and Camilleri (2015) conducted a controlled study to assess the accuracy of the Weber test as an aid in referral decisions for general practitioners. The study assessed 96 patients presenting with hearing loss to a local ears, nose, and throat department. It compared clinical findings on performing the Weber test with results from subsequent pure tone audiometry. Audiometry confirmed that 58 of the 96 patients (60 percent) had a degree of hearing loss. In detecting the presence of hearing loss, the Weber test had a sensitivity of 60 percent, specificity of 76 percent, and a positive predictive value of 80 percent. In detecting the presence of asymmetry, the Weber had a sensitivity of 78 percent and was most accurate at detecting conductive hearing impairment with a sensitivity of 72 percent and specificity of 88 percent. The Weber test is a useful tool for deciding whether to refer patients for further evaluation.

TECHNIQUE 10-7: **Assessing the Ears With an Otoscope**

Purpose: To assess the external auditory canal, middle ear, and eardrum
Equipment: Otoscope
An otoscope is a magnified light source to visualize the ear canal and tympanic membrane; consists of a handle, head, and different-sized disposable plastic ear specula (Fig. 10-9).

ASSESSMENT STEPS

> **SENC Patient-Centered Care** If the patient has an ear infection, this assessment may cause some discomfort. Tell the patient to let you know if he or she is experiencing pain.

1. Explain the technique to the patient.
2. Turn the light on for the otoscope and choose the largest and shortest speculum that fits comfortably in the patient's ear canal.
3. Ask the patient to sit up straight with the head tilted to the left side.
4. Hold the otoscope in your dominant hand with the handle either up or down, whichever is more comfortable for you.
5. With your other hand, use your fingers to grasp the right auricle and gently lift the auricle up and back to clearly visualize the external auditory canal.
6. Gently insert the speculum into the outer third (about one-half inch) of the ear canal (Fig. 10-10).
7. Look through the magnifying lens to assess the:
   - ☐ external ear canal
   - ☐ tympanic membrane
   - ☐ portions of the malleus (dense, whitish streak) assessed through the translucent tympanic membrane
   - ☐ umbo (the central depressed portion of the concavity on the lateral surface of the tympanic membrane)
   - ☐ cone of light (a triangular reflection when the light is focused on the malleus).
8. Gently move the light to get a full assessment of the tympanic membrane.
9. Ask the patient to tilt the head to the right side. Repeat steps 5, 6, and 7 on the left ear.
10. Document your findings.

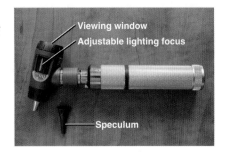

Fig. 10-9. Otoscope.

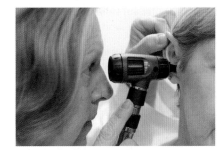

Fig. 10-10. Assessing the inner ear.

NORMAL FINDINGS

- External ear canal patent
- No inflammation or drainage
- Small amount of yellow, moist wax
- Tympanic membrane intact, pearly gray color; translucent; contour slightly conical
- Bony landmarks visible
- Cone of light present (Fig. 10-11)

    TIP You will see the cone of light in the anterior, inferior quadrant at the 7 o'clock location in the left ear and 5 o'clock location in the right ear.

ABNORMAL FINDINGS

- **Earwax (cerumen)** is a moist or dry, waxy substance that acts to protect the skin of the external ear canal from water damage, infection, trauma, and foreign bodies; usually asymptomatic but large amounts or impacted wax can cause conductive hearing loss and ear discomfort (Dinces, 2013).

SENC Safety Alert Impacted wax commonly obstructs the ear canal. There is a misconception that cerumen is related to poor hygiene; it is not. Impacted wax can be attributed to misguided attempts at cleaning. Using cotton swabs to clean the ear canal interrupts the self-cleaning mechanism and promotes accumulation of debris, pushing it in the opposite direction of the movement of the epithelium. Advise individuals not to use cotton swabs or any other equipment to clean their ears.

- **Otitis externa** is inflammation of the outer ear causing redness, inflammation, discharge, and pain; may be related to infection or swimmer's ear.
- **Otitis media** is inflammation of the inner ear causing pain, inflammation, pressure, and a build-up of fluid; bright, red bulging eardrum with diminished or no cone of light visible (Fig. 10-12).
- **Serous otitis media** is an accumulation of fluid in the middle ear caused by an obstruction of the eustachian tube; tympanic membrane will appear to be a yellowish color, with air bubbles, and bulging.
- **Otomycosis** is a fungal infection of the external auditory canal; black and white dots will be present on the eardrum or external canal.

    TIP Ear pain (otalgia) and ear drainage (otorrhea) are the most common individual complaints in which individuals seek medical care for the ears.

- **Scarred tympanic membrane** has less blood supply and appears to have white, dense, streaks and spotting; the individual may have had many ear infections during childhood.
- **Perforated tympanic membrane** is a ruptured tympanic membrane; a dark oval, hole will be present in the membrane (Fig. 10-13).

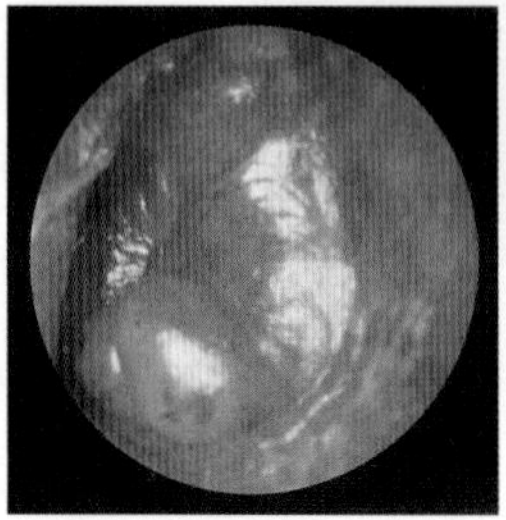

Normal Tympanic Membrane

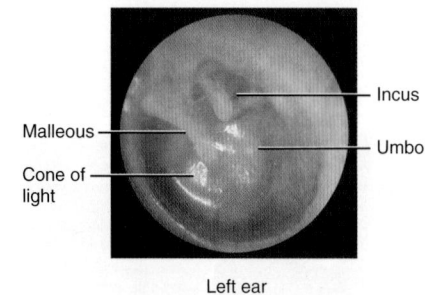

Fig. 10-11. Normal findings of the inner ear.

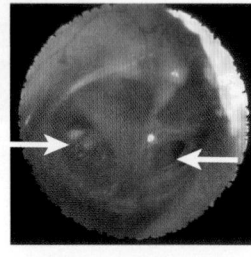

Fig. 10-12. Otitis media.

Fig. 10-13. Perforated tympanic membrane.

Healthy People 2020

Goal: Reduce the prevalence and severity of disorders of hearing and balance; smell and taste; and voice, speech, and language (HHS, 2010).

- Wear ear protection if you work with loud machinery or have social or recreational activities with loud noise, to prevent noise-induced hearing loss.
- Have a hearing test.

According to the National Institute for Occupational Safety and Health (NIOSH, 2016), occupational hearing loss is one of the most common work-related illnesses. Depending on the type of exposure and impairment, NIOSH estimates that there are between 5 and 30 million workers in the United States who are exposed to noise levels at work that put them at risk of hearing loss. An additional 9 million may be at risk due to exposure to ototoxic chemicals.

Individuals who have healthy ears and are not exposed to hazardous noises should be getting a hearing test every 3 years. Individuals should have their hearing tested annually if they:

- are regularly exposed to hazardous noise
- notice a change in hearing or develop tinnitus (ringing in the ears).

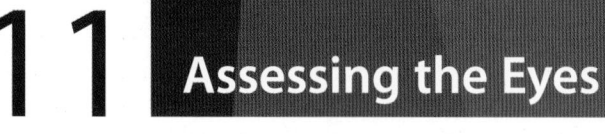

CHAPTER 11

Assessing the Eyes

INTRODUCTION

The eye is a complex organ that gives each person the ability to see and experience quality of life. Physiologically, sight occurs when the eyes and brain work together to detect, translate, and interpret incoming visible spectrum electromagnetic radiation (Shagam, 2010). Nurses assess a patient's visual acuity and external/internal structures. When assessing the eyes, you should always start from the outside of the eyes and examine the internal structures last (Gibbons, Amro, & Cox, 2009).

REVIEW OF ANATOMY AND PHYSIOLOGY

The external and internal structures of the eye work together to create vision (Fig. 11-1).

- Three cranial nerves control motor nerve activity of the eye:
  - ☐ Cranial nerve III: Oculomotor
  - ☐ Cranial nerve IV: Trochlear
  - ☐ Cranial nerve VI: Abducens
- Visual perception occurs as light waves travel through the cornea, anterior chamber, pupil, lens, and posterior chamber to the central fovea of the macula and are transformed into nerve impulses.
  - ☐ These impulses continue to travel through the optic nerve to the brain for interpretation of images.
  - ☐ The entire visual field is now interpreted and seen by the eye.

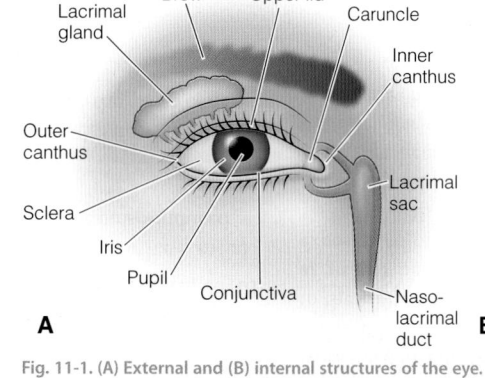

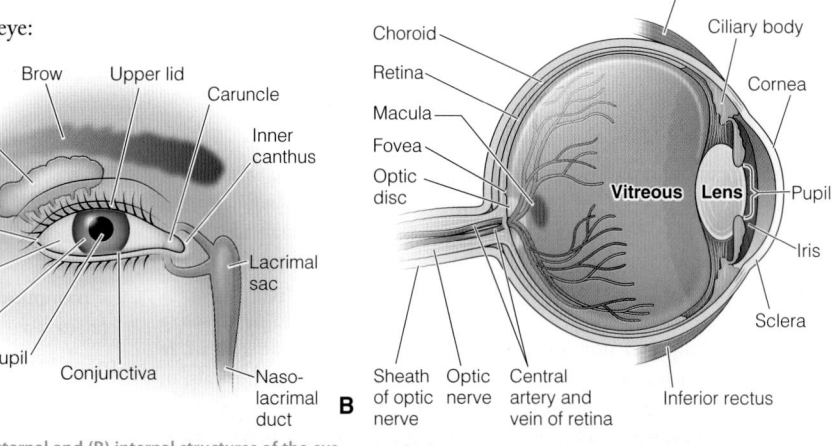

Fig. 11-1. (A) External and (B) internal structures of the eye.

- □ Eyes and brain are influenced by the parasympathetic and sympathetic nervous system.
- □ Eyes invert the image; the left side of what we see ends up in the right side of our brain, and vice versa. Optic pathways carry impulses from the retina to the occipital cortex; any damage on this pathway will cause a visual defect (Fig. 11-2).

Extraocular Structures

The following extraocular structures serve special functions for the eye (Fig. 11-1A).

- **Eyebrows and eyelashes:** specialized hairs protect the eyes.
- **Eyelids:** protect and lubricate the eyes
  - □ Small oil-producing glands line the inner edge keeping the eyes moist and clean
  - □ Tarsal plates: Firm lines of connective tissue within the eyelids that contain meibomian glands, which open on the lid margin and produce tear fluid
  - □ Palpebral fissure: Distance between the upper and lower lids
- **Conjunctiva:** thin membrane covering the front of the eye (bulbar conjunctiva) and inner eyelids (palpebral conjunctiva)
  - □ Produces mucous to lubricate the eye
  - □ Permits movement of the eyeball
- **Lacrimal glands:** the tear ducts that continually release tears and protective fluids to clean, lubricate, and moisten the eyes
  - □ Lacrimal sacs are the small pumps that drain the tears or fluid.
  - □ Tears and fluid drain into the nasolacrimal duct into the nose keeping the nasal mucosa moist.
  - □ Tear fluid: protects the conjunctiva and cornea from drying; produced from the meibomian gland, conjunctival gland, and lacrimal glands

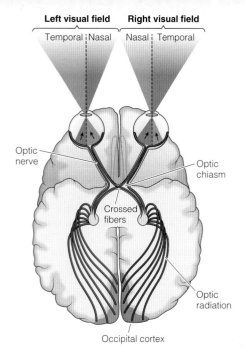

Fig. 11-2. Optic pathways.

Intraocular Structures

The following are the intraocular structures of the eye:

- **Sclera:** white avascular tissue that protects the eye and maintains the shape of the eye
- **Intraocular muscles:** six small muscles connect to the sclera to control eye movements, secure the eyeball in the sockets, and allow sight in different directions (Fig. 11-3).

☐ **Medial rectus:** moves the eye toward the nose

☐ **Lateral rectus:** moves the eye away from the nose

☐ **Superior rectus:** raises the eye

☐ **Inferior rectus:** lowers the eye

☐ **Superior oblique:** rotates the eye

☐ **Inferior oblique:** rotates the eye

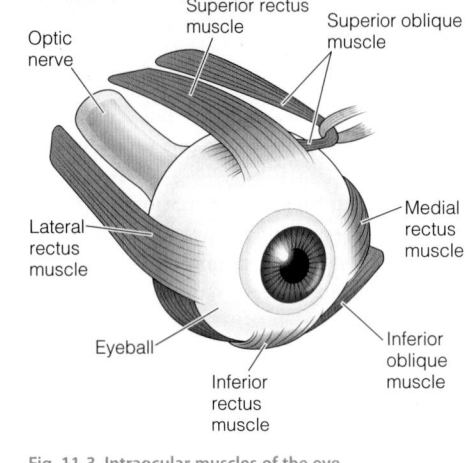

Fig. 11-3. Intraocular muscles of the eye.

■ **Aqueous humor:** water-like fluid that fills the anterior (space between cornea and iris) and posterior chambers (space between iris and front of the lens); helps to maintain the eyeball shape; a circulatory system assists to control the pressure within the eye.

■ **Choroid:** layer of blood vessels between the retina and sclera; supplies blood to the retina

■ **Iris:** composed of connective tissue and smooth muscle; colored part of the eye; color originates from microscopic pigmented cells of melanin; muscles within the iris control pupillary size allowing the pupil to contract and dilate and focus on near and distant objects

CULTURAL CONSIDERATIONS Eye color differs among people of various genetic backgrounds, with lighter eyes more prevalent in more Northern countries. Genetic background also influences the diameters of eyelids and eyebrows (Dillon, 2007).

■ **Lens:** transparent, biconvex structure that refracts light to be focused on the retina; changes shape and thickness to be able to focus on objects

■ **Pupil:** black part of the center of the eye; determines the amount of light that enters the eye; average diameter of 2 to 4 mm in bright light and 4 to 8 mm in the dark

■ **Posterior chamber:** space between the iris and the front of the lens; filled with aqueous humor that nourishes parts of the eye

■ **Cornea:** dome-shaped, avascular, transparent surface that covers the front part of the eye; covers the iris, pupil, and anterior chamber; allows light to enter and focus; considered to be the window of the eye; contains nerve endings responsible for tears, pain, and the blink reflex

■ **Fundus:** posterior section of the eye that includes the retina, choroid, fovea, macula, optic disc, and retinal vessels (Fig. 11-4)

■ **Macula:** yellow spot in the retina that is responsible for central vision; most sensitive area of the retina; fovea is the central indentation in the macula responsible for our highest visual acuity

■ **Optic disc:** bright spot on the retina where the optic nerve leaves the eye; optic nerve connects eye to brain, has about 1.2 million nerve fibers

■ **Retina:** multilayered, sensory portion that lines the back of the eye; contains millions of photoreceptors (rods and cones) that convert light rays into electrical impulses (central and peripheral vision) and transports these impulses to the optic nerve for interpretation in the brain; vision loss through damage to the retina.

■ **Retinal blood vessels, arteries, and veins:** supply blood to the retina

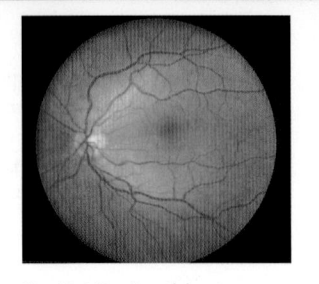

Fig. 11-4. Fundus of the eye.

- **Comprehensive dilated eye examination** is a painless procedure that allows the ophthalmologist or optometrist to examine the eyes and look directly at the retina and internal structures of the eye. During this examination, the patient has his or her eyes dilated with mydriatic eye drops. These drops are short-acting ciliary muscle paralytics that dilate the pupil (Fig. 11-5).

SENC Safety Alert Patients who go for eye examinations may have mydriatic eye drops put in their eyes to dilate the eye for assessment of the internal structures. If administered, mydriatic eye drops cause blurry vision and sensitivity to light. Sunglasses may be helpful when going outside in the sun. Patients should be instructed not to drive 1 to 2 hours after administration. Patients will need to have someone drive them home or take public transportation.

- **Tonometry** is a device to measure intraocular pressure (IOP); the device measures the outflow of the aqueous humor from the eye; creening test for glaucoma.

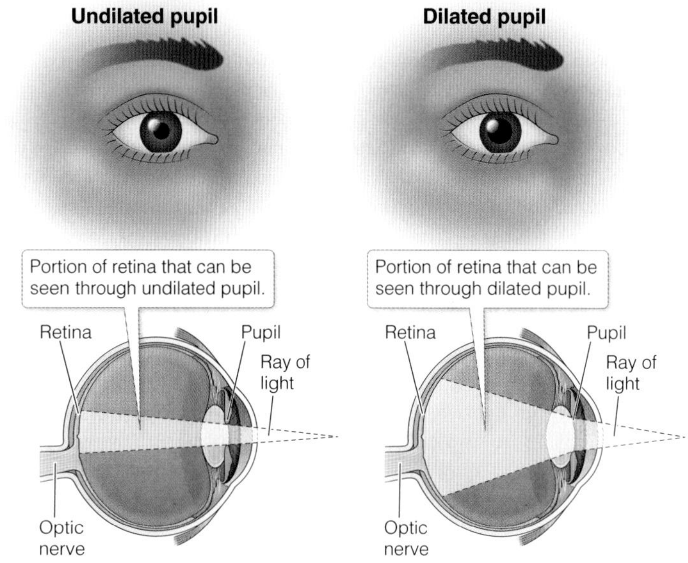

Undilated pupil   Dilated pupil

Portion of retina that can be seen through undilated pupil.

Portion of retina that can be seen through dilated pupil.

Retina   Pupil   Ray of light   Optic nerve

Retina   Pupil   Ray of light   Optic nerve

Fig. 11-5. Mydriatic eye drop eye dilation.

HEALTH HISTORY

Review of Systems

As part of the review of systems, it is important to do a focused review of the patient's ocular and surgical history. If the patient has complaints of eye pain, use the OPQRST or OLDCARTS mnemonic. Ask the patient the following questions.

Past Medical History

- Have you had any eye problems or eye diseases such as cataracts, glaucoma, or macular degeneration?
  - □ **Cataracts** are a clouding of the lens that causes blurry, decreased, or loss of vision.
  - □ **Glaucoma** is a buildup of intraocular pressure that damages the eye's optic nerve causing loss of peripheral vision.
  - □ **Macular degeneration** is a deterioration of the central part of the retina causing loss of central vision.

CULTURAL CONSIDERATIONS Open-angle glaucoma affects African Americans three to six times more often than Caucasians; it is six times more likely to cause blindness in African Americans than in Caucasians (Friedman, Kaiser, & Pineda, 2009).

- Did you have eye surgery? If so, what eye and what type of eye surgery? Were there any complications from the eye surgery?
  - ☐ Laser-assisted in situ keratomileusis (LASIK) is laser eye surgery to reshape the cornea to correct farsightedness, nearsightedness, or astigmatism.
  - ☐ Cataract surgery removes the cloudy lens and is replaced with an intraocular artificial lens.

Family History

- Do you have a family history of cataracts, congenital eye diseases, diabetes, macular degeneration, or glaucoma?
  - ☐ Patients who have family members with a history of diabetes are at greater risk of getting diabetes, and patients with diabetes are at great risk for retinopathy (a disorder of the retina) and blindness. Diabetics are 40 percent more likely to develop glaucoma and 60 percent more likely to develop cataracts (American Diabetes Association, 2013).

Health Promotion

- When was your last eye examination?
- Do you wear eye protection when needed? If so, when?

Current Vision History

- How is your vision?
  - ☐ There are two types of vision impairment: loss of visual acuity and loss of visual field.
  - ☐ **Loss of visual acuity** refers to the inability to see objects clearly. Visual acuity is assessed by having the patient read letters from a chart at a distance of 20 feet. The most common chart is the Snellen Chart (Box 11-1). Normal vision is 20/20, meaning that the patient has the ability to see from a distance of 20 feet what a person of normal vision should see at this distance (Venes, 2013, p. 42). The World Health Organization defines impaired vision as a visual acuity between 20/70 and 20/200 with the use of corrective lenses (World Health Organization, 2011).
  - ☐ **Loss of visual field** refers to the inability to see from side to side or up and down without moving the eyes or turning the head. Loss of visual field results from damage, injury, disease, or tumor that completely or partially obstructs areas on the visual pathway causing partial loss of vision. The patient may experience a blind spot in their field of vision. A normal visual field is approximately 160° to 170° in the horizontal plane; patients who have a visual field of 20° or less are considered legally blind (Shagam, 2010).
- Do you wear glasses?
- Do you wear contact lenses? Are they soft or hard? Do you sleep with them on? Do you have any problems with wearing contact lenses?
  - ☐ Redness and irritation are the most common problems with contact lenses.
- Do you have difficulty reading or seeing at a distance?
  - ☐ **Farsightedness (hyperopia):** difficulty focusing on near objects; visual image is focused behind the retina instead of on the retina.
  - ☐ **Nearsightedness (myopia):** distant objects appear blurred because the visual image becomes focused in front of the retina instead of on the retina.
- Do you have any drainage, redness or crusty eyelids?
- Do your eyes feel gritty or irritated?
  - ☐ May be indicative of a viral or bacterial infection, or dry eyes
- Do you have itching of the eyes?
  - ☐ May be indicative of allergies or dry eyes
- Have you experienced double vision?
  - ☐ Double vision, known as diplopia, may be related to a problem with the extraocular muscles, cranial nerves, or systemic disease.

BOX 11-1 **Tests to Assess Visual Acuity**

The Snellen Eye Chart is a quantitative measurement to assess visual acuity. In 1862, Herman Snellen, a Dutch ophthalmologist, designed this chart. The chart consists of eleven rows of the following capital letters: C, D, E, F, L, O, P, T, and Z. The block letters decrease in size with the largest letter on top and the smallest letters at the bottom. Each eye is assessed separately and then both eyes are assessed uncovered. The result is documented in a fraction: the numerator is the distance the patient stands from the chart which should be 20 feet (children stand 10 feet). The denominator identifies the last line the patient read correctly. Normal vision is 20/20.

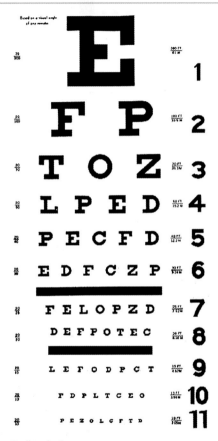

Snellen chart.

Continued

BOX 11-1 **Tests to Assess Visual Acuity—cont'd**

The Tumbling E chart has the capital letter "E" facing in different directions. The patient must see and determine which direction the E is pointing, either up, down, right, or left. The patient points his or her fingers in the direction of the "E." This is the chart to use if the patient has difficulty reading.

Another screening chart, the Rosenbaum Screening Card, is a hand-held card that provides distant visual acuity testing when held at a distance of 14 inches from the patient's face.

Tumbling E chart.

Hold card 14 inches from eye
Test vision in each eye separately (with/without corrective lenses)
Presbyopic patients should read through bifocal segment

(see back of card for Testing Central Visual Acuity information)

PUPIL GAUGE (mm.)

Rosenbaum screening card.

- Have you experienced blurry vision? If so, does it affect one or both eyes? Full vision or part of your vision? Do you have pain with the blurry vision?
  - □ Blurry vision may be a symptom of systemic disease, inflammation of the optic nerve, a hole in the retina, or a detached retina

SENC Safety Alert Sudden pain in an eye or changes in vision such as blurriness, double vision, or blind spots, could be signs of a serious eye disease or problem.

- Do you have difficulty seeing at night?
  - □ Night blindness is the inability to see well at night or in poor light; it is related to a disorder of the cells in the retina that are responsible for vision in dim light. Smoking tobacco may impair the ability to see at night (Venes, 2013).
- Do you have eye pain, either superficial or deep?
  - □ Superficial eye pain may be related to a foreign object in the eye or superficial injury. Deep eye pain may be more serious and may be related to a detached retina. Retinal detachment is separation of the retina from the tissues underneath it. Nearsightedness is risk

factor. Retinal detachment is a medical emergency (Chang, Lynm, & Golub, 2012).

- Have you seen white or dark specks in your vision?
  - □ Tiny spots or flecks in the field of vision, known as vitreous floaters, are a normal part of aging. Vitreous gel inside the eye rubs or pulls on the retina. It can occur intermittently or suddenly, though a sudden appearance of vitreous floaters and a blind spot in the vision may indicate a detached retina (*CareNotes*, 2014).
- Have you had flashing lights in your eyes? If so, when?
  - □ Flashing lights may be a sign of an oncoming ocular migraine headache or as serious as a detached retina.
- Do you have dry eyes or excessive tearing?
  - □ Dry, red, irritated eyes can manifest with several symptoms; patients who have LASIK refractive surgery have worsened dry eye problems (Bethke, 2013).
  - □ Chronic dry eyes may be related to aging, environmental factors, medications, or disease.
  - □ Excessive tearing may be related to eye irritation, allergies, or a tear drainage problem.

PREPARATION FOR ASSESSMENT

The eyes are assessed with the patient in the sitting position. The patient should inform you if he or she is experiencing any discomfort or pain during the examination.

Equipment Needed
Gauze
Gloves
Light source (e.g., penlight)
Ophthalmoscope
Pupil size measurement chart
Sterile cotton-tipped applicator

Sequence of Assessment
1. Inspect the eye.
2. Assess visual acuity.
3. Assess for color blindness.
4. Assess central vision.
5. Assess peripheral vision.
6. Assess ocular motility.
7. Assess for accommodation.
8. Assess pupil size and consensual response.
9. Assess internal structures using ophthalmoscope.

FOCUSED ASSESSMENT

TECHNIQUE 11-1: Inspecting the Eyes

Purpose: To assess the anterior eye structures
Equipment: Light source and Gloves

ASSESSMENT STEPS

1. Stand in front of the patient.
2. Inspect the eyelids.
  ☐ Observe that the eyelids open and close completely.
  ☐ Assess for any drainage.
3. Inspect the eyelashes for
  ☐ Distribution
  ☐ Drainage
  ☐ Crusting
4. Inspect the eyebrows.
  ☐ Assess symmetry.
  ☐ Assess distribution of hair and any scaly, flaky skin.
5. Inspect the cornea.
  ☐ Use a light source to inspect side to side the cornea for smoothness and clarity.
6. Inspect the lens.
  ☐ Use a light source to inspect side to side the lens of the eye for clarity.
  ☐ Use light source to inspect the color and round shape (Fig. 11-6).
7. Assess the sclera for color.
8. Inspect the conjunctiva.
  ☐ Use your thumbs to slide the bottom eyelids down to assess the mucosa of the lower conjunctiva (Fig. 11-7).
  ☐ Ask the patient to look up.
  ☐ Inspect the color of the mucosa.
9. Inspect the lacrimal duct.
  ☐ Wearing gloves, inspect and palpate the lacrimal duct for any swelling or excessive tearing (Fig. 11-8).

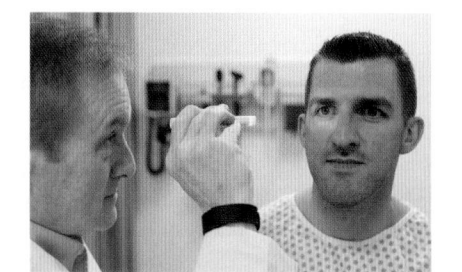

Fig. 11-6. Inspecting the eye, cornea, lens, and sclera using a light source.

10. Assess palpebral fissures.
   □ Assess the distance of the upper lid to the lower lid for symmetry (Fig. 11-9).
   □ Compare the palpebral fissures on each side of the face.
11. Inspect for abnormal involuntary eye movements.
12. Document your findings.

NORMAL FINDINGS

- Eyes symmetrical; no protrusion
- Upper and lower eyelids close completely; no redness or drainage; no drooping of an eyelid (ptosis); upper eyelid covers half of the iris.
- Eyelashes equally distributed; no drainage
- Eyebrows evenly distributed; no scaly or flaky skin; symmetrical
- Cornea clear with no opacities
- Lens transparent with no opacities
- Pupils equal in size
- Iris blue, green, brown, or hazel in color, smooth
- Sclera white
- Conjunctiva pink and moist
- Lacrimal ducts clear with no swelling
- Palpebral fissures equal bilaterally
- No abnormal involuntary movement

CULTURAL CONSIDERATIONS The most prominent characteristic of the Asian eyelid is the absent or very low lid crease and fuller upper eyelid (Saonanon, 2014).

ABNORMAL FINDINGS

- **Ptosis** is drooping of the eyelid caused by muscle or nerve dysfunction, injury or disease.
- **Blepharitis** is an inflammation and infection of the eyelid margins. The eyelid margin becomes red, crusty, and greasy due to too much oil being produced by the eye glands.
- **Blocked lacrimal duct** causes excessive tearing because tears cannot drain properly.

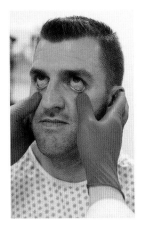

Fig. 11-7. Inspecting the conjunctiva.

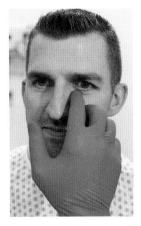

Fig. 11-8. Palpating the lacrimal ducts.

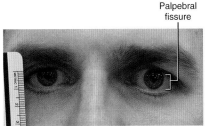

Palpebral fissure

Fig. 11-9. Assessing palpebral fissures.

- **Cataract** is opacity of the lens caused by aging, long-term exposure to ultraviolet light, metabolic disorders, trauma, or medications.
- **Conjunctivitis** is a bacterial or viral infection causing erythema of the sclera and yellow-green drainage of the conjunctiva.
- **Corneal abrasion** is a painful scratch to the clear surface of the eye, usually related to trauma to the eye.
- **Ectropion** is an everted eyelid (turns outward).
- **Entropion** is an inverted eyelid (turns inward).
- **Exophthalmos** is a protrusion of the anterior portion of the eyeball; common in hyperthyroidism; may cause patient to have dry eyes and difficulty closing the lids.
- **Hordeolum,** a stye, is an infection of a follicle of an eyelash that causes redness, inflammation, and a lump at the site.
- **Scleral jaundice** (Icterus) is a sign of elevated bilirubin in the blood; occurs with patients who have a liver disease.
- **Pterygium** is a gelatinous, abnormal growth of the conjunctiva; occurs more commonly on the nasal side of the eye.
- **Periorbital edema** is swelling in the tissues around the eye.

TECHNIQUE 11-2: **Assessing for Visual Acuity (CN II)**

Purpose: To measure a patient's vision to see details at near and far distances

Equipment: Snellen chart

TIP If the patient wears glasses or contact lenses, they should be worn during the vision assessment. Reading glasses should not be worn. Document if the patient has worn his or her glasses or contact lenses during the assessment.

ASSESSMENT STEPS

1. Explain the technique to the patient.
2. Place the chart at a comfortable height for the patient's height.
3. Have the patient stand 20 feet from the chart (Fig. 11-10).
4. Cover the left eye and have the patient start reading the lines out loud starting from the top and working down the chart. The patient reads the row from left to right.
5. Ask the patient to read each line. The patient can miss one or two letters and be considered to have vision equal to that line.
6. Repeat steps 4 and 5 by covering the right eye.
7. Repeat steps 4 and 5 with both eyes uncovered.
8. Document the last line that was correctly read for each assessment.

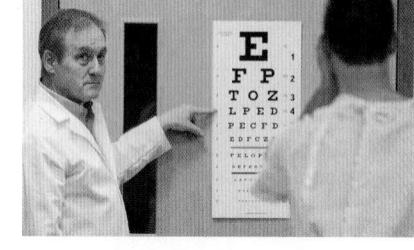

Fig. 11-10. Assessing visual acuity using a Snellen Chart.

TIP The results in a Snellen test are recorded using two numbers. The top number is the distance the patient is standing from the chart. The lower number indicates the distance at which an individual with normal eyesight could read the same last line that the patient correctly read. For example, 20/20 is considered normal. A result of 20/30 (-2) indicates that the last line the patient correctly read all letters correctly except for 2 letters at 20 feet away, can be read by an individual with normal vision from 30 feet away (NIH, 2015).

NORMAL FINDINGS

■ Normal distant visual acuity is 20/20; this means that the patient can read what a person with normal eyesight can read at 20 feet.

ABNORMAL FINDINGS

■ A higher denominator means poorer distant visual acuity.

■ **Nearsightedness,** known as **myopia,** is poor visual acuity; distant objects appear blurred because the images are focused in front of the retina rather than on it. The denominator is greater than 20.

■ **Farsightedness,** known as **hyperopia,** is the ability to see distant objects clearly, but objects nearby may be blurry.

■ **Presbyopia** is the inability to focus clearly on near objects; the patient holds the print farther away to focus; magnifying glasses are used to read.

■ **Legal blindness** is visual acuity of 20/200 or more; this means that the patient standing at 20 feet can see what a patient with normal vision can see at 200 feet or a visual field diameter less than 20 degrees; these patients can only see straight in front of them.

TIP An example of the medical abbreviations for documentation of the eyes is OS (left eye) 20/40 (-1), OD (right eye) 20/30 (-2), OU (both eyes) 20/40 (-2).

TECHNIQUE 11-3: **Assessing for Color Blindness**

Purpose: To assess the ability to distinguish colors

Equipment: Ishihara plates

There are 24 plates to look at. Plates 1–17 each contain a number, plates 18–24 contain one or two wiggly lines. To pass each test you must identify the correct number, or correctly trace the wiggly lines. This test is available online at http://colorvisiontesting.com/ishihara.htm

TIP Color blindness is a nerve cell dysfunction causing the eye to misinterpret colors; the most common colors affected are red, green, or blue; may be inherited or found in patients with suspected retinal or optic nerve disease.

ASSESSMENT STEPS

1. Explain the technique to the patient.

2. Ask the patient to look at the colored bars on the Snellen chart (if available).

3. Ask the patient to identify the embedded figures or numbers on each Ishihara plate within 3 to 5 seconds. (Fig. 11-11).

4. Document the patient's results.

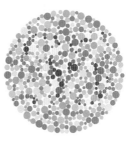

Fig. 11-11. Ishihara plate.

NORMAL FINDINGS
- The patient is able to correctly identify the colors or figures.

ABNORMAL FINDINGS
- The patient incorrectly identifies the colors or figures or does not see the colors or figures. This may indicate color blindness.

TECHNIQUE 11-4: **Using the Amsler Grid for Assessing Central Vision**

Purpose: To assess central vision
Equipment: Amsler grid
Reading glasses should be worn during this assessment. Instruct the patient to hold the Amsler grid the same distance from the eyes as if he or she was reading any type of reading material (Fig. 11-12).

ASSESSMENT STEPS
1. Explain the technique to the patient.
2. Have the patient cover the left eye.
3. Instruct the patient to focus on the dark dot in the center of the grid with the exposed right eye.
4. Ask if any of the lines are distorted, broken, or blurred.
5. Ask if there are any missing areas or dark areas in the grid.
6. Ask if he or she can see all the corners and sides in the grid.
7. Have the patient cover the right eye and repeat the test on the left eye.
8. Mark the areas on the Amsler Grid that the patient is not seeing correctly.
9. Document your findings.

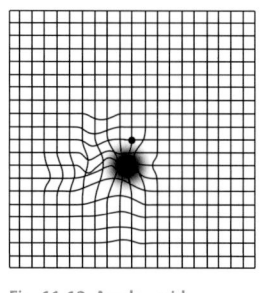

Fig. 11-12. Amsler grid.

NORMAL FINDINGS
- No lines look distorted, broken, or blurred.

ABNORMAL FINDINGS
- Lines look distorted, broken, or blurred.
- **Macular degeneration,** which is a breakdown of cells in the macula of the retina, causes loss of central vision.

TECHNIQUE 11-5: **Using Confrontation Test for Visual Field Testing (CN III, IV, and VI)**

Purpose: To assess peripheral vision, overall field of vision, and for blind spots
Equipment: None

■ **TIP** Visual defects commonly occur in the temporal fields.

ASSESSMENT STEPS

1. Face the patient.
2. Explain the technique to the patient. Instruct the patient to say "now" when he or she can see your fingers and state how many fingers he or she can see.
3. Cover your right eye; the patient covers his or her left eye with a hand.
4. Instruct the patient to look directly with his or her right eye into your uncovered eye.
5. Place your left hand with extended fingers behind the patient's field of vision. Now, move your fingers toward the patient's field of vision, stopping when the patient says "now" and states how many of your fingers he or she sees in the peripheral field.
6. At the time the patient says "now," estimate the angle the fingers are first seen.
7. Repeat assessing the field of vision from four different angles (Fig. 11-13):
   □ Superiorly
   □ Temporal
   □ Nasal
   □ Inferiorly
8. Assess whether the patient's peripheral vision corresponds with your visual fields.
9. Cover the opposite eye and repeat steps 3 through 7.
10. Document your findings.

NORMAL FINDINGS

■ The patient sees your fingers at the same time as you do and correctly states the number of fingers he or she sees.
■ Peripheral vision should be seen:
   □ Superiorly (50 degrees)
   □ Temporal (90 degrees)
   □ Nasal (60 degrees)
   □ Inferiorly (70 degrees)

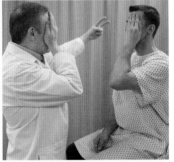

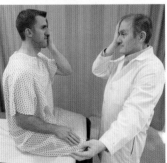

Fig. 11-13. Assessing visual field using confrontation test.

ABNORMAL FINDINGS

- This test is considered to be significant when the patient does not see your fingers at about the same time that you do; may be related to loss of peripheral vision or blind spots in the eye. The patient will need a referral to an ophthalmologist.
- **Scotoma** is an area of reduced or absent vision surrounded by an area of normal vision.
- **Hemianopia** is when half of the visual field is lost.

TECHNIQUE 11-6: Testing for Ocular Motility: Six Cardinal Positions of Gaze (CN III, IV, VI)

Purpose: To assess the functioning of the ocular muscles
Equipment: Penlight (optional)

ASSESSMENT STEPS

1. Explain technique to the patient.
2. Use your finger or hold an object in your hand (e.g., penlight) about 12 to 14 inches from the patient's face.
3. Instruct the patient not to move his or her head but to follow your finger or the object with just the eyes.
4. If the patient is unable to follow without moving his or her head, gently hold the patient's head in place.
5. Move the object in six different positions using a wide "H" or "star" pattern to assess the six cardinal positions (Fig. 11-14); pause between lateral and upward movements.
6. Document your findings.

   TIP Pausing in between changing positions allows you to watch for any involuntary movements of the eye.

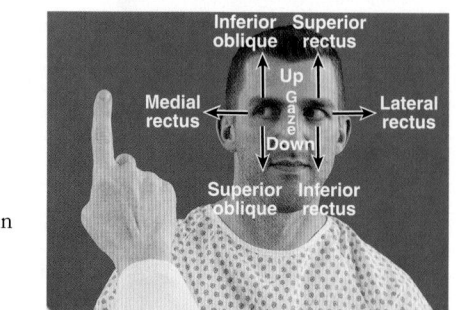

Fig. 11-14. Six cardinal positions of gaze.

NORMAL FINDINGS

- The eyes have a normal pattern of movement in each of the six cardinal directions. Mild nystagmus in the lateral angles is normal.

ABNORMAL FINDINGS

- Patient is not able to follow the pattern of movement in each of the six cardinal directions may indicate ocular muscle weakness; patient may experience double vision (diplopia) or uncontrolled eye movements.
  - □ **Diplopia** is a subjective complaint that may be related to a muscular dysfunction of the eye or neurological problem.
  - □ **Nystagmus** is an involuntary, cyclical movement of the eyes; occurs when the patient gazes or follows an object; may also occur if the patient has a fixed gaze in the peripheral field; may indicate a neurological disorder.

TECHNIQUE 11-7: **Testing for Convergence and Accommodation (CN II and CN III)**

Purpose: To assess the accommodation reflex of the eye
Equipment: Penlight (optional)

ASSESSMENT STEPS

1. Explain the technique to the patient.
2. Hold a penlight or your finger in front of the patient's eyes about 14 inches in front of his or her nose.
3. Instruct the patient to focus on your finger or object for 30 seconds.
4. Instruct the patient to follow your finger or object as you move it toward his or her nose (Fig. 11-15).
5. Assess for convergence and pupil size (pupils should constrict).
6. Document your findings.

NORMAL FINDINGS

■ Both eyes converge and both pupils constrict (accommodation) simultaneously to focus on a near object.

ABNORMAL FINDINGS

■ Pupils do not converge or constrict.

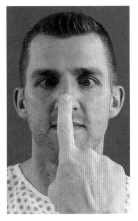

Fig. 11-15. Testing for convergence and accommodation.

TECHNIQUE 11-8: **Inspecting Pupil Size and Consensual Pupil Response (CN II and CN III)**

Purpose: To assess the pupillary light reflex that controls the diameter of the pupil, and to assess the integrity of the optic pathways (consensual pupil response)
Equipment: Penlight and Pupil-size measurement chart

1. Explain the technique to the patient.
2. Stand in front of the patient.
3. Use the penlight to inspect the pupils.
4. Assess color.
5. Assess shape of each pupil.
6. Assess symmetry.

7. Assess direct reaction. Shine light into the right eye pupil.

8. Assess consensual reaction. Put your nondominant hand between the patient's two eyes. Shine light into the left eye pupil and assess the right eye; right eye should constrict and have a consensual response (Fig. 11-16).

9. Repeat steps 7 and 8 in the left eye.

10. Measure the size of each pupil in millimeters (Fig. 11-17).

11. Document your findings.

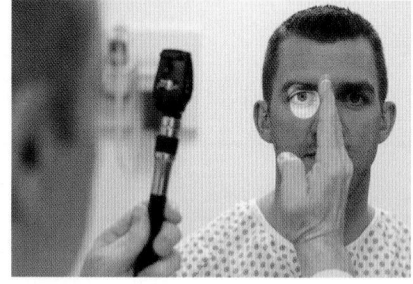

Fig. 11-16. Assessing consensual reaction.

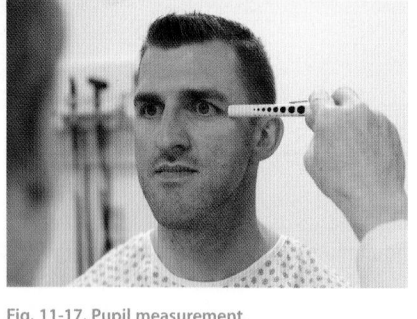

Fig. 11-17. Pupil measurement.

NORMAL FINDINGS

- Pupils constrict in response to light
- Both eyes have a consensual response on constricting to direct light.
- Pupil is round and black.
- Both pupils are equal size.
- Pupil diameter is 2 to 8 mm.

ABNORMAL FINDINGS

- Pupils are unequal in size or both dilated or constricted and fixed.
- **Anisocoria** is unequal size of the pupils; may be genetics, medications, or related to a neurological disorder (Fig. 11-18).

   TIP Occasionally, the pupil size may temporarily differ; if no other symptoms and pupillary reactions are normal, it is nothing to worry about.

- **Mydriasis** is bilateral dilated and fixed pupils; may be caused by eye drops, stimulation of sympathetic nerves, anesthesia, or central nervous system injury.
- **Miosis** is an abnormal constriction of the pupils; may be caused by a stroke, medications, or brain damage.
- **Horner syndrome** is a sign of a medical condition that affects one side of the face; drooping eyelid, constricted pupil (miosis).

   TIP Use the mnemonic PERRLA for Pupils are Equal, Round, and React to Light and Accommodation to document the assessment.

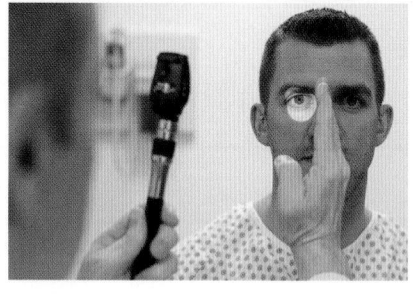

Fig. 11-18. Anisocoria and unequal pupil size.

ADVANCED ASSESSMENTS

The registered nurse does not routinely assess the internal structures of the eye but should know about why the assessment is performed. This technique requires practice to be able to perform a thorough and accurate assessment.

TECHNIQUE 11-9: **Assessing the Eyes With an Ophthalmoscope**

Purpose: To assess the internal structure of the eyes through a beam of light through the pupil that illuminates the internal structures of the eye
Equipment: Ophthalmoscope (Box 11-2)

■ **TIP** If you (the nurse) wear glasses or contact lenses, you do not have to take them off for this assessment. If the patient wears glasses or contact lenses, the patient must remove them.

SENC Safety Alert Remember to ask if the patient had eye surgery. Do not use the ophthalmoscope in the eye that had surgery because the eye is sensitive, and this may cause damage to the eye.

BOX 11-2 **Ophthalmoscopes**

Ophthalmoscopes work by redirecting bright light through a prism and into the eye. That light reflects off the retina and returns to the instrument in the form of a magnified image to assess the internal structures of the eye. There are two different types of ophthalmoscopes:

- A *standard ophthalmoscope* includes a light, a mirror with a single aperture through which the examiner views, and a dial holding several lenses that are selected to allow clear visualization of the structures of the eye.
  - When assessing with a standard ophthalmoscope, make sure the room is darkened or the lights dimmed to allow the eyes to be naturally dilated. When assessing the left eye, hold the standard ophthalmoscope in your left hand and use your left eye; when assessing the right eye, hold the standard ophthalmoscope in your right hand and use your right eye,
- *PanOptic ophthalmoscope* provides a panoramic view of the fundus that is five times larger than standard ophthalmoscopes (Welch Allen, 2013).
  - You do not need to use specific eyes or hands when using the PanOptic ophthalmoscope; it is recommended to use what is most comfortable for the healthcare provider.

Each ophthalmoscope has separate directions, so be sure to read the directions carefully, because there is a difference between the standard and PanOptic ophthalmoscope.

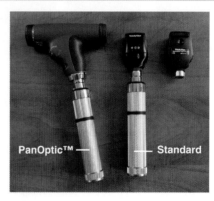

Ophthalmoscopes.

SENC Patient-Centered Care Shining a bright light directly into the pupil of the eye over an extended period of time can cause fatigue and discomfort. If necessary, allow short periods of rest during the assessment. Tell the patient to verbalize any discomfort.

ASSESSMENT STEPS

1. Explain the technique to the patient.
2. Turn on the light for the standard ophthalmoscope.
3. Dial the ophthalmoscope diopter power to "0."
   ▪ **TIP** A diopter is a unit of measurement of the optical power of the lens to converge or diverge light. Use your index finger to control the wheel to change the setting of the diopter to adjust your focus.
4. Check to make sure you can see clearly through the ophthalmoscope's viewing hole, the aperture.
5. Dim the lights so the room is darkened; this will make the pupils dilate to help visualize the internal structures.
6. Make sure the patient is seated comfortably; instruct the patient to look at a distant object or focal point over your shoulder.
   ▪ **TIP** Gently remind the patient not to stare or focus on a focal point because the pupil will constrict.
7. Gently place your nondominant hand on the patient's forehead or shoulder to stabilize.
8. Hold the ophthalmoscope in your right hand. Position the ophthalmoscope about 12 inches away and from a 15-degree lateral angle to the patient's line of vision (Fig. 11-19).
   ▪ **TIP** Try to keep your opposite eye open during the assessment while looking through the ophthalmoscope aperture.
9. Look through the aperture with your right eye and direct the light into the patient's right pupil and try to find the red reflex (Fig. 11-20), an orange, red glow in the pupil; assess for any opacities interrupting the red reflex.
   ▪ **TIP** The red reflex is a red reflection of light illuminating from the retina, the layer of tissue at the back of the inner eye. If you lose the reflection or cannot see this red reflection; try to reposition the ophthalmoscope.

SENC Safety Alert Patients with artificial eyes or cataracts do not have a red reflex. If the red reflex cannot be found, this may be a medical emergency, and the patient should be referred immediately to an ophthalmologist.

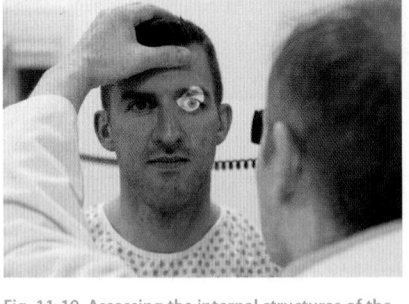

Fig. 11-19. Assessing the internal structures of the eye.

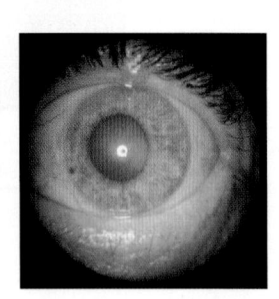

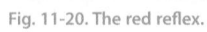

Fig. 11-20. The red reflex.

10. Slowly move toward the pupil maintaining the 15 degree lateral angle adjusting the lens disc focusing dial to positive (+) numbers to maintain clarity of viewing the anterior structures.

   ■ **TIP** If structures are blurry, adjust the lens disc for a sharper focus. If you or the patient is nearsighted, rotate the lens disc to the minus numbers; if you or the patient is farsighted, move the disc to the plus diopters.

11. Change the lens disc to minus (–) or red numbers as you assess the posterior structures: the internal eye structures will be more clearly visualized.

   SENC Safety Alert Be careful not to touch the pupil directly with the standard ophthalmoscope; the ophthalmoscope should only be close enough for assessment of the internal structures of the eye; you may have to go as close as the patient's eyelashes to clearly see the internal structures.

12. Look for a blood vessel, and follow the blood vessel to the optic disc.

13. Assess the optic disc for:
    ☐ Color: yellow/orange to creamy pink color
    ☐ Shape: round or oval
    ☐ Disc outline: sharp or cloudy
    ☐ Central physiologic cup (if present): brighter yellowish, white color
    ■ **TIP** You will recognize the central physiologic cup; the horizontal diameter is usually less than half the horizontal diameter of the optic disc.

14. Assess the retina:
    ☐ Arteries: light red; smaller diameter
    ☐ Veins: dark red; larger diameter
    ■ **TIP** You should see a paired artery and vein progressing to each quadrant of the fundus. An artery and vein may cross over, this is known as Arteriovenous (A-V) Crossing. Assess for any interruption in blood flow.
    ☐ Retinal background: red-orange uniform color

15. Instruct the patient to look directly into the light source to assess the macula: yellow, oval shaped with a highly pigmented darker, yellow center spot and the fovea, the center of the macula.

16. Repeat steps 8 through 15 on the left side.

17. Document your findings.

NORMAL FINDINGS (SEE FIG. 11-4)
- Optic disc: round; defined borders, color is a creamy yellow, yellow orange, or pink
- Physiologic cup: slightly depressed, lighter in color
- Cup-disc ratio: cup is less than half of the optic disc's diameter.
- Retinal arteries: light red, progressively narrower as they move away from the optic disc
- Retinal veins: darker red, progressively narrower as they move away from the optic disc
- Retinal background: consistent uniform red-orange color
- Macula: oval to round shape; darker yellow, highly pigmented

ABNORMAL FINDINGS

- **Gunn's Sign:** an arteriole is crossing a venue and impedes circulation; this may be seen in patients with hypertension (Cotton, 2011).
- **Cotton wool spots:** look like puffy white patches on the retina. They are caused by swelling of the surface of the retina, ischemia, and damaging nerve fibers; commonly seen in diabetic and hypertensive patients.
- **Diabetic retinopathy:** damage to the blood vessels of the retina; development of new vessels resulting from ischemia, lack of oxygen and poor circulation. This is a common complication of diabetes which eventually may lead to blindness.
- **Drusen bodies:** yellow deposits of normal cell metabolic by-products in the eye; seeing some drusen bodies is normal with aging; however, large amounts in the macula may be a sign of aging macular degeneration.
- **Papilledema:** optic disc swelling caused by increased intracranial pressure along the optic nerve. The optic disc appears swollen and loses its distinctive shape.

PATIENT EDUCATION

Healthy People 2020

Goal: Improve the visual health of the nation through prevention, early detection, timely treatment, and rehabilitation. The Healthy People 2020 vision objectives focus on evidence-based interventions to preserve sight and prevent blindness (HHS, 2010).

- **Encourage a comprehensive eye examination.** Many common eye diseases such as glaucoma, diabetic eye disease, and age-related macular degeneration often have no warning signs. A dilated eye examination is the only way to detect these diseases in their early stages.
- **Eat right to protect your sight.** A diet rich in fruits and vegetables, particularly dark leafy greens such as spinach, kale, and collard greens, is important for keeping your eyes healthy. Eye health benefits from eating fish high in omega-3 fatty acids, such as salmon, tuna, and halibut.
- **Wear protective eyewear.** Wear protective eyewear when playing sports, doing activities around the home, and protecting your eyes at work.
- **Protect your eyes from the sun's ultraviolet rays.** When purchasing sunglasses, look for ones that block out 99 to 100 percent of both UV-A and UV-B radiation.
- **Give your eyes a rest.** If you spend a lot of time at the computer or focusing on any one thing, you sometimes forget to blink and your eyes can get fatigued. Try the 20-20-20 rule: Every 20 minutes, look away about 20 feet in front of you for 20 seconds. This can help reduce eye strain.
- **Clean your hands and your contact lenses properly.** To avoid the risk of infection, always wash your hands thoroughly before putting in or taking out your contact lenses.

Assessing the Respiratory System

INTRODUCTION

The respiratory system is composed of organs and tissues that work together to help an individual breathe. The average adult takes 12 to 20 breaths per minute (bpm). Lungs mature by age 25 and after age 35 lung function begins to decline (American Lung Association, 2017). The major function of the lungs is gas exchange and the delivery of oxygen to all parts of the body. Total lung capacity is about 6 liters. The circulatory, musculoskeletal, and neurological systems work to maintain the respiratory system. Chronic disease, smoking, environmental factors, and developmental considerations need to be assessed during a respiratory assessment.

REVIEW OF ANATOMY AND PHYSIOLOGY

Upper Respiratory Tract

The upper respiratory tract includes the nose and the oropharynx (Fig. 12-1).

Nose

- The respiratory cycle begins as air enters through the nostrils.
- Air moves through the nasal cavity where it warms, humidifies, and is filtered.

Oropharynx

- This is the passageway between nose, sinuses, larynx, and trachea.
- The larynx contains the voice box and vocal cords; cartilage in the front of the larynx is called the Adam's apple.
- Major roles are speech, breathing, and the ability to talk; its closing mechanism prevents aspiration of liquids and solids during swallowing (Venes, 2013).
- No air exchange occurs in the oropharynx.

Lower Respiratory Tract

Trachea

- The trachea (windpipe) is composed of rings of cartilage lined with pseudostratified ciliated columnar epithelium.
- The function of the trachea is allowing air to flow into the bronchi of the lungs.

Bronchi

- There are two bronchi: the right and left main bronchi.
- Right bronchus is shorter, wider, and more vertical than the left bronchus.
- Left bronchus is smaller in size but longer in length.
- Their function is to warm and moisten air as it moves in and out of the respiratory tract.

  TIP Since the right bronchus is wider, objects are more easily aspirated into the right bronchus (Story, 2012).

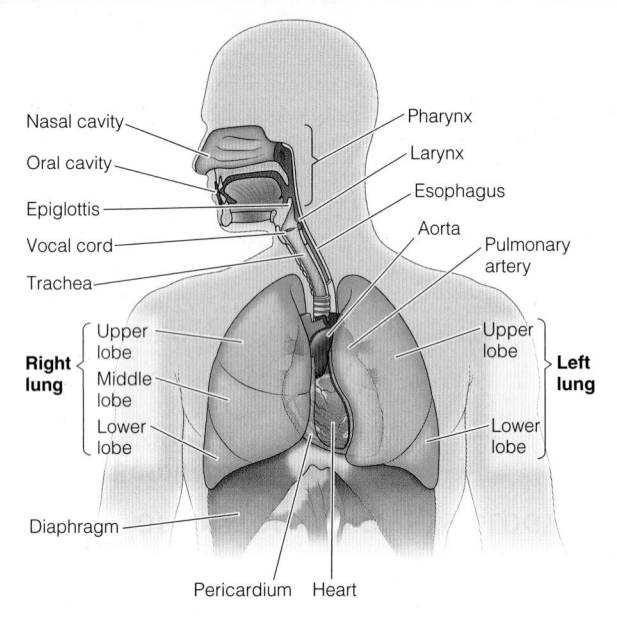

Fig. 12-1. Upper and lower respiratory tract.

Bronchioles

- Smaller branches of the bronchial tree
- Transitional airways that support gas exchange

Alveoli

- Smallest air sacs of the lungs
- Made up of squamous cells
- Secrete a surfactant, a substance that reduces the surface tension and keeps the alveoli moist
- Air is diffused through small capillaries into arterial blood (external respiration).

- Gases move across systemic capillaries; exchange of oxygen and carbon dioxide occurs at the cellular level (internal respiration).

Lungs

- Two cone-shaped, air-filled structures
- Right lung is larger and heavier, has three lobes divided by an oblique and horizontal fissure, and is about an inch shorter than the left lung.
- Left lung has two lobes divided by an oblique fissure and is longer and narrower than the right lung.
- They work with the heart to circulate oxygen throughout the body.

Acid-Base Balance

- The lungs control the blood pH through the release of carbon dioxide from the lungs; carbon dioxide is a waste product of oxygen metabolism.
- During each respiratory cycle, inhalation and exhalation, oxygen and carbon dioxide are exchanged at the alveoli tissue level; the lungs release carbon dioxide to maintain the acid-base balance.
- Changes in carbon dioxide influence the respiratory center in the brain by increasing or decreasing the respiratory rate to maintain the acid-base balance.

Pleura

- A serous membrane that forms a two-layer protective lining around the lungs
- There are two types of pleurae:
  - □ Parietal pleura lines and adheres to the thoracic wall; produces a serous fluid known as pleural fluid between the two pleurae to keep the area lubricated so the two layers can move easily.
  - □ Visceral pleura covers the outer surface of the lungs; it secretes a serous fluid that also lubricates the pleural cavity to help keep the lungs expanded.
- Pleural cavity is the area between the parietal and visceral layers that contains the pleural fluid.

Thoracic Cage

- Closed cavity consisting of bones, muscles, and cartilage of the thorax
- Protects internal organs and supports the upper body
- Consists of seven pairs of ribs that form the anterior and lateral parts of the thorax and join directly to the sternum; the cartilage of ribs 8, 9, and 10 articulates with the cartilage of rib 7, whereas the pairs of 11 and 12 are free floating and do not articulate anteriorly.
- Mediastinum is the space in the chest between the sternum and the vertebral column that houses the heart, trachea, esophagus, thymus gland, and major blood vessels. It does not include the lungs.
- Muscles of the thoracic cage are the internal, external, and accessory costal muscles.
- Accessory muscles of neck and chest assist the respiratory system in times of distress and during exercise; they respond from a command from the brain and nervous system.

Diaphragm

- A dome-shaped muscle that lies at the bottom of the chest cavity; it is the principal muscle of respiration.
- It separates the thoracic and abdominal cavities.
- During inhalation, the diaphragm contracts and the thoracic cage expands as air is drawn into the lungs, decreasing the air pressure in the thoracic cavity; during exhalation, the diaphragm relaxes and air flow re-enters the thoracic cavity, thereby increasing the air pressure in the thoracic cavity.
- The phrenic nerve controls the diaphragm; it originates from cranial nerves C3-C5.

Landmarking the Thoracic Cage

In performing any assessment, it is important to identify specific landmarks to help you reference your assessment findings (Fig. 12-2).

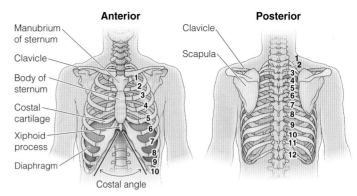

Fig. 12-2. Landmarking the thoracic cage.

Anterior Thorax

- Clavicle
- Manubrium
- Sternum
- Xiphoid process
- Costal angle

Posterior Thorax

- Vertebral column
  - □ Scapula
  - □ Cervical vertebrae (C1-C7)
  - □ Thoracic vertebrae (T1-T12)

Lobes of the Lungs (Fig. 12-3)

- Anterior lobes of the lung:
  - □ RUL
  - □ RML
  - □ RLL

□ LUL
□ LLL
- Posterior lobes of the lung
   □ RUL
   □ RLL
   □ LUL
   □ LLL

DIAGNOSTICS

- **Pulse oximeter** measures the oxygen saturation; this is the percent of arterial hemoglobin saturated with oxygen; a pulse oximeter reading should normally be higher than 95 percent (Fig. 12-4).
- Measuring **arterial blood gases** means measuring the levels of oxygen and carbon dioxide in the blood; sites are the radial, brachial, or femoral artery. The radial artery is the most common site.
- **Thoracentesis** is insertion of a needle into the thoracic cavity; the test is performed for analysis or removal of fluid from the pleural space for diagnostic or therapeutic purposes (Venes, 2013).
- **Bronchoscopy** is a diagnostic or therapeutic procedure that provides direct visualization of the larynx, trachea, and bronchial tree. A fiberoptic bronchoscope with a light is inserted through the patient's nose or mouth into the trachea or bronchi (Van Leeuwen & Bladh, 2015); this procedure is usually performed while the patient is anesthetized or under conscious sedation.
- **Lung biopsy** removes a small piece of lung tissue for analysis; the tissue can be removed during a bronchoscopy, needle biopsy, or surgery.
- The **Mantoux tuberculin skin test** is the standard method of determining whether a person is infected with *Mycobacterium tuberculosis*. This test is performed by injecting 0.1 mL of tuberculin-purified protein derivative (PPD) under the top layer of skin usually of the forearm. The skin is assessed for a reaction within 48 to 72 hours after administration (CDC, 2016).

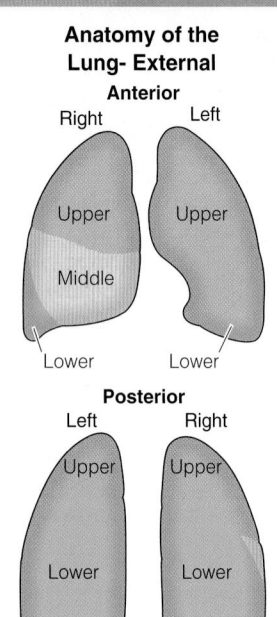

Anatomy of the Lung- External

Fig. 12-3. Lobes of the lungs.

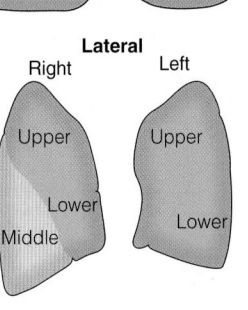

Fig. 12-4. Using a pulse oximeter.

HEALTH HISTORY

Review of Systems

Respiratory symptoms may be related to but not limited to several different causes, such as acute and chronic respiratory infections or disease, cardiac, metabolic, gastrointestinal, and even psychological problems. As with any assessment, the assessment findings must be reviewed in relation to the patient's history.

SENC Patient-Centered Care Active listening and therapeutic communication provide the patient with the comfort and ease to freely express his or her story. Be sensitive to a patient's privacy and only uncover the upper thorax area during the assessment. Be sure to explain the sequence of the assessment.

Ask the patient the following questions.

Past Medical History

■ Do you have any pulmonary disease (e.g., asthma, chronic obstructive pulmonary disease [COPD], cystic fibrosis)? When were you diagnosed? How are you being treated?

☐ **Asthma** is a reactive airway disease causing inflammation, increased mucus production, and narrowing of the bronchi; symptoms include cough, congestion, shortness of breath, and wheezing.

☐ **COPD** is an obstructive and progressive lung disease causing inflammation and destruction of the lung tissue; symptoms include shortness of breath and congestion. Smoking is the leading cause of COPD (American Lung Association, 2015).

☐ **Cystic fibrosis** is a hereditary disease of the exocrine glands; the body produces abnormally thick and sticky mucus that obstructs the lungs and digestive organs.

■ Have you had any acute or chronic respiratory infections (e.g., bronchitis, pneumonia)?

☐ **Bronchitis** is a viral or bacterial infection causing inflammation of the bronchi; the most common symptoms are fever, cough, and lung congestion.

☐ **Pneumonia** (PNA) is a viral, bacterial, or fungal infection of the lung causing inflammation and congestion in the alveoli of the lung; symptoms include fever, cough, congestion, and shortness of breath.

Medications

■ Do you take any medications to improve your breathing? Bronchodilators? Inhalers?

☐ Patients take oral medications and inhalers for many chronic lung diseases to improve airflow to the lungs.

Psychosocial Assessment

■ What is your occupation?

■ Have you been exposed to any environmental pollutants?

☐ Some occupations such as coal mining or working in factories may place patients at risk for inhalation of asbestos and chemicals that can cause pulmonary disease, lung cancer, or affect their breathing.

■ Do you smoke? How many cigarettes or packs per day? How many years?

☐ Smoking strips the lungs of their normal defenses and paralyzes the natural cleansing processes. Smokers usually have an early morning cough.

☐ Pack-year history is a quantitative measurement of a lifetime exposure to tobacco.

▐ **TIP** To calculate pack-year smoking history: Multiply the number of packs of cigarettes smoked each day times the number of years. For example, if the patient smokes 1 pack of cigarettes (20 cigarettes) daily for 25 years (20/20 x 25) = 25 pack-year history for smoking. If a patient smokes ½ pack (10 cigarettes) for 5 years (10/20 x 5) = 2.5 pack-year history for smoking.

- Are you exposed to secondhand smoke? If so, how often? How long?
  - ☐ Secondhand smoke is also known as environmental tobacco smoke. Secondhand smoke is a mixture of two forms of smoke that come from burning tobacco:
    - Sidestream smoke: smoke from the lighted end of a cigarette, pipe, or cigar. Sidestream smoke has higher concentrations of cancer-causing agents (carcinogens) than mainstream smoke (American Cancer Society [ACS], 2015).
    - Mainstream smoke: smoke exhaled by a smoker

Health Promotion

- If age appropriate, have you had the Pneumovax vaccination?
  - ☐ The pneumococcal polysaccharide vaccination (PPSV23) is recommended for all adults age 65 years and older and 19 years of age and older with high-risk medical conditions; information on these conditions may be found at the CDC website at http://www.cdc.gov/vaccines/vpd-vac/pneumo/vac-PCV13-adults.htm#recommendations

Breathing

- Do you ever feel short of breath? If so, when?
  - ☐ **Dyspnea** is an uncomfortable awareness of breathing; shortness of breath, with or without pain; related to air hunger.
  - ☐ **Cardiac dyspnea** is difficulty breathing related to an inadequate cardiac output.
  - ☐ **Expiratory dyspnea** is difficulty breathing associated with chronic obstructive lung disease; wheezing is usually present (Venes, 2013).
  - ☐ **Orthopnea** is difficulty breathing while lying in the supine position.
  - ☐ **Paroxysmal nocturnal dyspnea** is shortness of breath when the patient is asleep in bed; sits upright to attempt to relieve the shortness of breath; symptom of left ventricular heart failure.
- Is your shortness of breath affected by change of position?

- How many pillows do you sleep on at night?
  - ☐ Patients with respiratory distress or congestive heart failure with fluid in the lungs may be more comfortable sleeping on several pillows at night to improve their ability to breathe.
- How far can you walk without becoming short of breath?
- Do you use oxygen daily or as needed? If so, how many liters per minute?
- How severe would you rate your shortness of breath on a scale of 1 to 10?
- Does a certain position relieve your shortness of breath?

  SENC Safety Alert Patients having difficulty talking between breaths with an increased respiratory rate is a sign of respiratory distress.

Cough

- Do you have a cough? Describe your cough. When did it start or how long have you had it?
- Do you cough up any mucus (sputum)? If so, how much (i.e., "size of a dime or quarter or more?")? What color? Do you notice any blood in the sputum (hemoptysis)?
  - ☐ Nonproductive or dry cough has no sputum production.
  - ☐ Productive cough has mucus produced and expectorated.
  - ☐ Hacking cough is a persistent dry cough, as in many respiratory infections (Venes, 2013).
  - ☐ Chronic cough occurs daily for a minimum of 3 weeks.

Chest Pain

- Do you have chest pain?
  - ☐ There are noncardiac causes of chest pain.
  - ☐ Pleuritic chest pain is pain related to inflammation of the pleurae of the lung.

CULTURAL CONSIDERATIONS Ethnic differences in asthma prevalence, morbidity, and mortality are highly correlated with poverty, urban air quality, indoor allergens, lack of patient education, and inadequate medical care.

- In the United States, the populations that have high rates of poor asthma outcomes are African Americans, Hispanics, and Puerto Ricans. This burden has environmental, socioeconomic, and behavioral causes (Asthma and Allergy Foundation, 2016).
- African-American subjects are among those at greatest risk for asthma; it is unclear whether this increased risk solely represents differences in environmental exposures and health care or whether there is a predisposing genetic component (Rumpel et al., 2012).
- The risk of contracting tuberculosis (TB) among Hispanics/Latinos is more than four times the risk among non-Hispanics; also appears to be a significant problem among migrant workers.
- Tuberculosis (TB) is second only to HIV/AIDS as the greatest killer worldwide due to a single infectious agent (World Health Organization [WHO], 2014).

PREPARATION FOR ASSESSMENT

Read This First!

Begin in the front (anterior) or the back (posterior). *Example:* Start with inspection of the anterior, then move through palpation, percussion, and auscultation of the anterior before moving to the posterior. Because the anterior, posterior, and lateral lobes of the lung need to be assessed, you need to know that all four techniques are performed on one side before moving on to the lobes of the lungs on the other side.

Equipment Needed
Stethoscope

Sequence of Assessment
1. Inspection
2. Palpation
3. Percussion
4. Auscultation

Preliminary Steps
Completely inspect, palpate, percuss, and auscultate the anterior or posterior thorax. The lateral lobes may be assessed during the anterior or posterior assessment.

- Instruct the patient to sit on the side of the examining table.
- Advise the patient to breathe normally.
- Always compare findings at the same level on each side as you perform each assessment technique.
- Keep the anterior chest covered until you are assessing the anterior lungs; maintain modesty for all patients.

Mapping the Thoracic Cage
Mapping the thorax will help you landmark and stay organized with your assessment.

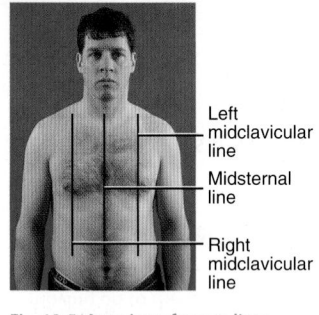

Left midclavicular line

Midsternal line

Right midclavicular line

Fig. 12-5. Anterior reference lines.

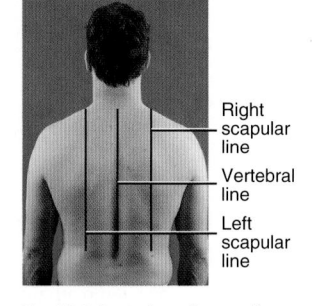

Right scapular line

Vertebral line

Left scapular line

Fig. 12-6. Posterior reference lines.

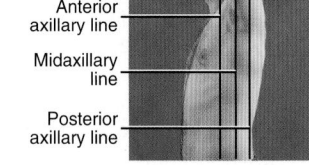

Anterior axillary line

Midaxillary line

Posterior axillary line

Fig. 12-7. Lateral reference lines.

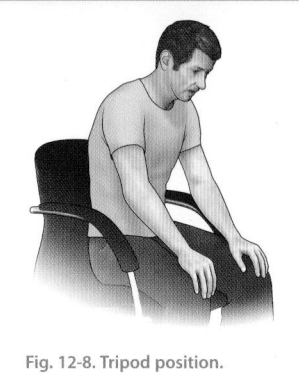

Fig. 12-8. Tripod position.

Anterior Reference Lines (Fig. 12-5)
- Right midclavicular line
- Midsternal line
- Left midclavicular line

Posterior Reference Lines (Fig. 12-6)
- Right scapular line
- Vertebral line
- Left scapular line

■ **TIP** Scoliosis and kyphosis, skeletal deformities, may limit thoracic cage excursion (see Chapter 16).

Lateral Reference Lines (Fig. 12-7)
- Anterior axillary line
- Midaxillary line
- Posterior axillary line

■ **TIP** Instruct a patient who is dyspneic to assume the position that is comfortable for him or her. Patients in respiratory distress may assume the tripod position to facilitate expansion of the lungs (Fig. 12-8).

TECHNIQUE 12-1: **Inspecting the Thoracic Cage**

Purpose: To inspect the size and shape of the thoracic cage

ASSESSMENT STEPS

1. Place the patient in the sitting position.

2. Inspect the anterior, posterior, and lateral thoracic cage for:
- ☐ size
- ☐ shape
- ☐ symmetry

☐ color
☐ respiratory rate and rhythm.

3. Document your findings.

NORMAL FINDINGS

- Transverse diameter is approximately twice the anteroposterior (AP) diameter; AP-to-transverse ratio is approximately 1:2, and the costal angle is less than 90 degrees (Fig. 12-9).
- Conical shape; smaller at the top and widens at the bottom
- Symmetrical; sternum is symmetrical; clavicles and scapula are the same height; chest movement is symmetrical.
- Skin color is uniform and intact; hair distribution is consistent with gender and ethnicity.
- Normal adult respiratory rate (eupnea) is 12–20 breaths per minute; even and smooth respirations; normal inspiratory-to-expiratory ratio (I: E) is 1:2; the expiratory phase is longer than the inspiratory phase.

■ **TIP** Do not tell the patient that you are taking the respiratory rate because this may change the breathing pattern.

ABNORMAL FINDINGS

- **Barrel chest:** anterior posterior-to-transverse ratio is 1:1, and the costal angle is greater than 90 degrees; increase in the costal angle may be a sign of chronic obstructive pulmonary disease (Fig. 12-10).
- **Pectus excavatum** (funnel chest): a congenital deformity; sternum is abnormally depressed or sunken into the chest (Venes, 2013).
- **Pectus carinatum** (pigeon breast): is a deformity of the chest; the sternum protrudes out from the chest.
- **Intercostal and accessory muscle retractions** may indicate problems with air movement; prolonged inspiratory phase may indicate upper airway obstruction; prolonged expiratory phase may indicate lower airway obstruction.
- **Abnormal respirations** (Table 12-1)
- **Abnormal skin color** (Table 12-2)
- **Pursed lip breathing** is breathing through the nose and exhaling through pursed lips; lips look like the patient is whistling; commonly seen in patients with chronic obstructive pulmonary disease to reduce the work of breathing.

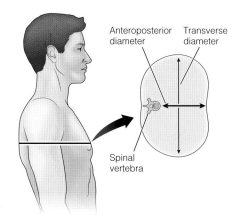

Fig. 12-9. Normal AP diameter.

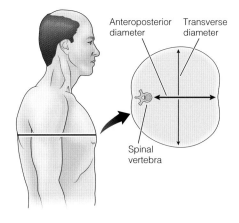

Fig. 12-10. Barrel chest.

TABLE 12-1 Abnormal Respiratory Rates and Rhythms

Type	Description
Bradypnea	Abnormally slow respirations, <12 breaths/minute
Tachypnea	Abnormally rapid respirations, >20 breaths/minute, usually shallow
Kussmaul Respirations	Respirations that are regular but abnormally deep and increased in rate
Biot Respirations	Irregular respirations of variable depth (usually shallow), alternating with regular or irregular periods of apnea (absence of breathing); also called ataxic breathing
Cheyne-Stokes Respirations	Gradual increase in depth of respirations, followed by gradual decrease and then a period of apnea; also called periodic respirations
Apnea	Absence of breathing

From Wilkinson, J. M., & Treas, L. S. (2015). *Fundamentals of nursing* (3rd ed.). Philadelphia, PA: F.A. Davis.

TABLE 12-2 Abnormal Skin Color Related to Respiratory Problems

Skin Color	Indication
White	Poor circulation Lack of oxygen Pallor
Blue	Cyanosis Lack of oxygen in the blood Respiratory infection Airway obstruction
Red	Vasodilatation Infection High blood pressure

TIP In dark-skinned patients, assess for color changes in the mucous membranes and the conjunctiva of the eye; cyanosis may be present as gray or whitish (not bluish) skin around the mouth, and the conjunctivae may appear gray or bluish. In patients with yellowish skin, cyanosis may cause a grayish-greenish skin tone. In general, mucosa may appear darker in people of Mediterranean, Asian, or African descent. (Sommers, 2011)

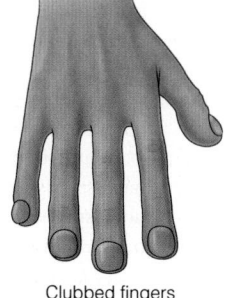
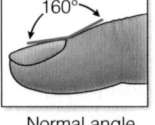
Normal angle of nail bed

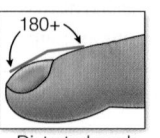
180+
Distorted angle of nail bed

Clubbed fingers

Fig. 12-11. Clubbing of fingernails.

- **Clubbing of nail plates** occurs with chronic lack of oxygen or hypoxia. The tips of the fingers and nails change in shape and size (Fig. 12-11).
  - ☐ The nailbeds soften. The nails may seem to "float" instead of being firmly attached.
  - ☐ The nail forms a sharper angle with the cuticle greater than 180 degrees.
  - ☐ The last part of the finger may appear large or bulging. It may also be warm and red.
  - ☐ The nail curves downward so it looks like the round part of an upside-down spoon (U.S. National Library of Medicine, 2016).

TECHNIQUE 12-2: **Palpating the Thorax**

Purpose: To assess surface characteristics or tenderness of the thoracic cage

  SENC Patient-Centered Care Tell the patient to let you know if she or he feels any tenderness, discomfort, or shortness of breath.

ASSESSMENT STEPS

1. Explain the technique to the patient.

2. Place the patient in the sitting position.

3. Using your finger pads, gently palpate the anterior, posterior, and lateral thoracic cage (Fig. 12-12) and assess:

  ☐ surface characteristics

  ☐ temperature

    ■ **TIP** Use dorsal surface of your hand to assess temperature.

  ☐ moisture

  ☐ tenderness

4. Document your findings.

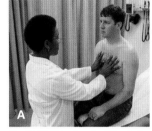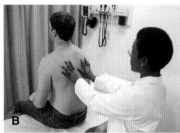

Fig. 12-12. Palpating the (A) anterior and (B) posterior thorax.

NORMAL FINDINGS

■ Surface is smooth and uniform

■ Warm skin

■ Skin dry

■ No tenderness

ABNORMAL FINDINGS

■ Irregular surface (lumps or masses)

■ Temperature cool, clammy

■ Tenderness

■ **Crepitus** (a light crackling or popping feeling under the skin caused by leakage of air into the subcutaneous tissue); sounds like Rice Krispies cereal popping under the skin

TECHNIQUE 12-3: **Palpating for Symmetrical Expansion**

Purpose: To assess symmetrical expansion of the thoracic cage

  SENC Patient-Centered Care Warm your hands by rubbing them together prior to placing on thoracic cage.

ASSESSMENT STEPS

1. Explain the technique to the patient.

2. Place the patient in the sitting position.

3. Place your warmed hands on the posterior chest wall with thumbs at level T (thoracic) 9 or T10.

4. Pinch up a small fold of skin between your fingers.

5. Instruct the patient to inhale deeply through the nose and to exhale through the mouth.

6. Observe chest expansion and the expansion of your hands and thumbs (Fig. 12-13).

7. Repeat steps 3 through 6 on the anterior chest wall at the xiphoid process.

8. Document your findings.

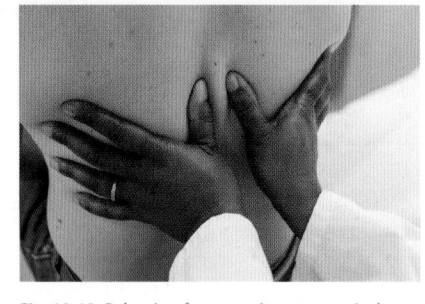

■ **TIP** Anterior symmetrical lung expansion should be assessed with the anterior thorax assessment. A good assessment always minimizes position changes for the patient.

Fig. 12-13. Palpating for posterior symmetrical expansion.

NORMAL FINDINGS

■ Thumbs move apart symmetrically with inspiration and return to the original position with expiration.

ABNORMAL FINDINGS

■ Asymmetrical expansion indicates decreased air movement in that side of the lung; may be related to pneumonia, airway obstruction, or pathology in the lung.

TECHNIQUE 12-4: **Palpating Tactile Fremitus**

■ **TIP** Do not palpate over scapula because bone changes the sound and alters the feel of the vibration.

Purpose: To palpate voice sound vibrations through the bronchi

ASSESSMENT STEPS

1. Explain the technique to the patient.

2. Place the patient in the sitting position.

3. Instruct the patient to repeat words such as "ninety-nine," "coin," "toy," or "boy" in a low-pitched voice.

4. Anterior: Starting just below the clavicle, use palmar base (ball of your fingers) or the ulnar side of your hands and palpate down the anterior lobes as the patient keeps repeating the same word.

5. Posterior: Starting just below the scapula, use palmar base (ball of your hands) or the ulnar side of your hands and palpate down the posterior lobes as the patient keeps repeating the same word (Fig. 12-14).

6. Document your findings.

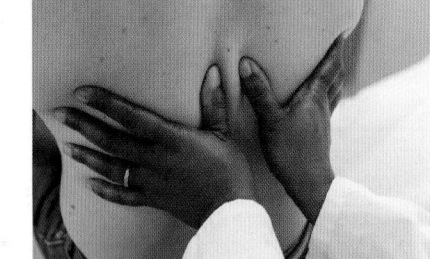

Fig. 12-14. Palpating for tactile fremitus.

TIP Chest wall thickness, voice pitch, and airway size can decrease the ability to palpate the sounds generated from the larynx.

NORMAL FINDINGS
- Palpable vibrations of sounds are felt equally on both sides of the lungs.

ABNORMAL FINDINGS
- The palpable vibration is not felt equally on both sides.
- **Increased fremitus** may indicate increased density of the lung tissue; may be related to fluid or pathology in the lung that is changing the density or compressing the lung tissue, such as pneumonia.
- **Decreased fremitus** may indicate the vibrations are obstructed with fluid (pleural effusion), decreased air movement (emphysema), obesity, or increased musculature.

TECHNIQUE 12-5: **Percussing the Thorax**

Purpose: To assess the presence of air in each lung and the density of underlying lung tissue

TIP Do not percuss over bony prominences.

ASSESSMENT STEPS

1. Explain the technique to the patient.
2. Place the patient in the sitting position.
3. Assess anterior lungs. Using the indirect percussion technique, percuss the intercostal spaces moving from the apex to the base on each side of the anterior lung fields, noting the tones of the percussion sounds (Fig. 12-15A).
4. Assess posterior lungs. Using the indirect percussion technique, percuss each side of the posterior lung fields moving from the apex to the base, noting the tones of the percussion sounds (Fig. 12-15B).
5. Instruct the patient to raise one arm at a time and percuss the lateral lung fields. Using the indirect percussion technique, percuss each side of the lateral lung fields moving from the apex to the base noting the tones of the percussion sounds (Fig. 12-15C).
6. Document your findings.

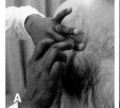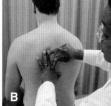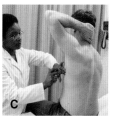

Fig. 12-15. Percussing the (A) anterior, (B) posterior, and (C) lateral thorax.

NORMAL FINDINGS
- Resonance is the low-pitched, clear, hollow sound that is percussed over healthy, air-filled lung fields.

ABNORMAL FINDINGS

■ **TIP** Lung consolidation (lung tissue is filled with liquid) occurs when the lung tissue that is normally filled with air has become filled with a dense, solid exudate or tissue; may occur in pneumonia.

■ **Dullness sounds** are soft and muffled and heard over areas of increased density; may be heard over solid mass or areas of increased consolidation such as pneumonia or pleural effusion (fluid between the layer of tissues that line the lungs) (Dugdale & Hadjiliadis, 2012).

■ **Hyperresonance** is a low-pitched, drumlike, accentuated percussion sound heard in the lungs when the bronchi and alveoli are overinflated as in emphysema or asthma.

TECHNIQUE 12-6: **Auscultating the Lungs**

Purpose: To assess airflow throughout all lobes of the lungs

Equipment: Stethoscope

PRELIMINARY STEPS

■ If the patient has a hairy chest or back, dampen the area with a warm wet cloth or apply a thin coat of Surgilube on the diaphragm of the stethoscope to decrease the friction.

■ While auscultating, note the pitch and characteristics of the sounds, and the duration and loudness of inhalation versus exhalation.

■ Never auscultate over bone.

■ **TIP** Never auscultate over the patient's clothing to ensure clarity of the sounds.

ASSESSMENT STEPS

1. Explain the technique to the patient.

2. Place the patient in the sitting position.

3. Warm the diaphragm of the stethoscope between your hands.

4. Instruct the patient to inhale and exhale through the mouth.

SENC Safety Alert The patient should breathe more deeply than normal. If the patient begins to feel lightheaded or starts to hyperventilate, allow the patient to rest.

5. Assess anterior lung fields. Start at the apex of the lungs. Place your stethoscope above the clavicle, then go to the 2nd ICS, and continue to auscultate down to the bases, noting what lobe of the lung that you are auscultating. Listen to one full inhalation and exhalation cycle (Fig. 12-16A).

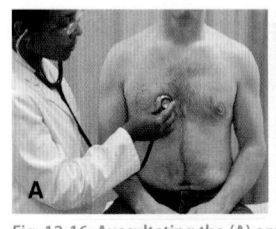

Fig. 12-16. Auscultating the (A) anterior, (B) posterior, and (C) lateral thorax.

TIP Closing your eyes helps you to focus and concentrate better to hear and differentiate normal from abnormal breath sounds.

6. **Assess posterior lung fields.** Start at the apex of the lungs. Place your stethoscope above the scapula, then go in-between the spine and the shoulder blades; continue to auscultate down to the bases, noting what lobe of the lung that you are auscultating. Listen to one full inhalation and exhalation cycle (Fig. 12-16B).

7. **Assess lateral lung fields.** Auscultate at the intercostal spaces moving from the apex to the base on right and left lateral lung fields noting breath sounds (Fig. 12-16C).

8. Document your findings.

NORMAL FINDINGS

- Bronchial breath sounds are heard over the trachea and larger bronchi; expiratory sounds are louder and last longer than inspiratory sounds and have a pause between them; high-pitched, hollow, tubular breath sounds.
- Bronchovesicular sounds are heard over the right and left bronchi; anteriorly over the mid-chest and between the scapula posteriorly; these are medium-pitched sounds.
- Vesicular sounds are heard throughout the periphery of the lungs; inspiration sound is longer and louder than expiration; soft, low-pitched, rustling sounds.

ABNORMAL FINDINGS

- It is abnormal to hear bronchial breath sounds when they are not in the normal locations.
- Breath sounds are diminished.
- Adventitious breath sounds are sounds not normally heard in a chest (Table 12-3).

TIP Some adventitious sounds are cleared with coughing; ask the patient to cough and then reassess the breath sound.

SENC **Safety Alert** A priority assessment for a patient who has/had an injury to the C-3 to C-5 vertebrae is the respiratory assessment; this cervical plexus innervates the diaphragm, the muscle that supports normal respirations.

TABLE 12-3 Adventitious Breath Sounds

Breath Sound	Description
Crackles (rales)	Produced by air passing over retained airway secretions or the sudden opening of collapsed airways Usually heard at the end of inspiration but may be heard on inspiration or expiration May be cleared by coughing Fine crackles are soft, high-pitched sounds; sounds like crunching, or a fine rubbing sound Course crackles are louder, low-pitched lung sounds (sounds like ripping open Velcro)
Wheezes	Caused by narrowed passageways in the trachea-bronchial tree by secretions, inflammation, obstruction, or a foreign body High-pitched, whistling or musical sound
Rhonchi (sonorous wheeze)	Rhonchi are louder, deeper, lower-pitched wheezes occurring in the upper bronchi; may be related to obstruction of the larger airways: commonly heard during exhalation; sounds like snoring.
Pleural Friction Rub	Caused by inflammation of the parietal and visceral pleurae that normally slide without friction Deep loud, harsh, leathery sound Painful; patient may have shallow respirations
Stridor	Heard loudest over the trachea during inspiration Indicates upper airway narrowing or obstruction Sign of respiratory distress Medical emergency

ADVANCED ASSESSMENTS
. . . .
Abnormal transmission of sounds requires further assessment.

TECHNIQUE 12-7: **Auscultating Bronchophony**

■ **TIP** Lung disease or some type of lung pathology may increase the resonance and clarity of voice sounds. These assessments are done when abnormal breath sounds are auscultated.

Purpose: To assess air flow through the lungs

Equipment: Stethoscope

ASSESSMENT STEPS

1. Explain the technique to the patient.

2. Place the patient in the sitting position.

3. Warm diaphragm of the stethoscope between your hands.

4. Instruct the patient to lean forward slightly.

5. Instruct the patient to repeat one of the words "ninety-nine," "coin," "toy," or "boy."

6. Auscultate the posterior lung fields moving from the apex to the base on each side of the posterior lung fields, noting the intensity of the sound and distinction of the word.

7. Document your findings.

NORMAL FINDINGS

■ The word "ninety-nine," "coin," "toy," or "boy" will become less distinct and muffled as you move to the lower chest.

ABNORMAL FINDINGS

■ The word "ninety-nine," "coin," "toy," or "boy" if clearly auscultated may indicate congestion in the lungs such as pneumonia.

TECHNIQUE 12-8: **Auscultating Egophony**

Purpose: To assess air flow through the lungs

Equipment: Stethoscope

Egophony is a change in timbre, pronunciation of sound, from "Ee to A" (Spira, 1995).

1. Explain the technique to the patient.
2. Place the patient in the sitting position.
3. Warm diaphragm of the stethoscope between your hands.
4. Instruct the patient to lean forward slightly.
5. Instruct the patient to repeat the letter "Ee."
6. Auscultate the posterior lung fields moving from the apex to the base on each side of the posterior lung fields, noting the distinct sound and clarity of the letter "Ee."
7. Document your findings.

NORMAL FINDINGS

- The letter "Ee" will become less distinct and muffled as you move to the lower chest.

ABNORMAL FINDINGS

- The letter "Ee" sound changes to the short letter "aaa" sound in areas of increased lung density or consolidation.

TECHNIQUE 12-9: **Auscultating Whispered Pectoriloquy**

Purpose: To assess air flow through the lungs

Equipment: Stethoscope

ASSESSMENT STEPS

1. Explain the technique to the patient.
2. Place the patient in the sitting position.
3. Warm diaphragm of the stethoscope between your hands.
4. Instruct the patient to lean forward slightly.
5. Instruct the patient to repeat the words "ninety-nine" or "one-two-three."
6. Auscultate the posterior lung fields moving from the apex to the base on each side of the posterior lung fields, noting the clarity of the spoken words.
7. Document your findings.

NORMAL FINDINGS

- The words "ninety-nine" or "one-two-three" are indistinct or faint.

ABNORMAL FINDINGS

- The words "ninety-nine" or "one-two-three" are clear and distinctly heard if there is lung consolidation such as pneumonia or increased tissue density, as with lung cancer.

TECHNIQUE 12-10: **Assessing Peak Expiratory Flow Rate**

Purpose: To assess lung functioning and forced expiratory volume of air in the lungs
Equipment: Peak flow meter

A peak flow rate is measured by a peak flow meter. A peak flow meter is a portable, inexpensive, handheld device used to measure how air flows from your lungs in one "fast blast." In other words, the meter measures your ability to push air out of your lungs (American Lung Association, 2017). Peak flow meters measure your peak expiratory flow rate (PEFR), a number that correlates with how open the lung's airways are (Fig. 12-17); when the airways in the lungs narrow, the PEFR decreases.

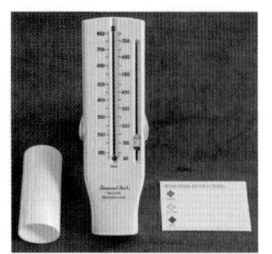

Fig. 12-17. Peak flow meter.

■ **TIP** Make sure the peak flow meter reads zero or its lowest reading.

This technique is performed in the standing position.

ASSESSMENT STEPS

1. Explain the technique to the patient, and demonstrate how to blow into the meter.
2. Instruct the patient to stand up straight or if unable to, the patient may sit.
3. Instruct the patient to take in a deep breath and hold it.
4. Place the peak flow meter in the mouth, with the tongue under the mouthpiece.
5. Instruct the patient to close the lips tightly around the mouthpiece and blow out as hard and fast as possible (Fig. 12-18).

    ■ **TIP** Instruct the patient that he or she should not bring the head forward while blowing out because it may decrease the airway volume; instruct the patient to blow as if blowing out candles on a birthday cake.

6. Repeat the process two more times.
7. Record the highest number obtained.
8. Document your findings.

    ■ **TIP** Do not average the numbers.

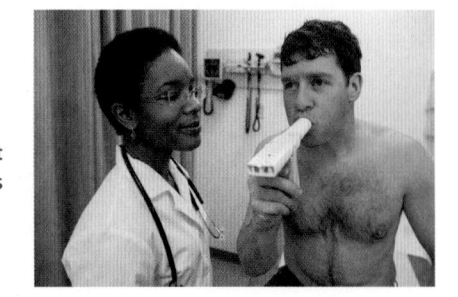

Fig. 12-18. Using a peak flow meter.

NORMAL FINDINGS

■ Based on an individual's age, height, sex, and race
■ **Green.** This is the good zone. The green zone is from 80 to 100 percent of your highest peak flow reading, or personal best. This is the zone you should be in every day. Measurements in this zone signal that air moves well through the large airways and that you can do your usual activities and go to sleep without trouble. (See Table 12-4.)

- **Yellow.** This is the caution or slow down zone. The yellow zone is from 50 to 80 percent of your personal best. Measurements in this zone are a clue that the large airways are starting to narrow. You may begin to have mild symptoms, such as coughing, feeling tired, feeling short of breath, or feeling like your chest is tightening.
- **Red.** This is the stop zone. The red zone is less than 50 percent of your personal best. Readings in this zone mean severe narrowing of the large airways has occurred. This is a medical emergency, and you should get help right away (Johns Hopkins Medicine, n.d.).

TABLE 12-4 Color Zones for the Peak Expiratory Flow Meter

Zone	Peak Expiratory Flow
GREEN: GO No asthma symptoms	80%–100%
YELLOW: CAUTION Airways are narrowing. If you remain in the yellow zone for several measures of peak expiratory flow, take your quick reliever. If you continue in the yellow zone, your asthma may not be under good control.	50%–80%
RED: Severe airway narrowing. Rescue medications are needed. Healthcare provider should be called.	Less than 50%

Adapted from National Heart, Lung, and Blood Institute. (2012). *National Asthma Education and Prevention Program*. NHLBI Expert Panel Report 3: Guidelines for Diagnosis and Management of Asthma.

PATIENT EDUCATION

Healthy People 2020

Goal: Promote respiratory health through better prevention, detection, treatment, and education efforts (HHS, 2010). The American Lung Association (2016) recommends the following:

- Do not smoke. Cigarette smoking is the major cause of pulmonary disease and lung cancer. Over time cigarette smoke destroys lung tissue and may trigger changes that grow into cancer.

- Avoid exposure to pollutants that can damage your lungs: secondhand smoke, outdoor air pollution, chemicals in the home and workplace, and radon can all cause or worsen lung disease.
- Prevent infection. Good hand and oral hygiene can protect you from the germs in your mouth leading to infections.
- Get vaccinated every year against influenza.

13

Assessing the Cardiovascular System

INTRODUCTION

The heart is the main pump of our body. The cardiac cycle transports blood through the lungs and to all the peripheral tissues of the body.

Knowledge of the structures and functions of the heart is essential to performing a cardiac assessment.

REVIEW OF ANATOMY AND PHYSIOLOGY

The Heart

- The heart is a cone-shaped, hollow muscular organ about the size of your fist. It is located left of the midline in the mediastinal cavity of the thorax between the third and sixth intercostal space; a small portion of the heart is located on the right of the sternum (Fig. 13-1).
- The heart works like a pump and beats about 100,000 times a day. An adult heart measures 5 inches in length, 3.5 inches in breadth, and 2.5 inches in thickness.

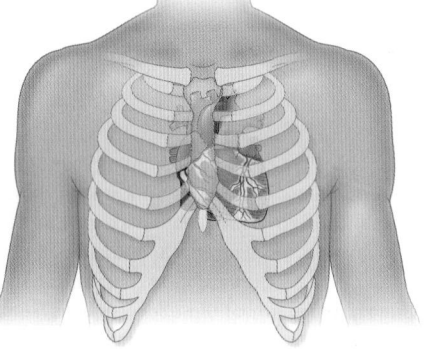

Fig. 13-1. Location of the heart.

- The widest part of the heart is the base (top of the heart) that lies upward toward the right shoulder.
- The apex (bottom) of the heart is narrower and points toward the left in the thoracic cavity.
- The posterior surface of the heart rests on the diaphragm.
- The precordium is the front of the chest wall.
- A muscular septum separates the heart into two lateral halves, the right and left sides of the heart. There is no communication between the right and left sides of the heart.
- Blood is supplied to the heart by the right and left coronary arteries. There are four layers of heart:
  □ Endocardium is the thin inner layer of the heart.
  □ Myocardium is the thick, middle, muscular layer of the heart.
  □ Epicardium is the thin, outer layer of the heart.

- Pericardium is the fluid-filled fibrous sac that surrounds the heart; the fluid helps to provide lubrication while the heart is contracting and relaxing; it is attached to the diaphragm (Fig. 13-2).

Cardiac Chambers

The heart is a double pump that is divided into four chambers:

- Right atria pumps blood to the right ventricle (deoxygenated blood).
- Left atria pumps blood to the left ventricle (oxygenated blood).
- Right ventricle pumps blood to the lungs (deoxygenated blood).
- Left ventricle pumps blood out to the aorta (oxygenated blood); does most work of the heart.
- The right side of the heart is responsible for pulmonary circulation (i.e., transporting blood into the pulmonary artery through the lungs).
- The left side of the heart is responsible for systemic circulation (i.e., pumping blood into the aorta to circulate to all the organs and tissues of the body).

Heart Valves

- Valves permit flow of blood in one direction through the heart.
- A healthy valve is pliable; it opens with little resistance and closes tightly to prevent retrograde blood flow. There is a set of valves on each side of the heart:

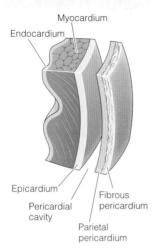

Fig. 13-2. Layers of the heart.

- Atrioventricular valves separate the atria from the ventricle and include the following:
  - Tricuspid valve separates the right atrium from the right ventricle.
  - Mitral valve separates the left atrium from the left ventricle.
- Semilunar valves separate the ventricles from the pulmonary and systemic circulation and include the following:
  - Pulmonic valve separates the right ventricle from the pulmonary artery.
  - Aortic valve separates the left ventricle from the aorta.
- Closure of the atrioventricular and semilunar valves creates the heart sounds S_1 and S_2.

Phases of the Cardiac Cycle

- The cardiac cycle is the start of one heartbeat to the start of the next heartbeat.
- One cardiac cycle is characterized by the electrical events required to stimulate cardiac contraction, the pressure changes that occur as blood flows from chamber to chamber and the opening and closure of the heart valves to ensure unidirectional flow of blood through the heart into the systemic and pulmonary circulation.
- Blood flows in a unidirectional flow through the cardiac system.
  - Blood in the right side of the heart (deoxygenated) is propelled to the lungs through the pulmonary artery.
  - Blood in the lungs drops off waste products and picks up oxygen.

☐ Oxygenated blood is propelled into the left side of the heart through the aorta to the systemic circulation (Fig. 13-3).

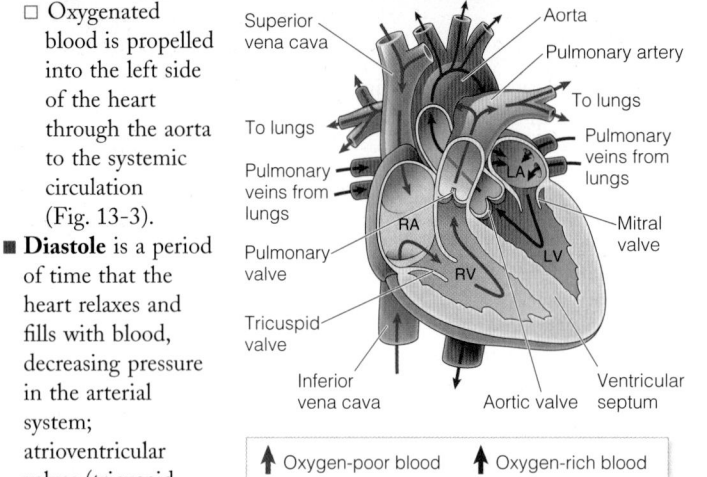

Fig. 13-3. Circulation of the heart.

■ **Diastole** is a period of time that the heart relaxes and fills with blood, decreasing pressure in the arterial system; atrioventricular valves (tricuspid and mitral) are open, and semilunar valves (pulmonic and aortic) are closed.

■ **Systole** is a period of time that the heart ventricles contract and push blood out into the arterial system; increasing pressure in the arterial system; atrioventricular valves (tricuspid and mitral) are closed, and semilunar valves (pulmonic and aortic) are open.

■ **Cardiac output** is the amount of blood the heart pumps out in 1 minute; heart pumps about 6 L/min.

Conduction System of the Heart

■ Atrial and ventricular contractions occur through a complex network of specialized cardiac muscle cells (myocytes).

■ Electrical impulses are initiated in the heart from the sinoatrial node, also known as the pacemaker of the heart, in the right atrium. The impulses then travel through the right atrium to the atrioventricular node located on the septum → Bundle of His in the septum → Purkinje fiber system (located in the ventricles) (Fig. 13-4).

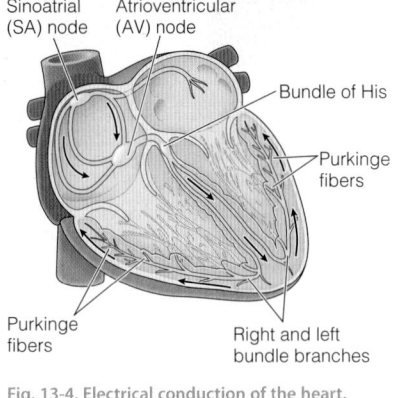

Fig. 13-4. Electrical conduction of the heart.

■ The cardiac cells (myocytes) are electrically polarized in their resting state; the inside of the cell is negatively charged. A membrane pump ensures the appropriate distribution of calcium, chloride, potassium, and sodium ions to keep the cell interior electronegative.

■ Depolarization is an electrical current moving from cell to cell that produces a positively charged wave through the myocardium; the interior of the cell becomes positively charged and initiates a contraction of the resting myocytes.

■ Depolarization and repolarization of the myocardium occurs as electrical impulses are traveling through the myocardium during the cardiac cycle; these can be traced on an electrocardiogram rhythm strip.

☐ P wave represents normal atrial depolarization (cell interiors become positively charged); atria are contracting.

☐ QRS represents electrical impulses traveling through the ventricular myocardium: ventricular depolarization; ventricles are contracting.

- ☐ T wave is ventricular repolarization; cells return to their normal polarity; atria and ventricles relax (Landrum, 2014) (Fig. 13-5).
- The electrical conduction system may encounter problems, making the heartbeat too fast (tachycardia), too slow (bradycardia) or be irregular (arrhythmias).

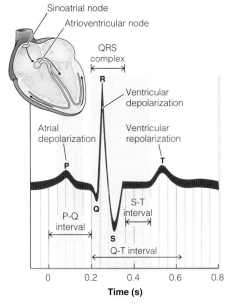

Fig. 13-5. Electrocardiogram.

Heart Sounds

Normal Heart Sounds

- Are created by the sudden closing of the atrioventricular (mitral and tricuspid) and semilunar (aortic and pulmonic) valves
- Caused by rapid deceleration of blood flow when the valves close at the beginning and end of each contraction
- There are two normal heart sounds.
  - ☐ First heart sound (S₁) is known as the "lub" sound; caused by turbulence and vibrations of taut atrioventricular valves immediately after closure along with the vibration of the adjacent walls of the heart and major blood vessels around the heart; lasts about 0.14 second (Hall, 2016); onset of systole; heard loudest at the apex of the heart.
  - ☐ Second heart sound (S₂) is known as the "dub" sound: the semilunar valves close causing blood to back up in the arteries, generating a short period of reverberation of blood back and forth between the walls of the arteries and valves. The vibrations create the second heart sound lasting about 0.11 seconds (Hall, 2016). This is the onset of diastole; heard loudest at the base of the heart (Fig. 13-6).

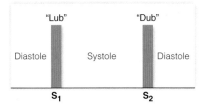

Fig. 13-6. S₁ [Lub] and S₂ [Dub] sounds.

Extra Heart Sounds
S₃ heart sound

■ **TIP** S₃ sound is heard best with the bell of the stethoscope with patient lying supine and then positioned in the left side-lying position (Reimer-Kent, 2013).

- S₃ is a faint, low-pitched extra heart sound that occurs directly after the S₂ heart sound (Fig. 13-7).
- Appears to be related to a sudden limitation of the movement of the ventricles (Chatterjee, 2012).

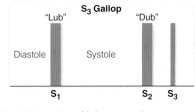

Fig. 13-7. Location of S₃ heart sounds.

- The rapid ventricular filling creates vibrations that can be auscultated; sounds like a horse's gallop; known as a "ventricular gallop"; ventricular rate greater than 90 BPM.
- S_3 can sound like "Kentucky" (Ken = S_1, tuck = S_2, ky = S_3), "sloshing-in" (S_1 = slosh, ing = S_2, in = S_3).
- This sound is normal in physically active young adults; abnormal in patients older than 40 years and associated with heart failure (Tseng, Yo, & Jaw, 2012); signals volume overload to the ventricle (Swartz, 2010).

S_4 heart sound

- S_4 is a soft, low-pitched sound that occurs at the end of diastole.
- Best heard over the apex of the heart with the bell of the stethoscope; position the patient in the left lateral position.
- Atria work hard to contract against a poorly compliant and resistant left ventricle that creates vibrations; may be due to scar tissue of hypertensive heart disease or coronary artery disease.
- S_4 occurs directly before the S_1 heart sound; thudlike quality sound (Fig. 13-8).

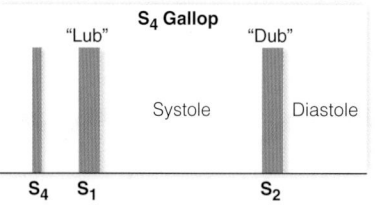

Fig. 13-8. Location of S_4 heart sounds.

- S_4 can sound like "Tennessee" (Ten = S_4, nes = S_1, see = S_2); "a-stiff-wall" (a = S_4, stiff = S_1, wall = S_2).
- S_4 is not heard if a patient is in atrial fibrillation since the S_4 relies on effective atrial contractions (Spiers, 2011).
- Abnormal S_4 sounds are louder and higher pitched; referred to as an "atrial gallop."

- S_4 may be normal in many healthy older adults without any cardiac problems due to decreased ventricular compliance with age (Chatterjee, 2012).

Heart Murmurs

- Heart murmurs are swishing or unusually prolonged sounds indicative of turbulent blood flow in the vascular system.
- Murmurs can occur during systole and diastole or anywhere in the cardiac cycle.
- Babies are born with heart murmurs or murmurs can develop sometime during a patient's lifetime.
- There are two types of heart murmurs:
  □ An innocent or physiological heart murmur is not caused by a heart problem; patient does not have symptoms. The heart sounds are produced as the blood flows through heart chambers and valves or when there is extra blood flow through the heart (i.e., during pregnancy) (Judd, 2014).
  □ An abnormal or pathological murmur is caused by age-related changes, heart disease or a heart problem such as heart valve disease; patients may have cardiac symptoms such as heart palpitations or shortness of breath.
- Some causes of heart murmurs are as follows (Fig. 13-9):
  □ Increased blood flow through a normal valve

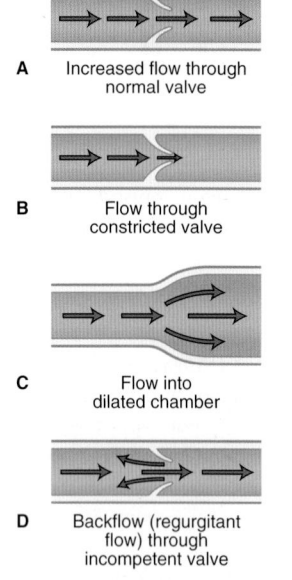

A — Increased flow through normal valve

B — Flow through constricted valve

C — Flow into dilated chamber

D — Backflow (regurgitant flow) through incompetent valve

E — Shunting

Fig. 13-9. Causes of heart murmurs.

- Blood flow through a constricted valve
- Flow into a dilated chamber
- Backflow (regurgitant flow) through an incompetent valve
- Shunting of blood through an abnormal hole in the heart; commonly these holes are congenital

■ Documentation of heart murmurs includes the following characteristics:
  - Intensity or loudness is determined by the quantity and velocity of blood flow; classified by the Levine grading scale (Table 13-1); documented as a fraction Grade IV/VI.
  - Timing or the placement in the cardiac cycle is the duration of time the murmur is heard during systole or diastole or both.
  - Quality of the sound can be described as:
    • harsh
    • rumbling
    • musical
    • blowing
    • grunting
    • squeaky.

TABLE 13-1 Six Grades of Heart Murmurs

Grade I	The murmur is only audible with a stethoscope while listening carefully for some time.
Grade II	Faint murmur but can be audible immediately with a stethoscope.
Grade III	Loud murmur readily audible; no palpable thrill
Grade IV	Loud murmur with a palpable thrill
Grade V	Loud murmur with a palpable thrill; murmur is audible with only the rim of the stethoscope touching the chest
Grade VI	Loud murmur with a palpable thrill; murmur can be heard with the stethoscope not touching the chest but lifted just above the area of the murmur

Source: Adapted from Chatterjee, 2012, and Silverman, 2008.

- Pitch or frequency is directly related to the velocity of blood flow and is described as:
  • high
  • medium
  • low.

■ Heart murmurs have different configurations (Fig. 13-10):
  - Crescendo: starts soft and gets louder
  - Decrescendo: starts loud and then gradually fades away
  - Crescendo and decrescendo: starts soft, gets louder toward the peak, and then gradually fades away
  - Plateau shaped: sound is the same from the beginning to the end of the murmur

■ Location of heart murmurs should be identified using precordium landmarks.

Ejection Sounds

■ Ejection clicks are high-pitched early diastolic sounds that occur at the moment of maximal opening of the aortic or pulmonic valves; occur with a dilated aorta or pulmonary artery or stenotic aortic or pulmonic valves (Jacobs, 1990).

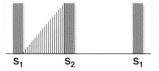
A *crescendo murmur* grows louder.

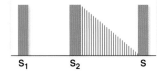
A *decrescendo murmur* grows softer.

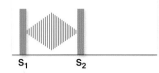
A *crescendo–decrescendo murmur* first rises in intensity, then falls.

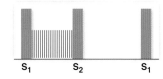
A *plateau murmur* has the same intensity throughout.

Fig. 13-10. Configuration of heart murmurs.

■ An ejection sound is a higher-frequency "clicky" sound reflective of increased cardiac output; it is heard after the S_1 sound best heard with the diaphragm of the stethoscope (Fig. 13-11).

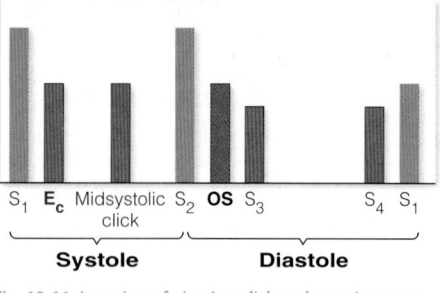

Fig. 13-11. Location of ejection click and opening snap.

■ Midsystolic ejection click is a cardinal finding of mitral valve prolapse; the mitral valve leaflets do not close properly.

Opening Snap (OS)

■ Opening snap is a loud, high frequency sound that occurs when a stenotic valve opens.
■ Stenosis of the mitral or tricuspid valve reduces the opening of the valve and blood flow through the valve creating a "snapping sound."
■ High-pitched diastolic sound auscultated after the S_2 heart sound (see Fig. 13-11).

Pericardial Friction Rub

■ High-pitched, muffled, grating, and leathery sound heard with each heart beat.
■ Caused by friction of the visceral and parietal layers of the pericardium.
■ May be indicative of pericardial sac inflammation (pericarditis); fluid may accumulate between the pericardial layers of the heart (pericardial effusion) (Fig. 13-12).

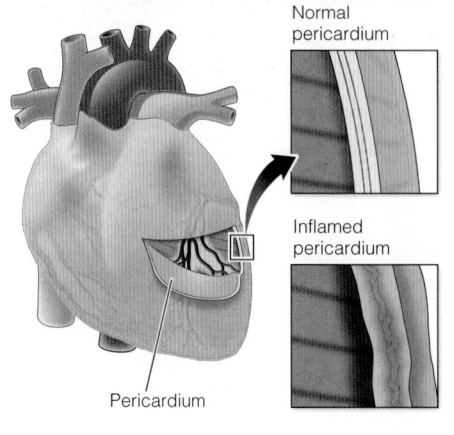

Fig. 13-12. Pericardial friction rub.

DIAGNOSTICS

The cardiac system can be assessed by laboratory and diagnostic testing.

■ **Lipid profile** is a group of blood tests that identify the amount of cholesterol in the bloodstream, a risk factor for coronary artery disease (CAD). The report will calculate the following:

  □ **Total Cholesterol Level:** Total cholesterol measures different types of cholesterol in the body. Cholesterol is a waxy, fat-like substance that is carried through the bloodstream. Cholesterol is made up of lipoproteins, which are composed of fat on the inside and proteins on the outside. Lipoproteins contain varying amounts of cholesterol, protein, and triglycerides.

  □ **Low-Density Lipoprotein (LDL-C):** LDL transports cholesterol from the liver to the walls of blood vessels; this is the cholesterol that builds up in the arteries. This is considered to be the "bad" cholesterol.

□ **High-Density Lipoprotein (HDL-C):** HDL transports cholesterol from tissues back to the liver where it is then broken down and eliminated from the body; this is the "good" cholesterol (Table 13-2).

TABLE 13-2 Normal and Abnormal Cholesterol Levels

Type of Cholesterol	Range Category
Low-Density Lipoprotein (LDL)	
Less than 70 mg/dL	Optional goal for an individual at high risk of a heart attack or death from a heart attack
100–129 mg/dL	Near optimal/above optimal
130–159 mg/dL	Borderline high
160–189 mg/dL	High
190 mg/dL and higher	Very high
High-Density Lipoprotein (HDL)	
Less than 40 mg/dL (men)	Low HDL (higher risk)
Less than 50 mg/dL (women)	Low HDL (higher risk)
40–59 mg/dL	The higher, the better
60 mg/dL and higher	High HDL (lower risk)
Triglycerides	
Less than 150	Desirable
150 to 199	Borderline-high risk
200 to 499	High risk
Greater than 500	Very high risk
Total Cholesterol	
Less than 200 mg/dL	Desirable
200–239 mg/dL	Borderline high (higher risk)
240 mg/dL and higher	High (more than twice the risk as desirable level)

Source: National Heart, Lung, and Blood Institute, 2012.

□ **Triglycerides:** Type of fat in the blood, end products of fatty foods, levels vary by age and sex (AHA, 2017). See Table 13-2 for normal and abnormal levels of cholesterol.

■ **TIP** American Heart Association (AHA) guidelines now recommend an integrated approach. The LDL range is no longer the primary factor for overall cardiovascular risk. The AHA recommends that all adults age 20 or older have their cholesterol and other traditional risk factors checked every four to six years, and work with their healthcare providers to determine their risk for cardiovascular disease and stroke (AHA, 2017).

■ **Creatinine kinase–MB** is an enzyme that is contained within cardiac muscle; this enzyme will increase when cardiac tissue is damaged due to decreased oxygenation; usually elevates 3 to 4 hours after cardiac tissue damage.

■ **Troponin Test** measures levels of proteins; these proteins are released when heart damage or tissue ischemia related to lack of oxygen in the heart tissue occurs; detectable a few hours to 7 days after the onset of symptoms of myocardial damage.

■ **Electrocardiogram (EKG)** provides vital information about the heart's electrical conduction system; records the electrical activity of the heart; helps diagnose abnormal heartbeats, heart rhythm, and tissue ischemia.

■ **TIP** Since the time of Einthoven's (1901) "electrocardiogram," the medical profession has used the letters EKG to represent the electrocardiogram. Some say that "ECG" is more correct. Medicine honors tradition, and EKG has been used for years (Dubin, 2000).

■ **Echocardiography** is a noninvasive ultrasound (US) that uses high-frequency sound waves of various intensities to help diagnose cardiovascular disorders. Procedure records the echoes created by the deflection of an ultrasonic beam off the cardiac structures and allows visualization of the size, shape, position, thickness, and movement of cardiac structures; this is the standard for establishing the cause of a heart murmur (Chatterjee, 2012).

- **Holter monitor** is an ambulatory test for 24 hours; the patient wears a monitor that records the cardiac electrical impulses; the monitoring is read and interpreted by a cardiologist.
- **Exercise stress test** monitors the heart function and rhythm while the patient is walking and running on a treadmill while under physical stress; the patient is hooked up to an EKG monitor during the test and is closely monitored; many aspects of your heart function can be checked including heart rate and abnormal heart rhythms, breathing, blood pressure, EKG, and how tired you become when exercising (Fig. 13-13). This test may help to identify coronary artery circulation and heart-related symptoms such as chest pain and shortness of breath.

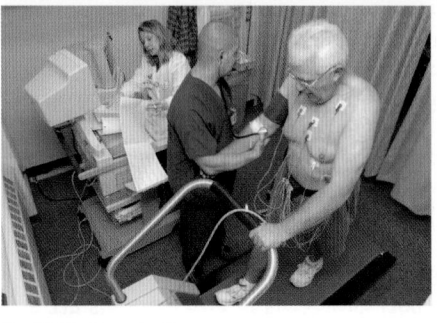

Fig. 13-13. Stress testing.

HEALTH HISTORY

The cardiac system influences the functioning of all organs. Remember to obtain a thorough past medical history related to the cardiac system.

Review of Systems

Use the **OLDCARTS** mnemonic (**O**nset, **L**ocation, **D**uration, **C**haracteristics, **A**ggravating/Alleviating factors, **R**elieving factors, **T**reatment, **S**everity) to identify attributes of a symptom.

Family History

- Do you have a family history of heart disease, rheumatic fever, or high blood pressure?
  - □ Cardiac conditions have familial tendencies. Creating and reviewing a genogram to review a family's history is a useful tool. Assessing the family history, risk factors, lifestyle behaviors, and symptoms is critical when assessing a patient with possible cardiac symptoms (Table 13-3).

  - □ Rheumatic fever is an inflammatory disease that can damage the heart and heart valves.

    TIP Acute rheumatic fever is no longer a nationally notifiable disease in the United States, and its annual incidence in the continental United States declined in the late 20th century (CDC, 2015).

- Did either of your parents or siblings die of a heart attack (myocardial infarction)?
  - □ Positive family history of first-degree relatives having a heart attack increases the chance of heart disease; if your father or brother had a heart attack before age 55, or mother or sister had one before 65, you are higher risk.

Medication History

- What medications do you take for your heart? Why are you taking them?
- Do you have any side effects?
  - □ Individuals sometimes do not know why they are taking medications, and this is a good time for patient teaching.

TABLE 13-3 Risk Factors for Coronary Artery Disease

Nonmodifiable Risk Factors

Age	Risk increases with age.
	For women, age becomes a risk factor at 55, after menopause because estrogen production decreases.
	Women who have gone through early menopause are twice as likely to develop heart disease as women of the same age who have not yet gone through menopause.
Sex	Incidence is greater in men than in women until women reach menopause.
Family History	
Race	Incidence is higher for African Americans under the age of 45 than in Caucasian men and women in the same age group.

Modifiable Risk Factors

Smoking	Smoking is a major cause of coronary heart disease.
Cholesterol	Serum cholesterol levels >200 mg/dL increase the risk for coronary heart disease.
High Blood Pressure	Uncontrolled high blood pressure increases the risk for coronary heart disease.
Physical Inactivity	People who are inactive are at greater risk for coronary heart disease.
Obesity	Being overweight or obese increases risk for coronary heart disease and high blood pressure.
Stress	
Diabetes and Prediabetes	Contributing factor for coronary heart disease

Source: National Heart Lung and Blood Institute, 2016.

□ Some common classifications of cardiac medications include Beta Blockers, Calcium Channel Blockers, Nitrates, Angiotensin-Converting Enzyme, and Statins used to lower cholesterol.

Health Promotion

■ What type of diet do you eat?
  □ A heart healthy diet:
    • includes fruits and vegetables
    • includes whole grains
    • is low in cholesterol and saturated and trans fats
    • is low in sodium.
■ Are you a smoker?
  □ Smoking and second-hand smoke are major risk factors for heart disease. Any amount of smoking damages the heart and blood vessels (NIH, 2016). Smoking increases the development of atherosclerosis, triggers myocardial infarction, and increases cardiovascular morbidity and mortality (Wang & Patterson, 2015, p. 97). If the patient is a smoker, smoking cessation is strongly encouraged to reduce a patient's risk for heart disease.
■ Do you exercise regularly? How often and for how long?
  □ Moderate exercise is recommended for at least 30 minutes 5 days a week, or more vigorous workouts at least 20 minutes three times a week.
■ Do you drink alcohol? If so, how often and how much?
  □ Alcohol may have some health benefits; the best-known effect of alcohol is a small increase in HDL cholesterol. The American Heart Association (2017) does not recommend drinking wine or any other form of alcohol to gain this potential benefit.
  □ Used in excess, alcohol could lead to heart failure, high blood pressure, and alcohol-related diseases such as cirrhosis of the liver.
■ Have you seen a cardiologist? If so, who, why, and when was your last visit?

■ Have you ever had an EKG or other diagnostic tests to assess your heart? If so, which ones?

Current Health Status

Chest Pain

▨ **TIP** Use the OPQRST or the OLDCARTS mnemonic to assess this symptom.

■ Have you experienced any chest pain or discomfort? If so, when?
■ How was the chest pain relieved?
  □ Angina pectoris is defined as sudden pain beneath the sternum, often radiating to the left shoulder and arm. Angina pain is precipitated when the oxygen supply to the heart is insufficient to meet oxygen demands (Lehne & Yaeger, 2016).
  □ Coronary heart disease is the leading cause of death in the United States.
  □ The most reported symptom of the cardiac system is chest pain. Even though chest pain may be related to various etiologies, chest pain must be thoroughly assessed because it could be indicative of a myocardial infarction, a heart attack (Box 13-1). Any patient who

---

BOX 13-2 **Seven Attributes of a Symptom**

1. **O**nset
2. **L**ocation
3. **D**uration
4. **C**haracteristic Symptoms
5. **A**ssociated Manifestations
6. **R**elieving/Exacerbating Factors
7. **T**reatment
8. **S**everity

---

complains of chest pain requires an in-depth pain assessment using the seven characteristics of pain assessment (Box 13-2).

Heart Palpitations

■ Have you experienced any heart palpitations?
  □ Heart palpitations are an increased awareness of the heart beating; patients describe a "fluttering" feeling or feel like their heart is racing; may be related to an irregular heart rate, fast heart rate, cardiac abnormality, fear, stress, or anxiety.

Color Changes

■ Have you noticed that your skin or lips look gray or blue?
  □ Central cyanosis is a bluish color that presents in the mucous membranes and skin with hypoxia (decreased oxygen in the blood).
  □ Peripheral cyanosis is a bluish color of the peripheral extremities related to decreased circulation and lack of oxygen in the blood.

Shortness of Breath (Dyspnea)

■ Do you experience shortness of breath? If so, when?
■ What relieves it?
■ What makes the shortness of breath better or worse?

BOX 13-1 **Common Symptoms of a Heart Attack**

• Uncomfortable pressure, squeezing, fullness, or pain in the center of the chest
• Discomfort in other areas of the upper body (jaw, arms, shoulder, abdomen)
• Shortness of breath with or without chest discomfort
• Breaking out in a cold sweat
• Nausea
• Dizziness

Source: American Heart Association, 2016.

- Does sleeping on more than one pillow at night relieve the shortness of breath?
- How many pillows do you sleep on at night?
  - Shortness of breath (SOB) has variations related to an individual's body shape, level of fitness, and age.
  - Ask the patient about his or her activity level when he or she is experiencing shortness of breath.
  - A symptom of congestive heart failure is shortness of breath due to increased fluid accumulation in the lungs.

Edema
- Do your legs, ankles, or feet get swollen?
- What do you do to help the swelling go down?
  - A symptom of congestive heart failure is edema of the lower extremities; it is caused by the heart's inability to adequately move blood forward; therefore, the blood backs up in the peripheral system causing edema in the dependent areas.

Nocturia
- Do you get up to use the bathroom at night? If so, how often?
  - Nocturia is excessive urination after going to bed at night; this may be a symptom of congestive heart failure. The kidneys are better perfused when the patient is lying down and sleeping using less oxygen demands; fluids shift and redistribute increasing the production of urine.

Fainting
- Have you ever fainted where you lost consciousness?
  - Syncopal episodes may be a sign of cardiac arrhythmias. It is important to differentiate whether the patient lost consciousness during the episode or just felt dizzy.

Risk Factors and Cultural Considerations
- Atherosclerotic cardiovascular disease (CVD) is a leading cause of mortality and morbidity worldwide, with coronary artery disease (CAD) being the single leading cause of death (Hamrefors, 2017).
- Heart disease is the number one killer of women, causing one in three deaths each year (AHA, 2016a). All individuals of any race have nonmodifiable risk factors; these are risk factors that cannot be changed such as gender, ethnic origin, or family history.
- Family history and genetics play an important role for increased risk of heart disease. Familial hypercholesterolemia is an inherited disorder whereby the body begins to produce abnormally high cholesterol levels at birth. One in 500 people in the United States may inherit this condition (CDC, 2014).
- Modifiable risk factors are those factors that a patient can change, related to weight, hypertension, diet, smoking, or exercise (see Table 13-3) to prevent heart disease.
- No ethnic group is spared the risk of coronary artery disease (Box 13-3).

SENC Evidence-Based Practice The Jackson Heart Study (2012) is the largest study in history to investigate the inherited (genetic) factors that affect high blood pressure, heart disease, stroke, diabetes, and other important diseases in African Americans. DNA has been obtained from every consenting participant in the Jackson Heart Study, and will be analyzed for many thousands of differences between people that may affect their health. These studies are likely to lead to the development of new treatments that do more good and less harm than treatments that are available today (Jackson Heart Study, 2012).

BOX 13-3 Cultural Considerations for Heart Disease

African Americans
- As of 2007, African-American men were 30 percent more likely to die from heart disease than were non-Hispanic white men.
- African-American adults of both genders are 40 percent more likely to have high blood pressure and 10 percent less likely than their white counterparts to have their blood pressure under control.
- African Americans also have the highest rate of high blood pressure of all population groups, and they tend to develop it earlier in life than others.
- Compared with whites, African Americans are at nearly twice the risk of having a first stroke and are more likely to die of stroke than are whites. (Centers for Disease Control and Prevention, n.d.)

Hispanic Americans
- In general, Hispanic-American adults are 20 percent less likely to have coronary heart disease than non-Hispanic white adults. They are also less likely to die from heart disease than non-Hispanic white adults.

- In 2010, Hispanics were 20 percent less likely to have heart disease, compared with non-Hispanic whites.
- In 2008, Hispanic men and women were 40 percent less likely to die from heart disease, compared with non-Hispanic whites. (Office of Minority Health, 2012a)
- The Hispanic population is between African-American and white populations for the risk of stroke. Hispanics are more likely to die of a stroke than are whites. (Centers for Disease Control and Prevention, n.d.)

Asian Americans
- Overall, Asian-American adults are less likely than white adults to have heart disease, and they are less likely to die from heart disease. In general, Asian-American adults have lower rates of being overweight or obese, have lower rates of hypertension, and are less likely to be current cigarette smokers.
- Asian Americans are 50 percent less likely to die from heart disease (Office of Minority Health, 2012b).

PREPARATION FOR ASSESSMENT

Equipment Needed
Stethoscope
Watch with a second hand

Preliminary Steps
- Good lighting is very important to closely inspect the precordium.
- Room temperature should be comfortable
- Patient should be supine with head-of-bed at 30 degrees (Reimer-Kent, 2013)

TIP Shivering and any muscular movement interfere with heart sound transmission, making it hard to accurately detect the distinct characteristics of the heart sounds (Buss & Thompson, 2010).

- A stethoscope with a bell is needed to auscultate the low-pitched sounds (diastolic murmurs, S_3 or S_4) and a diaphragm to auscultate the high-pitched sounds (systolic murmurs, S_1 and S_2) (Reimer-Kent, 2013).
- The environment should be quiet to clearly hear the heart sounds.
- Patient should be properly draped so that only the chest area is exposed.
- Assessment of the cardiac assessment requires the nurse to know the five essential landmarks of the precordium and auscultate heart sounds in this sequence (Table 13-4). These include:
  □ Right Sternal Border (RSB), Second Intercostal Space (ICS) (Aortic area)

TABLE 13-4 Accepted Abbreviations for Auscultation Landmarks

	Landmark Location	Abbreviation
Aortic Valve	Second Intercostal Space (ICS) Right Sternal Border (RSB)	2RSB
Pulmonic Valve	Second Intercostal Space (ICS) Left Sternal Border (LSB)	2LSB
Erb's Point	Third Intercostal Space (ICS) Left Sternal Border (LSB)	3LSB
Tricuspid Valve	Fourth Intercostal Space (ICS) Left Sternal Border (LSB)	4LSB
Mitral Valve	Fifth Intercostal Space (ICS) Left Midclavicular Line (MCL)	5LMCL

☐ Left Sternal Border (LSB), Second Intercostal Space (ICS) (Pulmonic area)
☐ Left Sternal Border (LSB), Third Intercostal Space (ICS) (Erb's Point)
☐ Left Sternal Border (LSB) Fourth Intercostal Space (ICS) (Tricuspid Valve)
☐ Left Sternal Border (LSB), Fifth Intercostal Space (ICS) (Mitral Valve) (Fig. 13-14)

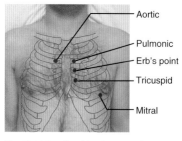

Fig. 13-14. Landmarking intercostal spaces.

TECHNIQUE 13-1: Inspecting Anterior Chest

Purpose: To assess the anterior chest for pulsations, symmetry, and heaves
Equipment: Tangential lighting

SENC Patient-Centered Care Maintain the patient's privacy and dignity during cardiac assessment and only expose the chest area.

ASSESSMENT STEPS

1. Explain the technique to the patient.
2. Adjust the head of the examination table so that the patient is lying supine with the head and chest elevated 30 degrees (Fig. 13-15).
3. Inspect the symmetry of the chest.
4. Inspect for surgical scars of the chest.

TIP Surgical scars of the chest may indicate that the patient had cardiac surgery or has an implantable defibrillator or pacemaker.

5. Inspect the anterior chest at the five landmark locations of the precordium for:
- □ pulsations
- □ lifts or heaves.

6. Document your findings.

Normal Findings

■ An apical pulsation may or may not be visible at the left fifth midclavicular line; no heaves or lifts; chest symmetrical.

Abnormal Findings

■ A *lift* (slight movement) or *heave* is a sustained, forceful, outward thrusting of the ventricle secondary to increased workload.

■ A right ventricular lift or heave is visualized at the sternal border; a left ventricular heave is seen at the apex.

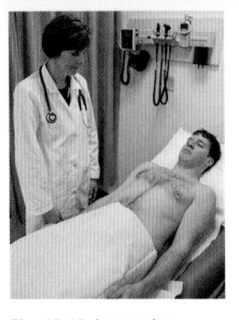

Fig. 13-15. Inspecting anterior chest with head of bed at 30 degrees.

TECHNIQUE 13-2: **Palpating the Precordium and Apical Pulse**

Purpose: To assess for vibrations and the apical pulse

The mitral area is located at or near the fifth intercostal space, just medial to the left midclavicular line; this area lies directly over the left ventricle and is referred to as the apical area, or point of maximal impulse (Buss & Thompson, 2010).

■ **TIP** Apical pulse may not be palpable in the following individuals:

■ **A patient who is obese**

■ **A patient with chronic obstructive pulmonary disease with a barrel chest**

■ **A patient with a thick chest wall or breast tissue**

■ **A patient who has fluid around the heart (this condition is called pericardial effusion)**

ASSESSMENT STEPS

1. Explain the technique to the patient.

2. Using the palmar surface of your right hand, gently palpate the five landmarks, feeling for pulsations or vibrations (Fig. 13-16).
- □ Right Sternal Border (RSB), Second Intercostal Space (Aortic Valve)
- □ Left Sternal Border (LSB), Second Intercostal Space (Pulmonic Valve)
- □ Left Sternal Border (LSB), Third Intercostal Space (Erb's Point)
- □ Left Sternal Border (LSB) Fourth Intercostal Space (Tricuspid Valve)
- □ Left Sternal Border (LSB), Fifth Intercostal Space (Mitral Valve)

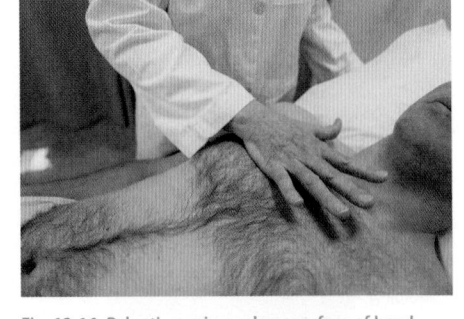

Fig. 13-16. Palpating using palmar surface of hand.

3. Ask the patient to turn slightly to the left lateral recumbent position, using your second and third finger pads of your dominant hand, palpate the apical pulse at the fifth left intercostal space at the midclavicular line noting the (Fig. 13-17):
   □ location
   □ amplitude.
   ■ **TIP** The left lateral position will push the apex beat further outward as the heart has a degree of mobility in the chest (Jevon & Cunnington, 2007). For a patient with an enlarged heart (cardiomegaly), the point of maximal impulse (PMI) will be lower and more laterally toward the axillary area.
4. While auscultating the apical pulse, use your other hand to palpate the carotid pulse or radial pulse; count and compare the beats per minute, and note (Fig. 13-18):
   □ amplitude
   □ beats per minute.
   ■ **TIP** Pulse deficit is the difference between the simultaneously counted apical heart rate and the carotid or radial pulse rate and may be indicative of atrial fibrillation. The carotid pulse is preferred over radial pulses because there is a palpable delay between ventricular contraction and more distal peripheral pulses (Reimer-Kent, 2013).
5. Document your findings.

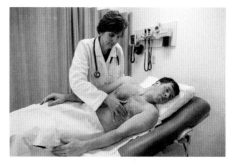

Fig. 13-17. Palpating the apical pulse.

NORMAL FINDINGS
■ No pulsations are felt at the five landmarks; apical pulse is palpated and auscultated at the fifth left intercostal space at the midclavicular line:
   □ Carotid or radial pulse is synchronous with the apical pulse.

ABNORMAL FINDINGS
■ Visible pulsations may indicate increased cardiac output:
   □ Heaves or lifts are forceful cardiac contractions that cause a slight to vigorous movement of sternum and ribs.
   □ Thrill is a palpable vibration caused by very turbulent blood flow; as increasing turbulence develops in moving fluid, a proportionate level of sound is produced (Hanifin, 2010); usually correlates with a loud cardiac murmur; feels like the throat of a purring cat.
   □ Pulsations felt at the five landmarks may indicate the following:
   • Right Sternal Border (RSB), Second Intercostal Space (ICS) (Aortic Valve): aortic aneurysm; a thrill may be indicative of aortic stenosis.
   • Left Sternal Border (LSB), Second Intercostal Space (ICS) (Pulmonic Valve): pulmonary hypertension; a thrill may be indicative of pulmonic stenosis.
   • Left Sternal Border (LSB), Third Intercostal Space (ICS) (Erb's Point): aortic and pulmonic anomalies
   • Left Sternal Border (LSB), Fourth Intercostal Space (ICS) (Tricuspid Valve): ventricular enlargement and defects

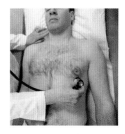

Fig. 13-18. Auscultating apical pulse and palpating radial pulse to determine a pulse deficit.

TECHNIQUE 13-3: **Auscultating Heart Sounds**

Purpose: To assess heart sounds
Equipment: Stethoscope with a bell and diaphragm
■ **TIP** Electronic stethoscopes can change filter frequency settings to toggle between bell and diaphragm modes; some have filtering devices to reduce distracting ambient noise (Shindler, 2007).

> **SENC Safety Alert** Prior to auscultating heart sounds, follow standard precautions and make sure to clean off the stethoscope to prevent any cross-contamination.

Listening for heart sounds requires an understanding of which valves should be open and which valves are closed during systole and diastole. Proper auscultation technique requires the following:

■ Listening and concentrating on one sound at a time during several cardiac cycles.
■ Use a sequence for auscultation, establish a pattern, and use it each time you auscultate (Spiers, 2011).
■ Do not rush while auscultating heart sounds.
■ Patients should be placed in a comfortable position. Heart sounds may be auscultated in the following positions:
  □ Supine
  □ Semi-Fowler's
  □ Fowler's
  □ Left side-lying position
■ The cardiac assessment requires both the bell and diaphragm to transmit the full spectrum of heart sounds.
■ Faint sounds require concentration and should be listened to for as long as necessary. This allows the ear to become attuned to the full intensity of that particular sound level (Shindler, 2007).
■ Extra sounds can be heard away from the valves; do not hesitate to expand your auscultatory sites to listen over the entire precordium.
■ Instruct your patient to breathe normally as you listen to heart sounds.

> **SENC Safety Alert** Never listen to heart sounds over the patient's clothes. The stethoscope should be touching the patient's skin. Auscultating over patient's clothing could cause artifact sounds and be misinterpreted as abnormal heart sounds.

■ **TIP** If the patient has a hairy chest, wet the patient's chest hair with a little warm water to decrease the sounds caused by friction of hair against the stethoscope.

ASSESSMENT STEPS
1. Explain the technique to the patient.
2. Place patient in a supine position with chest elevated 30 degrees.

3. Warm the stethoscope before placing on the precordium.
4. Using the second and third finger pads of your right or left hand, landmark each auscultatory site prior to placing the stethoscope on the skin (Fig. 13-19).

   ▮ **TIP** Closing your eyes while listening to the heart sounds may aide you in concentrating on the sounds.

5. Using the diaphragm of the stethoscope, auscultate the heart sounds ($S_{1[lub]}$ and $S_{2[dub]}$) at the five landmark sites (Fig. 13-20), listening for:
   □ S_1 and S_2 heart sounds
   □ rhythm of the heart sounds
   □ abnormal or extra heart sounds.

   ▮ **TIP** While interpreting the heart sounds, it is essential to understand from which part of the cardiac cycle they are being generated. This can be done by palpating the carotid artery simultaneously while auscultating the heart. The carotid upstroke corresponds to ventricular systole (Mangla & Gupta, 2012).

6. With the patient in the sitting position, ask the patient to lean forward; using the diaphragm of the stethoscope, auscultate the aortic and pulmonic valve areas listening for (Fig. 13-21):
   □ murmurs
   □ extra heart sounds.

   ▮ **TIP** Aortic valve murmurs are best heard when the patient is sitting up and leaning forward. Instruct the patient to inhale, exhale, and hold his or her breath, place the diaphragm on the second right sternal border.

7. Using the bell of the stethoscope, auscultate for low-pitched heart sounds at the five landmark sites.
8. Assist the patient to lie on his or her left lateral side. Using the bell of the stethoscope, auscultate the apical area listening for (Fig. 13-22):
   □ heart murmurs
   □ extra heart sounds.
9. Document your findings.

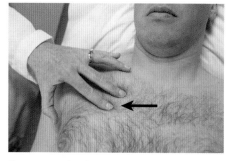
Fig. 13-19. Landmarking the 2nd ICS–auscultatory site.

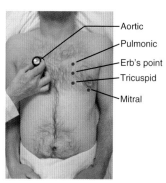
- Aortic
- Pulmonic
- Erb's point
- Tricuspid
- Mitral

Fig. 13-20. Auscultating with diaphragm of stethoscope at five landmarks.

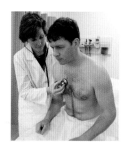
Fig. 13-21. Auscultating with patient sitting and leaning forward.

NORMAL FINDINGS

- S_1 and S_2 sounds heard; regular pattern
  - ☐ Split S_2 [dub] sound is a normal heart sound that is affected by respirations. During inspiration, the pulmonic valve closure is delayed due to increased venous return to the right side of the heart (Reimer-Kent, 2013). Towards the end of inspiration, the aortic valve closes 0.06 seconds earlier than the pulmonic valve causing the S_2 sound to physiologically split. This sound is heard at the pulmonic valve (Fig. 13-23).

ABNORMAL FINDINGS

- Extra or abnormal heart sounds are heard.
  - ☐ S_3, the third heart sound, may indicate congestive heart failure, aortic valve regurgitation, and be present after a myocardial infarction.
  - ☐ S_4, the fourth heart sound, may indicate thickening (hypertrophy) of the left ventricle, hypertension, aortic stenosis, or be heard after a myocardial infarction.
  - ☐ Murmurs may indicate increased turbulent blood flow related to obstructive or incompetent valves or abnormal heart conditions.
  - ☐ Opening snap may indicate mitral valve stenosis (Fig. 13-24).
  - ☐ Ejection clicks may be heard at valves with defective leaflets such as in mitral valve prolapse (Fig. 13-25).
  - ☐ Pericardial friction rubs result from inflammation of the pericardial sac surrounding the heart.

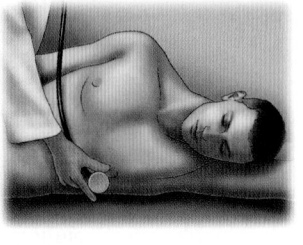

Fig. 13-22. Auscultating using bell–left lateral position.

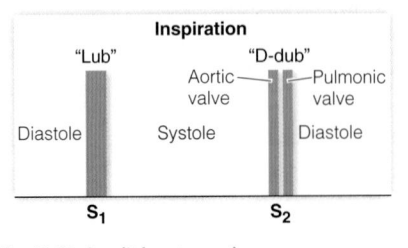

Fig. 13-23. S_2 split heart sound.

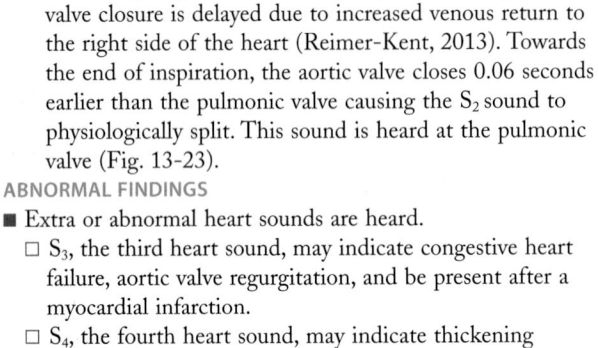

Fig. 13-24. Mitral valve stenosis.

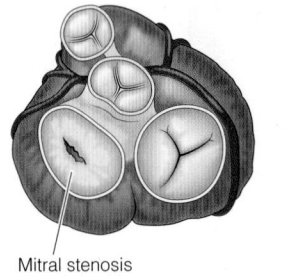

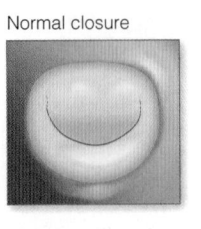

Normal closure

Prolapse closure

Mitral valve prolapse

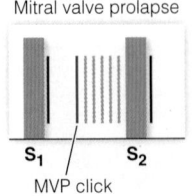

MVP click

Fig. 13-25. Mid-systolic ejection click and mitral valve prolapse.

PATIENT TEACHING

Healthy People 2020

Goal: Improve cardiovascular health and quality of life through prevention, detection, and treatment of risk factors for heart attack and stroke; early identification and treatment of heart attacks and strokes; and prevention of repeat cardiovascular events (HHS, 2010).

U.S. Preventive Services Task Force Recommendation

- The U.S. Preventive Services Task Force (USPSTF) strongly recommends screening men aged 35 and older for lipid disorders.
- The USPSTF recommends screening men aged 20 to 35 for lipid disorders if they are at increased risk for coronary heart disease.
- The USPSTF recommends screening women aged 20 to 45 for lipid disorders if they are at increased risk for coronary heart disease (U.S. Preventive Services Task Force, 2008).
- The USPSTF strongly recommends screening women aged 45 and older for lipid disorders if they are at increased risk for coronary heart disease.

American Heart Association

The American Heart Association recommends that all adults age 20 or older have their cholesterol and other traditional risk factors checked every four to six years. After that, people should work with their healthcare providers to determine their risk for cardiovascular disease and stroke (AHA, 2017b).

Potentially, more than half of the deaths and disability from cardiovascular disease can be delayed through public health initiatives and patient teaching to reduce the modifiable risk factors of cardiovascular disease (Gholizadeh, Davidson, Salamonson, & Worrall-Carter, 2010). Screening for normal lipid levels varies according to different professional organizations. Nurses should be aware that there are different guidelines.

Patient education should focus on:

- Reducing intake of saturated fats and cholesterol intake to 200 mg per day
- Red meats and sugary beverages and foods should be reduced.
- Increasing fiber by increasing whole grains, vegetables, beans, fruits, and nuts into our daily diet. Women should eat 25 grams of fiber per day and men 38 grams per day.
- Increasing physical activity to 35 minutes per day 7 days per week or 40 minutes of moderate to vigorous aerobic exercise three to four times a week (AHA, 2016b)
- Maintaining a healthy weight
- Moderating intake of alcohol:
  - ☐ Two drinks per day for men
  - ☐ One drink per day for women and older people (>65)
- Cessation of smoking

Assessing the Abdomen

INTRODUCTION

The abdomen is a complex and challenging region of the body that communicates with many different systems that can tell you about the overall health status of the patient. There are many vital organs contained in the abdominal cavity that require thorough assessment. Nurses have a key role in patient assessment, history taking, and management of care (Cole, Lynch, & Cugnoni, 2006).

It is critical that you assess and actively listen to your patient's self-report and abdominal complaints. A patient's complaints may be related to physiological or psychological alterations in their holistic integrity. Therefore, active listening and observation of the patient's nonverbal cues are essential during the health history and assessment. Nurses should use a systematic approach throughout the assessment.

REVIEW OF ANATOMY AND PHYSIOLOGY

Abdomen

- Has an oval form and is the largest cavity in the body (Fig. 14-1)
- Varies in size and shape, gender, and age
- Primary site for digestive organs and contains abdominal vasculature
- Covered by an endothelial serous membrane lining called the peritoneum; two types of peritoneum lining: the parietal peritoneum covers the walls of the abdominal cavity and the visceral peritoneum covers the organs
- The peritoneal cavity is the space between the parietal and visceral peritoneum.
- Mesentery is a double-layer membranous tissue connecting the intestines to the abdominal wall; contains blood vessels and nerves that supply the intestinal wall.

Abdominal Musculature

- The abdomen depends on muscles for support and protection.
- There are four pairs of abdominal muscles that support and protect the abdomen (Fig. 14-2):
  - External abdominal oblique
  - Rectus abdominis
  - Internal abdominal oblique
  - Transverse abdominis

Abdominal Viscera

- Viscera are the internal organs located in the abdominal cavity. There are two types of viscera:
  - The solid viscera of the abdomen are the adrenal glands, kidneys, liver, pancreas, spleen, ovaries, and uterus.

□ The hollow viscera are the gallbladder, small intestine, stomach, colon, and bladder.

Liver

- The liver is the heaviest and largest excretory organ in the body, weighing about 3 lbs.
- It occupies almost the entire right upper quadrant directly below the diaphragm.
- The liver is a highly vascular organ containing the hepatic artery that transports blood to the aorta.
- Three hepatic veins carry blood from the liver to the inferior vena cava.
- The liver plays a key role in metabolizing carbohydrates, proteins, fats, and drugs, producing bile, detoxifying harmful chemicals, and producing clotting factors.

DIAGNOSTICS

- **Aspartate aminotransferase (AST)** and **alanine aminotransferase (ALT)** are enzymes that exist in large amounts in the liver and myocardial cells and in smaller but significant amounts in skeletal muscle, kidneys, pancreas, and the brain. If damage to the liver occurs due to injury or pathology, there is a rise in these enzymes (Van Leeuwen & Bladh, 2015).
- **Ammonia (NH$_3$)** comes from two sources: removal of amino acids during protein metabolism and degradation of proteins by colon bacteria. The liver converts ammonia in the portal blood to urea, which is excreted by the kidneys. If the liver is severely compromised, especially in situations in which decreased hepatocellular function is combined with impaired portal blood flow, ammonia levels rise (Van Leeuwen & Bladh, 2015).
- **Bilirubin** is a by-product of heme catabolism from aged red blood cells (RBCs). Primarily produced in the liver, spleen, and bone marrow, an increase in bilirubin levels deposits a yellow pigment in the skin and sclera. The increase in yellow pigmentation is called jaundice or icterus (Van Leeuwen & Bladh, 2015).
- **Liver biopsy** is an excision of a tissue sample from the liver for microscopic analysis to determine cell morphology and the presence of tissue abnormalities. This biopsy is performed either percutaneously or after surgical incision (Van Leeuwen & Bladh, 2015). The nurse needs to assist the patient to maintain proper positioning during the procedure. After the biopsy a pressure dressing is applied. Monitor the patient for a change in vital signs and bleeding.

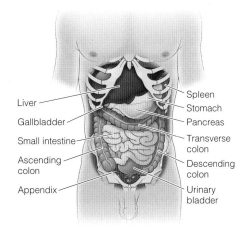

Liver
Gallbladder
Small intestine
Ascending colon
Appendix

Spleen
Stomach
Pancreas
Transverse colon
Descending colon
Urinary bladder

Fig. 14-1. Anatomy and physiology of the abdomen.

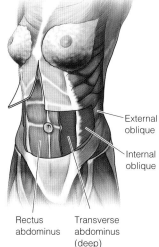

External oblique
Internal oblique

Rectus abdominus
Transverse abdominus (deep)

Fig. 14-2. Abdomen musculature.

Gallbladder

- The gallbladder is a pear-shaped organ (about 4 inches long) that is attached to the liver by connective tissue, blood vessels, and the hepatic duct.
- The gallbladder and biliary system collect, store, concentrate, and transport bile to the intestines to aid in digestion.
- Located in the right upper quadrant (RUQ), this organ contracts and releases bile into the common bile duct. Bile helps to digest fats.

DIAGNOSTICS

- **Ultrasound** of the liver and biliary system is a noninvasive test using high-frequency waves to evaluate the structure, size, and position of the liver and gallbladder. This procedure allows visualization of the gallbladder and bile ducts when the patient may have gallstones or impaired liver function (Van Leeuwen & Bladh, 2015).
- **Hepatobiliary iminodiacetic acid scan** is also known as HIDA scan. This is a nuclear medicine imaging study that tracks the production and flow of bile from the liver to your small intestine. It is primarily used to identify problems with the gallbladder, bile ducts, and liver.

Pancreas

- The pancreas is an irregularly shaped accessory organ of digestion.
- The head of the pancreas rests in the curve of the duodenum, and the tail extends laterally to touch the spleen.
- The pancreatic duct connects to the common bile duct that connects the pancreas to both the liver and the gallbladder.
- This organ has two primary functions. It has an endocrine function that secretes insulin and an exocrine function to release pancreatic juices.

DIAGNOSTICS

- Amylase and lipase are digestive enzymes that are sensitive indicators of pancreatic obstruction and pancreatic acinar cell damage.

Elevations of these enzymes may indicate obstruction, inflammation, or early pancreatic cancer.

- Glucose is a type of sugar that comes from ingestion of carbohydrate foods. Insulin is a hormone produced by the pancreas and released into the blood when glucose levels rise. This level has a direct link to the functioning of the islets of Langerhans in the pancreas that produce glucagon and insulin.

Stomach

- The stomach is a muscular, sac-like portion of the lower alimentary canal that permits digestion of food to take place gradually (Venes, 2013).
- It is approximately the size of an adult fist.
- There are three parts: the upper fundus, the body, and lower pylorus.
- Once food enters the stomach, hydrochloric acid is secreted and digests the food to create a substance known as chyme. The chyme is then propelled into the small intestine for further digestion.

DIAGNOSTICS

- **Esophagogastroduodenoscopy** is also known as an upper gastrointestinal (GI) endoscopy. A lighted, flexible scope or video scope is inserted through the patient's mouth and is passed through the esophagus and stomach, and to the duodenum of the small intestine. The procedure is done to assess the mucosa of the upper GI tract, to remove foreign bodies or polyps, and to aid in diagnosis of symptoms (Van Leeuwen & Bladh, 2015).

Spleen

- The spleen is a flat, oblong, soft, highly vascular, ductless organ measuring about 4 to 5 inches in length.
- It is situated in the left upper quadrant, extends into the epigastric region, and is protected by the ribcage.

- It is the largest lymph organ in the body with a major function in our immune system.
- As part of the reticuloendothelial system, the spleen filters blood; manufactures lymphocytes, monocytes, macrophages; stores erythrocytes and platelets; and produces erythrocytes during bone marrow depression.

DIAGNOSTICS
- **Complete blood count (CBC)** is able to assess portions of the reticuloendothelial system and the basic cells produced and maintained by the spleen. The CBC can include a differential of key cells in our blood system. The red blood cell (RBC) count calculates the number of erythrocytes and the size and shape of the RBCs. Platelet count is part of the CBC that can assess for bone marrow or bleeding disorders. The lymphocyte and monocyte counts can help identify problems with our immune function. Because the spleen is involved in maintaining the functioning of our overall immune system, the CBC with differential may help assess the functioning of this organ.

Small intestine
- The small intestine is a convoluted tube about 21 feet in length and is composed of three parts: duodenum (12 inches), jejunum (8 feet), and ileum (12 feet).
- It is contained in the central and lower part of the abdominal cavity and joins the large intestine at the ileocecal valve.
- The primary functions are completion of digestion and absorption of nutrients.

Large intestine
- The large intestine is a tubular-shaped organ about 5 feet in length that begins at the cecum and ends at the rectum.

- There are four segments of the large intestine: ascending, transverse, descending, and sigmoid colon.
- The primary function of the large intestine is the absorption of water and electrolytes.
- Peristalsis moves food and excretes the end products of digestion through the rectum.

Vermiform appendix
- A long, narrow, wormlike tube averaging 9 cm in length
- Located in the right lower quadrant about 2 cm below the ileocecal valve at McBurney's point (Fig. 14-3)
- Function unknown
- Sometimes fills with digestive materials from the cecum and becomes infected

DIAGNOSTICS
- **Stool analysis** is examination of feces for volume, odor, shape, color, consistency, and presence of mucus, pathogens, and substances (Van Leeuwen & Bladh, 2015).
- **Fecal occult blood test (FOBT)** is a test for hidden or occult blood in the stool. Hidden blood may come from any part of the digestive tract and is not seen by the patient. This noninvasive test is done annually on adults because it could be the first warning sign of colorectal cancer.

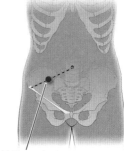

McBurney's point

Fig. 14-3. McBurney's point.

CULTURAL CONSIDERATIONS The rate of people getting colorectal cancer or dying from colorectal cancer varies by race and ethnicity. The year 2011 is the most recent year for which numbers have been reported: black people had the highest rate of getting colorectal cancer, followed by white Caucasian, Hispanic, Asian/Pacific Islander, and American Indian/Alaska Native people (Centers for Disease Control and Prevention [CDC], 2014).

- **Stool for culture** identifies the organism causing a patient's symptoms, usually diarrhea.
- **Barium enema** is a radiological examination and fluoroscopy with air or barium contrast. A rectal tube is inserted into the rectum to instill the barium. The patient holds the barium while a series of x-rays are taken. This test is useful to identify several different pathologies such as diverticula, tumors, polyps, rectal bleeding, or complaints of abdominal pain (Van Leeuwen & Bladh, 2015).
- **Sigmoidoscopy** uses a flexible fiberoptic scope to visualize the mucosa of the lower third of the large intestine. This noninvasive procedure is able to screen for colon cancer and polyps (abnormal growths) in the rectum and sigmoid colon.
- **Colonoscopy** uses a flexible tube with a camera (fiberoptic colonoscope) to inspect the inner lining of the mucosa of the large intestine, ileocecal valve, and terminal ileum for abnormalities. This procedure allows for tissue samples to be biopsied and polyps (abnormal growths) to be removed. This is the gold standard to detect colon cancer.
- **Virtual colonoscopy (CTC)** uses computed tomography to visualize a three-dimensional picture of the colon. CTC has emerged as an alternative to the traditional gold standard, optical colonoscopy, for screening asymptomatic adults and is considered the best radiological diagnostic test for imaging colorectal cancer (Patel, Patel, & Chang, 2016).

Kidneys and bladder

- Kidneys are bean-shaped organs (about 4 inches long) that lie in the back part of the upper abdomen.
- They are located on each side of the vertebral column (T12 to L3) (Fig. 14-4).
- The 12th rib forms an angle with the vertebral column on the back called the costovertebral angle.
- The right kidney is 1 to 2 cm lower than the left kidney due to the liver size and location in the abdomen.
- They excrete water-soluble waste.
- Ureters are two tubes that transport urine from the kidneys to the bladder.

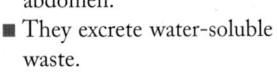

Kidney
Ureter
Bladder
Sphincter
Urethra

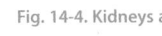

Fig. 14-4. Kidneys and bladder.

- Bladder is a hollow, muscular sac. It is the reservoir for holding urine located in the pelvic area; this organ collects urine excreted by the kidneys.

DIAGNOSTICS

- **Blood urea nitrogen (BUN)** is a nonprotein nitrogen compound formed in the liver from ammonia as an end product of protein metabolism. The compound is excreted by the kidneys. It is a reflection of the amount of urea produced and excreted. This value may be used to evaluate liver and renal function (Van Leeuwen & Bladh, 2015). If the kidneys are not working properly, the BUN level rises.

- **Creatinine** is the end product of muscle metabolism. This chemical waste is transported through the bloodstream and out of the body through the kidneys. If the waste products are accumulating and are not excreted by the kidneys, the creatinine level rises. This level is a reliable indicator that the kidneys are functioning properly.
- **Glomerular filtration rate (GFR)** assesses kidney functioning. This test estimates how much blood passes through the glomeruli of the kidneys in 1 minute (http://www.nlm.nih.gov/medlineplus/ency/article/007305.htm). This test assesses whether a patient has renal disease, renal insufficiency, or renal failure.
- **Bladder scan** is a portable ultrasound instrument used to identify how much urine is in the bladder. The scan is most often used to measure postvoid residual volume (PVR); this is urine retained in the bladder after voiding.

Reproductive organs
- In the female, the uterus, fallopian tubes, and ovaries are located in the pelvic portion of the pelvic cavity (Female Reproductive Assessment is discussed in Chapter 18).

Vasculature in the Abdominal Cavity
- The aorta is the largest artery in the body that bifurcates to form the right and left common iliac arteries (Fig. 14-5). The aorta transports oxygenated blood to the tissues of the body.

DIAGNOSTICS
- **Ultrasound** uses high-frequency sound waves to image the walls of the aorta. This noninvasive diagnostic test is most commonly used to measure the size of the aorta and to screen for aortic aneurysms.

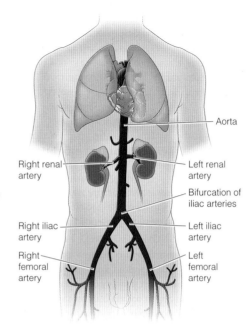

Fig. 14-5. Vasculature of abdomen.

Aorta

Right renal artery

Left renal artery

Bifurcation of iliac arteries

Right iliac artery

Left iliac artery

Right femoral artery

Left femoral artery

Major arteries
Major arteries include:
- aorta
- renal
- iliac
- femoral.

HEALTH HISTORY

Review of Systems

Use the **OLDCARTS** mnemonic (**O**nset, **L**ocation, **D**uration, **C**haracteristics, **A**ggravating/Alleviating factors, **R**elieving factors, **T**reatment, **S**everity) or **OPQRST** mnemonic **O**nset (O), **P**rovocation (P), **Q**uality (Q), **R**adiation (R), **S**everity (S), **T**iming (T) to identify attributes of a symptom.

Time must be spent interviewing your patient before the actual assessment. Patients with abdominal problems or pathology may have a wide range of symptoms (Cox & Steggall, 2009). Remember to ask your patient about past medical history, past surgical history, psychosocial history, and medication assessment. Medication assessment should include prescription, over-the-counter, and herbal remedies. Nurses must take into consideration that some topics such as discussing bowel and bladder habits may be a sensitive topic and embarrassing for the patient to share.

SENC Patient-Centered Care Actively listen to your patient's report. Provide compassionate care. Some patients are embarrassed to discuss their normal bowel and bladder functions. Through the art of genuine listening, you will enhance communicating with your patients and allow them openly and honestly discuss their health and psychosocial behaviors with you related to the abdomen.

A focused health assessment related to the abdominal assessment includes the following. Ask the patient the following questions.

Weight

- Have you gained or lost any weight recently? If so how much? Intentional or unintentional?

TIP If available, review previous weight to current weight. Calculate the body mass index (BMI) (see Chapter 5).

SENC Safety Alert Unintentional weight loss may be a sign of illness or metastatic disease.

Appetite

- Any change in your appetite?
  - □ Gastrointestinal dysfunction, mental health (i.e., depression), cognitive status (i.e., dementia), and finances are a few examples of factors that may affect the patient's appetite and ability to eat.
  - □ Anorexia is loss of appetite; this may be related to a pathological condition, mental health or cognitive impairment, side effects of medications, or dietary intolerances.
- What have you eaten in the last 24 hours?
  - □ Assess dietary intake.
  - □ Assess for food intolerances.
    - Lactose intolerance is due to a deficiency in intestinal lactase causing abdominal discomfort and diarrhea after ingestion of milk or milk products.
  - □ Assess cultural considerations for diet.

CULTURAL CONSIDERATIONS Lactose intolerance in adulthood is most prevalent in people of East Asian descent, affecting more than 90 percent of adults in some of these communities. Lactose intolerance is also common in people of West African, Arab, Jewish, Greek, and Italian descent (National Library of Medicine, 2014a).

Dysphagia (Difficulty Swallowing)

- Do you have any difficulty swallowing solid foods or liquids?
  - □ Assess if there are specific foods or liquids causing difficulty swallowing.
  - □ Assess if there is a pattern such as after every meal or intermittently throughout the day.
- Do you ever feel like you have a lump in your throat or the food does not go all the way down?
  - □ Oropharyngeal dysphagia could be due to a motor disorder affecting the pharyngeal muscles.

□ Some symptoms of dysphagia are: drooling, pocketing food in the mouth, coughing or gagging while eating.

Nausea and Vomiting

■ Have you been nauseous or vomited? If so, when did it start?
■ Is there a pattern (before or after meals)?
■ What color was the vomitus (emesis)? Did you notice any blood? Was there a foul odor to the vomitus? Types of vomit include:
□ Digested or undigested food may be related to gastritis or food poisoning.
□ Bilious: green-yellow bile related to a biliary obstruction
□ Black: vomit containing blood acted on by gastric digestion
□ Coffee-ground; appearance and consistency of coffee ground material; may have blood mixed in with the vomitus; if fecal odor, may indicate fecal material related to an intestinal obstruction (Venes, 2013)
□ Hematemesis: vomiting of blood may be related to gastrointestinal bleeding.
□ Projectile vomiting without nausea is a sign of central stimulation of the medulla; could be a sign of brain pathology or head trauma.

SENC Safety Alert A patient who has prolonged vomiting should be assessed for signs of dehydration (Box 14-1).

BOX 14-1 **Signs of Dehydration**

- Decreased skin turgor
- Decreased urine output
- Dark, concentrated urine
- Dry mouth and mucous membranes
- Dry eyes with no tear production
- Fatigue and weakness
- Headache
- Constipation
- Thirst

Indigestion or Heartburn

■ Do you experience heartburn (pyrosis)? If so, assess timing and duration.
■ Do you take any medication for indigestion? If so, is the medication effective?
■ Do you have any chest pain or indigestion after eating?
□ **Pyrosis** is indigestion/heartburn usually described as a "burning sensation" in the epigastric area radiating up to the throat.
□ **Dyspepsia** is a term that is used to describe a vague feeling of fullness and chest discomfort, indigestion, or burning in the chest or upper abdomen, especially after eating.
□ **Gastroesophageal reflux disease (GERD)** is motility disorder characterized by heartburn and reflux of gastric content into the lower esophagus.

Abdominal/Pelvic Pain

■ Ask the patient to describe the pain in his or her own words.
■ Use the OLDCARTS or OPQRST mnemonic to assess the pain.

SENC Safety Alert Abdominal pain could be a serious symptom and be a medical emergency. There are many causes of abdominal pain, and this large region containing major organs needs a thorough assessment.

□ Abdominal pain could indicate digestive, cardiac, renal disorders, or ectopic pregnancy.
□ Visceral pain is dull, gnawing, cramping, or burning; poorly localized; originates in the abdominal organs.
□ Parietal pain is steady, sharp, localized, and intensifies with movement; usually caused by inflammation of the parietal peritoneum.
□ Peritoneal pain caused by peritoneal inflammation (peritonitis) produces localized, sharp, or generalized abdominal tenderness.

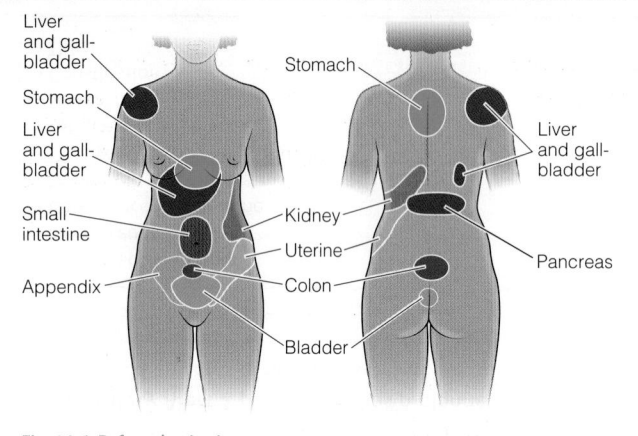

Fig. 14-6. Referred pain sites.

☐ Referred pain arises in one part of the abdomen but is perceived by the sensory cortex via nerve fibers remote from the site (e.g., gallbladder pain can be referred to the right shoulder) (Fig. 14-6).

Constipation or Diarrhea

TIP Normal bowel movements can occur as often as three times a day or as few as three times per week; every individual has a different bowel elimination schedule depending on diet, exercise, and lifestyle (Leviticus, 2011).

■ What are your normal bowel habits? Describe the color and consistency of your stool.

■ Do you feel that you are constipated?
  ☐ Ask about characteristics of being constipated or having diarrhea, such as color, consistency, size of stool.
  ☐ Perceived constipation is a state in which a person makes a self-diagnosis of constipation and ensures a daily bowel movement through use of laxatives, enemas, or suppositories.

■ Have you noticed a change in your bowel routine?

SENC Safety Alert Narrowing of stools or pencil-like stools may indicate some type of intestinal obstruction.

■ Did you notice blood in your stool?
■ Do you use laxatives? If so, how often?
  ☐ All shades of brown are considered normal: The foods you eat and the medications you take can change the color of your stools (Pico, 2012).
  ☐ Melena is black, tarry stool indicating lower gastrointestinal bleeding or colon cancer.
  ☐ Gray stools or clay-colored stools are common with hepatitis.
  ☐ Dark, nontarry stools are commonly seen in patients taking iron supplements.
  TIP Iron supplements have a tendency to cause constipation.
  ☐ Bright red stools indicate gastrointestinal bleeding or rectal bleeding.
  ☐ Blood and mucous in stools are associated with inflammatory bowel disorders.

Flatulence

■ Do you have any problems with gas (flatulence)?
■ Do you feel bloated?
■ Do you belch or burp?
  ☐ The average adult produces about one to three pints of gas each day, which is passed through the anus 14 to 23 times per day (Goldfinger, 2012).
  ☐ Flatulence and bloating can be influenced by our diet, how much air is swallowed (aerophagia) with eating, and some intestinal disorders such as irritable bowel syndrome.
  ☐ Common foods causing gas: beans, peas, lentils, cabbage, onions, high-fiber cereals, bananas, raisins, apricots, and milk products

Urination

- Do you experience frequency or urgency of urination?
- Do you have back pain?
- Do you experience painful or difficult urination (dysuria)?
- Is there a problem with incontinence?
- Ask men if they have difficulty or hesitancy starting the stream.
  - □ **Dysuria** is painful or difficult urination indicative of an inflammatory condition or pathology of the urinary tract.
  - □ **Renal colic pain** results from a kidney stone; the stone may partially or totally obstruct the ureter; it may remain in one place or travel down the urinary tract. A patient with acute renal colic usually experiences the sudden onset of severe pain originating in the flank and radiating to the groin or back.

Skin

- Have you experienced any change in your skin color or whites of the eyes?
  - □ Skin texture and color changes may be related to organ dysfunction such as liver, gallbladder, and kidney disease.
    - • **Jaundice:** yellow staining of body tissues and fluids resulting from excessive levels of bilirubin in the bloodstream or liver disease

Out-of-Country Travel

- Have you traveled out of the country?
  - □ Traveling outside the country to countries with poor sanitation poses the risk for acquiring food-borne illnesses and hepatitis A, B, and C.
  - □ Hepatitis A, B, C, is caused by a specific virus causing infection and inflammation of the liver. Symptoms may include abdominal pain, nausea, fatigue, and poor appetite.

SENC Safety Alert Individuals traveling out of the country should be vaccinated; international travel health clinics are up to date on the recommended vaccinations for travel abroad. Patients can check the CDC's Travelers' Health website for recommended versus required vaccinations at http://wwwnc.cdc.gov/travel/destinations/list.

CULTURAL CONSIDERATIONS Crohn's disease is a chronic disorder that primarily affects the digestive system; this condition typically involves abnormal inflammation of the intestinal walls. The inflamed tissues become thick and swollen, and the inner surface of the intestine may develop open sores (ulcers). Crohn's disease occurs more often in Caucasians (whites) and people of eastern and central European (Ashkenazi) Jewish descent than among people of other ethnic backgrounds (National Library of Medicine, 2014b).

PREPARATION FOR ASSESSMENT

Equipment Needed

Gloves
Stethoscope
Paper measuring tape (only used in advanced technique)
Pen or skin marker (only used in advanced technique)
Note: The order of the abdominal assessment is different from other assessments so that peristalsis is not stimulated by percussing and palpating.

Sequence of Assessment

1. Inspection
2. Auscultation
3. Indirect percussion
4. Palpation (light and deep)

TIP A cold room increases abdominal muscle tension. Throughout the assessment, observe the patient for nonverbal body language that may indicate discomfort.

Preliminary Steps
- Maintain privacy throughout the assessment.
- Explain all steps of the assessment to the patient and answer the patient's questions.
- Instruct the patient to empty his or her bladder.
- Ensure room is warm, well lit, and comfortable for the patient.
- Perform hand hygiene.
- Position patient in the supine position, with head on a pillow and arms by the side. If the patient is unable to flex knees, place a pillow under the knees.
- Expose the abdomen, place drape over the patient's symphysis pubis and chest area (Fig. 14-7).
- When examining a patient with a colostomy or ileostomy, remove bag only if needed.
- Warm the diaphragm of the stethoscope and your hands to avoid muscle tension during the assessment.
- If the patient states that he or she has abdominal pain, tell the patient that you will examine the painful abdominal area last.

Abdominal Mapping
Abdominal mapping is the process of dividing the abdomen into quadrants or regions. During the assessment, visualize the underlying structures for each quadrant or region. There are two types of abdominal mapping: four quadrant and nine regions.

Four-Quadrant Mapping
Four-quadrant mapping is the most commonly used method (Fig. 14-8).
1. Extend the midsternal line from the xiphoid process through the umbilicus to the pubic bone.
2. Draw a horizontal line at the umbilicus to form the following:
   □ Right Upper Quadrant (RUQ)
   □ Right Lower Quadrant (RLQ)
   □ Left Upper Quadrant (LUQ)
   □ Left Lower Quadrant (LLQ)

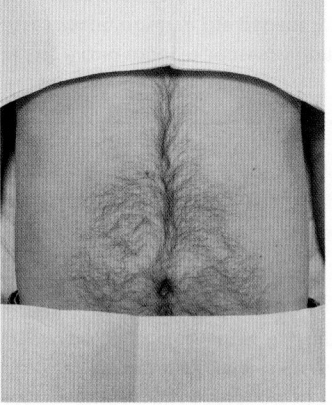

Fig. 14-7. Draping for abdominal assessment.

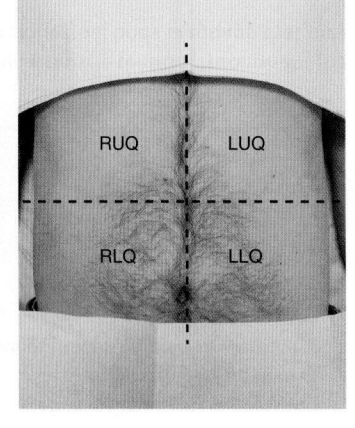

Fig. 14-8. Mapping the four quadrants of the abdomen.

The abdominal organ location for each quadrant may be viewed in Table 14-1.

Landmarking the Abdomen into Nine Regions
1. Extend the right and left midclavicular line to the groin.
2. Draw a horizontal line across the lowest edge of the costal margin.
3. Draw a second horizontal line at the level of the iliac crest. Creating these lines divides the abdominal area into nine regions (Fig. 14-9):
   □ Right hypochondriac
   □ Epigastric
   □ Left hypochondriac
   □ Right lumbar
   □ Umbilicus
   □ Left lumbar
   □ Right iliac
   □ Hypogastric
   □ Left iliac

TABLE 14-1 Organs in Each Abdominal Quadrant

Right Upper Quadrant (RUQ)	Left Upper Quadrant (LUQ)
Duodenum of small intestine	Left lobe of liver
Gallbladder	Stomach
Liver	Spleen
Head of pancreas	Body of pancreas
Right kidney	Left kidney
Right adrenal gland	Left adrenal
Hepatic flexure of colon	Splenic flexure of the colon
Part of ascending and transverse colon	Part of the transverse and descending colon

Right Lower Quadrant (RLQ)	Left Lower Quadrant (LLQ)
Cecum	Part of descending colon
Appendix	Sigmoid colon
Part of ascending colon	Left ovary and tube
Right ovary and tube	Left ureter
Right ureter	Left spermatic cord
Right spermatic cord	

Midline
Aorta
Uterus
Bladder

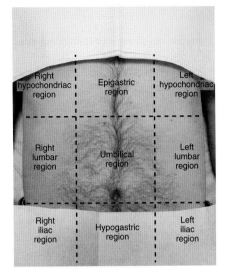

Fig. 14-9. Mapping the nine regions of the abdomen.

FOCUSED ASSESSMENT

TECHNIQUE 14-1: **Inspecting the Abdomen**

Purpose: To assess abnormalities in shape, skin, or movement of the abdomen

Inspection of the abdomen should be done in two positions: at the patient's side (Fig. 14-10A) and standing at the patient's feet (Fig. 14-10B).

ASSESSMENT STEPS

1. Assist patient to supine position.

2. Stoop by the patient's side so the abdomen is at eye level. Inspect the abdomen for:
- ☐ contour, size, and symmetry
- ☐ size and position of the umbilicus
- ☐ condition of skin: color, lesions, veins, hernias, hair distribution
- ☐ movements, pulsations, and peristalsis.

3. Inspect the abdomen by standing at the patient's feet:
- ☐ contour, size, and symmetry
- ☐ size and position of the umbilicus
- ☐ condition of skin: color, lesions, veins, hernias, hair distribution
- ☐ movements, pulsations, and peristalsis.

4. Document your findings.

NORMAL FINDINGS
- Contour (flat or rounded)
- Bilaterally symmetrical
- Umbilicus midline
- Skin smooth and intact without pulsations or visible peristalsis
- Peristalsis and aortic pulsations may be visible in very thin patients

ABNORMAL FINDINGS
- A scaphoid, distended, or protuberant abdomen is usually seen with an underlying pathology such as cancer, weight loss, hernia, or accumulation of fluid (Fig. 14-11).
- Increased peristaltic waves (ripple-like movement) are seen with intestinal obstruction.
- Pulsations are increased with the presence of aortic aneurysm.
  - ☐ An aneurysm is a weakening and outpouching of an artery.
- Abdominal distention is caused by fluid, fat, feces, flatulence, fibroids, or a fetus.
- Ascites is an abnormal accumulation of fluid in the peritoneal cavity.
- Diastasis recti is a bulging area in the abdomen occurring with the separation of the two halves of the rectus abdominis muscles in the midline at the linea alba (Fig. 14-12).

  TIP The bulge may appear only when the patient raises the head or coughs.

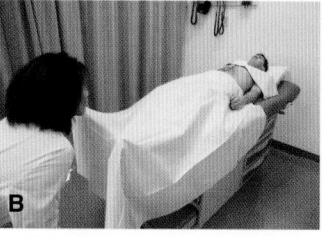

A

B

Fig. 14-10. Inspecting the abdomen.

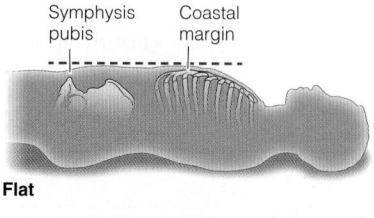

Symphysis pubis Coastal margin

Flat

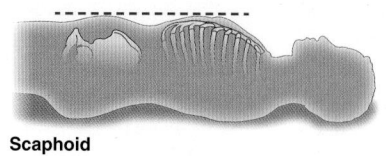

Scaphoid

Rounded

Protuberant

Fig. 14-11. Abdominal contours.

- Hernias may also be visible if the abdominal wall weakens and causes a loop of intestine or abdominal tissue to protrude through an opening in the peritoneum. Hernias are classified according to their location such as inguinal, epigastric, umbilical, incisional, or diastasis recti.
- Cullen's sign is superficial bleeding under the skin (ecchymosis) around the umbilicus and may indicate intra-abdominal bleeding (Fig. 14-13).

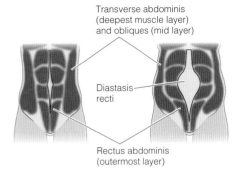

Transverse abdominis (deepest muscle layer) and obliques (mid layer)

Diastasis recti

Rectus abdominis (outermost layer)

Fig. 14-12. Separation of diastasis recti muscle.

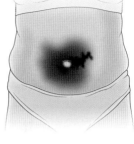

Fig. 14-13. Cullen's sign.

TECHNIQUE 14-2: Auscultating Bowel Sounds

Purpose: To assess a pattern of bowel sounds
Equipment: Stethoscope
■ **TIP** For a patient with a nasogastric tube, turn off the suction or pinch tube prior to auscultating.
ASSESSMENT STEPS
1. Auscultate bowel sounds by placing the diaphragm of the stethoscope on the abdomen at the ileocecal valve (RLQ) where bowel sounds are usually always present (Fig. 14-14).
   ■ **TIP** Listen for 3 to 5 minutes before documenting that there are no bowel sounds.
2. Note the quality or characteristics and frequency of the bowel sounds (Table 14-2).
3. Auscultate in all four abdominal quadrants (RLQ, RUQ, LUQ, LLQ).
4. Document your findings.
NORMAL FINDINGS
■ Five to 34 clicks or gurgles per minute; bowel sounds have an irregular pattern.
ABNORMAL FINDINGS
■ Hyperactive, high-pitched bowel sounds may indicate early bowel obstruction or increased peristalsis.
■ Hypoactive, soft, irregular sounds may indicating decreased peristalsis related to constipation.
■ No bowel sounds could indicate constipation or a paralytic ileus, no peristalsis movement.

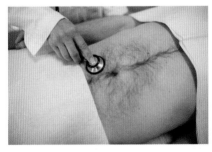

Fig. 14-14. Auscultating for bowel sounds starting at the ileocecal valve.

TABLE 14-2 Bowel Sounds

Normal	Hyperactive	Hypoactive	Absent
Borborygmus- loud gurgling or rumbling sounds made by the movement of gas through the intestines	Loud, high-pitched sounds Heard in patients with diarrhea, laxative use, gastroenteritis, early intestinal obstruction	Slow, decreased sounds Heard in patients with constipation, obstruction, medications	No sounds heard May indicate a paralytic ileus after surgery, bowel obstruction, peritonitis

Technique 14-2A: Auscultating Vascular Sounds

Purpose: To assess a normal pattern of blood flow in the abdominal vasculature

Equipment: Stethoscope

ASSESSMENT STEPS

1. With the bell of the stethoscope, press down firmly to listen over the aorta, renal, iliac, and femoral arteries (Fig. 14-15).
2. Auscultate over the liver (bell) for a venous hum, turbulent blood flow in the jugular venous system which may indicate liver disease or portal hypertension.
3. Document your findings.

   TIP Portal hypertension is an increase in pressure in the portal vein caused by an obstruction in the blood flow through the liver; the primary cause is cirrhosis of the liver (Iwakiri, 2014).

NORMAL FINDINGS

- No bruits over arteries

ABNORMAL FINDINGS

- Bruits are turbulent, blowing sounds heard over a partially or totally obstructed artery. Bruits are most commonly caused by a buildup of plaque in the artery.

SENC Safety Alert Bruits may be heard in patients with renal disease, hypertension, or peripheral vascular disease. Do not percuss or palpate an area where a bruit is heard. This may dislodge the obstruction causing the turbulent blood flow.

- Venous hum is a continuous medium-pitched sound caused by turbulent blood flow in a large vascular organ (Cox & Steggall, 2009).
- Friction rub is a grating sound heard over inflamed organs with serous surfaces; most commonly heard in the RUQ (liver) or LUQ (spleen).

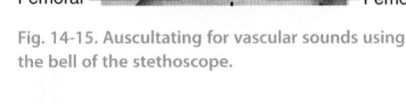

Fig. 14-15. Auscultating for vascular sounds using the bell of the stethoscope.

TECHNIQUE 14-3: **Percussing the Abdomen**

Purpose: To assist with identifying gas and solid or fluid-filled masses in the abdomen.

ASSESSMENT STEPS

1. Using indirect percussion, percuss over each quadrant and note the quality of sounds heard (Fig. 14-16).
2. Follow one of the two patterns for percussion (Fig. 14-17).
3. Document your findings.

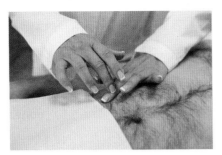

Fig. 14-16. Indirect percussion.

> **TIP** Tympany is high-pitched, hollow-quality, drum-like sound that is heard over air-filled viscera. Dullness is low-amplitude sound heard over fluid, organs, adipose tissue, or a distended bladder.

NORMAL FINDINGS

- Tympany in all four quadrants; dullness over organs

ABNORMAL FINDINGS

- Excessive, high-pitched tympanic sounds may indicate distention.
- Dullness may indicate increased tissue density such as organ enlargement or an underlying mass.
- Pain during percussion may indicate peritoneal inflammation.

> **TIP** If the spleen is enlarged, it expands anteriorly, downward, and medially, replacing tympany sounds of the stomach and colon with the dullness of a solid organ.

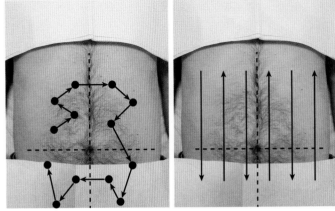

Fig. 14-17. Percussion patterns.

TECHNIQUE 14-4: **Palpating the Abdomen**

Purpose: To assess surface characteristics, tenderness, enlarged organs, or fluid in the abdominal cavity

Preliminary Steps:

- Warm your hands by rubbing them together prior to palpating the abdomen.
- If your patient is ticklish, have the patient rest his or her hand on top of your hand while you palpate (Cox & Stegall, 2009).
- Always palpate tender areas last.

Technique 14-4A: **Light Palpation**

Purpose: To feel for surface characteristics and assess for tenderness

ASSESSMENT STEPS

1. Using the finger pads of one hand, press down about ½ inch (Fig. 14-18).
2. Lightly palpate in a clockwise direction the entire abdomen.
3. Lift your fingers gently as you move to a different area.
4. Watch patient's facial expression for signs of pain or abdominal guarding.
5. Document your findings.

NORMAL FINDINGS

- No tenderness, smooth surface characteristics

ABNORMAL FINDINGS

- Tenderness is present; nodule or mass felt.

Technique 14-4B: **Deep Palpation**

Purpose: To assess for enlarged organs, masses, or tenderness

ASSESSMENT STEPS

1. Place your nondominant hand on top of your dominant hand (also known as bimanual palpation)
2. Deeply palpate; press down about 1.5 to 2 inches using a circular or a dipping motion in a clockwise direction (Fig. 14-19).
3. Lift your hands gently as you move to different areas.
4. Document your findings.

NORMAL FINDINGS

- No masses, enlarged organs, or tenderness

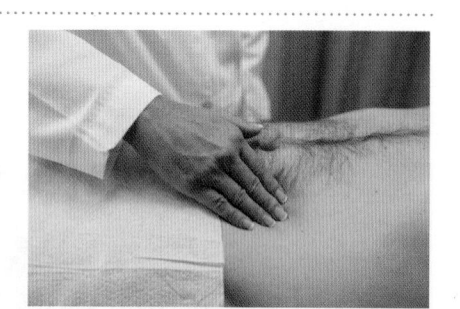

Fig. 14-18. Light palpation of the abdomen.

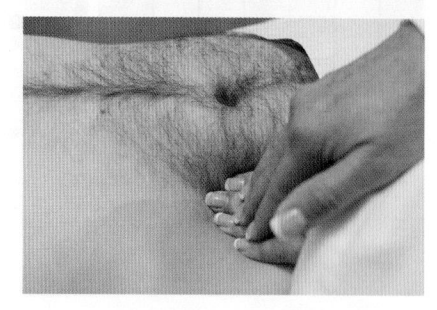

Fig. 14-19. Deep palpation of the abdomen.

ABNORMAL FINDINGS
- Masses are palpated.
- Enlarged organs
- Tenderness or pain is present

    TIP To check for rebound tenderness, press slowly on a tender area, then quickly "let go." Rebound tenderness is indicative of peritoneal inflammation.

Technique 14-4C: **Palpating the Bladder**

Purpose: To assess for a distended bladder

TIP A person with a distended bladder may have difficulty urinating or will release only small amounts of urine. It is normal for the patient to feel the urge to urinate during palpation.

ASSESSMENT STEPS
1. Ask the patient when she or he last emptied the bladder.
2. Lightly palpate for a distended bladder between symphysis pubis and umbilicus (Fig. 14-20).
3. Note the size and location of the bladder.
4. Document your findings.

NORMAL FINDINGS
- An empty bladder is not palpable.
- A partially filled bladder will feel firm and smooth.

ABNORMAL FINDINGS
- A distended bladder is palpated as a smooth, round, and firm mass extending as far up as the umbilicus.

    TIP Watch for nonverbal body language; tenderness or pain may indicate bladder infection.

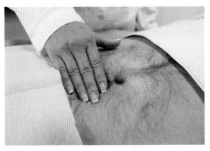

Fig. 14-20. Palpating the bladder.

ADVANCED TECHNIQUES

TECHNIQUE 14-5: **Percussing Costovertebral Tenderness**

Purpose: To assess tenderness or inflammation of the kidney

■ **TIP** You can do this assessment when the patient is already sitting up to minimize position changes.

You may use the indirect blunt percussion technique or the fist percussion technique to test for kidney inflammation.

SENC Safety Alert Do not percuss an organ transplant patient!

ASSESSMENT STEPS

1. Place patient in a sitting position; stand facing the patient's back.

2. To assess the kidney, place the palm of one hand over the 12th rib at the costovertebral angle on the back (Fig. 14-21).

3. Thump that hand with the ulnar edge of your other fist.

4. Document your findings.

NORMAL FINDINGS

■ Elicits no pain

ABNORMAL FINDINGS

■ Tenderness or pain may indicate kidney infection or presence of kidney stones.

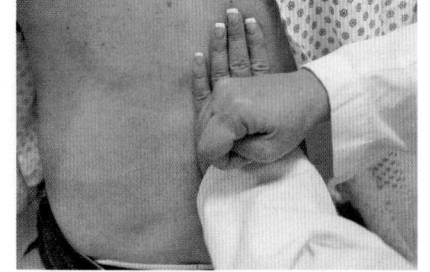
Fig. 14-21. Assessing for costovertebral tenderness using fist percussion.

TECHNIQUE 14-6: **Assessing for Ascites**

Ascites is an abnormal accumulation of fluid in the peritoneal cavity; some of the more common causes are liver disease and malignancies. A patient with ascites may complain of shortness of breath and abdominal discomfort due to the accumulation of fluid.

■ Ascitic fluid usually drops with gravity, whereas gas-filled loops of bowel float to the top, percussion gives a dull note in dependent areas of the abdomen where fluid is present.

■ Ascitic fluid is only detected after 500 mL of fluid has accumulated in the abdomen.

DIAGNOSTICS

■ A **paracentesis** is the procedure to remove fluid from the peritoneal cavity by inserting a needle into the cavity for diagnostic evaluation. This procedure is usually done when the patient is experiencing respiratory distress or abdominal pain.

■ **Ultrasound** of the abdomen usually is done to confirm diagnosis of ascites and during a paracentesis to identify pockets of fluid.

▪ **TIP** Patients who have ascites may experience respiratory distress when lying flat due to fluid pressure on the diaphragm. Place patient is semi-Fowler's or Fowler's position for comfort.

Technique 14-6A: Testing for Fluid Waves

Purpose: To assess for abnormal accumulation of fluid in the abdomen. (You will need someone to help you with this test, or if able, the patient may assist).

ASSESSMENT STEPS

1. Explain the technique to the patient.
2. Place patient in the supine position.

   ▪ **TIP** Lying in the supine position will make the fluid accumulate on the lateral sides of the abdomen.

3. Percuss the mid-abdomen; assess the percussion tone.
4. Percuss each lateral side of the abdomen; assess the percussion tone.
5. Ask your assistant or the patient to place the ulnar side of his or her hand and the lateral side of the forearm firmly along the midline of the abdomen (Fig. 14-22).

   ▪ **TIP** By having your assistant or patient place his or her hand and forearm midline on the abdomen, this will deter the movement of your tap across the patient's skin; only the fluid will move if present.

6. Place the palmar surface of your fingers and hand against one side of the abdomen.
7. Use your other hand to tap the other side of the abdomen (Fig. 14-23).
8. Assess the movement of fluid from one side of the abdomen to the opposite side.
9. Document your findings.

NORMAL FINDINGS

■ Percussion tones are tympanic.
■ No fluid is transmitted.

ABNORMAL FINDINGS

■ Ascites is present.
■ Percussion tone is tympanic at the mid-abdomen.
■ Dull percussion tones will be heard on the lateral sides where fluid is present.
■ You will feel movement of the fluid wave against your resting hand. This suggests that large amounts of fluid (ascites) are present in the abdomen.

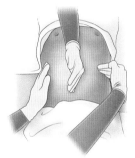

Fig. 14-22. Hand placement to assess for ascites.

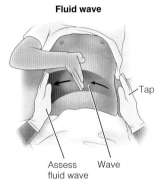

Fluid wave

Tap

Assess fluid wave

Wave

Fig. 14-23. Assessing for fluid wave.

PATIENT EDUCATION

Healthy People 2020

Goal: Reduce the number of new cancer cases, as well as the illness, disability, and death caused by cancer (HHS, 2010). There are three objectives specific to reducing colon cancer:

- Increase the proportion of adults who receive colorectal cancer screening based on the recent guidelines.
- Reduce invasive colon cancer.
- Reduce the colorectal cancer death rate.

Patient education should be ongoing throughout the assessment. Some key points to discuss with your patient are as follows:

- Maintaining a healthy weight; obesity increases the risk for colon cancer
- Eating a healthy diet high in vegetables, fruits, and whole grains; low in red and processed meats
- Limiting alcohol intake
- Increasing the intensity of an exercise regimen; participating in moderate-to-vigorous exercise for 30 minutes, 5 or more days per week

Colon Cancer Screening

Colorectal cancer is the third most common cancer diagnosed in both men and women in the United States, other than skin cancer (ACS, 2017a). The American Cancer Society (ACS) recommends that individuals be screened for colon cancer depending on their personal history or family history. The American Cancer Society (2017) believes that preventing colorectal cancer should be a major reason for getting screened.

- The ACS (2017b) recommends that beginning at age 50, both men and women at average risk follow one of these screening schedules:
  - ☐ Flexible sigmoidoscopy every 5 years
  - ☐ Colonoscopy every 10 years
  - ☐ Double-contrast barium enema every 5 years
  - ☐ Computed tomography virtual colonoscopy every 5 years
- The U.S. Preventive Service Task Force recommends screening for colorectal cancer (CRC) in adults, beginning at age 50 years and continuing until age 75 years. The decision to screen for colorectal cancer in adults aged 76 to 85 years should be an individual one, taking into account the patient's overall health and prior screening history (USPSTF, 2016).

CHAPTER 15

Assessing the Peripheral Vascular System and Regional Lymphatic System

INTRODUCTION

The body is a complex organ that requires many systems to function and interact together. The peripheral vascular system contains an intricate system of arteries and veins that transports oxygenated and deoxygenated blood throughout the circulatory system. This system also includes the lymphatic system that carries lymph fluid throughout our circulation. It is essential for nurses to know how to assess both of these systems.

REVIEW OF ANATOMY AND PHYSIOLOGY

Peripheral Vascular System

The peripheral vascular system is composed of large and small vessels that circulate blood throughout our body.

Arteries

- Cylindrical, tubular, thick blood vessels that transport oxygenated blood away from both the ventricles of the heart to tissues in every part of the body
- Several different sizes, with the larger arteries being the aorta and pulmonary artery
- Found in every part of the body and have three layers (Fig. 15-1):
  - ☐ Tunica adventitia is the strong outer covering; it is composed of connective tissue, collagen, and elastic fibers.
  - ☐ Tunica media is the middle layer; it is composed of smooth muscle and elastic fibers.
  - ☐ Tunica intima is the inner layer; it is composed of an elastic membrane lining and smooth endothelium.

Arterioles

- Arteries branch off into arterioles
- Smaller in diameter than arteries
- Transport smaller volumes of blood
- Surround the organs and tissues to ensure that all organs and tissues can receive oxygen
- Branch off to become capillaries

Capillaries

- Capillaries consist of a thin endothelial wall that is only one cell thick. They form an anastomosing network that brings the oxygenated blood into an intimate relationship with the tissue cells. This network allows oxygen and nutrients to shift out of the capillaries into the cells.

Veins

- Veins are larger than arteries and most veins carry deoxygenated blood back to the heart (Fig. 15-2); in fetal circulation, the pulmonary and umbilical vein transport oxygenated blood to the heart.

- A vein can range in size from 1 millimeter to 1 to 1.5 centimeters in diameter.
- Veins are composed of three layers:
  1. Tunica adventitia is the external layer that is made up of connective tissue.
  2. Tunica media is the middle layer that is made of smooth muscle.
  3. Tunica intima is the inner layer that is composed of elastic membrane lining and endothelial tissue.
- The majority of the larger veins have unidirectional valves that are arranged vertically in the direction of blood flow to prevent the backward flow.
- There are no valves in the small veins.
- The veins in the upper extremities, head, neck, and trunk carry deoxygenated blood to the right atrium of the heart.
- The veins of the lower extremities and trunk carry deoxygenated blood to the inferior vena cava.
- Blood is forced upward within the deep veins by contraction of the leg and thigh muscles, which intermittently compress the veins and propel the blood upward within the veins against gravity.

Venules

- A venule is a smaller blood vessel that transports deoxygenated blood.
- Collect blood from capillaries to form a vein.

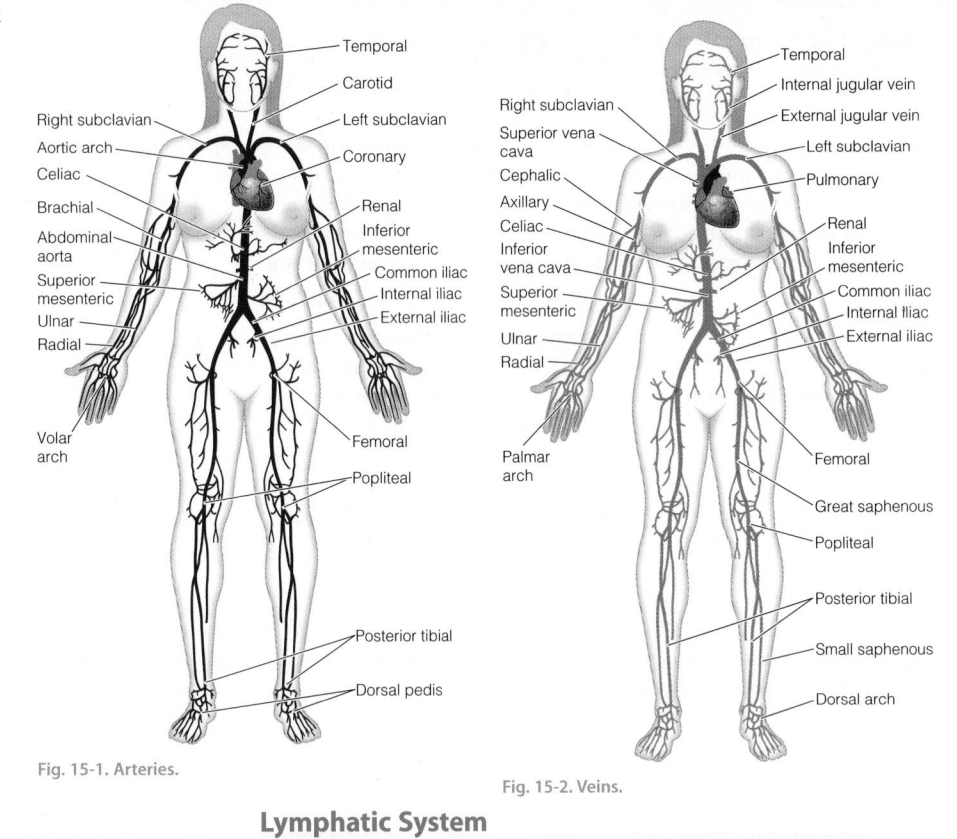

Fig. 15-1. Arteries.

Fig. 15-2. Veins.

Lymphatic System

- Lymphatic comes from the Latin word *lymphaticus*, meaning "connected to water." Lymph is clear fluid (Zimmermann, 2013).
- The lymphatic system is composed of lymphatic vessels and lymph nodes through which lymph fluid circulates throughout the body.

- The lymphatic system is a one-way upward flow system that returns lymph fluid via vessels to the cardiovascular system for eventual elimination of toxic by-products by end organs (i.e., kidney, liver, colon, skin, and lungs) (Fig. 15-3).
- There are two major ducts that the lymphatic vessels flow into:
  - Right lymphatic duct drains the right side of the head and neck, right arm, right side of the thorax, right lung and pleura, right side of the heart, and right upper section of the liver.
  - Thoracic duct transports about 4 liters of fluid per day; collects most of the lymph in the body and empties into the left subclavian vein; largest lymphatic duct on the body.

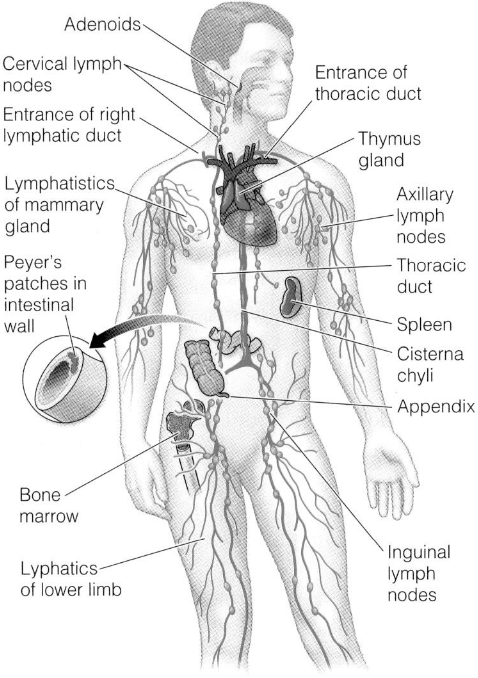

Fig. 15-3. Lymphatic system.

- Organs containing lymphatic tissue
  - The spleen is the largest lymphatic organ; filters blood.
  - The thymus and bone marrow produce lymphocytes.
  - The tonsils and adenoids are the initial line of defense as part of the immune system.
  - Appendix contains lymphatic tissue.
  - Lymph nodes are clusters of lymphatic tissue.
  - Peyer patches are raised clusters of lymphoid tissue in the small intestine.
- The functions of the lymphatic system are as follows:
  - Production of white blood cells (WBCs, i.e., lymphocytes) in the lymph nodes to help fight off invading bacteria.
  - Fluid and protein balance: as blood moves through the arteries and veins, 10 percent of the fluid filtered by the capillaries, along with vital proteins, becomes trapped in the tissues of the body; the lymphatic system collects this fluid and returns it to the circulatory system.
  - Immunity and spread of infection: the lymphatic system plays an integral role in the immune functions of the body: it is the first line of defense against disease.

Lymph fluid is a clear body fluid that contains a type of WBCs, along with proteins and fats; the lymph fluid seeps outside the blood vessels into the spaces around the body tissues and is then stored in the lymphatic system to flow back into the bloodstream; it moves unidirectionally within the lymphatic system with the assistance of valves and movement.

Lymph Nodes

- Lymph nodes are a network of fibers and irregular channels that slow down lymph flow; as lymph passes through the nodes, the fibers filter out bacteria, viruses, and cellular debris.
- Lymph nodes vary in shape and size; these nodes are covered by a fibrous capsule composed of connective tissue.

- There are about 450 lymph nodes present in the average young individual human body; approximately 60 to 70 lymph nodes are in the head and neck regions, 100 in the thorax and 250 in the abdomen and pelvis (Singh, 2014).

DIAGNOSTICS

There are several diagnostic scans that assist in diagnosing peripheral vascular insufficiencies, and blockages in the lymphatic system:

- **Computed tomography (CT scan), duplex ultrasound,** and **magnetic resonance angiography (MRA)** are noninvasive tests that can help the medical specialist map the blood flow in the affected areas. These tests may be considered if the patient's healthcare provider thinks that a procedure (revascularization) may be helpful to treat peripheral artery disease.
- An **angiogram** is an imaging x-ray that uses a special dye to visualize blood flow through arteries or veins. This test is ordered if an obstruction or blockage is suspected in the coronary or peripheral vascular system.
- In an **angioplasty,** a balloon is placed in the blocked area and inflated to break up the plaque, widen the diameter of the artery, and increase blood flow.

HEALTH HISTORY

Review of Systems

Use the **OLDCARTS** mnemonic (**O**nset, **L**ocation, **D**uration, **C**haracteristics, **A**ggravating/Alleviating factors, **R**elieving factors, **T**reatment, **S**everity) to identify attributes of a symptom.

The focused health history includes questions about pain, swelling, lumps, or edema, and skin changes of the extremities. Ask the patient the following questions.

Past Medical History

- Do you have any history of peripheral artery disease (PAD), heart disease, stroke, diabetes, high blood pressure (BP)?
  - □ Patients with a medical history of heart disease, stroke, diabetes, and high blood pressure have a higher risk of PAD.
- Do you have a high cholesterol level?
  - □ Cholesterol is a waxy, fatty substance that adheres to the inner lining of blood vessels; high levels of cholesterol cause plaque to build up in arteries.
  - □ **Peripheral arterial disease (PAD)** is a term used to describe narrowing or occlusion by atherosclerotic plaques of arteries outside of the heart and brain (Stöppler, 2014). PAD occurs with a buildup of fatty deposits and atherosclerotic vascular changes to the endothelial lining of blood vessels.
  - □ Patients can suffer from significant functional limitations in their daily activities and the most severely affected are at risk of limb loss (Andras & Ferket, 2014).
- Are you overweight?
  - □ Being overweight increases body fat, increasing the risk of fat accumulating in the arteries.

Family History

- Any family history of atherosclerosis, peripheral vascular disease (PVD), varicose veins, or diabetes?

Psychosocial History

- Do you sit for prolonged periods?
- Do you work? If so, do you sit for long periods of time?
- Do you travel for long periods of time on an airplane, car, or train? How many days per week do you exercise?
  - □ Less mobile patients are at risk for developing blood clots, decreased venous return (Muldoon, 2011).

- Do you smoke?
    - □ Nicotine can cause vasoconstriction in the upper and lower extremity vessels (Pamoukian & De Collibus, 2010); smoking increases the risk of PAD four times and accelerates the onset of symptoms by nearly 10 years (Bell, 2009).

Medications
- What medications are you taking?
    - □ Blood thinners such as aspirin are sometimes prescribed to thin out the blood.
    - □ Patients with atherosclerotic disease may be on medications to lower their cholesterol and vasodilators to dilate the arteries.
    - □ Oral contraceptives or hormone replacement therapy may increase the risk for blood clots.

Pain/Tingling or Numbness Sensations
- Do you experience any pain or leg cramps while walking? If so, how far until onset of pain or what activity precipitates the pain?
- Do you experience the pain in your extremities while sleeping?
- Do experience changes in sensation such as tingling or numbness in your extremities (paresthesia)?
    - □ **Intermittent claudication** is a symptom of PAD; cramp-like pain felt in the buttock, thighs, or calves during exercise or walking; due to decreased blood flow and oxygen (tissue ischemia) to the legs; may occur in both the upper and lower extremities. True claudication starts after a reproducible length of walking and resolves within a few minutes of rest (Bhattacharya, 2011).
    - □ Aching or burning in toes and feet during rest and especially while lying flat is a sign of ischemia (Ferri, 2014).

Edema or Swelling of an Extremity
- Have you noticed any swelling in your arms or legs? When is it better or worse?

BOX 15-1 Risk Factors for Lymphedema

- Family history of lymphedema
- Removal of lymph nodes
- Invasive surgery
- Radiation therapy
- Chemotherapy
- Morbid obesity

- Does it come and go or is it constant?
- What relieves the swelling?
- What does the extremity look like when it is swollen?
    - □ Edema is a localized or generalized condition in which body tissues contain an excessive amount of tissue fluid in the interstitial spaces; causes include cardiac, peripheral vascular, renal or liver disease, lymphedema or thrombosis.
    - □ **Lymphedema** is an accumulation of lymph fluid in the tissues. The most common cause is an obstruction of the lymphatic vessels. There are several risk factors for lymphedema (Box 15-1).
    - □ Unilateral edema may indicate the presence of a deep vein thrombosis (DVT).
        - • A thrombosis is a blood clot; blood clots can move throughout the bloodstream to the lungs (pulmonary embolism), heart, and the brain causing serious or fatal consequences.

Erectile Dysfunction
- Do you have a problem with erectile dysfunction?
    - □ Erectile dysfunction is a persistent or recurrent difficulty maintaining or achieving an erection sufficient for satisfactory sexual activity (Russell, Ecclestone, & Kavia, 2014).
    - □ Erectile dysfunction may be caused by decreased circulation and ischemia to the groin and lower extremities.

Lymph Node Enlargement

- Have you had any swollen lymph nodes?
- When did you first notice the swollen lymph node?
- Is the node painful or tender to touch?
- How long have you had it?
- Have you recently been sick?
  - □ Swollen lymph nodes usually occur as a result of exposure to a bacterium or a virus; less commonly, swollen lymph nodes are caused by cancer (http://www.mayoclinic.com/health/swollen-lymph-nodes/DS00880).
  - □ **Lymph node biopsy** is the gold standard for definitive diagnosis in patients with lymph nodes >1 cm (Scott, Kitt, & Derenge, 2016).

Skin Changes of the Extremities

- Have you had any skin color changes?
  - □ Changes in skin color, especially on feet (rubor, reddish-blue color when feet are in the dependent position) (Fig. 15-4), elevational pallor (pale skin) when raising up the affected extremity are signs of peripheral vascular insufficiency.
  - □ Redness and warmth of the skin may indicate infection/inflammation.
- Do your fingers or toes change colors in cold weather?
  - □ **Raynaud's phenomenon** is a result of cold-induced vasospasm of the small blood vessels in the fingers and toes, causing blanching, cyanosis, or redness of

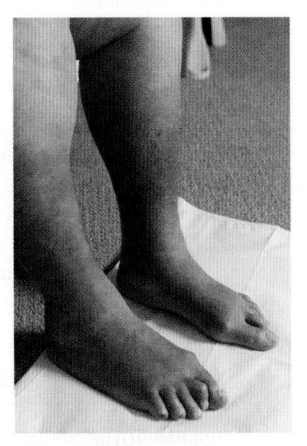

Fig. 15-4. Rubor (peripheral vascular insufficiency).

the hands and feet (Dunphy, Winland-Brown, Porter, & Thomas, 2015).

- Loss of hair on your extremities? Changes in the texture of your skin?
  - □ Decreased circulation causes hair loss on the affected extremity and rough, scaly, flaky skin.
- Do your extremities feel cool?
  - □ Decreased circulation causes coolness of the extremity.
- Do you have any wounds or skin ulcers? Are they healing?
  - □ Decreased circulation causes poor or delayed wound healing.

Risk Factors

- One in every 20 Americans over the age of 50 has PAD, a condition that raises the risk for heart attack and stroke (Advanced Heart and Vascular Institute, 2016).
- PAD affects 8 to 12 million Americans and increases the risk of mortality as much as 50 percent from heart attacks and strokes (Stephens, Hagler, and Clark, 2011).
- The most common cause of PAD is atherosclerosis.
- There are several risk factors for PAD (Box 15-2).

BOX 15-2 Risk Factors for Peripheral Vascular Disease

- A family history of peripheral artery disease, heart disease, or stroke
- Advancing age
- Smoking
- Diabetes
- Obesity
- High BP
- High cholesterol

CULTURAL CONSIDERATIONS
• PAD is more common in African Americans than any other racial or ethnic group (NIH, 2016).
• Diabetes and high BP are more common among African Americans, which places this race at higher risk for PAD. Diabetes is a high-risk factor for PAD in women (National Heart Lung and Blood Institute, 2016).

■ **Aneurysms** (a weakening of an arterial wall) can develop within the arterial system and can be life threatening. The three most common risk factors for aneurysms are:
  □ smoking
  □ high BP
  □ high cholesterol levels.

■ There is a genetic component to abdominal aortic aneurysms (AAAs); the prevalence in someone who has a first-degree relative with the condition can be as high as 25 percent.
  □ AAA affects as many as eight percent of people over the age of 65
  □ Males are four times more likely to have AAA than females
  □ AAA is the 17th leading cause of death in the United States (Cardiac Health, 2017).

CULTURAL CONSIDERATIONS
AAAs are less common in women and African Americans (Wedro, 2014).

PREPARATION FOR ASSESSMENT

Equipment Needed
Stethoscope
Gloves
Doppler stethoscope
Doppler gel
Measuring tape

Sequence of Assessment
1. Inspection
2. Palpation
The peripheral vascular and lymphatic systems assessment requires positional changes. Both system assessments are noninvasive and require little participation on the patient's behalf.

Preliminary Steps
Preparation for this assessment includes the following:
■ Ensuring a comfortable room temperature to prevent the arteries and veins from dilating and constricting
■ Assisting the patient to change positions as needed
■ Instructing the patient to remove clothing, footwear, socks, and jewelry
■ Draping of the patient
■ Performing hand hygiene
These assessments may be integrated throughout the comprehensive assessment to minimize the patient's positional changes or are performed as focused assessments depending on the patient's reason for seeking care.

TECHNIQUE 15-1: **Assessing the Lymph Nodes in the Head and Neck Region**

Purpose: To assess for enlarged lymph nodes and signs of inflammation or disease
Normally, lymph nodes are not palpated, but there are times that lymph nodes can be palpated. See Table 15-1 for differences between normal and abnormal lymph node characteristics.

ASSESSMENT STEPS

1. Explain the technique to the patient.
2. Ask the patient to sit up on the edge of the examination table.
3. Ask the patient to slightly flex his or her neck forward to relax the muscles.
4. Warm your hands by rubbing them together.
5. Using the finger pads of your index and middle fingers; gently palpate using circular motions, the ten facial and neck lymph nodes regions, using both hands to examine corresponding sides (Fig. 15-5):

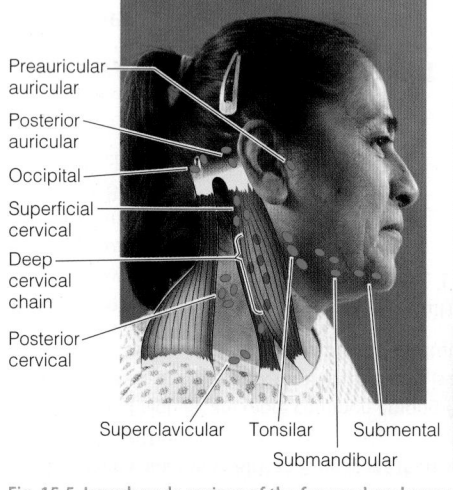
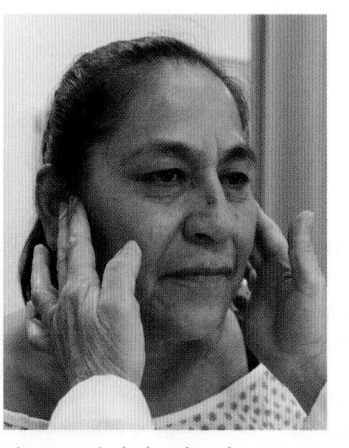

Preauricular-auricular
Posterior auricular
Occipital
Superficial cervical
Deep cervical chain
Posterior cervical
Superclavicular   Tonsilar   Submental
Submandibular

Fig. 15-5. Lymph node regions of the face and neck; assessing preauricular lymph nodes.

TABLE 15-1 **Normal Versus Abnormal Lymph Nodes**

Lymph Node Characteristics	Normal	Abnormal
Size	<1 cm	>1 cm and persistent for >4 weeks should be thoroughly evaluated
Consistency	Discrete	Rock-hard nodes are seen in malignancies
Mobility	Freely moveable (up or down or side to side) may occur with infection	Fixed or matted nodes
Tenderness	Nontender	Tender nodes indicative of inflammation

Source: bestpractice.bmj.com/best-practice/monograph/838/diagnosis.html

TIP Lymph node size varies according to their location. For example, inguinal lymph nodes may be as large as 2 cm in healthy individuals. The significance of enlarged lymph nodes must be viewed in the context of their location, duration, and associated symptoms, and the age and gender of the patient. As a general rule, lymph nodes measuring less than 1 cm are rarely of clinical significance (Best Practice, 2011).

☐ Preauricular (in front of the ears)
☐ Postauricular (behind the ears)
☐ Suboccipital (area between the back of the neck and head)
☐ Tonsillar (below the jaw bone)
☐ Submandibular (under the jaw on both sides)
☐ Submental (just below the chin)
☐ Superficial cervical (upper neck)
☐ Posterior cervical (on the side of the neck toward the back)
☐ Deep cervical chain (near the internal jugular vein)

TIP Use soft touch when palpating lymph nodes. If you palpate too deeply, you can move them.

6. Ask the patient to slightly flex her or his neck to the right and shrug the shoulders, palpate the left supraclavicular lymph nodes in the hollow area just above the clavicle.

7. Ask the patient to slightly flex his or her neck to the left and shrug the shoulders, palpate the right supraclavicular lymph nodes.

8. Document your findings.

NORMAL FINDINGS

■ No lymph nodes are palpated.
■ If palpated, the lymph node should be less than 1cm, discrete, moveable, and nontender.

ABNORMAL FINDINGS

■ Enlarged, greater than 1 cm, matted, hard, and tender may be signs of inflammation or a malignancy.

TECHNIQUE 15-2: **Assessing the Carotid Arteries**

Technique 15-2A: **Inspecting and Palpating the Carotid Arteries**

Purpose: To assess carotid artery circulation

TIP Palpating the carotid arteries may be more difficult in an obese patient; ask the patient to slightly turn his or her neck to the opposite side that you are trying to assess the pulse.

ASSESSMENT STEPS

1. Explain the technique to the patient.

2. Place the patient in a sitting or supine position.

3. Ask the patient to turn the head to the right side, inspect and palpate the left carotid artery for pulsations between the trachea and sternocleidomastoid muscle (Fig. 15-6).

4. Ask the patient to turn the head to the left side, inspect and palpate the right carotid artery for pulsations between the trachea and sternocleidomastoid muscle.

5. Note the following characteristics of the carotid pulses:

☐ rate

☐ rhythm

☐ amplitude

6. Document your findings.

NORMAL FINDINGS

- Visible symmetrical pulsations
- Pulse rate between 60 and 100 bpm
- Well-conditioned athletes 40 to 60 bpm
- Rhythm is regular
- Amplitude 2+

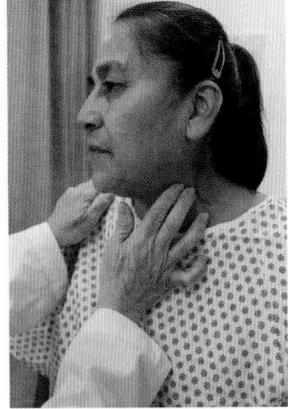

Fig. 15-6. Inspecting and palpating left carotid artery.

ABNORMAL FINDINGS

- No pulsations or asymmetrical pulsatile bulge may indicate decreased circulation or obstruction.
- Pulse rate less than 60 and greater than 100
- Rhythm: irregular with pauses; may be indicative of an irregular heart rate (arrhythmia)
- Amplitude: Absent (no heart rate), weak (decreased stroke volume), or bounding (increased stroke volume); may be indicative of changes in the circulatory system

   ▇ **TIP** A palpable vibration (thrill) may be felt while palpating a carotid artery. A palpable thrill over the carotid artery is an abnormal tremor accompanying a vascular murmur (Venes, 2013).

   SENC Safety Alert Do not vigorously palpate, massage, or palpate both carotid arteries at the same time. This causes an adverse reflex effect on the baroreceptors of the heart and may decrease the patient's heart rate and BP.

Technique 15-2B: **Auscultating the Carotid Arteries**

Purpose: To assess carotid artery flow for signs of obstruction

Equipment: Stethoscope

A bruit is an abnormal "swooshing" sound that blood makes when it rushes past an obstruction in an artery.

ASSESSMENT STEPS

1. Explain the technique to the patient.

2. Ask the patient to take a breath in and hold it.

> ▓ **TIP** It is important that you listen for a carotid bruit while the patient is holding her or his breath so that you do not get confused by the patient's tracheal breath sounds.

3. Using either the bell or the diaphragm of the stethoscope, auscultate the left carotid artery for a bruit as the patient holds her or his breath (Fig. 15-7).

4. Instruct the patient to breathe out.

5. Repeat steps 2 through 4 on the right carotid artery.

6. Document your findings.

NORMAL FINDINGS

■ No bruit heard

ABNORMAL FINDINGS

■ A swooshing sound (bruit) indicates turbulent blood flow.

■ Bruit may indicate partial obstruction of the carotid artery due to plaque in the artery.

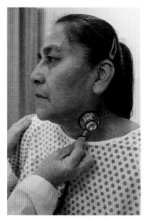

Fig. 15-7. Auscultating the left carotid artery.

TECHNIQUE 15-3: **Inspecting for Jugular Venous Distention**

Purpose: To assess for signs of increased central venous pressure (pressure in the right atrium of the heart)

Equipment: Penlight

The internal jugular veins are located deep beneath the sternocleidomastoid muscle, lateral to the carotid arteries. The veins are not normally visualized or protruding. Sometimes, the pulsations of the internal jugular veins are transmitted through the skin. The external jugular veins are lateral to the internal jugular veins and are superficial.

ASSESSMENT STEPS

1. Explain the technique to the patient.

2. Position patient in a sitting or semi-Fowler's (30- to 45-degree) position.

3. Ask the patient to turn his or her head to the left side.

4. Using a penlight, inspect the right side of the patient's neck for jugular vein distention (Fig. 15-8).

5. Note any pulsations.

6. Repeat steps #3 and #4 on the left side of the patient's neck.

7. Document your findings.

NORMAL FINDINGS

■ No visible pulsation or jugular vein distention

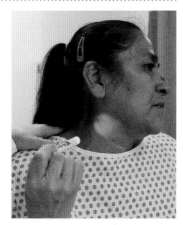

Fig. 15-8. Using penlight to assess jugular veins of the neck.

ABNORMAL FINDINGS
- Visible distention is a sign of venous pressure elevation, commonly seen in congestive heart failure and fluid overload.

TECHNIQUE 15-4: **Inspecting and Palpating the Upper Extremities**

Purpose: To assess for peripheral circulation
Equipment: Gloves (only if there are open areas or signs of bodily fluids), measuring tape
ASSESSMENT STEPS
1. Explain the technique to the patient.
2. Put on gloves (optional).
3. Position the patient in a sitting or supine position.
4. Inspect each arm from the shoulder to the fingertips for:
☐ symmetry
☐ color
☐ texture
☐ edema.
5. Closely inspect the fingernail beds of both hands for:
☐ color
☐ nail thickness
☐ profile sign (clubbing of the nail plates is discussed in Chapter 12).
6. Using the dorsal surface of your hand, palpate the temperature of each arm; compare the temperature of both arms.
7. Assess the epitrochlear lymph nodes by flexing the patient's left elbow to about 90°. Hold the patient's left hand in your left hand and palpate with your right hand behind the patient's left elbow between biceps and triceps muscle (Fig. 15-9); hold the patient's right hand in your right hand and palpate with your left hand behind the patient's right elbow between biceps and triceps muscle.
8. Assess the pulses in each arm by gently placing your second and third finger pads of your dominant hand on each of the following pulses (see Chapter 7):
☐ Radial pulse is palpated at the wrist on the radial artery.
☐ Brachial pulse is palpated at the medial side of the arm at the antecubital fossa space.
    TIP Ulnar pulse is not routinely palpated because it is not easily palpated nor felt.
9. Document your findings.

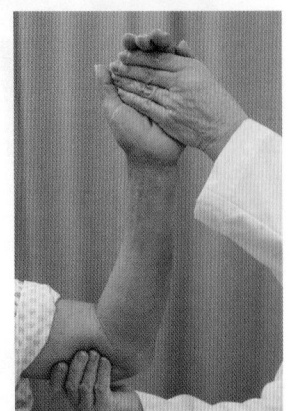

Fig. 15-9. Assessing epitrochlear lymph nodes.

- Arms are symmetrical
- Color is uniform
- No edema or ulcerations
- Fingernail beds pink
- Venous pattern normal
- Fingernails even thickness
- 160° angle of attachment
- Temperature warm to touch
- Epitrochlear nodes are not felt
- 2+ radial and brachial pulse

ABNORMAL FINDINGS

- Signs of altered peripheral circulation
- Discoloration, change in texture of skin, cool extremities, bilateral or unilateral edema
  - □ **Cellulitis** is a bacterial infection of the skin and subcutaneous tissues: the skin appears red and swollen; feels warm, hot, and tender (Fig. 15-10).
  - □ **Edema** is an accumulation of fluid seeping into the tissues; accumulation of fluid in the legs and feet is called peripheral edema. Any area that has edema should be assessed for pitting edema:
    - Gently apply pressure with your second and third finger pads on the edematous area and release the finger pressure.
    - Observe if an indentation remains embedded in the tissue area.
    - Pitting edema is graded on a score of +1 to +4 depending on the depth of the indentation (Fig. 15-11).
- **Ulcerations** (commonly occur with decreased circulation)
  - □ Tissue ischemia is a risk factor for the development of foot ulcers; it also contributes to delayed wound healing (Box 15-3).
- Enlarged epitrochlear nodes (may indicate an infection of the hand or forearm or some types of blood cancer)

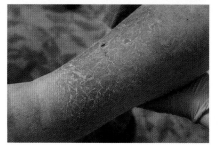

Fig. 15-10. Cellulitis.

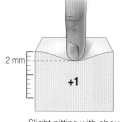

2 mm

+1

Slight pitting with about 2 mm depression that disappears rapidly; no visble distortion of the extreminty

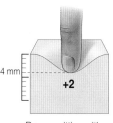

4 mm

+2

Deeper pitting with about 4 mm depression that disappears in 10 to 15 seconds; no visible distortion of the extremity

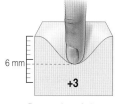

6 mm

+3

Depression of about 6 mm that lasts more than a minute; dependent extremity looks swollen.

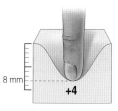

8 mm

+4

Very deep pitting with about 8 mm depression that lasts 2 to 3 minutes; dependent extremity is grossly distorted.

Fig. 15-11. Grading scale for pitting edema.

BOX 15-3 Signs of Tissue Ischemia

- Pain
- Pallor
- Change in color of skin
- Cool temperature

- Tingling or numbness
- Hair loss of extremity
- Nonhealing wounds or ulcerations

TECHNIQUE 15-5: **Assessing Capillary Refill Time: Blanch Test**

Purpose: To assess tissue perfusion

Equipment: Watch with a second hand

■ **TIP** Remove colored nail polish before performing this test for clear visualization of the color of the nailbed.

1. Explain the technique to the patient.
2. Hold the patient's hand higher than heart level.
3. Press down on the nailbed until the nailbed blanches (turns white).
4. Release the nailbed.
5. Note the amount of time for the pink color to return to the nailbed (Fig. 15-12).
6. Document your findings.

NORMAL FINDINGS

■ Pink color returns in less than 3 seconds.

ABNORMAL FINDINGS

■ Pink color return in greater than 3 seconds may indicate decreased perfusion or dehydration.

■ **TIP** Capillary refill may be influenced by cool environmental temperature, smoking, peripheral edema, and anemia.

SENC Evidence-Based Practice Dufault et al (2008) performed a research roundtable study, *Translating Best Practices in Assessing Capillary Refill*, to determine the strength, usefulness, and feasibility of empirical and clinical evidence evaluated in a systematic review assessing capillary refill. The study concluded that there are no nursing interventions that rely solely upon assessment of capillary refill; isolated performance of capillary refill assessment has been found to be of limited value. Practice implications include revision of nursing policies and procedures to indicate that capillary refill assessment is of limited diagnostic value.

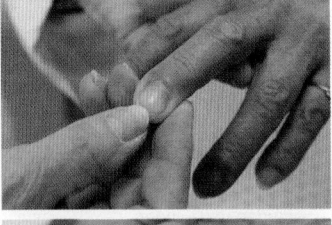
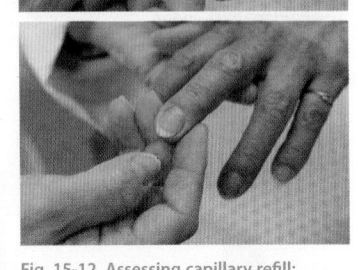

Fig. 15-12. Assessing capillary refill: blanching (top) and normal (bottom).

Because capillary refill assessment has limited value, future research needs to be directed toward evaluation and comparative analyses of alternate methods of assessing peripheral perfusion.

TECHNIQUE 15-6: Inspecting and Palpating the Lower Extremities

Purpose: To assess arterial and venous circulation
Equipment: Measuring tape, doppler ultrasonic stethoscope (optional), doppler gel, gloves
ASSESSMENT STEPS
1. Explain the technique to the patient.
2. Position the patient in the supine position.
3. Expose the lower legs from the groin to the feet making sure to keep the genitalia covered for privacy.
4. Inspect each leg from the groin to the toes for (Fig. 15-13):
    ☐ symmetry
    ☐ color
    ☐ texture
    ☐ edema
    ☐ venous pattern
    ☐ hair distribution
    ☐ ulcerations.

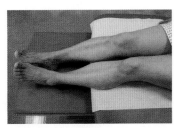

Fig. 15-13. Inspecting lower legs.

SENC Safety Alert Unilateral edema of a lower extremity may be a sign of DVT or inflammation of a vein. The Wells clinical decision assessment model (1995) encourages healthcare providers to look at three factors for screening for a DVT: signs and symptoms of DVT, risk factors and alternative diagnoses.

SENC Evidence-Based Practice Anthony (2013) examined the literature and supports the evidence that the Homan's sign is nonspecific and nonsensitive to screen for a DVT. The Homan's sign assessed for the presence of a DVT: if positive, the assessment elicits pain in the calf of the affected leg with dorsiflexion of the foot. Anthony supports previous research that the Homan's sign has no clinical value in screening for DVT, and nurses should not rely on it as a screening test (Cranley et al., 1976; Haeger, 1969; McLachlin et al., 1962; Tovey & Wyatt, 2003; Urbano, 2001; Vaccaro et al., 1986).

5. Closely inspect the toenail beds of both feet for:
    ☐ color
    ☐ nail thickness.

6. Using the dorsal surface of your hand, palpate the temperature of each leg; compare the temperatures of both legs (Fig. 15-14).

SENC Safety Alert If you are unable to feel a pulse, use the doppler ultrasonic stethoscope to try to hear a pulse. Palpate the extremity's temperature; if no pulse and extremity is cool to touch and the color is pale and mottled, notify the healthcare provider immediately. This could indicate an arterial or venous blockage.

7. Put on gloves.

8. Using your second, third, and fourth finger pads of your dominant hand, gently palpate the right and left inguinal groin areas near the saphenous vein to assess the inguinal lymph nodes (Fig. 15-15); assess the femoral pulses (Fig. 15-16).

    ☐ **Femoral pulse** is located in the groin area below the inguinal ligament, halfway between the symphysis pubis and the anterior-superior iliac spine.

9. Remove and discard gloves.

10. Assess the pulses in the right and left lower extremity by gently placing your second and third finger pads of your dominant hand. Assess the rhythm, amplitude, and symmetry of each of the following pulses:

    ☐ **Popliteal pulses** assessed by asking the patient to flex the right or left knee at approximately 120 degrees. Hold the back of the knee with both hands. Extend the index and middle fingers of your hands on the popliteal fossa and palpate the popliteal artery (Fig. 15-17).

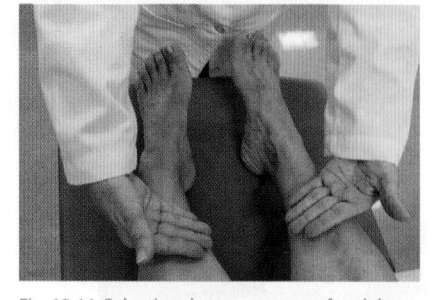

Fig. 15-14. Palpating the temperature of each leg.

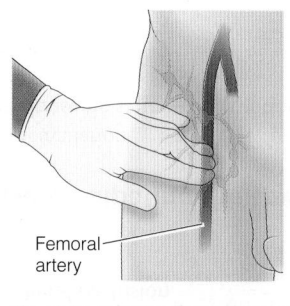

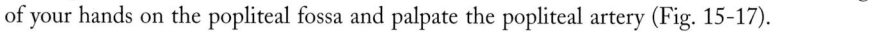

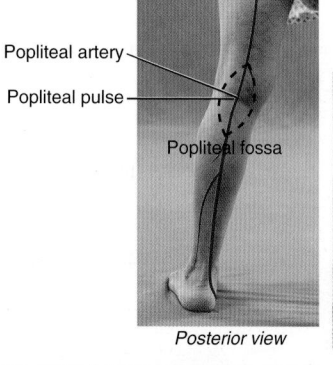

Fig. 15-15. Palpating inguinal lymph nodes.　Fig. 15-16. Palpating femoral artery.　Fig. 15-17. Palpating the popliteal pulse.

- ☐ **Dorsalis pedis pulse** is located on the dorsum part of the foot between the first and second toes (Fig. 15-18).
- ☐ **Posterior tibial pulse** is between the medial malleolus and the Achilles tendon (Fig. 15-19).

11. Ask the patient to sit up on the side of the examining table, after approximately one minute, inspect the veins of the legs in the dependent position for distention.

12. Document your findings.

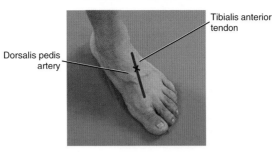
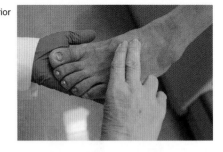

Fig. 15-18. Palpating the dorsalis pedis pulse.

NORMAL FINDINGS

- ■ Legs are symmetrical.
- ■ Color is uniform.
- ■ No edema or ulceration is present.
- ■ Toenails are pink with even thickness.
- ■ Temperature is warm to touch bilaterally.
- ■ Leg hair is evenly distributed; there are no ulcerations.
- ■ Inguinal lymph nodes are nonpalpable.
- ■ Pulses are 2+ symmetrical, regular femoral, popliteal, dorsalis pedis, and posterior tibial.
- ■ Venous pattern nondistended

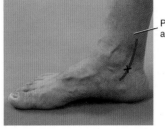
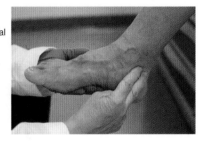

Fig. 15-19. Palpating the posterior tibial pulse.

ABNORMAL FINDINGS

- ■ Color: discoloration (cyanosis, bright red, pale, or rubor) may indicate arterial or venous insufficiency; rubor color is a red/bluish color when the legs are in the dependent position; indicates decreased circulation.
- ■ Texture: decreased texture; thick leathery skin (venous insufficiency), dry and shiny skin (arterial insufficiency)
- ■ Hair: loss of hair of one or both legs or feet (arterial insufficiency)
- ■ Temperature: cool skin (arterial insufficiency)
- ■ Toenails: thick (arterial insufficiency)
- ■ Arterial or venous insufficiency wounds (Table 15-2)
- ■ Presence of bilateral or unilateral edema
- ■ Presence of erythema: area of skin is warm to touch

TABLE 15-2 Signs of Arterial and Venous Insufficiency

Type of Ulcer	Appearance	Common Location	Description
Arterial	Appear "punched out"; round, smooth, well-defined borders	Feet Ankles Shin Heels Tips of toes	Pain is worse with activity and at night Loss of hair around area Base of ulcer is brown, black, yellow With/without necrotic tissue Minimal bleeding
Venous	Irregularly shaped, uneven edges; shallow wound	Below knee Inner legs Above ankles	Red or brown skin around ulcer Edematous with fluid drainage Coarse, shiny, tight skin Hemosiderin deposits (iron) Leg pain

- Pulses are diminished or absent (arterial insufficiency)
- **Varicose veins** (protruding veins of the lower extremities) resulting from incompetent valves; pooling of blood in the veins (Fig. 15-20)
- **Lymphedema** is an accumulation of lymphatic fluid in the interstitial tissue that causes swelling; may occur in one or both the arms or legs and other parts of the body; can develop if lymph nodes or lymph vessels are missing or not working properly; also seen as a side-effect after cancer treatments, surgery, or diseases (Fig. 15-21).

  TIP The dorsalis pedis and posterior tibial pulse sites can be difficult to locate as the position of these arteries can vary between individuals; it is reasonable to assume that vascular disease is present if pedal pulses cannot be found; take your time to thoroughly assess pedal pulses (Burland, 2012).

SENC Safety Alert If you are unable to palpate pulses, use a Doppler stethoscope to amplify the arterial pulsations (Fig. 15-22); it is important to accurately assess pulses to prevent documentation of false-negative results.

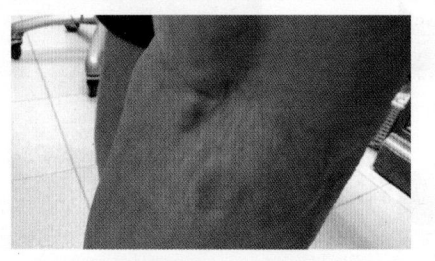

Fig. 15-20. Varicose veins.

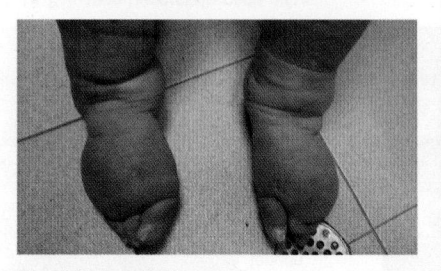

Fig. 15-21. Lymphedema.

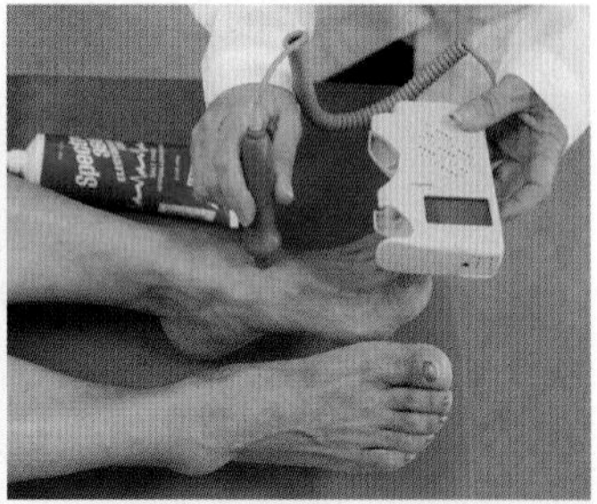

Fig. 15-22. Doppler stethoscope.

ADVANCED ASSESSMENTS

Advanced assessments are performed if insufficiency of blood flow is suspected to an extremity. See DavisPlus for the advanced assessments that might be performed.

PATIENT EDUCATION

Healthy People 2020

Goal: Reduce illness, disability, and death related to tobacco use and secondhand smoke exposure (HHS, 2010).

PVD can be prevented and controlled through modification of risk factors. Patients should be educated about PVD and signs of tissue ischemia. The following topics should be discussed with patients:

- Smoking increases the risk of PVD and DVT in women who take oral contraceptives and smoke; abstinence from smoking is strongly recommended.
- Diabetic patients should maintain glycemic control of their blood sugar levels; diabetics have a greater risk for delayed wound healing and decreased circulation; encourage patients to take very good care of the feet.
- Diet should be low in fat, low in sugar, and including at least five servings of fresh fruits and vegetables every day.
- Patients with hypertension should decrease salt intake and maintain good control of their BP.
- Encourage exercise 30 minutes a day on most days to improve circulation.
- Moderate exercise increases blood circulation, which can decrease the pain and appearance of varicose veins; exercise also slows or prevents the development of new varicose veins. All exercises should be performed gently and stopped immediately if there is any pain or discomfort. It is also important to elevate and rest the legs after performing exercises for varicose veins (Ninomiya, 2012).
- Patients should inspect their feet daily for signs and symptoms of sores and ulcers; use a mirror to check the soles of the feet.
- Patients with PVD should not walk barefoot to prevent risk of injury.
- Patients should be encouraged to wear supportive shoes.
- Patients with venous insufficiency should be encouraged to wear support hose during the day and take the hose off at night (Dunphy et al, 2015).

The U.S. Preventive Services Task Force (USPSTF) makes the following recommendations for AAA screening:

- One-time screening for abdominal aortic aneurysm (AAA) with ultrasonography in men ages 65 to 75 years who have ever smoked.
- Offer selective screening for AAA in men ages 65 to 75 years who have never smoked rather than routinely screening all men in this group.
- The USPSTF concludes that the current evidence is insufficient to assess the balance of benefits and harms of screening for AAA in women ages 65 to 75 years who have ever smoked.
- The USPSTF recommends against routine screening for AAA in women who have never smoked (U.S. Preventive Services, 2014).

Karen L. Gorton and Janice Thompson

INTRODUCTION

The musculoskeletal system is a complex system that provides structure, support, and protection to the human body, and gives the human body the ability to move in many directions. The skeletal system also provides the attachment points for ligaments and tendons. Movement occurs when the muscles contract, or shorten, in response to a neurological stimulus from the neurological system. Movement within the musculoskeletal system is generally voluntary. However, at times, movement will be involuntary such as a response to remove a hand from hot items, or a reflex.

REVIEW OF ANATOMY AND PHYSIOLOGY

Skeletal System

Bones of a variety of shapes, or classifications, exist within the skeletal system. The skeleton is composed of 206 bones and is divided into two regions for classification purposes (Fig. 16-1).

- The axial skeleton is composed of the head, vertebra, ribs, and sternum.
- The appendicular skeleton is composed of the upper and lower limbs, pelvis, clavicles, and scapulae.
- Bones are dense connective tissue that provides structure, protection, and the ability to move the body.
  - □ The outermost layer of bone is dense and compactly packed and is known as compact bone.
  - □ The innermost layer of bone, or trabecular bone, is more loosely packed and more porous (University of Chicago Medical Center, 2012).
  - □ Osteoblasts are cells within the bone that build the bone.
  - □ Osteoclasts are cells within the bone that remodel and remove bone tissue.
  - □ Osteocytes are cells within the bone that work to maintain healthy bone tissue.
  - □ The ends of the bones are known as the epiphyses, and the shafts of long bones are known as the diaphysis (Fig. 16-2).

Classification of Bones

Long Bones

- Long bones provide the framework for the arms and legs. The long bones are the:
  - □ femur
  - □ tibia
  - □ fibula
  - □ humerus
  - □ ulna
  - □ radius.

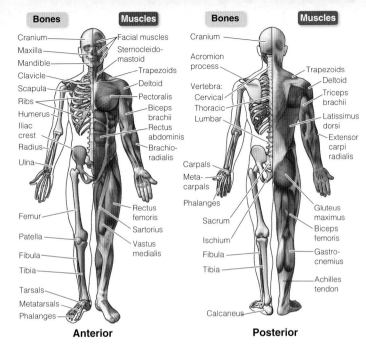

Bones	Muscles
Cranium	Facial muscles
Maxilla	Sternocleido-mastoid
Mandible	Trapezoids
Clavicle	Deltoid
Scapula	Pectoralis
Ribs	Biceps brachii
Humerus	Rectus abdominis
Iliac crest	Brachio-radialis
Radius	
Ulna	
Femur	Rectus femoris
Patella	Sartorius
Fibula	Vastus medialis
Tibia	
Tarsals	
Metatarsals	
Phalanges	

Anterior

Bones	Muscles
Cranium	Trapezoids
Acromion process	Deltoid
Vertebra:	Triceps brachii
Cervical	Latissimus dorsi
Thoracic	Extensor carpi radialis
Lumbar	
Carpals	
Meta-carpals	
Phalanges	
Sacrum	Gluteus maximus
Ischium	Biceps femoris
Fibula	Gastro-cnemius
Tibia	
Calcaneus	Achilles tendon

Posterior

Fig. 16-1. Skeletal system.

■ These bones may also be involved in the production of bone marrow/blood cells (Fig. 16-3).

Irregular/Short Bones

■ The irregular shapes of the bones in the ankle/foot and wrist allow motion to occur in more than one plane (Fig. 16-4).
■ The following smaller, irregular-shaped bones provide structure for the ankle, foot, and toes:

☐ Talus
☐ Calcaneus
☐ Navicular
☐ Cuneiform
☐ Cuboid
☐ Metatarsal
☐ Phalanx

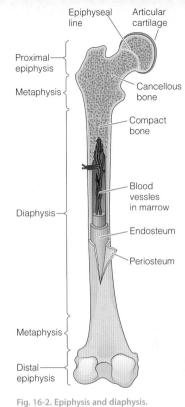

Fig. 16-2. Epiphysis and diaphysis.

Epiphyseal line
Articular cartilage
Proximal epiphysis
Metaphysis
Cancellous bone
Compact bone
Diaphysis
Blood vessles in marrow
Endosteum
Periosteum
Metaphysis
Distal epiphysis

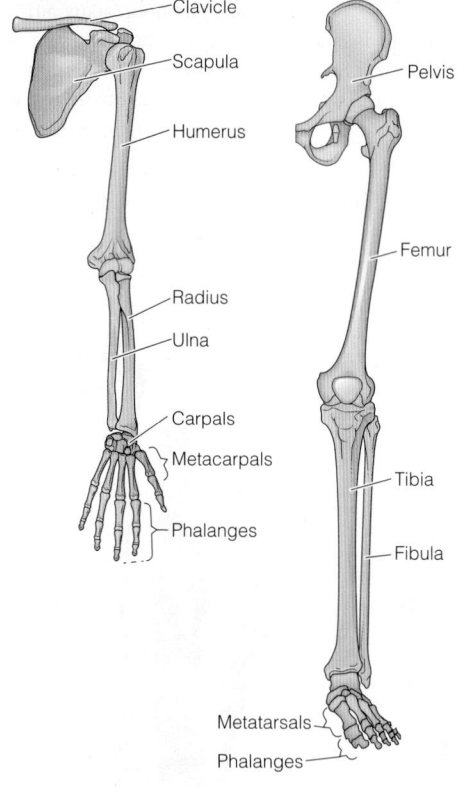

Fig. 16-3. Long bones of the arms and legs.

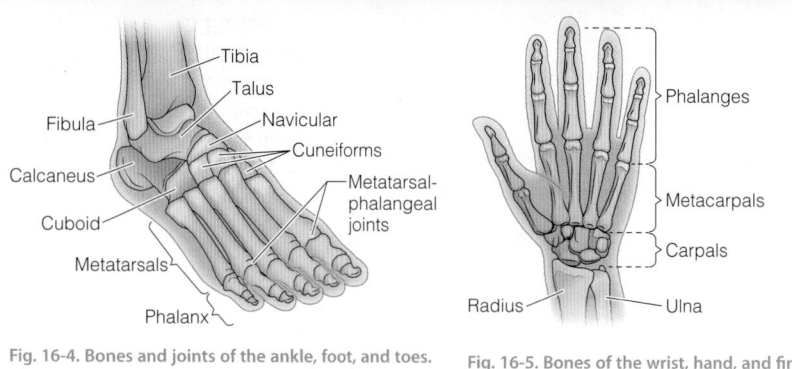

Fig. 16-4. Bones and joints of the ankle, foot, and toes.

Fig. 16-5. Bones of the wrist, hand, and fingers.

■ The following irregular bones provide structure for the wrist, hand, and fingers (Fig. 16-5):
  □ Carpals
  □ Metacarpals
  □ Phalanges

Joints

■ A joint is two or more bones coming together.
■ Some joints allow for no movement, some have limited movement, and other joints allow for great movement. The joints that move allow for functional movement of body parts.
■ Joints may be stabilized with ligaments.
■ Tendons may cross the joint to provide movement.
■ When those joints with limited movement are placed in sequence, the skeletal system can move in many directions as a whole that the individual joints are not able to attain.
■ Some joints are considered to be synovial, while others are considered to be nonsynovial.

- A synovial joint has a joint capsule that keeps the synovial fluid in the joint. The synovial fluid serves to lubricate and provide nutrients to the joint.
- A nonsynovial joint will not have synovial fluid or a joint capsule whose purpose is to keep synovial fluid in the joint (Laptiou, 2012).

■ The different types of joints are (Fig. 16-6):
- **Fused,** found primarily in the skull; these joints are irregular and flat.

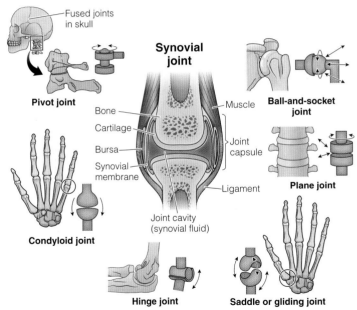

Pivot joint

Synovial joint

Bone
Cartilage
Bursa
Synovial membrane

Muscle

}Joint capsule

Ligament

Joint cavity (synovial fluid)

Ball-and-socket joint

Plane joint

Condyloid joint

Hinge joint

Saddle or gliding joint

Fig. 16-6. Different types of joints.

- **Ball and socket** allow for greater movement and are found in the shoulder and hip.
- **Hinge** are found in the elbow, fingers, knee, and toes.
- **Gliding** are found in wrist, hand, ankle, and foot.
- **Plane** are found primarily in the vertebrae.
- **Condyloid** are found primarily in the wrists.

Vertebrae

■ These 33 bones and cartilaginous segments compose the spinal column:
- Twelve thoracic
- Seven cervical
- Five lumbar
- Five sacral
- One coccyx
■ The two sacroiliac joints join the sacrum and ilium (Fig. 16-7).

Muscles

There are over 600 muscles in the human body to protect our bones and keep our blood circulating throughout the body (Martin & Saxena, 2015). Muscles are responsible for body movement and have a good blood supply.

■ There are three types of muscle:
- **Cardiac:** found only in the myocardium of the heart; cardiac muscles are involuntarily controlled and self-contracting.
- **Smooth:** found in blood vessels, vascular and gastrointestinal systems; this muscle is responsible for the contractility of hollow organs.
- **Skeletal:** found attached to the axial and appendicular skeleton to allow motion. Skeletal muscles are considered voluntary and are controlled by the somatic nervous system; the contraction of these muscles allows motion to occur around a joint.

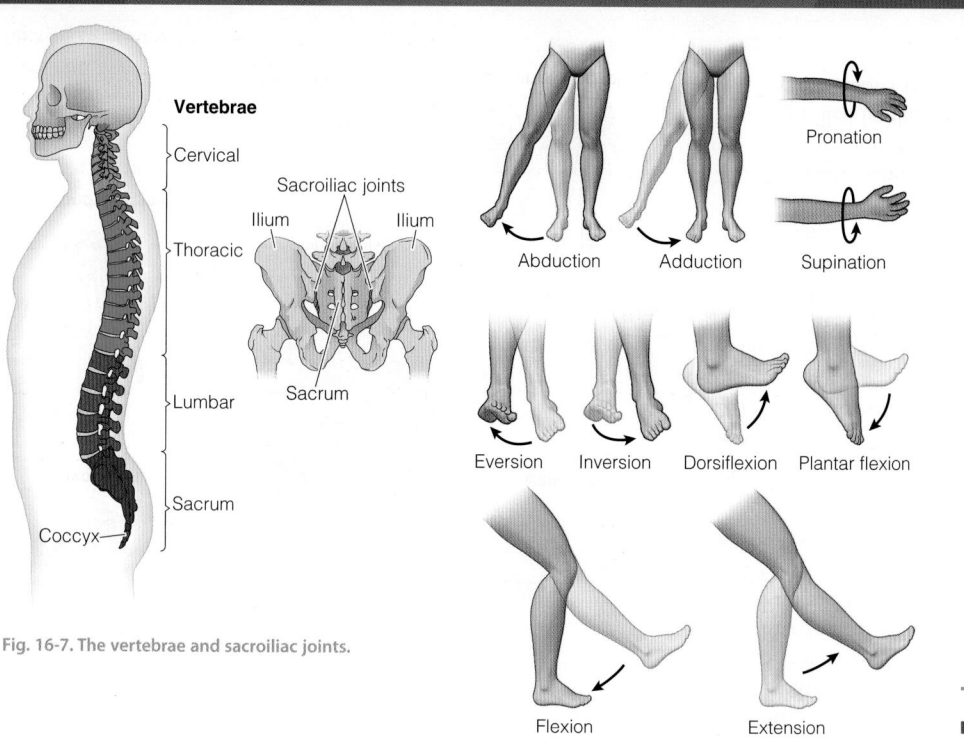

Vertebrae

Cervical

Sacroiliac joints

Ilium   Ilium

Thoracic

Sacrum

Lumbar

Sacrum

Coccyx

Fig. 16-7. The vertebrae and sacroiliac joints.

Abduction   Adduction   Pronation

Supination

Eversion   Inversion   Dorsiflexion   Plantar flexion

Flexion   Extension

Fig. 16-8. Movements of joints.

☐ **Abduction** is movement away from the midline.

☐ **Adduction** is movement toward the midline.

☐ **Pronation** is rotational movement away from anatomical neutral.

☐ **Supination** is rotational movement toward anatomical neutral.

☐ **Eversion** is moving away from the midline of the body.

☐ **Inversion** is moving toward the midline of the body.

☐ **Dorsiflexion** is upward flexion of the foot.

☐ **Plantar flexion** is downward flexion of the foot.

☐ **Flexion** is moving toward the body.

☐ **Extension** is moving away from the body.

☐ **Elevation** is movement that raises a body part in its plane (i.e., shoulder shrug).

Tendons and Ligaments

■ Tendons allow for the attachment of muscle to the bones. Tendons are formed by dense connective tissue at the ends of the muscle and are nonelastic (Fig. 16-9).

■ When a tendon is injured, it is called a **strain.**

■ Ligaments attach bone to bone and can provide additional support to the joint.

■ When a ligament is injured, it is called a **sprain.**

■ Motion within the musculoskeletal system occurs around joints. The contraction of the muscles causes the motion of the joint to occur normally. Movement actions are referenced from an anatomical neutral position. There are a variety of movements that can occur (Fig. 16-8). These movements are as follows:

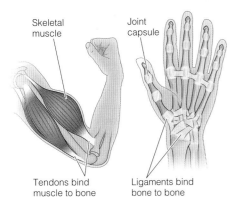

Skeletal muscle

Joint capsule

Tendons bind muscle to bone

Ligaments bind bone to bone

Fig. 16-9. Tendons and ligaments.

TIP Vertebral bodies of the spine are an example of a series of bones coming together and allowing only small motion at each joint, but overall, allowing for great motion.

DIAGNOSTICS

There are several types of diagnostic tests that the healthcare provider may order to assess the musculoskeletal system.

■ **Creatine phosphokinase (CPK)** is a blood test that shows increased CPK enzyme levels when muscle tissue is injured. Elevation of CPK can indicate muscular injury secondary to disease processes (muscular dystrophy, seizure disorder with active seizures); injury (crush type, many intramuscular injections); or strenuous exercise (marathon running) (Chen, 2015).

■ A variety of specialty radiology studies may be ordered to further evaluate bones, ligaments, and tendons. These include:

□ **X-rays** are commonly taken to assess bones and bony structures.

□ **Magnetic resonance imaging (MRI)** assesses soft tissue to determine the nature and severity of injury to tendons, ligaments, bones, and soft tissues.

SENC Safety Alert Patients who have had any type of joint replacements, electronic devices implanted in their body (pacemaker, insulin pump, infusion pump), or metal pieces in their body should not have MRI without informing their healthcare provider of their status. It is the nurse's responsibility to ask a patient if he or she could be or is pregnant. Pregnant women also should inform their healthcare provider of their status prior to undergoing MRI or x-ray exams.

■ **Computed tomography (CT)** scan may be used when a MRI is not possible due to metal in the region of injury to assess bones, ligaments, joints, and the axial skeleton.

■ **Dual-energy x-ray absorptiometry (DEXA)** scan is used to assess bone mineral density in patients who are at risk, or to determine risk for osteoporosis (a condition in which the bones become fragile and brittle).

HEALTH HISTORY

Review of Systems

Proper functioning of the musculoskeletal system is important for the performance of activities of daily living (ADLs) for each patient. A limitation in any component of the musculoskeletal system can have an impact on not only the quality of life for the patient, but the ability to live safely in one's own environment. It is important to gain an understanding of not only issues within the musculoskeletal system, but other health problems the patient may have. Use the OLDCARTS mnemonic (**O**nset,

Location, **D**uration, **C**haracteristics, **A**ggravating/**A**lleviating factors, **R**elieving factors, **T**reatment, **S**everity) to identify attributes of a symptom. Ask the patient the following questions.

Family History

- Is there any family history of musculoskeletal problems?
  - ☐ Congenital and genetic conditions may predispose the patient to a musculoskeletal condition.
    - Muscular dystrophies are a group of genetic disorders that result in muscle weakness over time. Different types of muscular dystrophy affect specific groups of muscles, have a specific age when signs and symptoms are first seen, vary in how severe they can be, and are caused by imperfections in different genes (CDC, 2016).

Past Surgical History

- Have you had surgery to correct/repair any joint, muscle, or ligament problem?
  - ☐ Surgery to correct/repair any joint, muscle, or ligament may limit the range of motion (ROM) in the affected area. The patient may also have some pain in this area if the surgery was recently completed. Also, there may be some decreased sensation in the area if superficial nerves were injured during the surgery.

Past Medical History

- Do you have any chronic diseases? Do you have any history of arthritis? Do you have a history of osteoporosis?
  - ☐ Chronic diseases may impact the patients' ability to perform ADLs and their mobility.
  - ☐ Myopathy may be focal or diffuse muscular dysfunction and weakness; patients experiencing muscle weakness may have difficulty performing ADLs.
- Arthritis affects joint health/functioning and can also cause increased pain.

- There are over 100 different types of arthritis that can affect joints in the body but osteoarthritis is the most common type of joint disorder in the world affecting people over the age of 65 (Prieto-Alhambra, Hunter, Arden, & Arden, 2014).
  - ☐ **Osteoarthritis (OA)** is a progressive disease; the protective cartilage at the ends of the bones wears down; affects the distal interphalangeal joints; often called "wear and tear arthritis" (Vincent, Vincent, & Watt, 2014).
  - ☐ **Rheumatoid arthritis** is a progressive, inflammatory, autoimmune disorder that affects the smaller synovial metacarpophalangeal and interphalangeal joints in the hands and feet; over a long-term period the joint(s) are destroyed causing a joint deformity.
- Decreased bone density may lead to increased risk for fractures.
  - ☐ **Osteoporosis** is a progressive disease; the bone matrix is not being replaced by new bone, and bone mass and density decrease.

CULTURAL CONSIDERATIONS

Caucasian women are more likely to have bone loss. Sometimes the tendency to have bone loss and thin bones is passed down through families (PubMed-Health, 2012). Risk factors for osteoporosis are:
- advancing age
- female
- Caucasian or Asian
- early menopause (before age 45)
- thin, small-framed body
- low calcium intake (Venes, 2013, p. 1695).

Nutrition

- Have you gained or lost any weight recently? If so, how much? Planned or unplanned?
  - ☐ Weight can cause increased stress on the joints if a patient is overweight. Some patients with chronic musculoskeletal pain may experience weight loss due to anorexia.

- Being overweight may cause increased stress on the joints of the spine, hip, knee, ankle, and foot.
- Unplanned significant weight loss may be one indicator of a more serious underlying condition.

Pain Assessment

- How much pain do you have now? How much pain do you have during activities?

  TIP Back pain is one of the five most common reasons to seek care and is the most common musculoskeletal condition treated in emergency rooms; the incidence of lower back pain increases with age. Individuals with chronic back pain are more likely to experience depression and a decrease in their quality of life (Alpert, 2014).

- Use OLDCARTS or OPQRST mnemonic to evaluate the pain. Assess for areas of pain. Ask the patient to point to the area with the greatest pain with one finger in one spot.
  - Muscle pain or myalgia may be related to overuse of a group of muscles, infections, muscle injury, and medications.

- Having the patient specifically locate the pain by pointing to the location will help you narrow your assessment to that area. The nature of the pain may provide insight into the problem. For example, burning may indicate nerve or vascular involvement. Aching may indicate chronic problems, or joint problems. A sharp pain may indicate a newer injury.

  TIP Patients taking atorvastatin, a statin medication to lower cholesterol, were twice as likely to report symptoms of muscle pain (myalgia) as compared with those taking placebo (Foster, Kalvaitas, Stott, & Volansky, 2012). Ask your patient what medications are being taken because myalgia could be a side effect.

- Is any numbness or tingling present?
  - Numbness or tingling may indicate nerve or vascular problems in the area; this may be an indication that tissue is not being perfused at the cellular level.

- Is there any swelling in the area? If yes, ask what the patient has done to make the swelling improve and what makes the swelling worse?
  - Swelling may be present due to an acute injury or chronic problem. If activity makes the swelling worse, it may indicate a problem within the joint.
- Have you experienced any change in your skin color? Have you felt your skin temperature to the affected area to be cool or warmer than normal?
  - Skin discoloration or bruising may indicate the severity of the injury to muscles, tendons, and/or ligaments.
  - Purple coloration is indicative of newer damage, and yellow/greenish coloration is indicative of resolving damage.
  - Erythema (redness) may indicate inflammation or infection.
  - Pale and cool skin may indicate decreased circulation.
  - Surgical scars may indicate repair of injury or joint in the area.

CULTURAL CONSIDERATIONS In patients with darker skin, the assessment of the color, or absence of, may be a bit more difficult as the changes can be quite subtle. In a darker-skinned person, red or purple coloration may not be noted as such. Rather, discoloration may be noted as an area of deeper color when compared to the surrounding tissue. It will also be important to assess skin temperature in patients who are darker skinned as it is not as easy to note visual cues related to alteration in function of the musculoskeletal system.

Risk Factors

Each person is unique in body image and appearance. Genetics and culture are passed from generation to generation and need to be taken into consideration. Gender alone can place individuals at risk.

- Women are more likely to develop rheumatoid arthritis (RA) than men. Risk factors for RA include:
  - smoking cigarettes
  - family history
  - age between 40 and 60 years.

- Osteoarthritis (OA) is another disease of the joints. More women are affected by it than men. Osteoarthritis is more likely to occur in older adults with a history of:
  - ☐ joint injuries
  - ☐ obesity or malnutrition
  - ☐ sedentary lifestyle
  - ☐ engaging in contact sports in the past.

- The length of participation and type of contact sport both contribute to the increased risk; however, people with no history of contact sport participation can also develop osteoarthritis.

SENC Patient-Centered Care You will also want to note if there is any special treatment provided to the patient by family or friends. You can ask the patient about values or beliefs that may affect the condition and treatment of it, make traditional treatment difficult for the patient, or even not allow the patient to undergo treatment.

PREPARATION FOR ASSESSMENT

Equipment Needed
Gloves
Paper Tape Measure

Sequence of Assessment
1. Inspecting
2. Palpating
3. Assessing ROM
4. Assessing strength

Preliminary Steps
To prepare the patient for an assessment of the musculoskeletal system, you will need the following:
- An area with good lighting
- Enough space to have the patient move around
- A sturdy chair
- An examination table

As a healthcare provider, you will need to:
- explain the procedure to the patient in clear, easy-to-understand language
- perform hand hygiene
- while interviewing the patient, remember that there may be a connection between the musculoskeletal system and the neurovascular system. The "five P's" will help you focus on specific musculoskeletal symptoms or injuries:
  - ☐ **P**ain
  - ☐ **P**aralysis
  - ☐ **P**aresthesia
  - ☐ **P**allor
  - ☐ **P**ulselessness

SENC Safety Alert Numbness and tingling may be a serious symptom that needs to be further assessed; nurses should notify the patient's healthcare provider.

TIP Always compare sides for all musculoskeletal assessments.

TECHNIQUE 16-1: **Inspecting Gait**

Purpose: To assess the ability of the patient to ambulate.

When a patient has a specific musculoskeletal body part that is causing problems, the nurse can focus the examination to this specific area after assessing the gait. How well the patient ambulates and the patient's pattern of ambulation will provide the nurse with clues related to the patients' complaint.

■ **TIP** During this assessment, inspecting and palpating are done separately as you can inspect the patient's gait, posture, and some ROM as the patient, or you, enters the room.

SENC Safety Alert When assessing gait and posture in some patients, you may need to provide them with something to hold onto while they perform the requested activities. Geriatric patients and some patients with neurologic conditions may not have the best balance, placing them at risk for falls.

ASSESSMENT STEPS

1. Explain the technique to the patient.
2. Have the patient walk away from you first and then back toward you. This allows for both anterior and posterior observation of gait.
3. Inspect any differences in leg swing and arm swing.
4. Assess the patient's ability or inability to control any joints. Are they limping, unable to move a lower extremity joint through the functional ROM?
5. Assess if the patient uses any assistive devices.
6. Document your findings.

■ **TIP** Some of the more common assistive devices are a walker, rolling walker, cane, or crutches. Use of the type of assistive device should be documented in the nursing note.

NORMAL FINDINGS

■ Gait length is approximately 1.5 m for adults without musculoskeletal problems.
■ Arm swing with gait should be contralateral.
■ The left arm should swing forward as the right leg swings forward. There should be no loss of balance with each step.

ABNORMAL FINDINGS

■ Alterations from normal gait such as limping, decreased motion, absent motion, or excessive motion within the lower and upper extremities
  □ Limping may indicate muscle weakness; bone pain; injured muscle, tendon, or ligament; bone length difference; or long-standing deformity.

- Alterations in motion: decreased may indicate lack of motion in a joint secondary to swelling or bony injury. Absence of motion may indicate a joint that is frozen or fused. Excessive motion may indicate a joint that has lost much of the ligamentous or bony support that limits motion.

- **Ataxia** is an unsteady gait that may be used to compensate for an injury or pain in the extremities. This may also indicate a problem with cerebellar function.

- **Scissors,** or **diplegic gait,** is most commonly seen in cerebral palsy. The legs cross the midline in a swinging fashion to compensate for lack of motion.

- **Shuffling gait** may indicate a problem with balance, Parkinson's disease, or decreased lower extremity strength.

  ▪ **TIP** A patient who has Parkinson's disease may have the presence of a shuffling gait; this is a key characteristic symptom of the disease.

- Increased numbness and tingling may cause the individual to slap the foot to the surface when walking as he or she may not feel the heel strike phase of gait. For individuals with neuropathy, this may or may not occur.

- **Foot drop** is a weakness or paralysis of the muscles of the lower leg or the inability to control plantar flexion of the ankle; it may indicate peroneal nerve injury or muscle or neurological disorders. In this condition, the patient is unable to use the muscles to bring the foot into the neutral position (Fig. 16-10A). This is where the foot is at 90 degrees to the lower leg, much like the letter *L*.

  ▪ **TIP** Note if the patient using an ankle-foot orthosis or some other splint. The ankle-foot orthosis, or other splint, serves to hold the ankle in a normal position (Fig. 16-10B).

SENC Safety Alert Use of accessory devices such as cane, walker, or crutches will impact gait. Be sure that the patient uses the device correctly, with placement in the hand that is opposite of the involved lower extremity for a cane or one crutch. If you are in doubt about proper use, consult with a physical therapist.

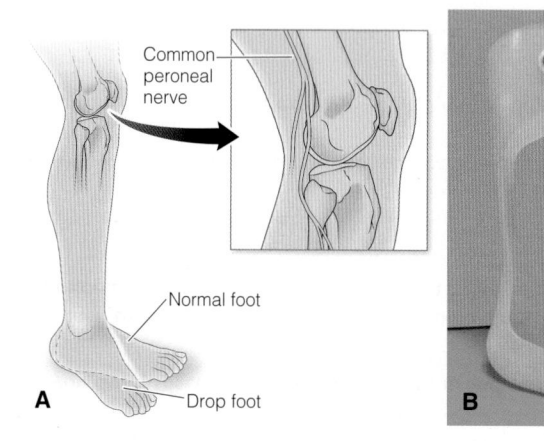

Fig. 16-10. (A) Foot drop. (B) Ankle foot orthosis.

TECHNIQUE 16-2: **Inspecting Posture**

Purpose: To assess alignment of muscle and joints within the musculoskeletal system

Posture and overall functioning of the musculoskeletal system are evaluated on the ambulatory patient as he or she moves into the examination room or within the hospital room, his or her house, or in the healthcare providers' office.

TIP If a patient is not able to perform all the ROM activities in a standing position, have the patient sit.

ASSESSMENT STEPS

1. Explain the technique to the patient.
2. Inspect the patient's posture while the patient is walking (Fig. 16-11), assessing the following:
   - ☐ Is the head centered on the axial skeleton?
   - ☐ Is there an alteration in balance, ability to ambulate or stand?
   - ☐ Have the patient sit in a chair and get up from a chair; note any difficulties the patient may have in lowering or raising his or her body.
3. Ask the patient if he or she has any back or neck pain that would prevent performing some ROM activities.

SENC Safety Alert If the patient has an alteration in balance, it is very important to provide measures to assure stability when the patient performs the actions noted below.

TIP Ask the patient if he or she is experiencing any numbness or tingling. If so, or if it happens when performing these activities, stop and assess the new symptoms before moving to the next step.

4. Inspect the patient's posture.
   - ☐ Are the shoulders level and even?
   - ☐ Is the head sitting centered on the axial skeleton?
   - ☐ Is there pain with sitting?
   - ☐ Inspect the location of the head in relation to the trunk.
   - ☐ Is the head sitting forward?
   - ☐ Is the head tipped to one side?
   - ☐ Is the neck fixed in a flexed or extended position?
5. Ask the patient to rotate (turn) the head to the right and then to the left.
6. Ask the patient to tip the head to the right and then to the left.
7. Ask the patient to flex the neck, or touch the chin to the chest.
8. Ask the patient to extend the neck, or look to the ceiling.
9. Ask the patient to stand. Again, assess the ease or difficulty in changing positions from sitting to standing.

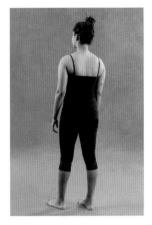

Fig. 16-11. Inspecting good posture.

10. Ask the patient to bend forward at the waist; inspect the spinal curvature (Fig. 16-12).

11. Ask the patient to bend at the waist to the left side and then to the right side as you note if these motions are symmetrical and fluid.

12. Ask the patient to bend backward and then forward from the waist as you assess the ROM.

NORMAL FINDINGS

■ When standing, feet should be shoulder width apart.

■ When sitting and standing, the patient should be upright, looking forward with the head centered on the axial skeleton.

■ Shoulders should be even and not sloped forward (Fig. 16-13).

■ When standing, weight should be distributed evenly on both lower extremities.

■ ROM of the neck and back should be symmetrical, fluid, and without pain.

ABNORMAL FINDINGS

■ Numbness or tingling may indicate a problem with a nerve or the circulation to the area.

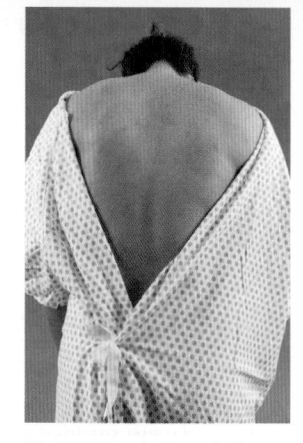
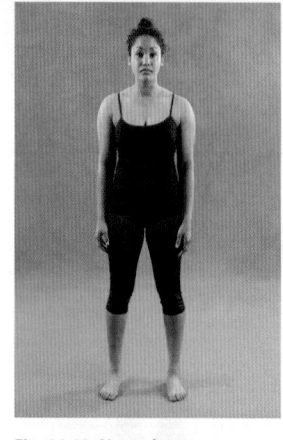

Fig. 16-12. Inspecting spinal curvature.

Fig. 16-13. Normal posture.

■ Head not centered on the axial skeleton may indicate muscular tightness (head held toward area of tightness), muscle weakness (head unable to be held up in stable manner), or spinal column injury (compression fractures may alter normal alignment).

■ Limitations in ROM in the neck may indicate muscular tightness or limitations to muscular weakness.

■ Shoulders that are not level may indicate an injury (old or new) to one of the upper extremities or a deformity affecting the vertebrae.

■ Motion of the trunk that is not fluid and symmetrical may indicate muscular tightness, muscular weakness, pain, or bony structure problems.

■ **TIP** Documentation of the differences in motion is important. For example, a patient with a cervical disc injury may have limited neck motion in rotation to one side.

TECHNIQUE 16-3: Inspecting and Palpating the Vertebral Column

Purpose: To assess for abnormalities in the structure of the vertebral column.

ASSESSMENT STEPS

1. Explain the technique to the patient.

2. Ask the patient to stand.

3. Facing the patient's back, inspect the alignment of the vertebral column and assess for:
- ☐ How straight is the vertebral column when the patient is standing?
- ☐ Is there any noted deviation in the anterior-posterior plane?

4. Ask the patient to bend at the waist and assess whether the vertebral column is straight.

5. Facing the patient's back, using two or three finger pads, starting at the top of the vertebral column, palpate the vertebral column assessing for (Fig. 16-14):
- ☐ areas of tenderness
- ☐ noted deviations in the lateral plane.
  - • This would be noted as a deviation from a straight line that the vertebral column should maintain.
- ☐ protrusions, something being more prominent along the vertebral column, or depressions, like a pit or hole, may indicate dysfunction within the vertebral column.

6. Document your findings.

NORMAL FINDINGS

- ■ The vertebral column is straight when the patient is standing and flexed forward.
- ■ No deviation noted in anterior-posterior plane
- ■ No areas of tenderness
- ■ No deviation in the lateral plane
- ■ No protrusions or drop-offs within the vertebral column

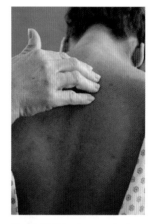

Fig. 16-14. Palpating vertebral column.

ABNORMAL FINDINGS

- **Scoliosis** is an abnormal curvature of the spine that occurs in a lateral manner; it may look like a *C* or *S* on visualization and be palpable (Fig. 16-15A).
- **Kyphosis** is a curvature of the spine that looks like a slouching, or hunchback, posture; this can lead to problems with the contents of the thorax. This occurs in the thoracic spine (Fig. 16-15B).
- **Lordosis** is a curvature of the spine that looks like an arched lower back: it is an increased inward curvature of the lumbar spine (Fig. 16-15C).
- Areas of tenderness may indicate a problem with the bony structure or the ligaments within the vertebral column.
- Protrusions or depressions may indicate a displacement of one vertebral body on another vertebral body.

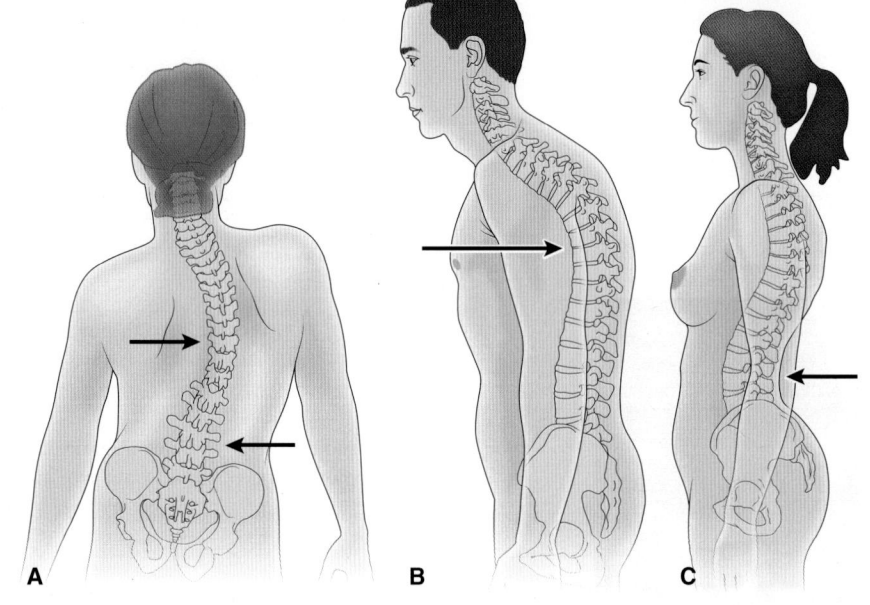

Fig. 16-15. (A) Scoliosis. (B) Kyphosis. (C) Lordosis.

TECHNIQUE 16-4: **Inspecting and Palpating the Upper Extremities**

Purpose: To determine if there are any abnormalities within the upper extremity.

ASSESSMENT STEPS

1. Explain the technique to the patient.
2. Inspect the upper extremity on the right side then the left side; compare the right to the left side.
3. Using two or three finger pads, gently palpate the upper extremity on the right side:
   ☐ Shoulder
   ☐ Elbow

☐ Wrist

☐ Hand/fingers and joints

4. Assess for:

☐ tenderness

☐ depressions

☐ bulges

☐ changes in temperature.

5. Repeat steps 3 and 4 on the left side.

6. Document your findings.

NORMAL FINDINGS

With the patient standing, inspection of the upper extremity should find:

■ symmetry between left and right upper extremities

■ no forward rounding of the shoulder

■ straight upper arms

■ slight bending in the elbows

■ wrists in line with the lower arm and palms facing the upper leg

■ some slight flexion of the fingers

■ no findings of tenderness/pain; depression or protrusions; increased warmth; increased joint size or missing fingers.

ABNORMAL FINDINGS

■ Forward rounding of the shoulders may indicate tightness of muscles across the anterior thorax and a weakness of the muscles of the posterior thorax.

■ Non-straight upper arm may indicate a fracture (old or new) or a significant muscle tear.

■ A straight, or hyperextended elbow may indicate lack of bony structure or muscle tone to hold it in a slightly flexed position.

■ A flexed elbow that is unable to be straightened may indicate a serious problem with the joint.

■ If the wrist is out of line with the lower arm, there may be a new or old bony injury causing limitations to the motion.

■ When the palms do not face the upper leg, there may be some bony limitation to ROM within the wrist joint.

■ Fingers that are more than slightly flexed may indicate some sort of disease process that limits ROM.

■ Areas of tenderness or pain may indicate an injury to bone, muscle, tendon, or ligament.

■ Depressions may indicate a dislocated joint, significant muscle injury, or joint subluxation.

■ Protrusions may also indicate a dislocated or subluxed joint, a displaced fracture, the buildup of calcium within the muscle, a type of arthritis, or a tumor.

□ **Bouchard's nodes** are bony enlargements on the proximal interphalangeal joints (PIP) joints; commonly seen in osteoarthritis or rheumatoid arthritis (Fig. 16-16A).

□ **Heberden's nodes** are bony enlargements on the distal interphalangeal joints (DIP); commonly seen in osteoarthritis (Fig. 16-16B).

■ Increased warmth in the joints may be an indication of infection or disease process within that joint.

■ Missing fingers may indicate old trauma, or disease process.

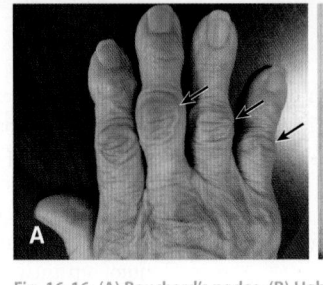
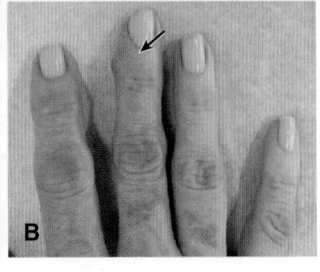

Fig. 16-16. (A) Bouchard's nodes. (B) Heberden's nodes.

TECHNIQUE 16-5: **Assessing Range of Motion and Muscle Strength of the Upper Extremities**

Purpose: To assess strength and limitations in ROM in the upper extremities

ASSESSMENT STEPS

1. Explain the technique to the patient. You will ask the patient to perform specific motions independently first and then against resistance.

2. Ask the patient to perform the following ROM activities of the right and left upper extremity.

□ **Shoulder motion**

• **Flexion:** movement of the upper extremity as a whole, forward, with thumb facing forward when starting. Have the patient lift both arms toward the ear (Fig. 16-17A).

• **Flexion against resistance:** movement of the upper extremity as a whole, forward, with thumb forward, to the ear. Place your palm on the anterior aspect of the elbow and provide resistance as the patient attempts this motion (Fig. 16-17B).

Fig. 16-17. Shoulder motion. (A) Flexion. (B) Flexion against resistance.

• **Extension:** movement of the upper extremity as a whole, backward. The thumb should be facing forward when starting (Fig. 16-18A).

• **Extension against resistance:** movement of the upper extremity as a whole, backward. The thumb should be facing forward when starting. Place your palm on the posterior aspect of the elbow and provide resistance as the patient attempts this motion (Fig. 16-18B).

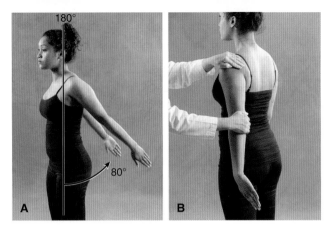

Fig. 16-18. Shoulder motion. (A) Extension. (B) Extension against resistance.

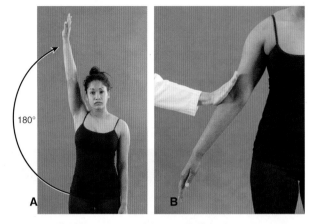

Fig. 16-19. Shoulder motion. (A) Abduction. (B) Abduction against resistance.

- **Abduction:** movement of the upper extremity as a whole away from anatomic neutral position (0°) toward the ear (180°); ask the patient to move the right arm away from the body up to 180°; repeat on the left side (Fig. 16-19A).
- **Abduction against resistance:** movement of the upper extremity as a whole away from anatomic neutral position toward the ear. Place your palm on the lateral aspect of the elbow and provide resistance as the patient attempts the motion (Fig. 16-19B).
- **Adduction:** movement of the upper extremity as a whole away from the ear toward the waist and then across the midline in front of the naval (Fig. 16-20A).
- **Adduction against resistance:** movement of the upper extremity as a whole away from the ear toward the waist and then across the midline in front of the naval. Place your palm on the medial aspect of the elbow and provide resistance as the patient attempts the motion (Fig. 16-20B).

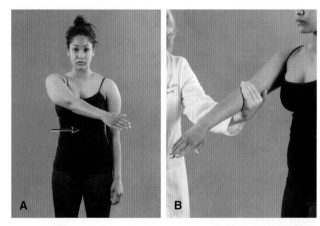

Fig. 16-20. Shoulder motion. (A) Adduction. (B) Adduction against resistance.

- **Internal rotation:** ask the patient to pretend to tuck a shirt into the waistband in the front and in the back. This is a functional assessment of the patients' ability to perform internal rotation (Fig. 16-21A).
- **Internal rotation against resistance:** as the patient holds the upper arms at the side with the elbow flexed to 90 degrees, place your palm against the patient's palm and provide resistance as the patient moves his or her hand toward the opposite hip or naval (Fig. 16-21B).
- **External rotation:** ask the patient to rub the back of his or her head with the right hand and then the left hand (Fig. 16-22A).
  ▨ **TIP** This is also a functional assessment of the patient's ability to perform external rotation.
- **External rotation against resistance:** as the patient holds the right upper arm at the side with the elbow flexed to 90 degrees, place your palm on the back of the patient's hand and provide resistance as the patient moves his or her hand toward the starting point for internal rotation (Fig. 16-22B).

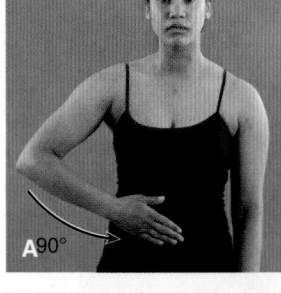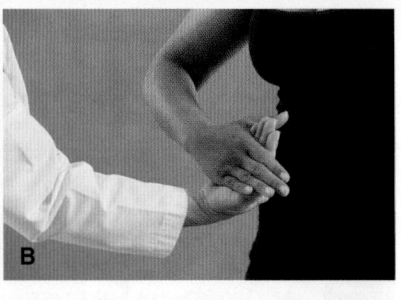

Fig. 16-21. Shoulder motion. (A) Internal rotation. (B) Internal rotation against resistance.

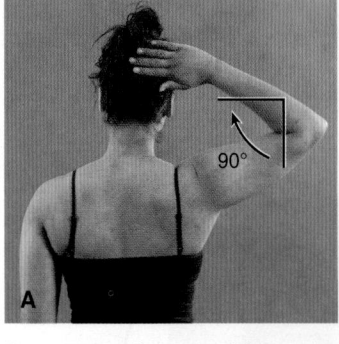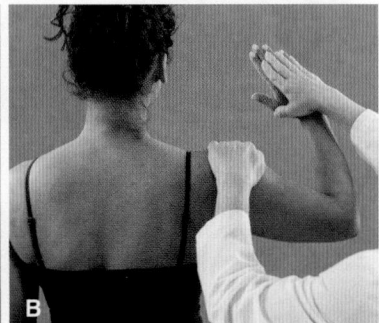

Fig. 16-22. Shoulder motion. (A) External rotation. (B) External rotation against resistance.

☐ **Elbow motion**
- **Flexion:** move the right hand to the shoulder from the anatomic neutral position; repeat using the left hand (Fig. 16-23A).
- **Flexion against resistance:** movement of the hand to the shoulder from anatomic neutral. Place your palm on the patient's right forearm and resist as the patient performs the above motion; repeat using the left elbow motion (Fig. 16-23B).
- **Extension movement:** move the hand from the shoulder to anatomic neutral position (Fig. 16-24A).
- **Extension against resistance:** move the hand from the shoulder to anatomic neutral. Place your palm on the posterior aspect of the patient's forearm and resist as the patient performs the motion (Fig. 16-24B).
- **Pronation:** with the elbow flexed to 90 degrees, move the hand from palm facing up to palm facing down (Fig. 16-25A).
- **Pronation against resistance:** with the elbow flexed to 90 degrees, move the hand from palm facing up to palm facing down. Hold the patient's hand and resist the motion to determine the strength (Fig. 16-25B).

- **Supination:** with the elbow flexed to 90 degrees, movement of the hand from palm facing down to palm facing up (Fig. 16-26A)
- **Supination against resistance:** with the elbow flexed to 90 degrees, movement of the hand from palm facing down to palm facing up. Hold the patient's hand and resist the motion to determine strength (Fig. 16-26B).

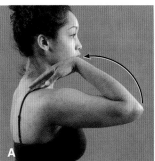
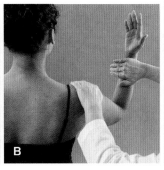

Fig. 16-23. Elbow motion. (A) Flexion. (B) Flexion against resistance.

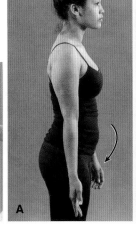
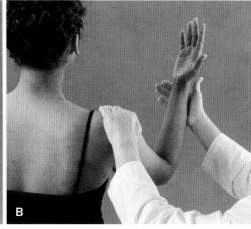

Fig. 16-24. Elbow motion. (A) Extension. (B) Extension against resistance.

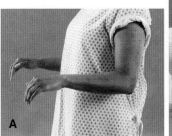
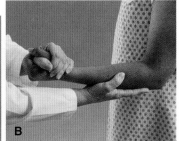

Fig. 16-25. Elbow motion. (A) Pronation of hand. (B) Pronation of hand resistance.

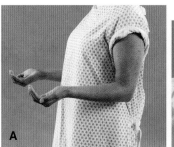
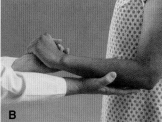

Fig. 16-26. Elbow motion. (A) Supination of hand. (B) Supination of hand resistance.

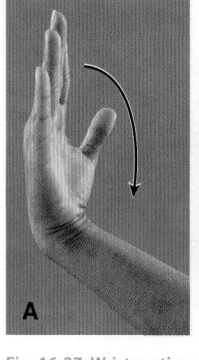
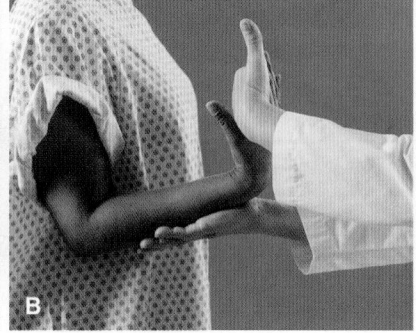

Fig. 16-27. Wrist motion. (A) Flexion. (B) Flexion against resistance.

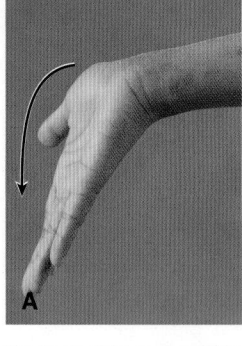
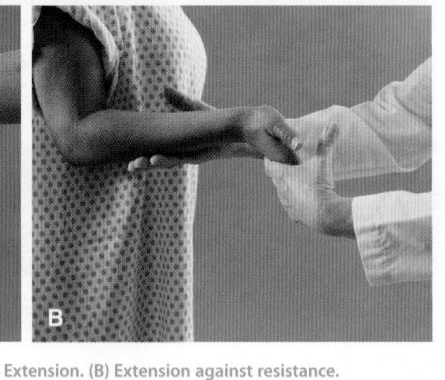

Fig. 16-28. Wrist motion. (A) Extension. (B) Extension against resistance.

☐ **Wrist motion**
- **Flexion:** move the palm toward the forearm (Fig. 16-27A).
- **Flexion against resistance:** place your palm on the patient's palm and resist the patient's motion to determine strength (Fig. 16-27B).
- **Extension:** movement of the palm from the forearm (Fig. 16-28A).
- **Extension against resistance:** place your palm on the posterior aspect of the patient's hand and resist the movement of the palm from the forearm (Fig. 16-28B).
- **Radial deviation:** movement of the hand toward the radial head (Fig. 16-29A)
- **Radial deviation against resistance:** place your palm over the thumb of the hand and resist movement of the hand toward the radial head (Fig. 16-29B).

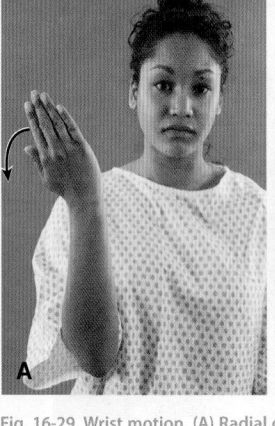
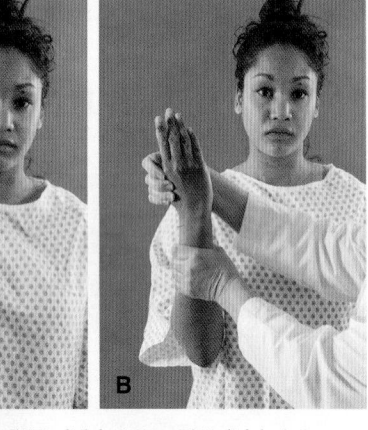

Fig. 16-29. Wrist motion. (A) Radial deviation. (B) Radial deviation against resistance.

- **Ulnar deviation:** movement of the hand toward the ulnar head (Fig. 16-30A)
- **Ulnar deviation against resistance:** place your palm over the medial aspect of the hand and resist movement of the hand toward the ulnar head (Fig. 16-30B).
- **Tinel's sign** is performed to assess for carpal tunnel syndrome; with the patient's right palm facing up, tap on the median nerve (on the thumb side of the hand) (Fig. 16-31); if the patient complains of tingling or pain radiating to the thumb, index finger, or middle finger, perform the Phalen's test (Bostock, 2012). Repeat this assessment on the left hand.
- **Phalen's test:** Ask the patient to flex both wrists with the fingers extended and pointing downward and press them together for one full minute; ask the patient if he or she feels any tingling or numbness in the palmar aspect of the fingers (Fig. 16-32).

☐ **Finger motion**
- **Flexion:** movement of the fingers toward the palm into a fist-like position (Fig. 16-33A).
- **Flexion against resistance:** have the patient attempt to squeeze two of your fingers one hand at a time (Fig. 16-33B) and then bilaterally (Fig. 16-33C).
- **Extension:** movement of the fingers out of the fist-like position into a straight and slightly flared position (Fig. 16-34A).
- **Extension against resistance:** movement of the fingers out of the fist-like position into a straight and slightly flared position. Have the patient try to open his or her fist against your palm that is over their fingers (Fig. 16-34B).

3. Document your findings.

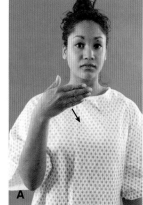
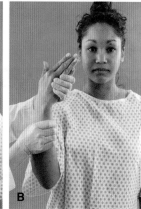

Fig. 16-30. Wrist motion. (A) Ulnar deviation. (B) Ulnar deviation against resistance.

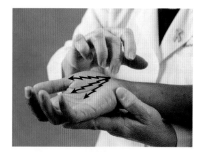

Fig. 16-31. Tinel's sign.

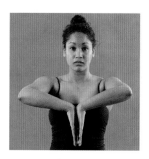

Fig. 16-32. Phalen's test.

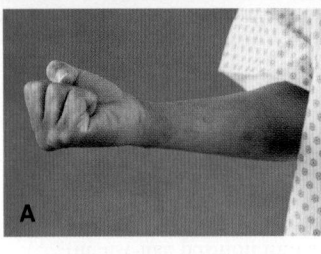
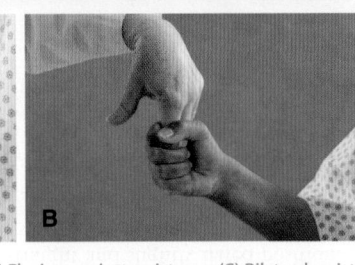
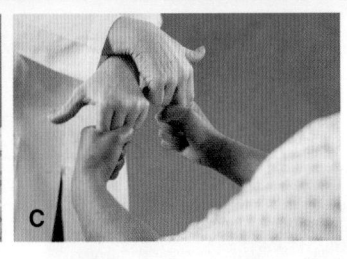

Fig. 16-33. Finger motion. (A) Flexion. (B) Flexion against resistance. (C) Bilateral resistance.

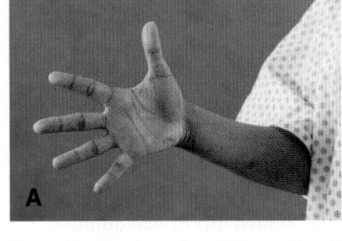
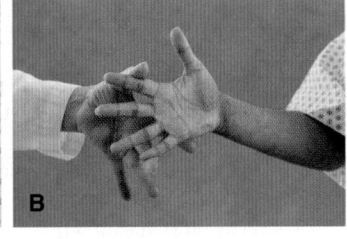

Fig. 16-34. Finger motion. (A) Extension. (B) Extension against resistance.

NORMAL FINDINGS

- All motions should be symmetrical when compared to the same motion of the right and left upper extremities (Tables 16-1, 16-2, 16-3).
- The fingers should be able to flex fully, as demonstrated by making a closed fist, and extending as demonstrated by having the fingers flare out in a straight manner.
- Tinel's Sign: no pain, tingling, or numbness sensation felt in the wrist, hand, and fingers
- Strength of extremities: strength is graded on a scale of 0 to 5 (Table 16-4). It is the measurement of the muscles' ability to contract and work against a load.

TABLE 16-1 Expected Range of Motion of the Shoulder

Motion	Degrees	Motion	Degrees
Flexion	180	Adduction	10–20
Extension	45–60	Internal Rotation	70–90
Abduction	150	External Rotation	90

TABLE 16-2 Expected Range of Motion at the Elbow and Forearm

Motion	Degrees	Motion	Degrees
Flexion	145	Pronation	70
Extension	0	Supination	85

TABLE 16-3 Expected Range of Motion of the Wrist

Motion	Degrees	Motion	Degrees
Flexion	90	Radial deviation	20
Extension	70	Ulnar deviation	50

TABLE 16-4 Grading Strength of Muscle

Score or Grade	Contractibility Noted
0	Unable to contract muscle in a gravity eliminated position
1	Able to contract muscle slightly
2	Able to move joint in a gravity eliminated position
3	Able to move joint against gravity
4	Able to move joint with some resistance through range of motion
5	Able to move joint with full resistance through range of motion

ABNORMAL FINDINGS

- Anything less than expected full ROM can be considered to be an abnormal finding. This may be due to a new injury, old injury, surgical procedure, disease, or neurological problem.
- If a Tinel's or Phelan's test produces pain or tingling sensations, this may indicate carpal tunnel syndrome.
  - □ **Carpal tunnel syndrome** is compression of the median nerve; a nerve that runs from the forearm to the palm of the hand; may be caused by repetitive movements.
- Strength of less than 4 of 5. This indicates muscular weakness. The weakness may be due to injury or deconditioning.
- Pain when meeting resistance: this may indicate injury to the muscle. Document the motion and the strength grade. For example, elbow flexion 4/5 with pain.

TECHNIQUE 16-6: Inspecting and Palpating the Lower Extremities

Purpose: To assess for any abnormalities within the lower extremity

■ **TIP** When assessing the lower extremity, it is recommended that each extremity be fully exposed for this assessment.

ASSESSMENT STEPS

1. Explain the technique to the patient. You will ask the patient to perform specific motions independently first and then against resistance.

2. Inspect the lower extremity on the right side then the left side; compare the right side to the left side.

3. Using your finger pads, gently palpate the right and left lower extremities:

□ Hip
□ Knee
□ Ankle
□ Foot
□ Toes

■ **TIP** Palpation of the lower extremities may be done with the patient on the examination table in a sitting or supine position.

4. Assess the presence of:
- ☐ tenderness
- ☐ depressions
- ☐ bulges
- ☐ changes in temperature.

5. Document your findings.

SENC Safety Alert For the older patient or patient who does not demonstrate good balance, the use of an examination table is preferred. The patient will need to sit and lay on the table to complete the assessment of the hips, knees, and ankles. For other patients, sitting on the table will allow for improved assessment of the knee, ankle, and foot.

NORMAL FINDINGS

- No pain/tenderness; depressions or protrusions; swelling; increased joint size or missing digits
- When the patient is standing, he or she should be bearing weight on both lower extremities equally. There should be no forward flexing at the hip, and the upper leg should be straight.
- The knees should be slightly flexed and pointed forward.
- The ankle should be perpendicular to the straight lower leg.
- The foot should be straight forward, in line with the knee, and a slight arch should be noted on the medial aspect of the foot.

ABNORMAL FINDINGS

- The inability to bear weight equally on both lower extremities may indicate the presence of pain in one of the extremities.
- A shortened extremity may indicate a bony injury or be resultant from a disease or surgical procedure.
- Forward flexion at the hip may indicate problems within the hip joint, tightness of the muscular structure around the hip, or a problem with the lower back.
- A nonstraight upper leg may indicate a significant bony or muscular injury in the past. If the patient is able to bear weight, the injury is most likely old.
- Knees that are straight may indicate a laxity in the ligaments supporting the knee or a problem with the bony structure of the knee.
- Knees that are more than slightly flexed may indicate increased bony buildup within the joint; a disease process; a loose body that locks the joint in this position; or an old injury. Sometimes the knee will appear rotated inward or outward. This is an indication of bony rotation above or below the knee.
- Lower legs that are not straight may indicate an injury to the bones or muscles. The ability to bear weight on this type of lower leg deformity indicates that it is not a new injury.
- **Generalized edema** in the lower extremity may indicate a circulatory problem. Note this in the documentation and inform the healthcare provider.

- Ankles that are not perpendicular to the lower leg indicate a lack of ROM within the ankle joint. This may be caused by tight tendons, bony deformity within the ankle joint or old injury, or surgery that caused a loss of normal joint function.
- A foot without a slight arch may be indicative of problems with the following: plantar fascia injuries, fallen arches, and old bony injuries.
- **Hallux valgus** (bunion) is a lateral deviation and an enlarged joint of the great toe (Fig. 16-35).
- **Hammertoe** is a permanent contracted toe deformity; the proximal interphalangeal joint of the second, third, or fourth toe may be affected (Fig. 16-35).

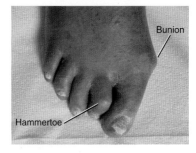

Fig. 16-35. Bunion and hammertoe.

TECHNIQUE 16-7: **Assessing Range of Motion and Strength of the Lower Extremities**

Purpose: To assess strength and limitations in ROM in the lower extremities

TIP Always remember to compare one side with the other side.

ASSESSMENT STEPS

1. Explain the technique to the patient, and tell the patient you will be assessing each lower extremity separately, and he or she will have to perform specific motions without assistance.
2. Ask the patient to perform the following ROM activities without and with resistance of each lower extremity; assess any differences in symmetry of motion and the fluid nature of the motion.
   - ☐ **Hip motion**
     - **Flexion:** movement of the hip forward and toward the anterior aspect of the body (Fig. 16-36A).
     - **Flexion against resistance:** movement of the hip forward, toward the anterior aspect of the body. Place your palm on the anterior aspect of the upper thigh and resist the motion (Fig. 16-36B).
     - **Extension:** movement of the hip backwards away from the anterior aspect of the body (Fig. 16-37A).

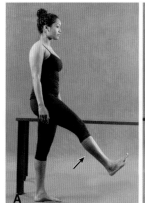
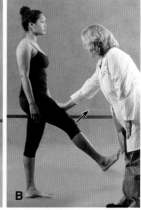

Fig. 16-36. Hip motion. (A) Flexion. (B) Flexion against resistance.

- **Extension against resistance:** movement of the hip backward, away from the anterior aspect of the body. Place your palm on the posterior aspect of the upper thigh and resist the motion (Fig. 16-37B).
- **Abduction:** movement of the lower extremity away from the midline of the body (Fig. 16-38A).
- **Abduction against resistance:** movement of the lower extremity away from the midline of the body. Place your palm on the lateral aspect of the thigh and resist the motion (Fig. 16-38B).
- **Adduction:** movement of the lower extremity toward the midline of the body (Fig. 16-39A).
- **Adduction against resistance:** movement of the lower extremity toward the midline of the body. Place your palm on the distal one third of the medial aspect of the upper thigh and resist the motion (Fig. 16-39B).

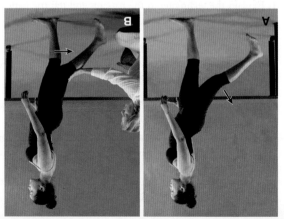

Fig. 16-37. Hip motion. (A) Extension. (B) Extension against resistance.

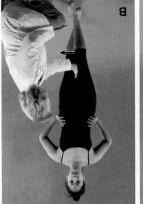
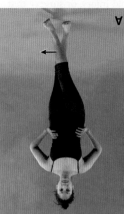

Fig. 16-38. Hip motion. (A) Abduction. (B) Abduction against resistance.

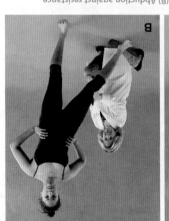
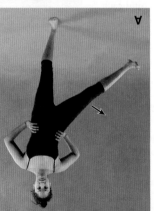

Fig. 16-39. Hip motion. (A) Adduction. (B) Adduction against resistance.

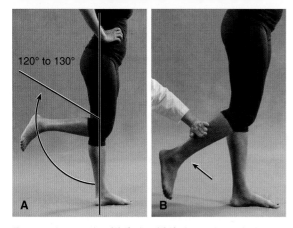

Fig. 16-40. Knee motion. (A) Flexion. (B) Flexion against resistance.

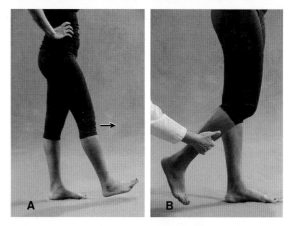

Fig. 16-41. Knee motion. (A) Extension. (B) Extension against resistance.

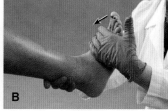
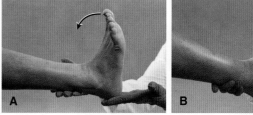

Fig. 16-42. Ankle motion. (A) Dorsiflexion. (B) Dorsiflexion against resistance.

☐ **Knee motion**
- **Flexion:** movement of the heel toward the buttocks (Fig. 16-40A).
- **Flexion against resistance:** movement of the heel toward the buttocks. Place your palm on the anterior aspect of the distal one third of the lower leg and resist the motion (Fig. 16-40B).
- **Extension:** movement of the lower extremity toward the anterior aspect of the body (Fig. 16-41A).
- **Extension against resistance:** movement of the lower extremity toward the anterior aspect of the body. Place your palm on the anterior aspect of the distal one third of the lower leg and resist the motion (Fig. 16-41B).

☐ **Ankle motion**
- **Dorsiflexion:** movement of the sole of the foot away from the floor, toward the knee (Fig. 16-42A).

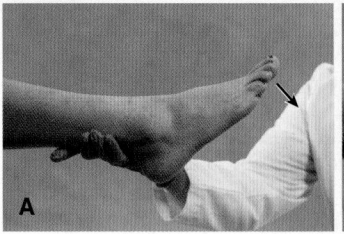
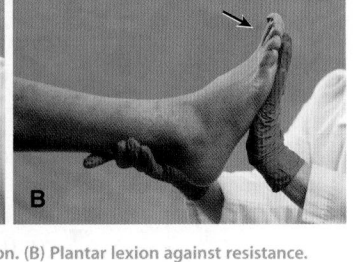

Fig. 16-43. Ankle motion. (A) Plantar flexion. (B) Plantar lexion against resistance.

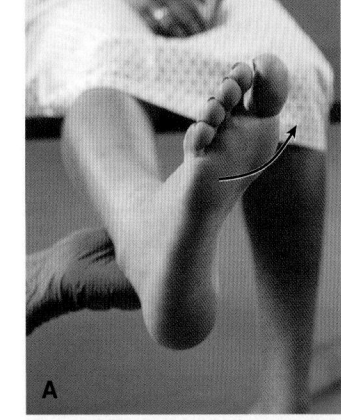
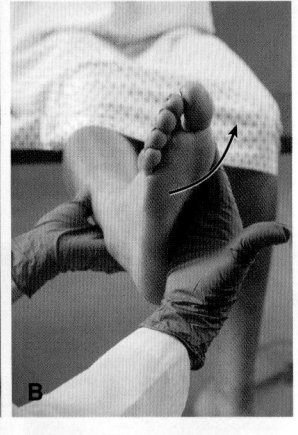

Fig. 16-44. Foot motion. (A) Inversion. (B) Inversion against resistance.

- **Dorsiflexion against resistance:** movement of the sole of the foot away from the floor, toward the knee. Place your palm on the top of the foot and resist the motion (Fig. 16-42B).
- **Plantar flexion:** movement of the sole of the foot toward the floor, away from the knee (Fig. 16-43A).
- **Plantar flexion against resistance:** movement of the sole of the foot toward the floor, away from the knee. Place your palm on the sole of the foot and resist the motion (Fig. 16-43B).

☐ **Foot motion**
- **Inversion:** movement of the great toe/foot toward the midline of the body (Fig. 16-44A).
- **Inversion against resistance:** movement of the great toe/foot toward the midline of the body. Place your palm on the medial aspect of the foot and resist the motion (Fig. 16-44B).
- **Eversion:** movement of the great toe/foot away from the midline of the body (Fig. 16-45A).
- **Eversion against resistance:** movement of the great toe/foot away from the midline of the body. Place your palm on the lateral aspect of the foot and resist the motion (Fig. 16-45B).

3. Document your findings.

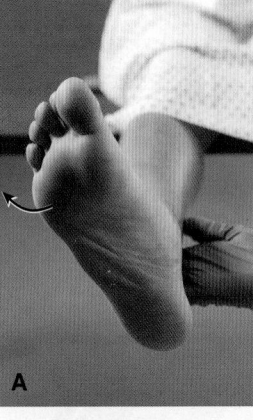
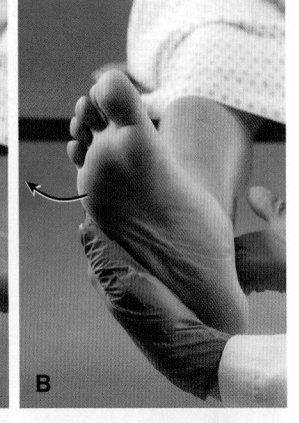

Fig. 16-45. Foot motion. (A) Eversion. (B) Eversion against resistance.

NORMAL FINDINGS

- The ROM of each joint is symmetric when compared with the opposite limb (Tables 16-5, 16-6, 16-7).
- Motion is fluid and without restrictions.
- Motion is without pain.
- The patient should demonstrate strength of at least 4/5 in all of the motions in the lower extremities.
  - □ Strength of extremities: Strength is graded on a scale of 0 to 5 (see Table 16-4). It is the measurement of the muscles' ability to contract and work against a load.

ABNORMAL FINDINGS

- The ROM of each joint is not symmetric to the opposite limb.
- Motion is not fluid. This may indicate a muscular strain.
- Limitation in ROM may indicate a problem in the joint or with the muscular strength.
- Pain is present with ROM activities. This may indicate injury to the muscle or joint.
- Alteration in strength with findings of 3/5 or less in one or more of the motions may indicate an injury to the muscle.
- Limitations in ROM against resistance may indicate a problem in the joint such as a loose body or a tendon getting caught when movement is attempted.
- Ability to resist at 4/5 or 5/5 for part of the ROM, but at a level of 3/5 or less for another part of the ROM. This may indicate that one of the muscles that performs the movement may be injured.

TABLE 16-5 Range of Motion of the Hip

Motion	Degrees	Motion	Degrees
Flexion	120	Abduction	40–50
Extension	20–20	Adduction	10–20

TABLE 16-6 Range of Motion of the Knee

Motion	Degrees	Motion	Degrees
Flexion	130–150	Extension	0 to –3

TABLE 16-7 Range of Motion of the Ankle

Motion	Degrees	Motion	Degrees
Plantar Flexion	50	Inversion	30
Dorsiflexion	20	Eversion	15

PATIENT EDUCATION

Healthy People 2020

Goal: Prevent illness and disability related to arthritis and other rheumatic conditions, osteoporosis, and chronic back conditions (HHS, 2010).

This can be accomplished by patients working together with their healthcare providers to maintain a level of wellness, or to improve their current level of wellness in respect to the musculoskeletal system.

- Encourage eating a healthy diet that includes foods rich in calcium, vitamin D, magnesium, and phosphorus.
- Encourage maintaining, or achieving, a healthy body weight.
- Encourage regular physical exercise and exercises that strengthen the core.
- Encourage good posture and good body mechanics.
- Encourage stretching exercises such as yoga, which builds muscle strength, increases flexibility, and improves posture.

Work-related musculoskeletal disorders including those of the neck, upper extremities, and lower back are one of the leading causes of lost workday injury and illness. Maintaining good posture and proper alignment of the spinal column while sitting and standing will prevent strain on the back. Workers in many different industries and occupations can be exposed to risk factors at work, such as lifting heavy items, bending, reaching overhead, pushing and pulling heavy loads, working in awkward body positions, and performing repetitive task movements. Musculoskeletal disorders are one of the most frequently reported causes of lost or restricted work time. Exposure to these known risk factors for musculoskeletal disorders increases a worker's risk of injury (Prevention of Musculoskeletal Disorders in the Workplace, n.d.). Integrate teaching moments about principles of ergonomics (the study of workplace design).

Assessing the Neurological System

Kimberly Foisy and Janice Thompson

INTRODUCTION

The human sensory-neurological system is one of the most complicated systems of the human body. Assessing the neurological system is a challenging and complex task. A thorough baseline neurologic assessment includes evaluation of mental status, cranial nerve function, motor function, sensory function, and reflexes (Vacca, 2014). Knowledge of the basics of the examination, especially those components that are effective in screening for neurological dysfunction, is essential for all nurses (Oommen, 2011).

REVIEW OF ANATOMY AND PHYSIOLOGY

The neurological system consists of the brain, spinal cord, and a complex network of neurons. Neurons are specialized cells that transmit information from different parts of the body. The system is responsible for sending, receiving, and interpreting messages.

Central Nervous System

Brain
- Largest part of the central nervous system (CNS)
- Contains gray matter and white matter
- The meninges are the connective tissue membranes that protect and cover the brain and spinal cord.
- The brain is composed of four cavities known as ventricles: the ventricles are filled with cerebral spinal fluid that bathes and cushions the brain. There are three parts of the brain (Fig. 17-1):
  - □ **Cerebrum** is the largest portion of the brain; it composes about two thirds of the brain mass. It is divided into two hemispheres.

- The cerebral cortex is the outer covering of the cerebrum; center for humans highest level of functioning; it is divided into four lobes of the brain.
  - Frontal lobe is located in the front part of the brain; main functions are to perform high-level cognitive functions such as reasoning, abstraction, and concentration. Provides for storage of information. Controls voluntary eye movement. Broca's area is located here and is critical for motor control of speech.
  - Parietal lobe is located in the middle part of the brain: its main function is to integrate sensory information.
  - Temporal lobe is located below the frontal and parietal lobe. The main functions are sense of smell and sound, processing complex stimuli. Wernicke's area is located here and is critical for language comprehension.
  - Occipital lobe is located in the posterior lower aspect of the brain; the main function is to interpret visual stimuli and sense of light.

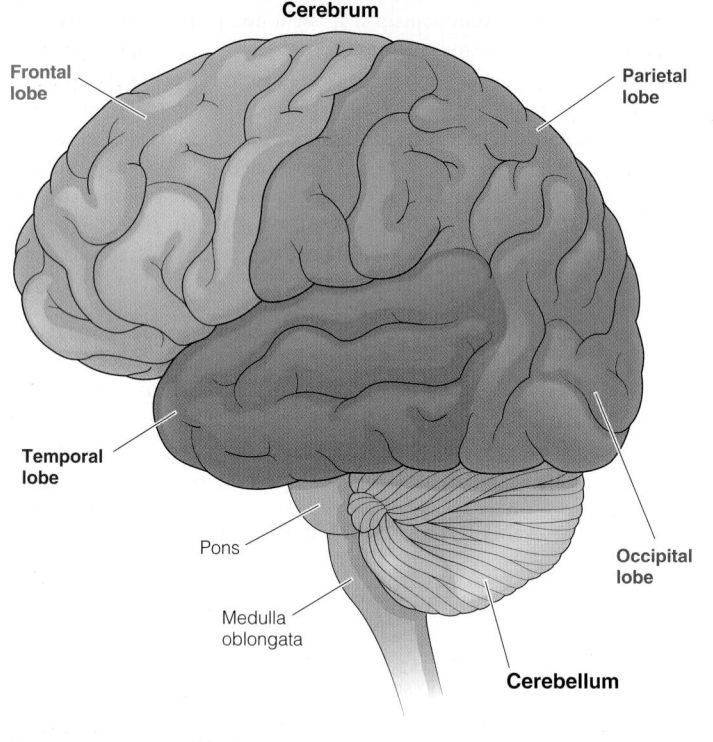

Cerebrum

Frontal
lobe

Parietal
lobe

**Temporal
lobe**

Pons

Occipital
lobe

Medulla
oblongata

Cerebellum

Fig. 17-1. Major areas of the brain.

□ **Cerebellum** is located in the back of the brain. It has the following functions:
- Links sensory input with motion
- Responsible for coordination of movement, speech, and senses

- If cerebellum is damaged, a person experiences problems with balance and coordination (University of Minnesota Ataxia Center, 2014).

□ **Brainstem** is located in the posterior part of the brain; connects the cerebrum to the spinal cord. It has the following functions:
- Central core of the brain
- Controls the involuntary behaviors such as breathing, heart rate, coughing
- Transmits impulses from spinal cord to brain
- The brainstem includes three vital parts:
  - Medulla oblongata transmits information for the coordination of head and eye movement, and also contains the centers for cardiac, vasomotor, and respiratory systems.
  - Pons relays messages between the cortex and the cerebellum; contains the pneumotaxic center that controls respiratory function.
  - Midbrain serves as the center for the cerebral hemispheres and the lower brain and as the center for auditory and visual reflexes.

Pathways of Central Nervous System

There are two pathways of the CNS:
- Sensory pathways allow sensory data to become conscious perceptions.
- Motor pathways transmit impulses from the brain to the muscles.

These pathways receive sensory information and control motor function. The fibers cross over; therefore, the left cerebral cortex receives information and controls motor function to the right side of the body, and vice versa.

Peripheral Nervous System

The peripheral nervous system (PNS) is made up of cranial nerves, spinal cord and nerves, and the autonomic nervous system.

Cranial Nerves

- Cranial nerves are nerves that emerge directly from the brain.
- There are traditionally 12 pairs of cranial nerves (Table 17-1).
- Only the first and the second pairs emerge from the cerebrum.
- The remaining 10 pairs emerge from the brainstem (Fig. 17-2).

Spinal Cord and Nerves

- The spinal cord is part of the central nervous system; it is the primary connection between the brain and the body; protected by vertebral column.

- The spinal cord measures approximately 45 cm long.
- Surrounded by cerebral spinal fluid that cushion the vertebrae
- The term *spinal nerve* generally refers to a mixed spinal nerve, which carries motor, sensory, and autonomic signals between the spinal cord and the body.
- Humans have 31 left-right pairs of spinal nerves, each roughly corresponding to a segment of the vertebral column (Fig. 17-3):
  - □ Eight cervical spinal nerve pairs (C1-C8)
  - □ Twelve thoracic pairs (T1-T12)

TABLE 17-1 Name, Number, and Function of Cranial Nerves

Name	Number	Function
Olfactory	CN I	Sensory: Smell
Optic	CN II	Sensory: Sight
Oculomotor	CN III	Motor: Opening eyelid; moving eye superiorly, medially, and diagonally; constricting pupils
Trochlear	CN IV	Motor: Moving eye down and laterally
Trigeminal	CN V	Motor: Chewing and jaw opening and clenching Sensory: Conveying sensory data from eyes (cornea), nose, mouth, teeth, jaw, forehead, scalp, and facial skin
Abducens	CN VI	Motor: Moving eye laterally
Facial	CN VII	Motor: Closing eyes, closing mouth, moving lips and other muscles of facial expression, salivation and lacrimation (secreting saliva and tears) Sensory: Tasting on anterior tongue
Acoustic	CN VIII	Sensory: Hearing, equilibrium
Glossopharyngeal	CN IX	Motor: Swallowing, gag sensation, secretion of saliva Sensory: Tasting on posterior tongue
Vagus	CN X	Motor: Palate, pharynx, larynx (speaking and swallowing) Sensory: Sensations in pharynx and larynx Sensorimotor: Cardiovascular, respiratory, and digestive systems
Spinal accessory	CN XI	Motor: Contracting muscles of neck and shoulders
Hypoglossal	CN XII	Motor: Tongue movement, articulating with tongue, swallowing

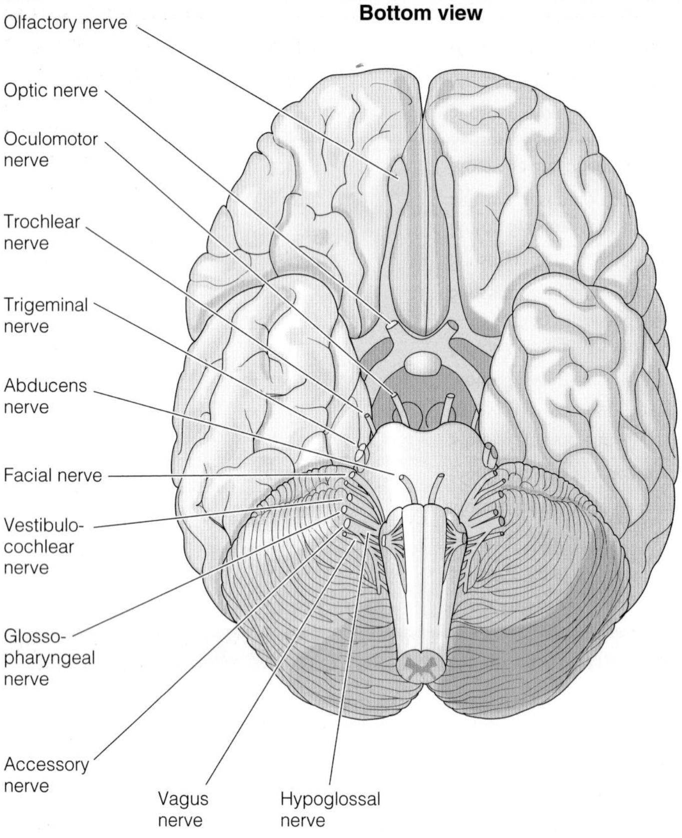

Bottom view

Olfactory nerve

Optic nerve

Oculomotor nerve

Trochlear nerve

Trigeminal nerve

Abducens nerve

Facial nerve

Vestibulo-cochlear nerve

Glosso-pharyngeal nerve

Accessory nerve

Vagus nerve

Hypoglossal nerve

Fig. 17-2. Bottom view of the cranial nerves.

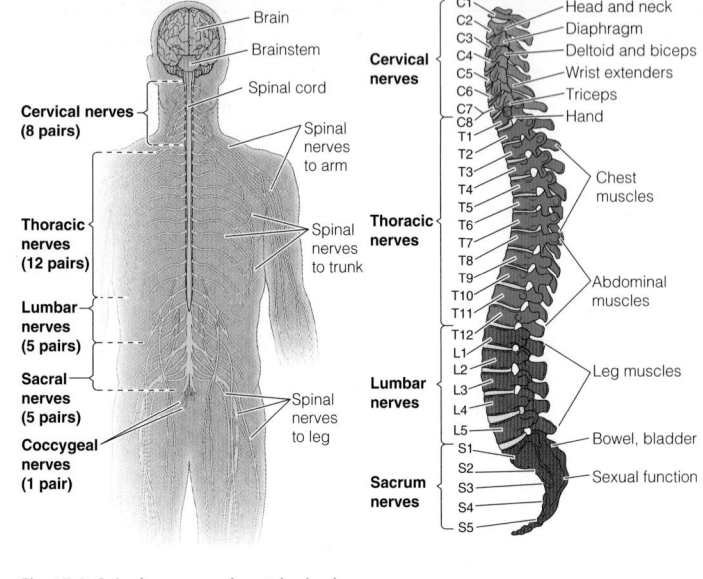

Brain

Brainstem

Spinal cord

Cervical nerves (8 pairs)

Spinal nerves to arm

Thoracic nerves (12 pairs)

Lumbar nerves (5 pairs)

Sacral nerves (5 pairs)

Coccygeal nerves (1 pair)

Spinal nerves to trunk

Spinal nerves to leg

C1
C2
C3
C4
C5
C6
C7
C8

T1
T2
T3
T4
T5
T6
T7
T8
T9
T10
T11
T12

L1
L2
L3
L4
L5

S1
S2
S3
S4
S5

Cervical nerves

Thoracic nerves

Lumbar nerves

Sacrum nerves

Head and neck

Diaphragm

Deltoid and biceps

Wrist extenders

Triceps

Hand

Chest muscles

Abdominal muscles

Leg muscles

Bowel, bladder

Sexual function

Fig. 17-3. Spinal nerves and vertebral column.

☐ Five lumbar pairs (L1-L5)
☐ Five sacral pairs (S1-S5)
☐ One coccygeal pair

Autonomic Nervous System

■ It is composed of two divisions:
☐ The sympathetic nervous system controls the excitatory response, "fight or flight."
☐ The parasympathetic system controls visceral functions, "rest-and-digest."

- The autonomic nervous system is the part of the nervous system that controls involuntary actions, such as the beating of your heart and the widening or narrowing of your blood vessels. Functions are to maintain and restore internal homeostasis.
  - ☐ Controls activities of smooth muscles
  - ☐ Controls activities of the glands of internal organs and blood vessels
  - ☐ Returns sensory information to the brain

DIAGNOSTICS

Diagnostic tests for the neurological system are numerous and complex. The major diagnostics will be mentioned here.

- **Computed tomography (CT scan):** structural imaging study; it is used to diagnose cerebral hemorrhage, tumors, and inflammatory disorders
- **Electroencephalogram (EEG):** sensors are attached to the head to measure electrical activity of the brain; used to diagnose seizure activity and neurological disorders
- **Lumbar puncture:** insertion of a needle into the subarachnoid space of the vertebrae to withdraw cerebrospinal fluid for analysis, administer medications, or measure pressure of cerebrospinal fluid
- **Magnetic resonance imaging (MRI):** structural imaging study, creates a clearer picture of the tissue; used for diagnosing neurological diseases, spinal cord injury, and cerebral infarction
- **Positron-emission tomography (PET scan):** a computer-based nuclear medicine imaging study to evaluate the brain's function by evaluating metabolism, blood flow, oxygen use, glucose metabolism, and chemical processes within the brain; a dye is injected with radioactive tracers; useful for early detection of dementias, Parkinson's disease, and amyotrophic lateral sclerosis
- **Cerebral angiography:** dye is injected in the femoral arteries to assess cerebral circulation; used to detect stenosis, occlusions, or aneurysms.

HEALTH HISTORY

SENC Patient-Centered Care Assessment of the patient should include family members or other identified support or significant others who may provide additional information or be involved in the plan of care of the patient (American Association of Neurologic Nurses, 2009).

Review of Systems

A complete review of systems is essential in obtaining a complete neurological assessment and history. Many times you may uncover an important fact that you did not assess or your patient failed to mention in another part of the assessment.

Use the OLDCARTS mnemonic (**O**nset, **L**ocation, **D**uration, **C**haracteristics, **A**ggravating/Alleviating factors, **R**elieving factors, **T**reatment, **S**everity) to identify attributes of a symptom.

TIP Observe the following while obtaining a review of systems:
- Is the patient dressed appropriately?
- What is the patient's affect and mood?
- Is the patient able to communicate with you?
- Are the patient's gait and balance normal?

General Health

- How have you been feeling? Have you had a fever?
  - ☐ **Meningitis** is an inflammation and infection of the meninges caused by a virus, fungus, or bacteria. It is most common in young adults living in the college setting. The swelling associated with meningitis often triggers the "classic" signs and symptoms of this condition, including headache, fever, altered mental status, and a stiff neck (Putz, Hayani, & Zar, 2013).

☐ Observe the patient's affect (mood, emotions, or feelings) and general behavior throughout the assessment.

Family and Social History

■ Tell me about any medical or surgical neurological history within your immediate family.
  ☐ Familial history will help to assess stroke, seizures, or neurological genetic conditions.
■ Any recreational drug, alcohol, or tobacco use?
  ☐ Lifestyle risk factors such as recreational drug use, moderate alcohol intake, and smoking increase a patient's risk for stroke and injury.
■ Are you using any over-the-counter medications or herbal remedies?
  ☐ Medications and herbal remedies that affect blood pressure and relieve pain may increase the risk of stroke or have side effects such as dizziness or headache.

Health Promotion
Nutrition

■ Are you on any special diet?
  ☐ High cholesterol increases the risk for stroke by causing plaque buildup in arteries.
■ What did you eat in the past 24 hours?
  ☐ There are some foods and food additives that may cause headaches because they dilate the blood vessels or increase blood flow to the brain. Some of the more common foods and beverages that are considered headache triggers are:
    • Cold foods such as ice cream or ice cold beverages; brain freeze is sometimes called an ice cream headache.
    • Monosodium glutamate (MSG) is a food additive that also enhances flavor; commonly found in Chinese/Asian foods, meat tenderizers, and soy sauce.
    • Red wine or alcohol containing preservatives such as sulfites
    • Deli or processed meats containing preservatives/additives such as nitrites/ nitrates; these foods may also have a high sodium content.
    • Coffee, tea, and beverages containing caffeine
    • Chocolates and aged cheeses containing the amino acid tyramine

Exercise

■ Do you exercise? If so how often and what type?
  ☐ Contact sports can increase risk for traumatic brain injury. Long-term memory and temporary short-term memory loss are proven with concussion and traumatic brain injury from contact sports.

▨ **TIP** The Centers for Disease Control and Prevention (CDC, 2016) created two free online courses, *Heads Up On Concussions*, one for healthcare providers and another for youth and high school sports coaches, parents, and athletes. These courses provide important information on preventing, recognizing, and responding to a concussion. These courses can be found at www.cdc.gov/headsup/resources/index.html.

Sleep and rest patterns

■ How many hours do you sleep per night?
  ☐ Sleep deprivation can reduce blood flow and metabolism in the brain and affect cerebral function. The cognitive functions particularly affected by sleep deprivation are: executive attention, decision making, and higher cognitive abilities (Goel, Rao, Durmer, & Dinges, 2009).
  ☐ Sleep apnea can result in decreased cognitive function from hypoxia.
  ☐ Increased somnolence (drowsiness) may be a symptom of an underlying neurological disorder such as increased intracranial pressure.

Stress

- How do you deal with stress?
  - □ Stress influences the sympathetic nervous system by signaling the adrenal glands to release cortisol and adrenalin; this initiates the "fight or flight" response.
  - □ Symptoms of stress may include: headaches, dizziness, feeling faint, tachycardia, and hyperventilation.

Skin

- Have you had any loss of sensation?
  - □ Loss of sensation may feel like numbness, tingling, or the inability to feel.
    - **Neuropathy** is loss of sensation that may feel like numbness, tingling, or the inability to feel; this is most often felt in the extremities.
    - **Neuropathies** occur when nerves of the peripheral nervous system are damaged, caused by peripheral vascular disease, tissue ischemia, and diabetes. Symptoms may include tingling, numbness, a burning sensation, pain, or muscle weakness.
    - **Transient ischemic attack (TIA),** is temporary loss of blood flow to the brain; may last only a few minutes. The patient may experience the following symptoms: loss of sensation, numbness, difficulty speaking, double vision, dysphagia, dizziness, and motor or sensory deficits.
- Have you had a rash?
  - □ A deep red or pink-colored rash that does not fade when pressure is applied could indicate meningitis (Fig. 17-4).

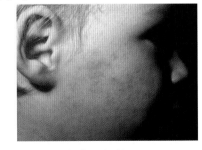

Fig. 17-4. Rash of meningitis.

Head, Ears, Eyes, Nose, Throat

- Have you had any change in your senses (vision, smell, hearing, taste, touch)?
  - □ Any changes in senses could indicate cranial nerve damage.
- Have you had headaches? If so, how often?
  - □ Headaches, specifically pressure headaches, could indicate intracranial bleeding or disease pathology (Table 17-2).
- Do you get dizzy or experience vertigo? If so, what were you doing when you felt dizzy? How long did it last?
  - □ Dizziness is feeling lightheaded, faint, and weak.
  - □ Vertigo feels like the area around the individual is spinning or moving.
- Have you ever had a seizure?
  - □ A seizure is a symptom of a medical or neurological disorder; abnormal electrical activity in the brain produces abnormal body movements such as mild to severe twitching, jerking of the muscles, changes in level of consciousness, and rigidity of the body.
- Have you had any difficulty talking or any changes in your speech?
  - □ **Dysphasia** denotes a *partial* impairment of language and speech impacting the ability to communicate (Worral et al., 2016); the damage is less severe and occurs in the left side of the brain that contains the language center.
  - □ **Aphasia** is a complete impairment of comprehension and expression in the verbal, written, and signed modalities (Worrall, 2016). The damage is more severe and occurs in the left side of the brain that contains the language center. Patients who experience damage to the right side of the brain may have additional difficulties beyond speech and language issues (American Speech-Language Hearing Association, 2015). Patients with aphasia may have difficulty with:
    - speech
    - understanding language
    - reading and writing.

TABLE 17-2 Types of Headaches

Type of Headache	Definition	Cause
Migraine	Throbbing or pulsing head pain often confined to one side of the head with sensory sensitivity, such as light, sound, and movement; may occur with or without an aura.	Evidence shows this may be due to dysfunction in brainstem or familial genetics (Fishman et al., 2010)
Tension	Episodic generalized pain. Feels like pressure around the circumference of the head with absence of nausea, vomiting, photophobia. Predisposing factors are stress, eye strain, and poor posture.	Not understood; evidence supports stress-related (Fishman et al., 2010)
Cluster	Unilateral one sided burning, stabbing, piercing pain. May have swelling or redness around affected eye; occurs the same time daily; occurs in males 3:1 over females	Cause is unknown; may be related to a disorder or dysfunction of posterior hypothalamus, or trigeminal nerve
Chronic Daily	Headache is accompanied by neck stiffness and muscle contraction. Most severe upon awakening; exacerbated by activity and exertion	Most common cause is overuse of analgesic medications
Increased or Decreased Cerebral Spinal Fluid Headache	Pressure, generalized headache, presents on waking and exhibits some relief over the day; visual disturbances present	Benign lesion Increased CSF can cause increased ICP Decreased can be post lumbar puncture, vigorous Valsalva such as lifting, straining, and coughing

Adapted from Wright, K. (2015). *Guide to headaches and migraines: Symptoms; causes; treatment; prevention.* Glasgow, Scotland: Geddes and Grosset; and Fishman, S., Ballantyne, J., Rathmell, J. P., Bonica, J. J., & Ovid. (2010). *Bonica's management of pain* (4th ed.). Baltimore, MD: Lippincott, Williams & Wilkins.

- [ ] **Receptive aphasia** is damage to Wernicke's area of the brain; unable to understand language in written or spoken form (i.e., you do not understand someone speaking or writing in a foreign language).
- [ ] **Expressive aphasia** is caused by damage to the Broca's area; unable to communicate language in written or spoken form; however, patient knows what he or she wants to say. Different types of aphasia and speech deficits are associated with transient ischemic attack or stroke (Table 17-3).

■ Have you had any difficulty with swallowing (dysphagia)?
- [ ] **Dysphagia** is difficulty swallowing food or liquids.

SENC Safety Alert Patients with dysphagia have increased risk for aspirating food or liquids as the contents pass through the trachea and into the lung. These individuals are at high risk for aspiration pneumonia. Patients should always be instructed to eat slowly and be in an upright position when eating and drinking. Patients who have difficulty swallowing are put on aspiration precautions. A speech therapist assesses patients for dysphagia and makes recommendations for the type of diet the patient should eat to prevent aspiration.

TABLE 17-3 Aphasia and Speech Deficits

Type of Aphasia/Speech Deficits	Definition	Indication
Visual-Receptive	Disorder of central language processing; inability to recognize spoken words	Injury to parietal-occipital area
Expressive Aphasia	Inability to express words; nonverbal	Injury to inferior frontal brain area
Global Aphasia	Impaired comprehension and expression of speech	Commonly seen with left; middle, cerebral artery infarction
Apraxia	Partial or complete inability to articulate using the tongue, lips, and lower jaw	Lesion in Broca's area
Dysphonia	Difficulty in speaking; hoarseness or whisper	Paralysis of soft palate
Dysarthria	Inability to articulate	Motor deficit of tongue or speech muscles

Respiratory

■ Have you had any difficulty with breathing (dyspnea)?
  □ **Hypoxia,** defined as lack of oxygen supply to the brain, can result in changes to mental status.

Cardiovascular

■ Do you have any cardiovascular problems?
  □ Cardiovascular disease increases the risk for stroke, by contributing to plaque buildup in the arteries and high blood pressure.
■ Cerebral vascular accident (CVA), also known as a "stroke," occurs for two reasons:
  □ Ischemic stroke is an occlusion of oxygenated blood flow to the brain. The leading cause is a blood clot impairing or occluding an artery in the brain.
  □ Hemorrhagic stroke is leaking of blood from an artery in the brain.

CULTURAL CONSIDERATIONS

• Racial disparities in stroke death continue to widen in the United States where African Americans are twice as likely to die from stroke as Caucasians, and their rate of first strokes is double that of Caucasians.

• Hispanic populations in the United States have a different occurrence of stroke risk factors than their Caucasian counterparts. Hispanics are more likely to suffer a stroke at a younger age (average age of 67) compared to 80 for non-Hispanic Caucasians. Stroke and heart disease account for one in four deaths among Hispanic men and one in three deaths among Hispanic women (American Stroke Association, 2015a).

■ Do you have an irregular heartbeat?
  □ **Atrial fibrillation** increases the risk for stroke by contributing to formation of blood clots in the atrium of the heart. This clot can dislodge and become entrapped in cerebral arteries.
■ Do your hands become numb or change color in response to cold?
  □ **Paresthesia** is numbness or tingling of the extremities related to decreased circulation. Chronic paresthesia is often a symptom of an underlying neurological disease or traumatic nerve damage, disorders affecting the central nervous system, or a tumor or vascular lesion causing pressure on the brain or spinal cord (National Institute of Neurological Disorders and Stroke, 2014).

Gastrointestinal

- Do you have any nausea or vomiting?
  - ☐ Nausea and projectile vomiting (forcible ejection of stomach contents through the mouth) can indicate increased intracranial pressure.
- Have you had any loss of bowel or bladder function?
  - ☐ Bowel or bladder impairment/incontinence may indicate spinal cord damage, or a compressed nerve.

Musculoskeletal

- Do you have any loss of sensation, numbness, or muscle weakness? Do you have any difficulty walking?
  - ☐ Can be associated with many neurological disorders
  - ☐ **Myasthenia** is lack of muscle strength or muscle tone.
  - ☐ **Myasthenia gravis** is a chronic autoimmune neuromuscular disorder that causes weakness of the voluntary muscle groups. Symptoms include chronic muscle fatigue, dysphagia, drooping eyelid, and slurred speech (Myasthenia Gravis Foundation of America, 2010).
  - ☐ **Multiple sclerosis (MS)** is an inflammatory nervous system disease; the myelin of the nerve cells of the brain and spinal cord are damaged causing decreased nerve transmission and communication between the brain and body; a patient may not be able to walk depending on the amount of damage to the nerves.

CULTURAL CONSIDERATIONS Multiple sclerosis occurs in most ethnic groups, including African Americans, Asians, and Hispanics/Latinos, but is more common in Caucasians of northern European ancestry (National Multiple Sclerosis Society, 2015).

Endocrine

- Do you have diabetes or thyroid disease?
  - ☐ Diabetes can increase the chance of peripheral neuropathies. Long-term hyperglycemia contributes to nerve damage and loss of sensation in peripheral nerves.
  - ☐ Low levels of the thyroid hormone may contribute to symptoms of fatigue, dizziness, lethargy, and a flat affect.

Hematological

- Do you have any blood disorders?
  - ☐ Coagulation disorders can cause the blood to thicken, and this increases the risk for blood clots; this can increase the risk for stroke.

CULTURAL CONSIDERATIONS The uniqueness and individuality of each person needs to be considered when performing a neurological assessment. Ethnicity, gender, employment, and area of residence needs to be noted.

- Some neurological disorders are more common in one ethnicity than another.
- African-Americans are more impacted by stroke than any other racial groups within the American population. African-Americans are twice as likely to die from stroke as Caucasians, and their rate of first strokes is almost double that of Caucasians.
- Hispanics are more likely to suffer a stroke at a younger age—average age of 67—compared to 80 for non-Hispanic Caucasians.
- American Indians and Alaska Natives are 2.4 times more likely to have a stroke than their Caucasian counterparts; stroke is the sixth leading cause of death among this population.
- Asian-Americans are less likely to die from a stroke. They tend to have lower rates of being overweight or obese and lower rates of high blood pressure than all other racial groups.
- Native Hawaiians and Pacific Islanders have been shown to have higher prevalence of major stroke risk factors—specifically high blood pressure, diabetes, and obesity. (National Stroke Association, 2017)

PREPARATION FOR ASSESSMENT

Equipment Needed
- Coffee beans
- Cotton wisp
- Flashlight
- Gloves
- Object with soft and sharp areas
- Ophthalmoscope
- Other scents
- Pupil scale chart
- Reflex hammer
- Snellen chart
- Teaspoon
- Tongue blade
- Tuning fork
- Water

Sequence of Assessment
1. Inspection/observation
2. Neurological assessments (major categories):
   - ☐ Level of consciousness and mental status
   - ☐ Cranial nerve function
   - ☐ Motor system
   - ☐ Sensory system
   - ☐ Reflexes

Preliminary Steps
- The patient should be in an examination gown in order to complete the full assessment.
- If the patient wears eyeglass or hearing aids, have the patient keep them on during the assessment.
- A comatose patient cannot cooperate with the assessment. Your assessment will rely on observation and reflex responses.
- Perform hand hygiene.

FOCUSED ASSESSMENT

TECHNIQUE 17-1: Assessing Level of Consciousness and Mental Status

Purpose: To assess level of consciousness

ASSESSMENT STEPS
1. Assess the patient's ability to arouse and respond to questions.
2. Assess the patient's orientation to person, place, time, and situation.
   TIP Always assess orientation to facts that can be confirmed through secondary resources.
3. Ask the patient the following questions:
   - ☐ What is your name? (orientation to person)
   - ☐ Where are you now? What city are you in? (orientation to place)

☐ What year is it? What season is it? What month is it? What day of the week is it? (orientation to time)

☐ What brings you here to see the healthcare provider? (orientation to situation)

4. Document your findings.

NORMAL FINDINGS

■ Alert and oriented to person, place, time, and situation

ABNORMAL FINDINGS

■ May indicate brain lesion, stroke, dementia, psychological problem, or medication side effect

■ Disorientation or confusion

■ Lethargic: difficulty maintaining mentation or mentation is sluggish; patient is arousable and able to answer questions.

■ Obtunded (decreased alertness): able to only keep the patient awake by verbal or tactile stimuli; patient is confused when awake

■ Stupor: patient is unresponsive to verbal stimuli with decreased responsiveness to painful stimuli; nonverbal if he/she opens eyes

■ Comatose (deep unconsciousness): lack of response to any stimuli

☐ May be a medical emergency related to a serious injury, pathological disease, or illness

TIP The Mini-Mental State Examination is a valuable tool to assess cognitive impairment (Table 17-4).

TABLE 17-4 Sample Items from the Mini-Mental State Examination (MMSE)

Orientation to Time	What is the date?
Registration	Listen carefully. I am going to say three words. You say them back after I stop. Ready? Here they are: *apple* (pause) *penny* (pause) *table* (pause) Now repeat those words back to me. (Repeat up to five times, but score only the first trial.)
Naming	What is this? (Point to a pencil or pen.)
Reading	Please read this and do what it says. (Show examinee the stimulus form.) Close your eyes.

Reproduced by special permission of the Publisher, Psychological Assessment Resources, Inc., 16204 North Florida Avenue, Lutz, Florida 33549, from the Mini-Mental State Examination, by Marshal Folstein and Susan Folstein, Copyright 1975, 1998, 2001 by Mini Mental LLC, Inc. Published 2001 by the Psychological Assessment Resources, Inc. Further reproduction is prohibited without permission of PAR, Inc. the MMSE can be purchased from the PAR, Inc. by calling (813) 968-3003.

TABLE 17-5 Glasgow Coma Scale

Observation	Response Elicited	Score
Eye response	Opens spontaneously	4
	Opens to verbal command	3
	Opens to pain	2
	No response	1
Motor response	Reacts to verbal command	6
	Identifies localized pain	5
	Flexes and withdraws from pain	4
	Assumes flexor posture	3
	Assumes extensor posture	2
	No response	1
Verbal response	Is oriented and converses	5
	Is disoriented but converses	4
	Uses inappropriate words	3
	Makes incomprehensible sounds	2
	No response	1

SENC Evidence-Based Practice The Glasgow Coma Scale (GCS) (Table 17-5) is an evidence-based assessment of mental status. This scale is widely used and recognized among all interdisciplinary professionals. The scale is based on a score of 3–15. This is a more objective way to assess the patient's level of consciousness. The scale evaluates eye response, motor response, and verbal response and assesses by checking, observing, and stimulating. A score of 15 is the highest score indicating the patient is awake, alert, and oriented. Three, the lowest score, indicates the person is not responding with a poor prognosis. Instructions and video for the new structured responses for the GCS can be accessed at www.glasgowcomascale.org/.

TECHNIQUE 17-2: Assessing Cranial Nerve Function

Purpose: To assess the function of the 12 pairs of cranial nerves
■ **TIP** Each cranial nerve has a right and left side, and each patient's side is assessed separately. Nurses should always compare the responses of each side.

Technique 17-2A: Assessing Sense of Smell (CN I)
Purpose: To assess the sense of smell
Equipment: Coffee beans, other available scents
■ **TIP** Make sure the patient's nostrils are patent and not clogged or congested.

ASSESSMENT STEPS
1. Explain the technique to the patient.
2. Ask the patient to close her or his eyes and occlude the right nostril (Fig. 17-5).
3. Hold one of the available scents under the unoccluded left nostril, and ask the patient to sniff the scent.
4. Ask the patient to identify the scent.
5. Ask the patient to occlude the left nostril.
6. Hold a different available scent under the unoccluded right nostril.
7. Ask the patient to identify the scent.
8. Document your findings.

NORMAL FINDINGS
■ Able to state the correct scent on each side

ABNORMAL FINDINGS
■ **Anosmia:** inability to smell or identify the correct scent, indicating loss of function to olfactory nerve

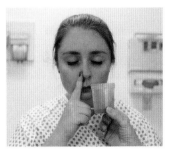
Fig. 17-5. Occluding right nostril.

Technique 17-2B: **Assessing for Visual Acuity (CN II)**
See Chapter 11, Technique 11-2 for assessment of visual acuity.

Technique 17-2C: **Testing for Ocular Motility: Six Cardinal Positions of Gaze (CN III, CN IV, CN VI)**
See Chapter 11, Technique 11-6 for assessment of ocular motility.

Technique 17-2D: **Inspecting Pupil Size and Consensual Pupil Response (CN II and CN III)**
See Chapter 11, Technique 11-8 for inspection of pupil size and consensual pupil response.

Technique 17-2E: **Assessing Sensation (CN V)**
Purpose: To assess sensation of the skin
Equipment: Cotton wisp, object with sharp and dull side
ASSESSMENT STEPS

1. Explain the technique to the patient.
2. Tell the patient that every time he or she feels the light wisp of cotton to say "now."
3. Ask the patient to close his or her eyes.
4. Standing in front of the patient, touch the patient lightly with the wisp of cotton on the following areas of the face (Fig. 17-6):
   ☐ Forehead
   ☐ Right cheek
   ☐ Left cheek
   ☐ Jaw

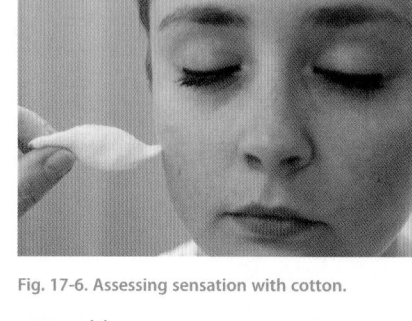
Fig. 17-6. Assessing sensation with cotton.

5. Now, touch the patient lightly with the wisp of cotton on the following areas of the upper and lower extremities:
   ☐ Upper arm bilaterally
   ☐ Forearm bilaterally
   ☐ Thigh bilaterally
   ☐ Lower shin bilaterally
6. Ask the patient to open his or her eyes.
7. Explain the next assessment for identifying sharp and dull sensations.
8. Take an object with sharp and dull sides. Demonstrate on the patient's skin what "sharp and dull" will feel like.
9. Advise the patient to close his or her eyes.
10. Using the object and following steps 4 and 5, alternate patterns between sharp (Fig. 17-7A) and dull (Fig. 17-7B).
11. Document the findings.

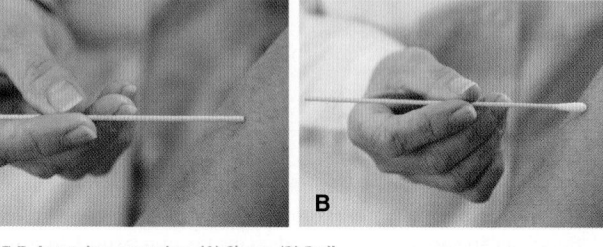
Fig. 17-7. Assessing sensation. (A) Sharp. (B) Dull.

■ Light, sharp, and dull sensations are felt at all sites.

ABNORMAL FINDINGS

■ Light, sharp, or dull sensations are not felt at a site; this may indicate a peripheral nerve disorder.

Technique 17-2F: **Assessing Jaw Movement (CN V)**

Purpose: To assess the motor portion of CN V

ASSESSMENT STEPS

1. Explain the technique to the patient.

2. Advise the patient to open his or her eyes.

3. Ask the patient clench his or her teeth (to test motor component).

4. Palpate the temporal and masseter muscles (Fig. 17-8), just above the mandibular angle; ask the patient to open and close his or her jaw and move the jaw side to side.

5. Document your findings.

NORMAL FINDINGS

■ Patient can clench teeth tightly.

■ Masseter muscles bulge when teeth are clenched.

■ On palpation, both masseter muscles feel equal in size and strength.

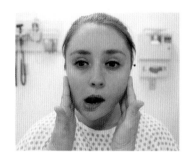

Fig. 17-8. Assessing jaw movement.

ABNORMAL FINDINGS

■ Temporomandibular disorders may cause muscle weakness; the patient cannot clench jaw and move jaw side to side.

■ Unilateral jaw muscle weakness may indicate a lesion impinging on CN V.

■ Trigeminal neuralgia is facial pain caused by inflammation or compression of CN V.

Technique 17-2G: **Assessing Cranial Nerve VII (Facial Nerve)**

Purpose: To assess facial movements

ASSESSMENT STEPS

1. Explain the technique to the patient.

2. Stand in front of the patient.

3. Assess the patient's ability to perform the following facial movements. Ask the patient to:

    □ smile

    □ frown

    □ puff out his or her cheeks

    □ close eyes and try to open eyes against resistance (Fig. 17-9).

4. Document your findings.

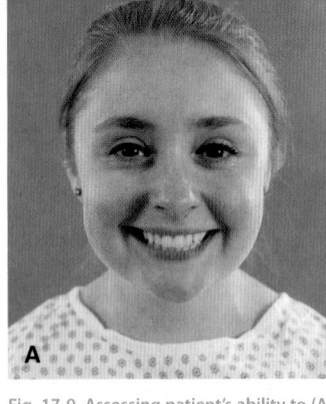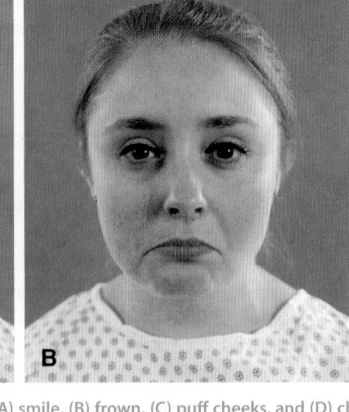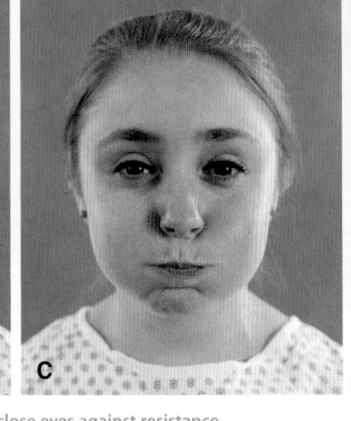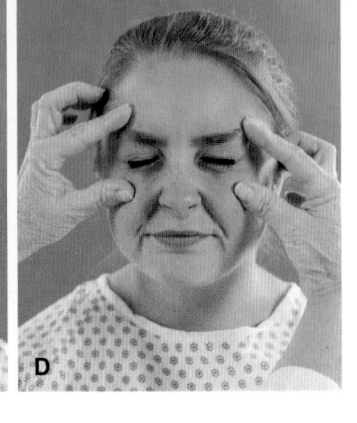

Fig. 17-9. Assessing patient's ability to (A) smile, (B) frown, (C) puff cheeks, and (D) close eyes against resistance.

NORMAL FINDINGS
- Patient is able to smile, frown, and puff out cheeks.
- Muscles are symmetrical.
- Eyes do not open against resistance.

ABNORMAL FINDINGS
- Asymmetrical muscles while smiling, frowning, or puffing out cheeks
  □ Drooping of one side of face and/or mouth can indicate stroke.
  □ Bell's palsy is inflammation of the facial nerve of unknown cause resulting in muscle weakness or paralysis on one side of the face.
- Eyes open against resistance.

Technique 17-2H: **Conducting the Whispered Voice Test (CN VIII)**
See Chapter 10, Technique 10-4 for conducting the whispered voice test.

Technique 17-2I: **Assessing Cranial Nerve IX (Glossopharyngeal Nerve) and Cranial Nerve X (Vagus Nerve)**
Purpose: To assess pharyngeal sensation and function, and the presence or absence of a gag reflex
Equipment: Gloves, tongue blade, teaspoon, water

1. Explain the technique to the patient.
2. Put on gloves.
3. Ask the patient to open his or her mouth.
4. Gently touch the posterior aspect of tongue or pharynx with the tip of the tongue blade to initiate a gag reflex (Fig. 17-10A).
5. If gag reflex is absent, assess for pharyngeal sensation by asking the patient to close the eyes.
6. Instruct the patient to lift the right or left hand to the side at which the patient feels the tip of the tongue blade. If the tip is felt on the correct side, this indicates positive pharyngeal sensation (Fig. 17-10B).
7. Touch the tongue blade to the right side of the pharynx.
8. Remind the patient to lift the arm on the side where the patient is feeling the sensation.
9. Touch the tongue blade to the left side of the pharynx.
10. Remind the patient to lift the arm on the side he or she is feeling the sensation.
11. Assess vocal quality by asking the patient to say "ah, ah, ah."
12. Assess the bilateral symmetry of the elevation of the soft palate and central location of uvula.
13. Ask patient to swallow a teaspoon of water.
14. Assess the movement of the throat.
15. Document your findings.

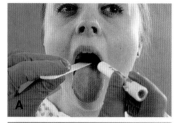

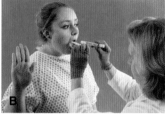

Fig. 17-10. (A) Assessing gag reflex. (B) Pharyngeal sensation.

NORMAL FINDINGS
- Positive gag reflex
- Positive pharyngeal sensation bilaterally
- Clear voice
- Ability to swallow

ABNORMAL FINDINGS
- Absent gag reflex
- Absent or unilateral pharyngeal sensation may indicate dysphagia.
- Difficulty with swallowing indicates dysphagia.
- Coarse raspy voice indicates poor pharyngeal function.

TIP Patients who have dysphagia will need to be referred for further diagnostic evaluation. Usually, a referral is made to the speech therapist for a swallow study.

Technique 17-2J: **Assessing Cranial Nerve XI (Spinal Accessory Muscle)**

Purpose: To assess the strength of the sternocleidomastoid and trapezius muscles

ASSESSMENT STEPS

1. Explain the technique to the patient.
2. Have the patient sit on the end of the bed or examining table.
3. Stand in front of the patient.
4. Ask the patient to shrug shoulders against resistance as the examiner pushes down on shoulders assessing the strength of both shoulders (Fig. 17-11A).
5. Ask the patient to turn his or her head to the right side against the resistance of your hand; assess the strength of the right side of the face (Fig. 17-11B).
6. Ask the patient to turn his or her head to the left side against the resistance of your hand; assess the strength of the left side of the face.
7. Document your findings.

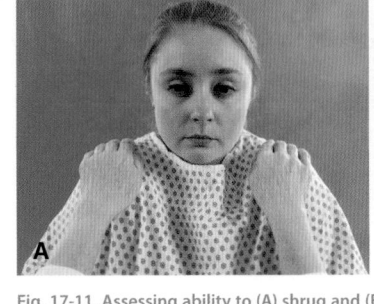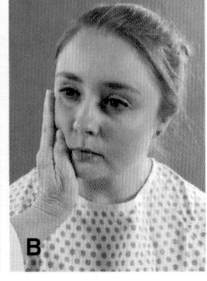

Fig. 17-11. Assessing ability to (A) shrug and (B) turn head against resistance.

NORMAL FINDINGS

■ Ability to shrug both shoulders against resistance using equal strength on both sides.
■ Turn head both ways against resistance with equal strength on each side.

ABNORMAL FINDINGS

■ Inability to shrug shoulders or turn head against resistance may indicate paralysis or lesion to the accessory nerve (Hickey, 2014).

Technique 17-2K: **Assessing Cranial Nerve XII (Hypoglossal Nerve)**

Purpose: To assess movement of tongue

ASSESSMENT STEPS

1. Explain the technique to the patient.
2. Ask the patient to stick out tongue and inspect the tongue for:
   □ symmetry
   □ alignment.
3. Ask the patient to move the tongue from side to side.
4. Document your findings.

NORMAL FINDINGS

■ Tongue symmetrical and midline without tremor.
■ Tongue moves smoothly from side to side.

ABNORMAL FINDINGS

■ Tongue is not midline or has tremors; this can indicate paralysis or stroke, or a lesion of cranial nerve XII (Hickey, 2014).

TECHNIQUE 17-3: **Assessing the Motor System**

Purpose: To assess cerebellar function, specifically muscle strength, tone, movement, and symmetry of muscles

Assessing the motor system requires four areas of the nervous system to work together:

1. Cerebellar system: posture and rhythmic movement

2. Motor system: muscle strength

3. Sensory system: position sense and vibrations

4. Vestibular system: balance and coordination

Technique 17-3A: **Assessing Muscle Strength of the Upper and Lower Extremities**

See Chapter 16, Technique 16-5 and Technique 16-7 for in-depth assessment of muscle strength of the upper and lower extremities.

Purpose: To assess muscle strength in the upper and lower extremities

ASSESSMENT STEPS

1. Explain the technique to the patient. You will ask the patient to perform specific motions independently first and then against resistance.

2. Ask the patient to perform ROM activities of the right and left upper extremities, including the shoulder, elbow, wrist, and fingers, with and without resistance.

3. Ask the patient to perform ROM activities of the right and left lower extremities including the hip, knee, ankle, and foot with and without resistance.

4. Document your findings.

NORMAL FINDINGS

■ Muscles will be symmetrical, and muscle tone and resistance will be equal on both sides.

ABNORMAL FINDINGS

■ **Hypotonia:** decreased tone and may be seen in neuromuscular disorders and cerebellar lesions

■ **Flaccidity:** loss of muscle tone

■ **Hypotonia:** decreased muscle tone and strength; may be seen in neuromuscular disorders and with cerebellar lesions.

■ **Hypertonia:** increased muscle tone and may be result of injury to upper motor neurons

■ **Rigidity:** muscles are contracted and tense; associated with Parkinson's Disease and neuromuscular injuries or diseases

■ **Spasticity:** increased motor tone causing stiffness and tight muscles

■ **Hemiparesis:** loss of muscle tone, strength to unilateral side of body; can involve upper extremity, lower extremity, or both; indicative of stroke or neurological injury or disease.

■ **Paraplegic:** absence of movement and sensation in lower extremities, indicative of spinal cord injury/lesion at or below thoracic spine level

■ **Quadriplegic:** absence of movement and sensation in upper and lower extremities, indicative of spinal cord injury/lesion at or below cervical spine 1

- **Decorticate posturing:** consists of internal rotation and adduction of the arms with flexion of the elbows, wrists, and fingers; plantar flexion of the feet with internal rotation of the legs; both legs are stiffly extended; indicates severe brain injury (Fig. 17-12A)
- **Decerebrate posturing:** consists of arms stiffly extended, adducted, and hyperpronated with hyperextension of the legs and plantar flexion of the feet; legs are stiffly extended; indicates more serious damage in midbrain and brainstem (Fig. 17-12B)

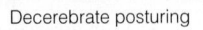
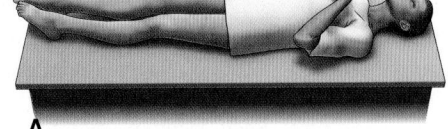
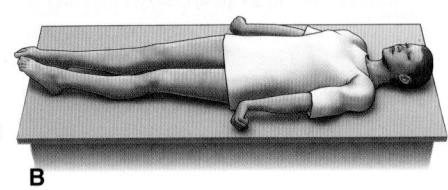

Fig. 17-12. (A) Decorticate and (B) decerebrate posturing.

Technique 17-3B: **Assessing Gait**

Purpose: To assess balance, coordination, muscle strength, and tone

ASSESSMENT STEPS

1. Explain the technique to the patient.
2. Identify a specific distance that you want the patient to walk to in the room.
3. Ask the patient to walk from you first and then back toward you. This allows for both anterior and posterior observation of gait, balance, and posture.
4. Ask the patient walk on his or her toes and return walking toward you on his or her heels; this allows you to assess balance (Figs. 17-13A, 17-13B).
5. Instruct the patient to walk heel-to-toe away from you and back toward you; this is called tandem walking. While tandem walking, assess for muscular weakness (Fig. 17-13C).
6. Ask the patient to hop on the right foot and then alternate to the left foot; this assesses position sense and cerebellar function.
7. Ask the patient to do a shallow knee bend; this assesses muscle weakness.
8. Document your findings.

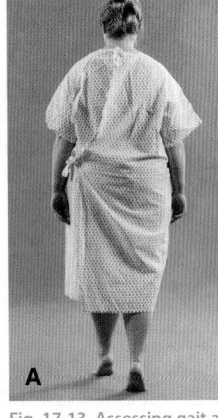
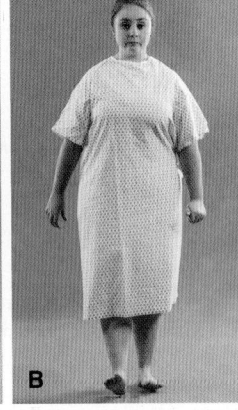
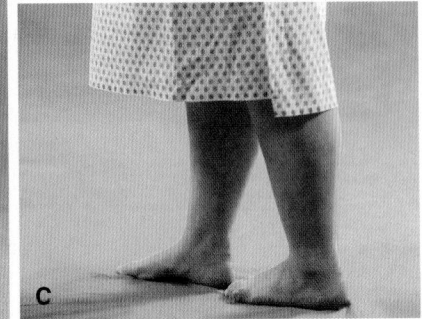

Fig. 17-13. Assessing gait and balance while patient (A) walks on toes, (B) walks on heels, and (C) tandem walks.

- Gaits, hopping, and knee bends are stable, smooth, and coordinated.

ABNORMAL FINDINGS
- Gaits lack stability, smoothness, and coordination.
- Ataxia is defective muscle coordination; may be related to loss of position sense, drugs, alcohol, or cerebellar disease.
- Inability to walk on toes may indicate plantar flexion weakness. Inability to walk on heels may indicate dorsiflexion foot weakness. Inability to walk on both heels and toes may indicate muscular weakness, poor position sense, or vertigo.

Technique 17-3C: **Heel-to-Shin Test**

Purpose: To assess coordination of lower extremity motor movement and position sense

> **SENC Safety Alert** Patient should be in the supine position to prevent a fall.

ASSESSMENT STEPS
1. Explain the technique to the patient.
2. With the patient in the supine position, ask the patient to place the heel of the right leg on the left knee and slowly run it down the shin to the left ankle; assess smoothness and coordination (Fig. 17-14).
3. Repeat step 2 on using the left leg.
4. Have the patient close his or her eyes, and repeat steps 2 and 3; this assesses position sense.
5. Document your findings.

NORMAL FINDINGS
- Movement of leg is smooth and coordinated

ABNORMAL FINDINGS
- Heel does not stay on the shin or moves from side to side while running down the shin may indicate cerebellar disease or loss of motor coordination.

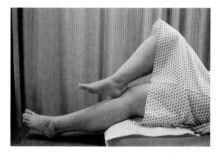

Fig. 17-14. Heel-to-shin test.

Technique 17-3D: **Finger-to-Nose Test**

Purpose: To assess cerebellar function, coordination, and point-to-point movements
Equipment: Pen with cap

ASSESSMENT STEPS
1. Explain the technique to the patient.
2. Stand in front of the patient. Give the pen cap to the patient. Hold the pen about 12 inches away from the patient at eye level and instruct the patient to recap the pen using the right hand; repeat using the left hand. (Fig. 17-15A)
3. Now, hold your index finger in front of the patient at eye level.

4. Ask the patient to touch the tip of your index finger and then touch the tip of the nose with his or her right index finger (Fig. 17-15B).

5. Repeat several times while you are moving your finger a few inches in each direction up, down, right, and left, each time the patient attempts to touch your finger by extending his or her arm.

6. Repeat steps 3 and 4 with the patient's left index finger.

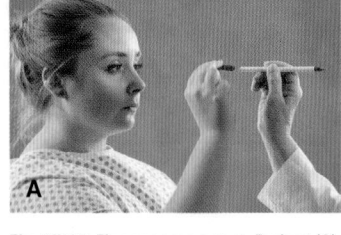 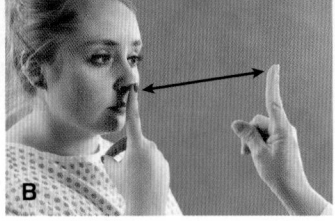 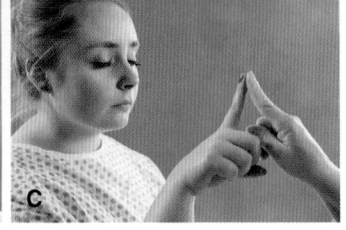

Fig. 17-15. Finger-to-nose test. Patient (A) recapping pen, (B) touching finger to nose, and (C) touching finger to finger with eyes closed.

7. Ask the patient to close his or her eyes (Fig. 17-15C), and using his or her right index finger, have the patient touch your finger several times; repeat using the left index finger with eyes closed.

8. Document your findings.

NORMAL FINDINGS

■ Patient is able to put the cap on the pen accurately and smoothly.
■ Patient touches the nurse's finger and nose accurately and smoothly in all locations.
■ Patient touches the nurse's finger accurately and smoothly in the one location with eyes closed.

ABNORMAL FINDINGS

■ Patient's finger is unsteady and unable to cap the pen or touch the moving target, indicating difficulty with coordination and decreased cerebellar functioning.
■ Patient is unsteady and unable to touch the stationary finger with the eyes closed; may indicate cerebellar disease.
■ **Dysmetria** is the inability to perform point-to-point movements due to over or under projecting the finger to touch an object.

Technique 17-3E: **Assessing Rapid Alternating Movements**

Purpose: To assess coordination of the muscles

ASSESSMENT STEPS

1. Explain and demonstrate the technique to the patient.

2. Upper extremities: ask the patient to place both hands palm down on his or her thighs (Fig. 17-16A).

3. Lift both hands and place both hands palm up on his or her thighs (Fig. 17-16B, Fig. 17-16C).

4. Ask the patient to repeat these alternating movements for 10 seconds.

5. Observe the alternating movements for speed and smoothness.

6. Lower extremities: ask the patient to rapidly pat your hand using the ball of the right foot for 10 seconds (Fig. 17-17); observe speed and smoothness.

7. Repeat step 6 on the left foot.

8. Document the findings.

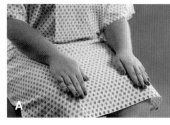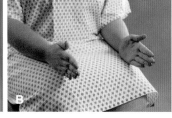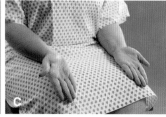

Fig. 17-16. Assessing rapid alternating movements of upper extremities.

NORMAL FINDINGS

■ Coordinated and smooth movement of both hands
■ Coordinated and smooth movement of both feet

ABNORMAL FINDINGS

■ **Dysdiadochokinesis** is uncoordinated, slow, and clumsy movements; may be a sign of cerebellar disease, Parkinson's disease, or multiple sclerosis.

  □ **Parkinson's disease** is a progressive movement disorder caused by decreasing amounts of dopamine being produced in the brain; this causes a person to be unable to control movement normally (Parkinson's Disease Foundation, 2017). Primary motor signs of Parkinson's disease include the following:

  • Tremor of the hands, arms, legs, jaw, and face
  • Bradykinesia or slowness of movement
  • Rigidity or stiffness of the limbs and trunk
  • Postural instability or impaired balance and coordination

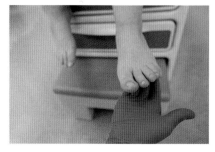

Fig. 17-17. Assessing rapid alternating movements of lower extremities.

Technique 17-3F: **Pronator Drift**

Purpose: To assess motor function and proprioception

This assessment can be performed standing or sitting.

ASSESSMENT STEPS

1. Explain the technique to the patient.
2. Ask the patient to extend both arms out with palms up.
3. Ask the patient to close his or her eyes and observe the patient's arms for change in position for 20 to 30 seconds (Fig. 17-18).
4. Document your findings.

   ▮ **TIP** When the patient closes his or her eyes, proprioception (sense of relative position) alone maintains the position of the arms.

NORMAL FINDINGS

■ **Negative pronator drift:** arms should remain in the extended position without drifting.

ABNORMAL FINDINGS

■ **Positive pronator drift:** an arm does not remain raised, the palm may pronate or drop slightly (Fig. 17-19); may indicate an abnormality in the corticospinal tract, the upper motor neurons in the brain and spinal cord that mediate voluntary muscle movement

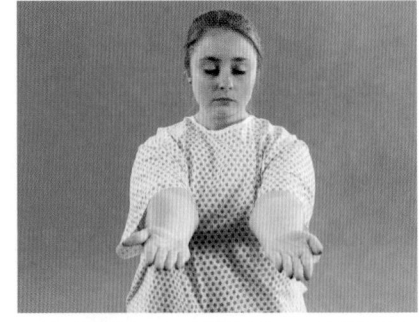

Fig. 17-18. Assessing for pronator drift.

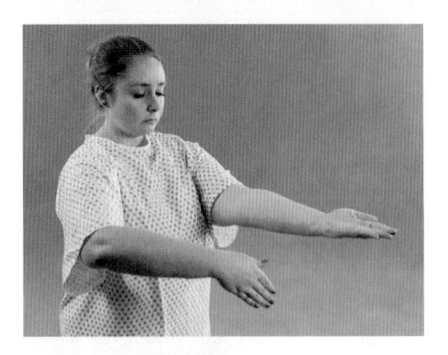

Fig. 17-19. Positive pronator drift.

Technique 17-3G: **Romberg Test**

Purpose: To assess position sense and cerebellar function, balance, and coordination

ASSESSMENT STEPS

1. Explain the technique to the patient.
2. Ask the patient to stand with feet together and arms at sides and look straight ahead for 30 seconds without any support (Fig. 17-20A).
3. Assess for any swaying to either side or loss of balance.
4. Now, with the patient in this position, stand on the side of the patient and extend your hands in the front and back of the patient for patient safety.
5. Ask the patient to close her or his eyes and continue to stand in this position for 30 seconds; observe for swaying and balance (Fig. 17-20B).
6. Document your findings.

   SENC Safety Alert Keep your hands in front and back of the patient in case the patient starts to sway or fall.

NORMAL FINDINGS

■ **Negative Romberg's test:** Maintains position without swaying or loss of balance, with and without opening eyes.

ABNORMAL FINDINGS

■ **Positive Romberg's test:** Swaying or loss of balance with or without eyes open may indicate cerebellar dysfunction, or lesions in the cerebellum or spinal cord.

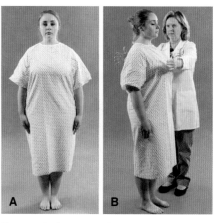

Fig. 17-20. Performing Romberg test with patient's (A) eyes open and (B) closed with nurse in safety position.

TECHNIQUE 17-4: **Assessing Sensory Function**

Purpose: To assess for loss in function to sensory nerves

The following techniques will be used when the examiner has detected sensory loss or it is known that the patient has spinal cord disease.

Technique 17-4A: **Assessing Graphesthesia**

Purpose: To assess the sensation of touch or tactile stimulation

ASSESSMENT STEPS

1. Explain the technique.
2. Have patient extend right arm and turn palm face up toward ceiling.

3. Ask patient to close eyes.

4. Write a letter or number on the right palm and ask the patient to state which letter or number was written (Fig. 17-21).

5. Repeat steps 2, 3, and 4 on the left palm.

6. Document your findings.

NORMAL FINDINGS

■ Patient is able to state letter or number correctly on each side.

ABNORMAL FINDINGS

■ Patient is unable to feel and state the letter or number.

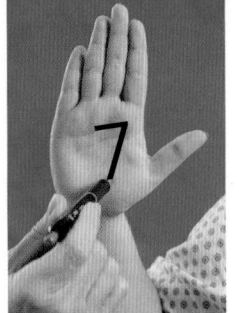

Fig. 17-21. Assessing graphesthesia.

Technique 17-4B: **Assessing Stereognosis**

Purpose: To assess the perception of a shape of an object

Equipment: Two different objects (i.e. coin, paper clip)

ASSESSMENT STEPS

1. Explain the technique.

2. Ask patient to close eyes.

3. Put a small object in the palm of the patient's right hand (Fig. 17-22).

4. Ask the patient to identify the object.

5. Using a different object, repeat steps 2 and 3 using the left hand.

6. Document your findings.

NORMAL FINDINGS

■ Patient is able to perceive and identify the shape of the object.

ABNORMAL FINDINGS

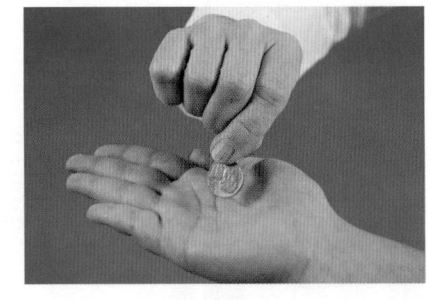

Fig. 17-22. Assessing stereognosis.

■ **Tactile Agnosia** is the inability to process sensory information and to perceive and recognize an object by touch; caused by lesions in the brain's parietal lobe.

ADVANCED ASSESSMENTS

Advanced assessments can be performed to verify a finding the examiner may have found during the general neurological assessment. The following assessments will help the examiner to focus in on the area of involvement within the neurological system.

Deep Tendon Reflexes

A reflex arc is a neural pathway. When a reflex is initiated, a sensory neuron is stimulated and travels through the spinal cord to stimulate a motor neuron, creating a reflex movement. Reflexes are involuntary responses. Assessment of deep tendon reflexes reveals the intactness of the reflex arc at specific spinal levels. The inability to elicit a reflex may indicate level of injury or CNS involvement. When assessing deep tendon reflexes, tendons and muscles are involved:

- Tendons are attached to skeletal muscles and have receptors that are sensitive to stretch.
- Striking a tendon stretches the attached muscle.
- The muscle contracts to elicit the reflex.

   TIP The reason that we strike a tendon to elicit a reflex is that the tendon is hard, and striking it stretches the tendon, which then stretches the attached muscle (Braddom & Braddom, 2015).

Preliminary Steps

- The patient will need to be relaxed in order to elicit a reflex.
- To elicit a true reflex, distract the patient by talking with him or her.
- While assessing reflexes, always compare the grading of the right and left sides.
- Deep tendon reflexes are graded on a scale of 0 to +4 (Table 17-6).

TABLE 17-6 Deep Tendon Reflexes	
Scale	Tendon Reflex Grading
0	Absent
1+	A slight response but diminished
2+	Normal response with average strength
3+	A very brisk or exaggerated response; may or may not be normal
4+	A tap elicits a repeating reflex (clonus); always abnormal

Adapted from Walker H. K. (1990). Deep tendon reflexes. In: H. K. Walker, W. D. Hall, & J. W. Hurst (eds.), *Clinical methods: The history, physical, and laboratory examinations* (3rd ed.). Boston: Butterworths.

- Deep tendon reflexes may also be increased, decreased, or absent in various conditions.
- Hyperactive indicates overresponsive response. This could indicate lesions of the corticospinal system.
  - □ **Clonus** is a repetitive, rhythmic, uncontrolled reflex response caused by several neurological disorders.
- Hypoactive indicates decreased response. This could indicate a dysfunction of some component of the reflex arc.
- They are often absent in deep coma, narcosis (stupor), heavy sedation, and deep sleep.
- Exaggeration of the deep tendon reflexes may occur in psychogenic disorders, and in anxiety, fright, and agitation.

   TIP Testing deep tendon reflexes should not hurt the patient.

TECHNIQUE 17-5: **Assessing the Triceps Reflex**

Purpose: To assess the integrity of sensory and motor pathways at the level of Cervical 6 and Cervical 7
Equipment: Reflex hammer
ASSESSMENT STEPS
1. Explain the technique to the patient.
2. Patient should be in a sitting position; encourage the patient to relax the left arm.
3. Using your left hand, flex the patient's left arm between 45 and 90 degrees.
4. Encourage the patient to relax so the forearm is hanging loose.
5. With either side of the reflex hammer, strike the patient's triceps tendon, just above the olecranon process (Fig. 17-23).
6. Assess the reaction of the left forearm.
7. Repeat steps 2 through 6 on the right side and compare reactions.
8. Document your findings.

NORMAL FINDINGS
■ Contraction of the triceps muscle; extension of the forearm (2+).

ABNORMAL FINDINGS
■ Hypoactive, hyperactive, or no contraction and extension of the forearm.
■ Disorders in the sensory limb will prevent or delay the transmission of the impulse to the spinal cord. This causes the resulting reflex to be diminished or completely absent.
■ Hypoactive reflexes with clonus may indicate multiple sclerosis or spinal cord injury.
■ Absent reflexes can indicate degenerative disease.

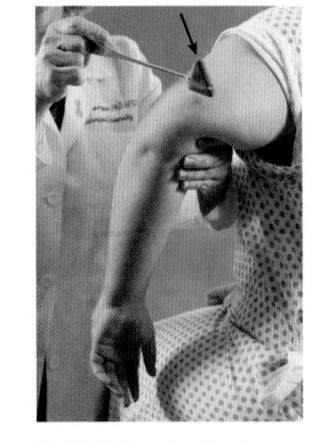

Fig. 17-23. Assessing the triceps reflex.

TECHNIQUE 17-6: **Assessing the Biceps Reflex**

Purpose: To assess the integrity of sensory and motor pathways at the level of Cervical 5 and Cervical 6
Equipment: Reflex hammer
ASSESSMENT STEPS
1. Explain the technique to the patient.
2. Patient should be in a sitting position with his or her arm resting on the lap, elbow is flexed, and right hand slightly pronated.

3. Encourage the patient to relax and look straight ahead.
4. Using your thumb of your nondominant hand, stretch the biceps tendon.
5. Strike your thumb with the reflex hammer as it is stretching the right biceps tendon (Fig. 17-24).
6. Assess the reaction of the right forearm for flexion.
7. Repeat steps 2 through 6 on the left side and compare reactions.
8. Document your findings.

NORMAL FINDINGS
■ Biceps muscle contracts; flexion of the forearm (2+).

ABNORMAL FINDING
■ Hypoactive, hyperactive, or no contraction of the biceps muscle; no flexion of the forearm.

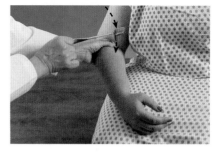

Fig. 17-24. Assessing the biceps reflex.

TECHNIQUE 17-7: **Assessing the Brachioradialis Reflex**

Purpose: To assess the integrity of sensory and motor pathways at the level of Cervical 5 and Cervical 6
Equipment: Reflex hammer

ASSESSMENT STEPS
1. Explain the technique to the patient.
2. The patient should be in a sitting position with right arm relaxed and forearm slightly pronated resting on the lap.
3. Tap the right forearm directly, about 2 to 3 cm above the wrist (Fig. 17-25).
4. Assess the reaction of the right forearm.
5. Repeat steps 2, 3, and 4 on the left side and compare reactions.
6. Document your findings.

NORMAL FINDINGS
■ Brachioradialis muscle contracts; flexion of the elbow and supination of the forearm (2+).

ABNORMAL FINDINGS
■ Hypoactive, hyperactive, or no contraction of the brachioradialis muscle; no flexion of the elbow or supination of the forearm.

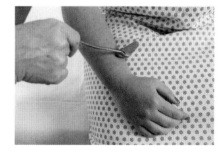

Fig. 17-25. Assessing the brachioradialis reflex.

■ **TIP** To distract the patient while testing reflexes of lower extremities, have the patient hold both hands together and pull hands against each other and look straight ahead while eliciting this reflex (Fig. 17-26).

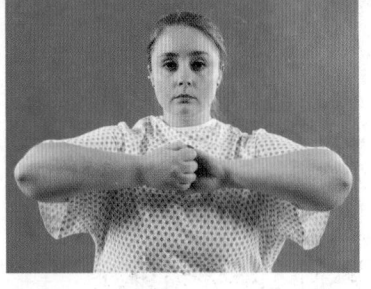

Fig. 17-26. Position for testing reflexes of lower extremities.

TECHNIQUE 17-8: **Assessing the Quadriceps Reflex (also known as Patellar Tendon Reflex)**

Purpose: To assess the integrity of sensory and motor pathways at the level of Lumbar 2, Lumbar 3, and Lumbar 4
Equipment: Reflex hammer

SENC Safety Alert This is also called the knee-jerk reflex. Do not stand directly in front of the patient during this assessment, because the knee will quickly extend forward in a normal response and could hit you. Always stand to the side of the patient.

ASSESSMENT STEPS
1. Explain the technique to the patient.
2. Have the patient sit on the edge of the examination table and instruct the patient to look straight ahead.
3. Let the lower legs dangle freely off the edge of the examination table.
4. Stand on the right side of the patient and place one hand on the lower thigh just above the right knee and palpate the patella tendon.
5. Tap the right patella tendon directly just below the right patella (Fig. 17-27).
6. Assess the reaction of the right knee for extension of the lower leg.
7. Repeat 4, 5 and 6 on the left side and compare reactions.
8. Document your findings.

NORMAL FINDINGS
■ Contraction of the quadriceps muscle; extension of the lower leg (2+).

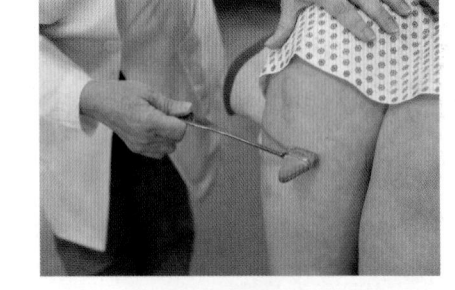

Fig. 17-27. Assessing the quadriceps reflex.

■ Hypoactive, hyperactive, or no contraction of the quadriceps muscle; no extension of the lower leg.

TECHNIQUE 17-9: **Assessing the Achilles Reflex**

Purpose: To assess the sensory and motor pathways of Sacral 1 and Sacral 2.
Equipment: Reflex hammer
ASSESSMENT STEPS
1. Explain the technique to the patient.
2. This reflex can be tested with the patient supine on the examination table or sitting up with the feet dangling.
3. Hold the right foot in dorsiflexion and tap the Achilles tendon (Fig. 17-28).
4. Assess the reaction of the right foot and toes.
5. Repeat steps 3, 4, and 5 on the left side and compare reactions.
6. Document your findings.
NORMAL FINDINGS
■ The foot plantar flexes against your hand (2+).
ABNORMAL FINDINGS
■ Hypoactive, hyperactive, or no plantar flexion is observed.

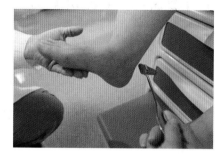

Fig. 17-28. Assessing the Achilles reflex.

TECHNIQUE 17-10: **Assessing the Plantar Reflex**

Purpose: To assess the sensory and motor pathways of Lumbar 4 to Sacral 2.
Equipment: Reflex hammer
ASSESSMENT STEPS
1. Explain the technique to the patient.
2. Using the handle of the reflex hammer, stroke the lateral side of the patient's sole of the left foot upward toward the great toe (Fig. 17-29).
3. Assess the response of the toes.
4. Repeat steps 2 and 3 on the right side and compare reactions.
5. Document your findings.

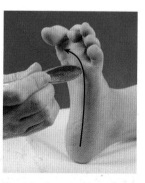

Fig. 17-29. Assessing the plantar reflex.

NORMAL FINDINGS
- Plantar flexion of the great toe and the other toes flex toward the heel of the foot, away from the patient's head, flexor-plantar response.

ABNORMAL FINDINGS
- Babinski's reflex occurs when the great toe extends upward and the other toes fan out, indicating neuron disease of the corticospinal tract (Hickey, 2014).
- A sluggish plantar flexion response may be related to neurological impairment or depression related to drugs.

PATIENT EDUCATION

Healthy People 2020

Goal: Improve cardiovascular health and quality of life through prevention, detection, and treatment of risk factors for heart attack and stroke; early identification and treatment of heart attacks and strokes; and prevention of repeat cardiovascular events (HHS, 2010).

In order to accomplish this goal, nurses need to encourage the patient to control modifiable risk factors that can lead to a stroke:

- Hypertension
- High cholesterol
- Cigarette smoking
- Diabetes
- Exercise/physical health
- Obesity

Teach the patient the warning signs of a stroke. The American Stroke Association (2015) has developed the mnemonic **F.A.S.T.** as an easy way to remember the sudden signs of stroke:

- **F**ace drooping: Does one side of the face droop or is it numb? Ask the person to smile. Is the person's smile uneven?
- **A**rm weakness: Is one arm weak or numb? Ask the person to raise both arms. Does one arm drift downward?
- **S**peech difficulty: Is speech slurred? Is the person unable to speak or hard to understand? Ask the person to repeat a simple sentence, like "The sky is blue." Is the sentence repeated correctly?
- **T**ime to call 9-1-1: If someone shows any of these symptoms, even if the symptoms go away, call 9-1-1 and get the person to the hospital immediately. Check the time so you'll know when the first symptoms appeared.

INTRODUCTION

Women's health continues to be a growing specialty that requires gender-specific assessments. The female reproductive system undergoes multiple physiological changes during the life span. Cyclically, a woman experiences constant hormonal changes during the reproductive years with significant changes occurring in puberty, pregnancy, lactation, and menopause. Women have unique healthcare considerations affecting their quality of life. In the United States, 1 in 4 women dies from heart disease and is more likely than men to have a condition called "broken heart syndrome." This is a recognized heart problem related to extreme emotional stress that can develop into heart muscle failure (NIH, 2014).

Nurses need to be knowledgeable in performing health assessments and to identify risk factors related to gender-specific medical conditions and cancers. Based on current incidence rates, a woman has about a 1 in 8 chance of developing invasive breast cancer at some time during her life (breastcancer.org, 2017).

Mental health illnesses and safety issues continue to be influenced by one's external environment and relationships. Nearly 1 in 4 women (22.3 percent) aged 18 and older in the United States has been the victim of severe physical violence by an intimate partner in her lifetime (CDC, 2015a). More than one-third of women in the United States (36% or approximately 42 million women) have experienced rape, physical violence, and/or stalking by an intimate partner at some point in their lifetime (Black et al., 2013). Intimate partner violence (IPV), sexual trauma, and posttraumatic stress are essential issues to recognize and address in

women's health care (Wipf, 2015). IPV includes actual or threatened physiological, physical, emotional, verbal, sexual, or economic abuse (prevented from working or controls money), including stalking between individuals in a current or former relationship. This can occur between heterosexual, same sex, bisexual, and transgendered couples. Women at risk for IPV include young age, women with disabilities, substance abuse, marital/relationship difficulties, and economic difficulties (Moyer, 2013).

US Preventive Services Task Force (USPSTF) recommends all women 14–46 be screened routinely for IPV and referred to services if screen is positive (Moyer, 2013). One of the best methods found to screen for IPV is the HITS screening tool (Moyer, 2013). Each question is scored and scores greater than 10 indicate possible IPV (see Chapter 3, Box 3-2 for HITS screening tool).

Sexual assault is a major public health problem in the United States, defined by a range of different types of assault, including rape, attempted rape, coercion, forced pornography, unwanted fondling, any genital or oral contact by a person or an object against one's will, accomplished by some type of force or coercion. Lifetime estimates of rape in the United States are as high as 1 in 5 women, and 1 in 10 women will experience rape by an intimate partner (Black et al., 2013). Women who have been sexually assaulted have complex healthcare needs. It is recommended that victims of sexual assault receive comprehensive care, consisting of a health and history assessment, prophylactic treatment for sexually transmitted infections, HIV post-exposure prophylaxis, pregnancy prophylaxis, forensic evidence collection, and psychological follow-up (U.S. Department of Justice, Office on Violence Against Women, 2013). Over the years specialized programs have been developed to improve healthcare delivery to patients who have been sexually assaulted. Every effort should be made for a sexually assaulted patient to receive care within a healthcare system with specialized services so that they receive comprehensive care from trained nurses and doctors, including a medical forensic examination with evidence collection. A medical forensic examination includes an interview with the patient, the documentation of the assault, photographs of the injuries, an assessment of the physical and mental health, and a lengthy evidence collection process. The process can take several hours to complete. In addition, all patients should be given post-exposure prophylactic medications to prevent STIs, HIV, and pregnancy (Workowski, 2015).

Human trafficking is a form of modern-day slavery, widespread throughout the world with women and children disproportionately affected. Human trafficking deprives people of their human rights and freedom. Trafficking includes sexual acts, being forced to commit as well as be in forced labor situations as domestic servants (nannies or maids); sweatshop workers; janitors; restaurant workers; manicurists; agricultural and farm workers; fishery workers; hotel or tourist industry workers; drug trade, child soldiers, beggars, and organ harvesting. Many of the victims have been tricked, kidnapped, forced, coerced, or even sold by their families. Human traffickers are at risk for injuries, STIs including HIV, malnutrition, dental issues, pregnancy, occupational health exposures, PTSD, depression and anxiety.

Nurses need essential knowledge about these life, safety, reproductive, and hormonal changes to be able to discuss and educate their patients.

REVIEW OF ANATOMY AND PHYSIOLOGY

Breasts

■ Breasts are mammary glands that change in size, shape, weight, and function for each individual during different life stages, including puberty, pregnancy, lactation, and menopause. Breasts are composed of skin, subcutaneous tissue, and breast tissue.

TIP Women know their normal appearance and size of their breasts; sometimes one breast may be larger than the other.

■ Milk-producing gland
■ Lie over the pectoral muscles of the chest and are attached to the chest wall by Cooper's ligaments
■ Breasts extend from the second through sixth ribs and are divided into four quadrants (Fig. 18-1) including the tail of Spence; the tail of Spence is the lateral corner and axillary extension of the breast.

External Surface Anatomy

■ Areola is a dark pigmented disk about 1 to 2 cm round that surrounds the nipple; contains small sebaceous glands (Montgomery's glands); the areola also contains hair follicles; hair may

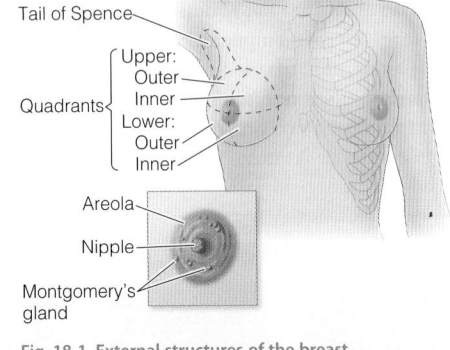
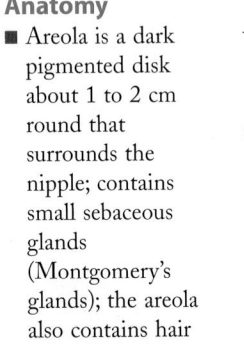

Fig. 18-1. External structures of the breast.

grow from the areola; areola color varies from pink, red, brown, to dark brown.

- The nipples are protuberant and round; located at the center of the areola and breast; may be flat or inverted. They are a highly sensitive area that contains milk glands, nerve endings, and smooth muscle fibers that contract and become erect based on temperature, stimulation, or lactation.

Internal Anatomy

- Contains three types of tissue
  □ Fatty
  □ Fibrous: provides support to breasts
  □ Glandular: Contains 15 to 20 lobes per breast; each lobe has 20 to 40 lobules that contain milk-producing acini cells (Fig. 18-2)
- Amount and size of the three types of tissue vary depending on the production of two female hormones, progesterone and estrogen.

TIP Female hormones, estrogen and progesterone, influence the development of the female breasts and reproductive system, high-pitched voice, and wide hips in women. Estrogen and progesterone are produced by the hypothalamus, anterior pituitary gland, and ovaries.

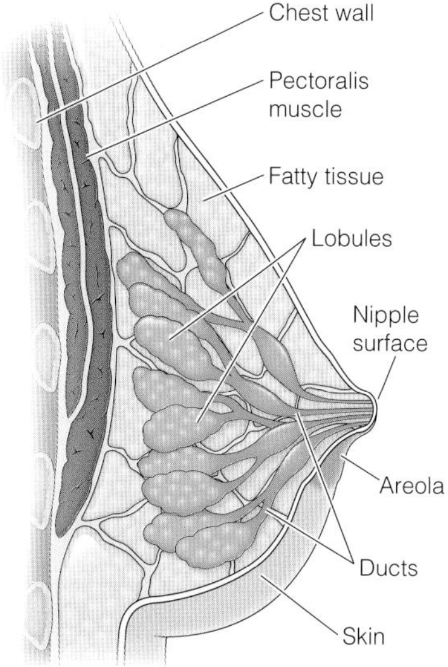

Chest wall
Pectoralis muscle
Fatty tissue
Lobules
Nipple surface
Areola
Ducts
Skin

Fig. 18-2. Internal structures of the breast.

- The internal mammary and lateral thoracic arteries provide the blood supply to the breasts.

Lymphatic System

- Each breast has lymphatic vessels and nodes that lie directly below the surface of the skin (Fig. 18-3).
- The lymphatic circulation moves toward the upper outer quadrant of each breast and toward the axillary nodes.
- Breast infection or disease may cause enlargement of the lymph node(s).

SENC Safety Alert If a woman has breast cancer, the axillary lymph nodes are one of the first places the cancer may spread (metastasize).

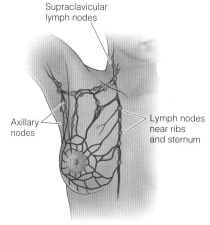

Supraclavicular lymph nodes
Axillary nodes
Lymph nodes near ribs and sternum

Fig. 18-3. Lymphatic vessels and nodes.

External Genitalia

- Vulva is the external genitalia organ that consists of the following (Fig. 18-4):
  □ Mons pubis is a round, fleshy elevation composed of subcutaneous fatty tissue over the pubic bone that becomes covered with pubic hair during puberty.

☐ Labia majora and minora are cutaneous folds made up of skin and adipose tissue.

☐ Clitoris is part of the vulva that contains nerve fibers; sensitive and enlarges during sexual stimulation.

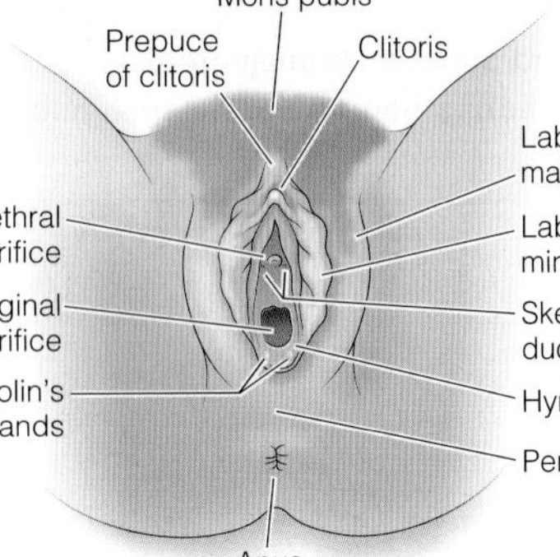

■ Skene's glands are located on the anterior wall of the vagina; related to female ejaculation.

■ Bartholin's glands are two pea-sized glands located near the beginning of the vagina; produce clear mucus that lubricates the area during sex.

■ Urethra is a hollow tube that is a passageway for urine to exit the body.

■ Perineum is the area between the vagina and rectum.

Internal Reproductive Organs

■ Vagina is a hollow, muscular, expandable canal measuring about 2 to 4 inches in length; extends from the external genitalia to the cervix (Fig. 18-5). Normal bacteria flora maintains the pH of the vagina between 4 and 5, thereby reducing infectious bacteria growth.

■ Uterus is a hollow muscular organ shaped like a pear; lies between the bladder and the rectum; during pregnancy the fetus grows and develops within the uterus. It is made of two segments; fundus,

Fig. 18-4. External female genitalia.

located at the top, and isthmus which is the lower portion of the uterus. The position of the uterus can be anteverted, retroverted, or midline.

■ Cervix is part of the lower uterus and is a canal that is made up of columnar epithelium that secretes mucous and is located inside the vagina. The opening of the cervix is called the external os and is located in the vagina.

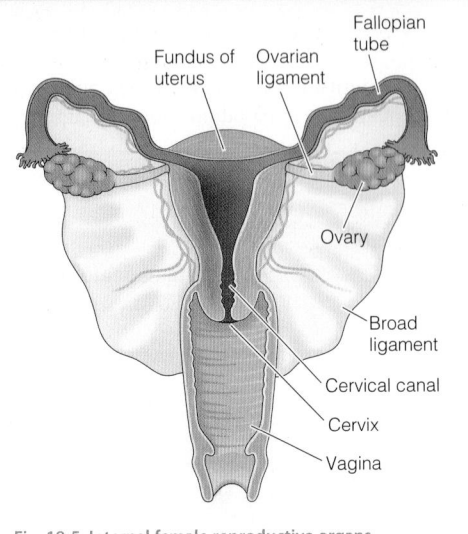

Fig. 18-5. Internal female reproductive organs.

■ Fallopian tubes are tube-like structures measuring 10–12 cm that initiate from the left and right sides of the fundus; the end of each tube branches out close to each ovary; use ciliary and muscular waves to move a mature egg toward the uterus.

■ Ovaries are almond-shaped organs, they measure approximately 3–4 cm in length, 2 cm in width, and 1–2 cm thickness, and located on each side of the uterus; produce the female hormones of estrogen and progesterone and contain female eggs.

Menstrual Cycle

A women's reproductive years begin at puberty or menarche (usually occurs around age 12) and ends with menopause (around age 50). The overall period of puberty lasts 3–5 years and is influenced by a variety of factors, including heredity, ethnicity, health, nutritional status, childhood infections, and environmental exposures (Pierce & Hardy, 2012). During the reproductive years the body undergoes complex hormonal and physiological changes in preparation for conception. The four hormones involved in the menstrual cycles include follicle-stimulating hormone (FSH), estrogen, luteinizing hormone (LH), and progesterone. The menstrual cycle is comprised of two major phases: the follicular phase and the luteal phase. The follicular phase begins on the first day of menses and ends on the day before the luteinizing hormone surges and can last between 14–21 days. During this phase an egg in the ovary is getting mature to be released from the ovary and the lining of the uterus thickens and becomes ready for a fertilized egg (conception). The luteal phase begins with ovulation, an egg is released from the ovary and ends at the onset of the next menses and lasts 13 to 15 days. Ovulation occurs in the middle of the menstrual cycle and occurs when an ovary releases a matured egg. The egg will travel down the fallopian tube and if semen is present then fertilization occurs. If fertilization does not occur, the body undergoes cyclic hormonal changes known as the menstrual cycle whereby the thickened part of the endometrium lining that was preparing for the implantation of the fertilized egg of the uterus is shed. Cervical mucus changes during the menstrual cycle; most often the cervix produces a whitish discharge that maintains the flora and pH of the vagina and closer to ovulation the cervix produces clear sticky mucous that facilitates semen to navigate through the cervix and towards the released egg. The changes in the hormones throughout the menstrual cycle can also bring about changes in mood, breast tenderness, fluid retention, cramping, weight gain, diarrhea, and constipation.

BOX 18-1 Symptoms of Menopause

Dry skin
Hair thinning/loss
Hot flashes
Mood changes
Insomnia
Irregular menstrual periods
Irritability
Sweating/night sweats
Vaginal dryness
Weight gain

Menopause

The permanent cessation of menstrual activity normally occurs in women in the United States between the ages of 45 and 55, with the mean age of 51 (North American Menopause Society, 2016).

- **Perimenopause** may occur several years prior to menopause; the hormones, estrogen and progesterone, fluctuate causing some woman to experience symptoms of menopause (Box 18-1).
- **Menopause** occurs when the woman has no menstrual activity for a period of 12 months (Venes, 2013); estrogen and progesterone levels decrease contributing to menopausal symptoms.
- **Postmenopause** is the period of time after menopause when menopausal symptoms start to diminish; women have a greater risk of osteoporosis, cardiovascular disease, and urinary incontinence.

DIAGNOSTICS

Diagnostics of the breasts and internal reproductive organs aid in diagnoses of disease pathology. Some of the more commonly used diagnostics for women's health assessment are as follows:

- **Mammogram** is one of the best screening tests to detect breast cancer; it is a film x-ray of the internal structures and tissues of the breasts.

SENC Safety Alert Breast cancer is the second leading cause of death in women. Women should know how their breasts normally look and feel and report any breast changes promptly to their healthcare provider.

■ **Needle biopsy** is the insertion of a needle directly into the suspicious breast tissue; the tissue sample then is assessed for cytological pathology.

■ **Sonogram** is a breast ultrasound that uses sound waves to take pictures of breast tissue; used to differentiate between solid and cystic masses and guides location for needle biopsy.

■ **Papanicolaou test** also known as Pap smear, is a screening test to detect abnormal cervical cells including cervical cancer; the cervical

smear captures cell changes on the cervix that might become cervical cancer.

■ **Human papillomavirus (HPV) test** is recommended to be used along with the Pap test for screening women aged 30 years and older for the HPV infection which can put a woman at higher risk for cervical cancer (CDC, 2015b).

■ **Vaginal specimens** are obtained in women with vaginal discharge; the specimen identifies the organisms causing the symptoms; commonly collected for sexually transmitted infections (STIs) or vaginal drainage of unknown etiology.

HEALTH HISTORY

Review of Systems

Use the OLDCARTS mnemonic (**O**nset, **L**ocation, **D**uration, **C**haracteristics, **A**ggravating/Alleviating factors, **R**elieving factors, **T**reatment, **S**everity) to identify attributes of a symptom. Use the OPQRST mnemonic (**O**nset, **P**rovoking, **Q**uality, **R**adiation, **S**everity/Symptoms, **T**iming/Triggers) when describing pain symptoms.

A focused health assessment related to women's health includes the following. Ask the patient the following questions.

Menstrual History

■ What age did you start to menstruate?
  □ Menstruation can begin as early as age 8 and as late as age 14.
  □ The first menstrual period is called menarche.
■ What date did your last menstrual period begin?
TIP It might be helpful to show the patient a calendar to recall the date.
■ Is your menstruation cycle regular or irregular? Do you miss cycles? If so, how often? Every woman of childbearing age who has a

complaint of irregular or absent menstrual cycles should be tested for pregnancy.
  □ A regular menstrual cycle occurs about 24 to 38 days and lasts up to 7 days. The cycle is from day one of bleeding to day one of the next cycle of bleeding.
  □ Menstrual cycles that are longer than 38 days or shorter than 24 days are abnormal (ACOG, 2017)
  □ **Amenorrhea** is the absence of menses.
    • Primary amenorrhea is defined in women who are age 15 years and older and have not had a menstrual cycle.
    • Secondary amenorrhea is the absence of a menstrual cycle for more than three months in girls or women who previously had regular menstrual cycles or for six months in girls or women who had irregular menses (Welt & Barbieri, 2017).
  □ **Metrorrhagia:** uterine bleeding at irregular intervals most often associated with dysfunctional ovaries
■ What is the usual number of days of bleeding?
  □ The average number of days of bleeding is about 3 to 7 days.

TIP The menstrual cycle is usually expressed as X/Y. X = Duration: How many days does menstruation last? Y= Cycle: How often does menstruation occur? For example, 7/28 means menstruation lasts for seven days and occurs every 28 days (Clifford, Yau, Kelly & Hallam, 2012, p. 125).

■ What absorbent products do you use?

■ How would you describe the amount of flow? Do you experience lighter or heavier vaginal bleeding during menstruation? Ask about the onset of any changes in bleeding, amount, duration, and frequency.

  □ The total amount of blood loss may be less than 80 mL for the whole menstrual period; this amount may vary in different women and from period to period in the same woman.

  □ Heavy menstrual flow is defined as blood loss greater than or equal to 80 mL per menstrual cycle (Beebeejaun & Varma, 2013); bleeding usually lasts seven or more days.

  □ Heavy menstrual bleeding is a subjective report; and women vary in their perceptions of what is acceptable blood loss and when they should seek help (Hoaglin et al., 2013).

SENC Safety Alert A woman is considered to have heavy menstrual bleeding if she needs to change her tampon or pad every hour or more often or if she passes clots the size of a quarter or larger (CDC, 2015c).

  □ **Menorrhagia:** excessive or prolonged duration of menses; may pass many clots with menstrual flow

  □ **Oligomenorrhea:** decreased or light menses

■ Do you have menstrual cramps? If so, how bad? What medication do you take for the cramps?

  □ **Primary dysmenorrhea** is defined as menstrual pain occurring with ovulatory menstrual cycles; it is accompanied by a range of systemic symptoms such as lower abdominal pain that may radiate to the lower back or legs, headache, nausea, vomiting, diarrhea, irritability, fatigue, and depression (Arora, Yardi, & Gopal, 2014).

TIP Dysmenorrhea is diagnosed when the pain is so severe as to limit normal activities, or require medical attention.

Abnormal Vaginal Bleeding

■ Do you experience spotting or bleeding in between your menstrual cycle?

  □ Midcycle spotting or bleeding can occur during ovulation.

  □ Pelvic inflammatory disease and infection of the uterus, fallopian tubes, or ovaries may cause bleeding.

  □ Polycystic ovarian syndrome (PCOS) is an endocrine disorder in women of reproductive age that can cause irregular menstrual cycles; other PCOS symptoms may include unwanted hair growth on the face, chest, and back (hirsutism), weight gain, oily skin, and infertility.

■ Do you have premenstrual symptoms?

  □ **Premenstrual syndrome (PMS)** is a group of symptoms occurring 1 to 2 weeks prior to menstruation; changes in hormones, stress, diet, and alcohol may be factors involved (HHS, 2017) (Box 18-2).

■ Do you experience bleeding after sexual intercourse (postcoital bleeding)?

BOX 18-2 Premenstrual Symptoms

Nausea
Vomiting
Tender breasts
Fatigue
Bloating
Gastrointestinal symptoms (e.g., constipation, heartburn, or diarrhea)
Insomnia
Irritability
Mood swings

☐ Bleeding after sexual intercourse may be related to friction of the cervical mucosa.

SENC Safety Alert Postcoital bleeding refers to spotting or bleeding unrelated to menstruation that occurs during or after sexual intercourse; it can be a sign of a serious symptom and should be reported to the healthcare provider (Shahini, Kone, Ceka, Petrela, & Haxhihyseni, 2013).

Menopause

- At what age, did you start menopause? Do you experience any menopausal symptoms (see Box 18-1)?
- Do you take any medications or over-the-counter (OTC) medications to help relieve symptoms?
  ☐ Estrogen and progesterone hormone replacement therapy may be prescribed by the healthcare provider.
  ☐ Nonprescription remedies such as soy, black cohosh, and vitamin E are available at local pharmacies and health food stores.
- Has menopause affected your quality of life?
  ☐ Hormonal changes at menopause as well as other physiological, psychological, sociocultural, interpersonal, and lifestyle factors contribute to midlife sexual problems (Shifren & Gass, 2014).
  ☐ Depression, anxiety, and decreased sense of well-being are common psychological symptoms that may affect daily living.
- Do you have any spotting or bleeding?
  ☐ Bleeding during menopause could be a sign of a serious problem and needs to be reported to the healthcare provider.

Contraceptive History

Contraception can be categorized as hormonal or barrier methods that provide control over the timing and prevention of pregnancy, menstrual cycle and some hormonal conditions such as PMS. A contraceptive history should include current method, compliance with method, failure, or inability to use method appropriately and side effects.

- What is your present contraceptive method?
  ☐ Birth control pills are a form of hormonal contraception preventing pregnancy. Varying birth control pills will include varying amounts of estrogen and progestin.
  ☐ Transdermal patch is a combined hormonal contraceptive containing both progestin and estrogen that is applied to the skin; hormones are released daily, resulting in a steady state of systemic hormones, resulting in ovulation suppression.
  ☐ Nuvaring is a hormonal bendable ring that is inserted into the vagina. Has a local effect of ovulation suppression and thickening of the uterus which protects against pregnancy.
  ☐ Diaphragm is a barrier method, dome-shaped cup that is inserted in the vagina to cover the cervix. Spermicide is often recommended to be applied inside the cup to allow for additional contraceptive protection.
  ☐ Intrauterine devices (IUDs) are small, "T" shaped devices that are placed into the uterus and are a long-acting, reversible method of birth control. IUDs prevent sperm from reaching or fertilizing an egg. IUDs also prevent a fertilized egg from attaching to the uterus and developing into a fetus. IUDs are either copper or plastic, have a local hormone that slowly releases progestin and may suppress ovulation.
  ☐ Female condom is a flexible pouch that is inserted into the vagina prior to intercourse; barrier contraceptive.
  ☐ Male condom is thin, flexible penile sheath made of synthetic or natural materials; barrier contraceptive.
  ☐ Spermicide acts as a barrier and inhibits sperm motility in the vagina and function. Surfactant designed to dissolve lipids in the sperm cell membrane, thus inactivating or killing the sperm. Spermicide is often used with other barrier methods to enhance the effectiveness of contraception.

TIP The male condom is 98 percent effective as a contraceptive if used every single time with sex and if used correctly (Planned Parenthood, 2017). Both the female and male condoms protect against STIs.

- ☐ Rhythm method uses abstinence from sexual intercourse during the time of ovulation, and involves tracking changes in body temperature and cervical mucous.
- ☐ Posttubal ligation is a surgical procedure that blocks both fallopian tubes; permanent form of birth control.

TIP When assessing the type of contraceptive method the patient is using, assess her satisfaction, consistency of use, side effects, and length of time used. If a patient does not like the method, she may not use this method as directed.

- ■ Have there been any failure problems of this form of contraception in the past?

Obstetric History
(See Chapter 22.)

Family and Medical History

- ■ Do you have a family history of breast disease?
  - ☐ Roughly 5 percent of breast cancers are due to an inherited mutation in *BRCA1* or *BRCA2*; women with such mutations have a significantly increased risk of breast or ovarian cancer, often at an early age (Mayor, 2013).

TIP The American Cancer Society (ACS, 2015a) recommends that a woman with the *BRCA1* or *BRCA2* gene mutation should have a mammogram and magnetic resonance imaging annually.

- ■ Have you had any previous breast disease?
  - ☐ **Fibrocystic breast disease** is benign painless lumps or thickening of tissue that are felt in a woman's breast; often associated with hormonal changes during a woman's menstrual cycle.
  - ☐ **Breast cysts** are fluid-filled lumps in the breast; may or may not be painful.
  - ☐ **Fibroadenomas** are solid, round, rubbery lumps filled with fibrous and glandular tissues; these lumps move easily when pushed; more common in younger women.
- ■ Have you had any type of breast surgeries?
  - ☐ **Mastectomy** is the surgical removal of one or both breasts.
  - ☐ **Breast reduction surgery** removes breast tissue and skin to reduce the size of the breasts.
  - ☐ **Breast augmentation** is a surgical procedure to increase the size of one or both breasts.

SENC Safety Alert Prophylactic surgery to remove both breasts (called bilateral prophylactic mastectomy) can reduce the risk of breast cancer in women. A woman can be at very high risk of developing breast cancer if she has a strong family history of breast and/or ovarian cancer, a disease-causing mutation in the *BRCA1* gene or the *BRCA2* gene, or a high-penetrance mutation in one of several other genes associated with breast cancer (National Cancer Institute, 2013).

SENC Evidence-Based Practice Jin (2013) researched the most common reasons women chose contralateral prophylactic mastectomy and found a desire to decrease their risk of contralateral breast cancer, desire to improve survival, and peace of mind. No definitive data to date have shown a survival benefit for contralateral prophylactic mastectomy in women without a genetic predisposition.

Breast Examinations

- ■ Have you had a clinical breast examination (CBE)? If so, when?
  - ☐ The CBE is an examination of your breasts by a health professional such as a doctor, nurse practitioner, nurse, or physician assistant. The healthcare provider carefully palpates your breasts and underarms for any changes or abnormalities (such as a lump)

(Susan G. Komen Foundation, 2016). This examination is performed in the supine position and sitting up.

TIP It is recommended that healthcare providers have special training in CBE to identify abnormal from normal findings. Trained and experienced healthcare providers can find breast abnormalities that a woman might not have felt herself and can detect lumps as small as a pea (about 1 centimeter) (United Breast Cancer Foundation, 2015).

■ Do you perform breast self-examination (BSE)?
  □ BSE is palpating your own breasts for lumps or changes in the shape and size of the breasts (Box 18-3).
  □ Risk factors for breast cancer are related to lifestyle, environment, and genetic factors (Box 18-4).
■ Have you had a mammogram? If so, when?
■ Do you have any breast concerns, such as:
  □ Lumps
  □ Pain in one or both breasts
    • Mastalgia is breast pain that usually is correlated to a woman's menstrual cycle.
  □ Tenderness; if so, is it during a specific time of the month?
    • Hormonal changes can cause breast tenderness.
  □ Nipple discharge: both abnormal and normal nipple discharge can be clear, yellow, white, or green in color; blood nipple discharge is never normal.
  □ Physiologic nipple discharge is usually bilateral; mainly caused by repeated manipulation, pregnancy, or medications.
  □ Pathologic nipple discharge is usually unilateral, spontaneous, and persistent (Wong Chung et al., 2016).

TIP Always have the patient identify the timing and location of the breast concern. Assess whether there is a pattern that correlates with her menstrual cycle and if the discharge is:

■ unilateral or bilateral

■ color

BOX 18-3 Warning Signs for Breast Cancer

• Lump
• Thickening or dense tissue felt inside the breast or underarm area
• Swelling, warmth, inflammation, or color changes
• Change in the size or shape of the breast
• Dimpling or puckering of the skin
• Itchy, scaly sore or rash on or around the nipple
• Retraction of the nipple or other parts of the breast
• Nipple discharge
• Pain in an area of the breast

BOX 18-4 Risk Factors for Breast Cancer

• Family history of one or more first-degree relatives
• Inherited mutations in the *BRCA1* and *BRCA2* genes
• Advancing age
• Obesity in advancing age
• Moderate levels of alcohol
• Combined hormonal therapy of estrogen and progesterone
• Physical inactivity
• Increased breast tissue density
• Long menstrual period (periods that start early and/or end later in life)
• Oral contraceptives
• Never having children
• Having a child after age 30

Adapted from American Cancer Society. *Cancer facts and figures 2016*; CDC, 2016, What Are the Risk Factors for Breast Cancer?

- amount
- frequency
- consistency
- relationship to menstruation
- associated factors and symptoms.

Ask the healthcare provider if a sample of the nipple discharge should be sent out for analysis.

Skin Changes
- Note the specific location, type (i.e. rash, redness, dimpling), texture, and any discomfort.

Axillary Changes
- Location
- Note any lumps or tenderness
- Date discovered
- Changes in size or tenderness
- Relationship to menstruation
- Associated factors and symptoms

Gynecological History
The five main types of cancer affecting a woman's reproductive organs are: cervical, ovarian, uterine, vaginal, and vulvar. As a group, they are referred to as gynecologic cancers (CDC, 2017) (Fig. 18-6).

TIP Ovarian cancer is the fifth leading cause of cancer death in women aged 35 to 74 years. The most common symptom reported is abdominal

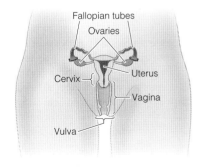

Fig. 18-6. Five types of gynecological cancers.

Labels: Fallopian tubes, Ovaries, Cervix, Uterus, Vagina, Vulva

---

BOX 18-5 **Risk Factors for Ovarian Cancer**

- Personal or family history of breast, ovarian, or colon cancer
- *BRCA1* and *BRCA2* gene mutation
- Increasing age
- Obesity
- Nulliparity
- Undesired infertility
- Start of menstruating before age 12
- Menopause after age 50
- Menopausal hormone replacement therapy

American Cancer Society. (2016). *What are the risk factors for ovarian cancer?* Retrieved from http://www.cancer.org/cancer/ovariancancer/detailedguide/ovarian-cancer-risk-factors
Ovarian Cancer National Alliance. (2016). Risk Factors. Retrieved from http://www.ovariancancer.org/about/risk-factors/

bloating. Risk factors for ovarian cancer are similar to those for breast cancer (Box 18-5).

Ask the patient:
- Did you ever have gynecological symptoms (past and present)?
  - ☐ Vaginal bleeding or itching
  - ☐ Genital sores
  - ☐ Abdominal or pelvic pain
  - ☐ Bloating
  - ☐ Painful urination
  - ☐ Pain or bleeding with intercourse
- Have you had gynecological surgeries or procedures (biopsy, laparoscopy, hysterectomy)?
- Have you experienced problems getting pregnant?
  - ☐ **Infertility** is a disease defined by the failure to achieve a successful pregnancy after 12 months or more of appropriate, timed unprotected intercourse or therapeutic donor insemination (Practice

Committee of the American Society for Reproductive Medicine, 2013).

- Do you have any vaginal discharge? If so, ask about the following:
  - ☐ Onset, duration, frequency, volume, and odor of discharge.
  - ☐ Characteristics (color, scant, profuse, thick, thin, frothy, malodorous) and any relation to menstrual cycle.
    - Normal vaginal discharge is clear; may turn white or yellow when exposed to the air; no odor, pain, or itching, and color and amount of drainage may change during the menstrual cycle.
    - Abnormal vaginal discharge may be related to infections and have a distinctive color, odor, and associated symptoms. Some examples can be viewed in Table 18-1.
- Have you ever had vaginal infections or STIs? Lesions?
- What is the date of your last pelvic examination and Pap smear?
- Do you use external products such as douches?
  - ☐ If so, frequency, method, type of solutions, reasons, and time you douched?

SENC Safety Alert Douching is not recommended because this washing depletes the vagina of normal healthy bacteria and mucus, increasing the risk of vaginal, uterine, ovarian, and fallopian tube

infections (HHS, 2015). Patients should be educated about the health concerns.

CULTURAL CONSIDERATIONS Douching has been a common practice for various cultural backgrounds. African-American women douche more often than women of other races. In some parts of the world, douching is a routine cleansing method, while other women douche after menstruation, sexual relations, or to prevent infection (Stewart, 2014).

Pelvic Pain

- Do you experience any lower abdominal or pelvic pain?
  - ☐ Use the OPQRST or OLDCARTS mnemonic.
  - ☐ Ask about the patterns of pain in relation to menstruation and physical or sexual activity, associating factors (nausea and vomiting), and alleviating factors.

CULTURAL CONSIDERATIONS Assessing the female organs is embarrassing and can be difficult for women. Keep in mind that it is essential for you to be aware of cultural considerations.

- Certain cultures only allow same-sex healthcare providers, and women may ask for their husbands or significant others to be present during the assessment. It is essential to respect all cultural considerations.

TABLE 18-1 Examples of Abnormal Vaginal Drainage

Vaginal Disorder	Cause	Color and Odor of Vaginal Drainage	Other Symptoms
Bacterial Vaginosis	STI Overgrowth of vaginal bacteria flora	Thin, white, yellow, or grayish Fishy odor	Genital itching, redness, dysuria
Candidiasis	Fungal infection caused by yeast: Candida	Thick, white, curd-like	Genital itching, burning, dysuria
Chlamydia	STI Organism is a bacterium: Chlamydia trachomatis	Bleeding after sexual intercourse Discharge with foul odor	Dysuria, abdominal pain, genital itching or burning
Trichomoniasis	STI Organism is a parasite: Trichomonas vaginalis	Clear, white, yellow-green Frothy discharge	Genital itching, burning, redness, dysuria

- There are some cultures, such as the Hispanic culture, in which it is believed to be inappropriate to touch the breasts. Please take a patient's culture into consideration and ask permission to examine or expose the breasts.
- Breast cancer in African-American women and in women of ethnic groups living in countries of low socioeconomic status, is virtually unknown; breast cancer incidence is rapidly increasing in underdeveloped countries (Williams, Olopade, & Falkson, 2010).
- The human papillomavirus (HPV) is the most common cause of cervical cancer. The number of new cervical cancer cases has been declining steadily over the past decades. Incidence rates have declined over most of the past several decades in both Caucasian and African-American women.
- In 2013, Hispanic women had the highest rate of getting cervical cancer, followed by black, white, American Indian/Alaska Native, and Asian/Pacific Islander women. Black women were more likely to die of cervical cancer than any other group (CDC, 2017). For women in many countries in Africa, Asia, and Latin America, cervical cancer is often detected late, when there is little hope for successful treatment (Saslow, 2013).

Military Health: Women Veterans

Women have served in every U.S. military conflict since the American Revolution (ACOG, 2013) and are now the fastest growing cohort within the community of veterans (U.S. Department of Veterans Affairs, 2012). Nurses should ask women if they have ever served in the military.

As a growing population, these women have healthcare needs that may be related to their time in the military. In 2012, the Department of Veterans Affairs developed the Women Veterans Task Force. This task force identified that women veterans represent a unique patient population with specific medical, psychiatric, and psychosocial care needs. Women veterans may not be ready to disclose their physical or emotional concerns. Although this reluctance must be respected, any important educational resources, including hotline and crises information, should be provided as well as any communication strategies normally used during the patient encounter by nurses (e.g., text messaging, social media, e-mail) (Conard, Armstrong, Young, & Hogan, 2015). Civilian nurses can provide meaningful therapeutic listening and advocacy skills, health assessment, and interventions to assist women with their mental and physical health issues.

PREPARATION FOR ASSESSMENT

- Exposing the breasts for examination may be embarrassing for the patient.
- Provide privacy and ensure the room is warm and comfortable.
- Maintain the modesty and dignity of the patient at all times.
- Talk to the patient and explain what you are doing during the assessment to help the patient to relax.
- Encourage the patient to ask questions during the assessment.
- Perform hand hygiene.

Equipment Needed

Gloves
Gown
Drape

Sequence of Assessment

1. Inspecting
2. Palpating

FOCUSED ASSESSMENT

TECHNIQUE 18-1: **Inspecting the Female Breasts**

Purpose: To assess the breasts for size, shape, color, and abnormalities

A patient who has had a mastectomy or breast augmentation requires the same full assessment (Fig. 18-7).

Inspect the breasts in four different positions:
- Seated with the arms hanging by each side
- Seated with the arms placed over the head
- Seated with the hands on the hips
- Standing and leaning forward

ASSESSMENT STEPS

1. Explain the technique to the patient and tell her to let you know if she is uncomfortable in any position during the assessment.
2. Ask the patient to sit up with both arms at her side (Fig. 18-8).
3. Assist the patient to lower the gown to her waist.
4. Inspect the breasts for:
   ☐ symmetry
   ☐ size of breasts.

SENC Safety Alert If you notice that one breast is larger than the other, ask the patient if this is normal for the patient; if not normal, this may be indicative of an abnormal growth.

SENC Patient-Centered Care A woman may be sensitive and embarrassed if she thinks her breast size is abnormal; breast size can affect a woman's self-image and her self-esteem. A caring patient-centered approach will make the patient feel more comfortable.

TIP Pendulous breasts are longer, larger, and hang down the chest wall (Fig. 18-9).

5. Inspect the skin for:
   ☐ color
   ☐ contour (dimpling or retraction)
   ☐ edema

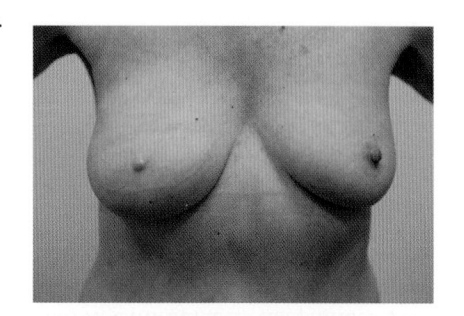

Fig. 18-7. Patient with right mastectomy.

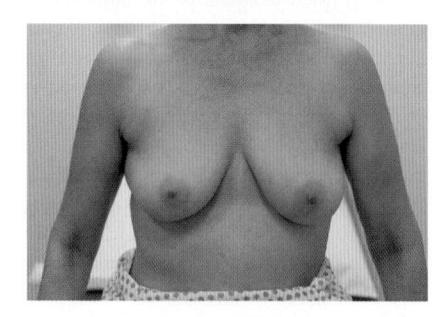

Fig. 18-8. Inspecting breast sitting up with arms by the side.

□ lesions
□ ulcerations
□ texture of skin
□ vascularity
□ venous patterns.

6. Inspect the areola for:
□ shape
□ color
□ hair
□ visible lumps

7. Inspect the nipples for:
□ size
□ position
□ shape
□ discharge
□ crusting
□ presence of accessory nipples

▪ **TIP** A supernumerary nipple is an accessory or additional nipple and is a common congenital malformation; most commonly located on the embryonic milk line.

□ eversion or inversion of nipples (Fig. 18-10).

▪ **TIP** Ask the patient if the everted or inverted nipple is normal for her or new. An inverted nipple can be manually pulled out. A retracted nipple caused by breast cancer cannot be pulled out.

8. Inspect breast for signs of retraction, such as (Fig. 18-11):
□ dimpling
□ puckering
□ furrows (a groove in the skin).

9. Ask the patient to raise her arms over her head and inspect the lower aspect of the breasts for (Fig. 18-12):
□ symmetry
□ skin changes
□ nipple deviations.

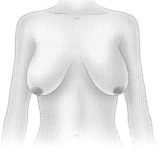

Fig. 18-9. Pendulous breasts.

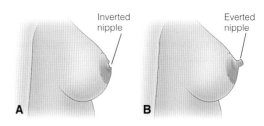

Fig. 18-10. (A) Nipple inversion. (B) Nipple eversion.

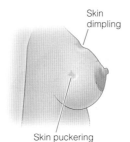

Fig. 18-11. Signs of breast retraction.

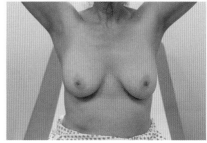

Fig. 18-12. Inspecting breasts with the arms raised up.

10. Inspect the axilla for:
  □ hair distribution
  □ skin texture
  □ protrusion of lumps or masses.
11. Ask the patient to press her hands against her hips contracting the pectoral muscles and inspect again for (Fig. 18-13):
  □ symmetry
  □ skin changes
  □ retraction areas
  □ nipple deviations.
12. Ask the patient to stand and bend forward and inspect from the front (Fig. 18-14A) and laterally (Fig. 18-14B) for:
  □ symmetry
  □ skin changes
  □ nipple deviations.
13. Document your findings.

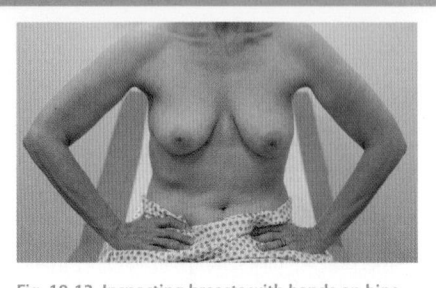

Fig. 18-13. Inspecting breasts with hands on hips contracting pectoral muscles.

NORMAL FINDINGS

■ Breasts are symmetrical; size varies per individual.
■ Color of skin is uniform; no dimpling, retractions, edema, or lesions; texture smooth.
■ Areola is round or oval, uniform color, Montgomery tubercles present.
■ Nipples are centered, round, without discharge or crusting; color varies from pink to dark brown; everted or it may be normal for one or both nipples to be inverted.
■ Venous patterns are the same in both breasts.
■ Striae are stretch marks related to aging or pregnancy.
■ **Supernumerary nipple** is an additional nipple somewhere along the mammary line, which runs from underneath the axilla down toward the groin. The extra nipple can be small, having the appearance of a mole, and can also have mammary glands and produce milk during the lactation period. They are considered normal.

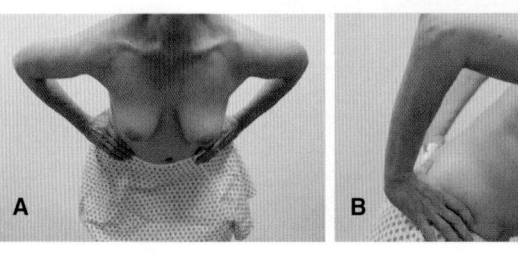

Fig. 18-14. Inspecting breasts while standing and bending forward. (A) Front. (B) Laterally.

ABNORMAL FINDINGS

- Asymmetrical breast or one abnormally large breast may indicate an abnormal growth.
- Erythema and signs of inflammation may indicate an infection.
- **Mastitis** is redness and inflammation of the breast tissue often occurring in the postpartum period when breastfeeding.
- Signs of breast tissue retraction, lumps, or dimpling may indicate an abnormal growth or be a sign of breast cancer.
- Unilateral venous pattern may indicate increased blood flow related to a malignancy.
- **Peau d'orange** is pitting, dimpling, or swelling seen in inflamed skin that overlies inflammatory carcinoma of the breast (Venes, 2013) (Fig. 18-15).

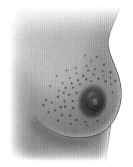

Fig. 18-15. Peau d'orange.

TECHNIQUE 18-2: **Palpating the Female Breasts**

Purpose: To assess for lumps, density of breast tissue, or breast masses
Equipment: Gloves (if needed)

▧ **TIP** Nurses need to be aware that breast tissue is not evenly distributed.

There are several different techniques to assess for lumps. It is important that the nurse has a systematic search pattern to thoroughly assess each breast, the tail of Spence, and axillary lymph nodes.

- **Circular pattern for palpation** starts by palpating the areola first and moving in a circular motion from the areola to the outer perimeter of the breast (Fig. 18-16A).
- **Radial spoke pattern for palpation,** also known as the wedge pattern, divides the breast into wedges; starts at the periphery of the breast and palpates toward the nipple (Fig. 18-16B).
- **Vertical strip pattern for palpation** starts at the sternum palpating up and down in straight lines toward the outer perimeter of the breast, ending up in the axillary area (Fig. 18-16C).

SENC **Safety Alert** If there are any signs of drainage or ulceration, gloves should be worn during palpation.

SENC **Evidence-Based Practice** Several methods have been utilized for clinical breast examination. There is a need to develop a standardized method to improve clinician performance. The vertical strip is the recommended method. The vertical strip method is superior for ensuring that all breast tissue is examined, because it is better for the examiner to track which areas have been examined, and the entire nipple-areolar complex is included (Barton, 1999; Freund, 2000, Breast Cancer.org, 2014).

ASSESSMENT STEPS

1. Explain the technique to the patient.
2. Assist or ask the patient to assume the supine position on the examination table.
3. Ask the patient to take her right arm out of the gown sleeve and raise it above her head, keeping the left breast covered (Fig. 18-17).

   ▓ **TIP** You can place a pillow under the side being assessed to help spread breast tissue.

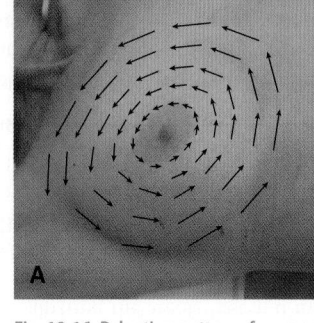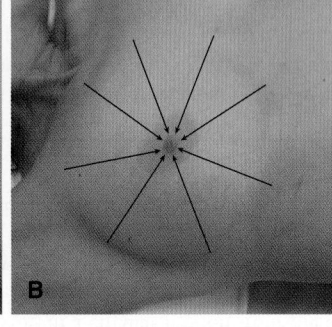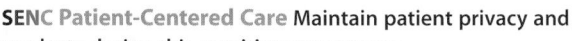

Fig. 18-16. Palpation patterns for assessing breasts. (A) Circular. (B) Radial spoke. (C) Vertical strip.

SENC Patient-Centered Care Maintain patient privacy and modesty during this sensitive assessment.

   ▓ **TIP** The bimanual technique for breast palpation is better to use for a woman with large pendulous breasts (Fig. 18-18).

4. Standing on the patient's right side, using the three finger pads of your dominant hand (Fig. 18-19), palpate the right breast and corresponding axillary area using both light and deep firm circular motions following one of the three methods assessing for:

   ☐ Tissue density
   ☐ Lumps: If a lump, mass, or increased tissue density is palpated, note:
   • shape (round, oval, irregular)
   • consistency (hard, soft, gel-like)
   • location (use a clock face to identify location, i.e., 1 o'clock)
   • size (measured in centimeters)
   • moveable or fixed
   • tenderness.
   ☐ Tenderness or nontender

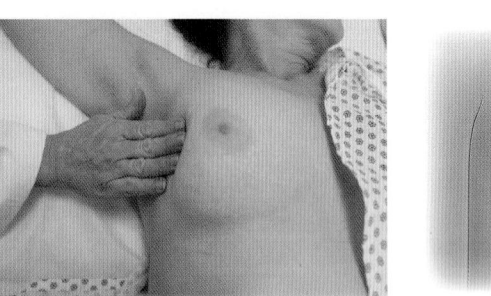

Fig. 18-17. Palpating the breast in supine position with right arm raised over the head.

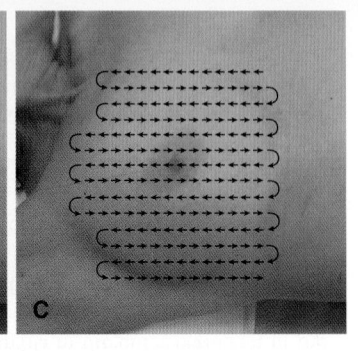

Fig. 18-18. Bimanual technique to palpate pendulous breasts.

TIP Raising the arm permits greater distribution of the breast tissue, allowing for you to examine the breast more evenly.

SENC Safety Alert It is critical to assess all the tissue areas, nipple, and areola so that you do not miss any abnormalities.

5. Assist the patient to put her right hand back in the gown sleeve.

6. Repeat steps 3 through 5 on the left side.

SENC Safety Alert Wear gloves if any past medical history of nipple drainage or reports of nipple drainage.

7. Gently palpate the nipple and compress the nipple and areola between your thumb and index finger to assess for any discharge (Fig. 18-20). If discharge is present, assess the:
- ☐ amount
- ☐ color
- ☐ odor
- ☐ consistency.

8. Document your findings.

NORMAL FINDINGS
- No tenderness, lumps, or increased tissue density
- No nipple discharge
- Firmness in the lower curve of each breast is normal.
- **Nipple discharge** is normally seen in a pregnant woman and one who is breastfeeding an infant.

ABNORMAL FINDINGS
- Tenderness or pain may indicate infection or inflammation.
- Lumps or masses may be benign or cancerous and need further evaluation by the healthcare provider.
- Nipple discharge may need to be sent for diagnostic assessment especially if there is bloody discharge or milky discharge outside the postpartum or non-lactation period.
- **Paget's disease,** a type of breast cancer, may occur in the areola area; the areola is bumpy, persistently itchy, red, or scaly; patient may complain of tingling sensation.

TIP If nipple discharge is present notify the healthcare provider; a sample is usually collected for cytology.

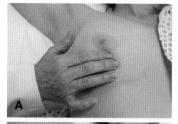

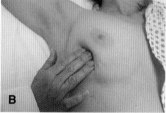

Fig. 18-19. (A) Light palpation. (B) Deep palpation.

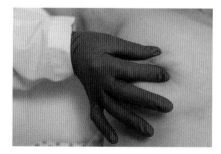

Fig. 18-20. Palpating the nipple.

TECHNIQUE 18-3: Palpating Lymph Nodes

Purpose: To assess for enlarged lymph nodes
Equipment: Gloves

> **SENC Safety Alert** Assessing lymph nodes is very important because breast cancer can metastasize to the lymphatic regions causing swelling and enlarged lymph nodes.

ASSESSMENT STEPS

1. Explain the technique to the patient.
2. Position the patient in a sitting position with her arms down by her sides.
3. Using the three finger pads of your dominant hand, gently palpate the cervical nodes (on the neck), supraclavicular nodes (above the collarbone), and infraclavicular nodes (behind the collarbone) bilaterally using firm circular motions. (See Chapter 15.)
4. Put on gloves.
5. Ask the patient to slightly hold up her right arm. Using the three finger pads of your dominant hand, palpate deeply the following right axillary lymphatic regions using firm circular motions on the skin (Fig. 18-21A). Palpate the four axillary areas and assess for (Fig. 18-21B):
   □ texture of breast tissue (soft or hard)
   □ enlarged lymph nodes
      • singularity or multiple node
      • size of node(s)
      • mobility of nodes (fixed or matted)
      • tenderness or nontender

> **TIP** Lymph nodes are better felt with gentle palpation; it is normal to feel soft and nontender nodes.

7. Repeat step 5 on the left side.
8. Document your findings.

> **TIP** If the patient is in a sitting position, support her arm while palpating the axilla nodes.

NORMAL FINDINGS

■ No swelling, tenderness, or lumps

ABNORMAL FINDINGS

■ Enlarged nodes may indicate infection or breast cancer metastasis.

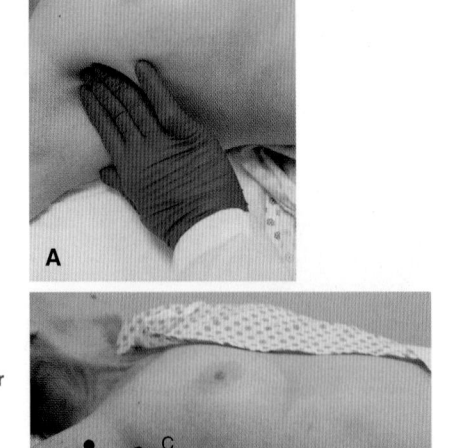

Fig. 18-21. (A) Palpating the right axillary lymph nodes. (B) Four axillary locations.

ADVANCED ASSESSMENTS

The role of registered nurses (RNs) is inspection of the external genitalia. More commonly, the midlevel provider or physician or forensic nurse performs the inspection and palpation of the internal genitalia. Nurses who work in specialty units such as labor and delivery may receive the training needed for internal assessments. Depending on the state board's scope of practice, RNs are allowed to perform speculum pelvic internal examinations on and collect specimens from women. Some states require a special course or training to be completed prior to performing this assessment. It is every nurse's responsibility to know and understand his or her state's legal scope of practice for RNs.

The nurse has the role of preparing and positioning the patient for the examination. The nurse will also be involved in collecting and sending specimens to the lab. It is essential for nurses to be familiar with the techniques and equipment needed for assessing the genitalia. Nurses have the essential role of providing support to the patient during the examination.

SENC Patient-Centered Care It is normal for women to be anxious prior to the examination. Provide comfort and reassurance as needed. Encourage the patient to verbalize any concerns about the examination. Reinforce to the patient that the examination should not be painful. Explain to the patient what she should expect as part of the assessment, and provide reassurance.

Preparation for Examination of External and Internal Genitalia

SENC Safety Alert A woman should not have sexual intercourse, douche, or use vaginal creams or sprays 24 hours prior to an internal examination and Pap smear or vaginal cultures because this can alter the results.

- Ensure privacy.
- Encourage the patient to void prior to the assessment.
- Make sure the examination room is a comfortable temperature.
- Prepare the examination room with all the necessary supplies and equipment.
- While preparing the setup, explain the instruments and encourage the patient to ask questions (Fig. 18-22).

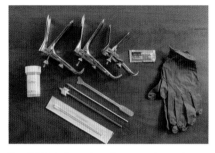

Fig. 18-22. Equipment used to assess internal genitalia.

- Preferably, the examination table should be facing away from the entry door.
- Ask the patient to undress from the waist down, but tell her that she may leave her socks on; provide a gown, draping, and privacy for the patient.
- Tell the patient that she can sit at the end of the examination table until the healthcare provider is ready to perform the assessment; the healthcare provider will assist the patient into the lithotomy position (Fig. 18-23).
- When the healthcare provider is ready to begin, assist the patient into the lithotomy position by having the patient move her buttocks down to the end of the examination table; ask the patient to place the heels of her feet into the stirrups; assist the patient as needed for comfort and safety. Provide a sheet over her legs and knees for privacy until the assessment begins.

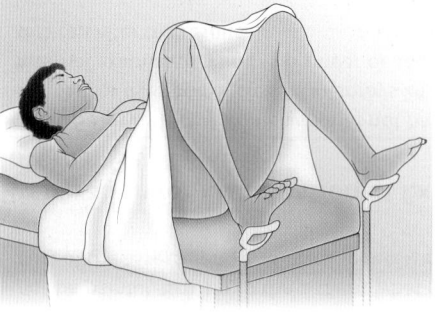

Fig. 18-23. Lithotomy position.

■ **TIP** The stirrups can be cold and un-comfortable, apply covers to the stirrups if available.

■ Patient may be lying flat or in a semi-Fowler's position. A semi-Fowler's position may be preferred as this will allow the patient to make eye contact with the provider.

SENC Safety Alert Nurses need to always be alert to signs of sexual abuse. The woman may have feelings of anxiety, shame, or anger, which may interfere with her ability to make choices that are self-protective. Be alert to signs of injuries, bruising or tears of the external and internal genitalia. If injuries are identified, ask the patient about them in a nonjudgmental way with open-ended questions.

TECHNIQUE 18-4: **Inspecting the Female External Genitalia**

Purpose: To assess for inflammation, lumps, lesions, or abnormalities.

Equipment: Light source, handheld mirror (optional)

SENC Safety Alert STIs present with symptoms of drainage, lesions, or warts. You should be aware of the different presentations of STIs (see Chapter 19).

ASSESSMENT STEPS

1. Explain the technique to the patient.

2. Show and demonstrate the instruments that will be used for the procedure and offer the use of a mirror to explain findings.

3. Prepare all slides and specimen container for use with patient's name and date.

4. Fully drape the patient and assist the patient to be in the lithotomy position; assist the patient to place her feet in the stirrups; ask the patient if she is comfortable.

5. Offer the patient a mirror to also observe the examination.

SENC Patient-Centered Care Offering a mirror to the patient will encourage the patient to see her external genitalia; encourage her to ask questions and use this time as a teaching moment.

6. Position stool and light source so that good visualization can occur.

7. Make sure the patient is able to voice any concerns or discomfort; let the patient be able to see you during the examination so that you can make eye contact with the patient; this helps to alleviate fear and anxiety.

8. Perform hand hygiene and put on gloves.

9. Talk to the patient as you are performing the steps of the assessment.

10. Inspect the skin color of the labia majora and minora.

11. Inspect the following external genitalia for redness, swelling, or lesions:
    □ Mons pubis
    □ Labia majora
    □ Labia minora
    □ Perineum for hair distribution

12. Using your dominant gloved hand, gently separate the labia majora to inspect the urethral meatus for developmental abnormalities, discharge, lesions, warts, and abscess (Fig. 18-24).

13. Inspect the clitoris and vestibule for size, color, presence of lesions, and discoloration or masses.

14. Inspect the perineum of swelling, ulcers, condylomata (warts), or changes in colors.

15. Inspect urethral meatus for position.

16. Inspect the vaginal orifice for discharge, protrusion of the walls, and condition of the hymen.

17. Inspect the perineum and anus for color and shape.

18. Remove and discard gloves.

19. Document your findings.

SENC Safety Alert Be alert to signs of infection for patients who have external genitalia piercings.

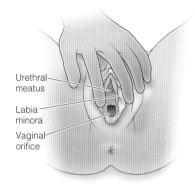

Fig. 18-24. Inspecting the urethral meatus while separating the labia majora.

NORMAL FINDINGS
- Labia majora and labia minora are uniform color, symmetrical, wrinkled skin; may have nontender, yellow, sebaceous cysts that are less than 1cm in diameter.
- Skin over mons pubis is smooth with even hair distribution.
- Pubic hair is evenly distributed and shaped like an inverse triangle; no lice or nits.
- Clitoris is approximately 1.5 to 2.0 cm long.
- Urethra is a slit-like opening; midline; no swelling, redness, or discharge.
- Bartholin's glands are at 4 and 8 o'clock; no redness or inflammation.
- Skene's glands are at 1 and 11 o'clock; no redness or inflammation.
- Perineum is smooth and skin color is uniform; if present, episiotomy scar is healed without inflammation.
- Anus is dark brown; puckering of skin; no swelling, inflammation, or protrusions.

ABNORMAL FINDINGS

- Labia majora and labia minora are bruised, swollen, inflamed, have lesions or lumps, a rash, or warts.
- No pubic hair or sparse pubic hair may be related to aging, endocrine disease, nutritional deficiencies, or genetic factors.
- **Pediculosis pubis** is the presence of lice or nits.
- Urethra is swollen, red, or inflamed; discharge is present.
- **Urethra caruncle** is benign fleshy outgrowths at the urethral meatus; most common lesion of the female urethra, occurring primarily in postmenopausal women (Rickley, 2012).
- Fungal infections, candidiasis, or yeast infections commonly occur in the groin areas and external genitalia.
- Perineum is with a tear, redness, or fissure; if present, episiotomy is red and inflamed.
- Hemorrhoids are venous protrusions of dilated veins; may be inflamed, red, and swollen.

PATIENT EDUCATION

Women's health care has had some controversial recommendations. Essential health assessments may vary depending on healthcare provider preference, the patient's age, family history, risk factors, and personal preference. Women should never be shy or afraid to discuss their health and preventative screenings with their healthcare provider.

Breast Self-Examination

Breast cancer is the most commonly diagnosed cancer in women in the United States, and the second leading cause of death from cancer in American women. Breast cancer mortality can be effectively reduced through screening and awareness (ACOG, 2016). Teaching breast self-awareness and breast self-exam can save lives. Women should be alert to breast self awareness: knowing what is the normal look and feel of their breasts. Breast self-exam (BSE) is a step-by-step approach a woman can use to look at and feel her breasts (SusanGKomen.org, 2017). Nurses are on the front lines to spread the word and make a difference. Reinforce to each woman that most breast problems or changes are benign. Early detection of breast cancer can greatly improve a woman's chance to survive. In recent years, controversy exists about the value of BSE and whether it reduces mortality rates in women. Recommendations include:

- The USPSTF (2016) recommends against teaching breast self-examination (BSE).
- The National Breast Cancer Foundation (2016) recommends adult women of all ages to perform breast self-exams at least once a month.
- The American Cancer Society (2015) does not recommend routine breast self-examination (BSE), neither do they recommend against routine BSE. A woman may choose to perform regular BSE or occasional BSE, or she may choose to not perform BSE at all.
- Women should be told about benefits and limitations of BSE. They should report any new symptoms to their healthcare provider.

  It is essential that nurses feel comfortable with their own knowledge of BSE to share it with a patient. Nurses should:

- assess the patient's understanding of breast self-awareness
- assess the patient's understanding of breast self-exam
- assess how and when the patient is doing BSE.

Encourage women to conduct a BSE regularly so they know how their breasts look and feel. Since the vertical strip palpation method is preferred, show the patient a picture of this method and simulate on a breast model. Pamphlets are available from many organizations.

SENC Safety Alert Women who have had a mastectomy (removal of the breast) should continue to perform BSE. Instruct the woman to begin her assessment on the unaffected side and then do incisional BSE.

Teaching Points for Breast Self-Examination

- The best time to perform a BSE is 7 to 9 days after menses, when the breasts are least likely to be swollen or tender due to hormonal changes.
- Pregnant women and menopausal women should identify a day each month to do BSE. The key is to remember to do the examination regularly.

There are several positions in which a woman can perform BSE:

- Standing in front of a mirror
- Standing while taking a shower
- Lying down on a flat surface such as a bed

TIP Explain to the patient that lying down on a flat surface with a pillow under the side being examined helps to spread the breast tissue evenly over the chest wall.

Mammograms

Nurses need to educate women about the importance of having screening mammograms. The American Cancer Society (ACS, 2016) recommends the current guidelines for women at average risk for breast cancer to have a mammogram:

- Women ages 40 to 44 should have the choice to start annual breast cancer screening with mammograms if they wish to do so.
- Women age 45 to 54 should get mammograms every year.
- Women 55 and older should switch to mammograms every 2 years, or can continue yearly screening.
- Screening should continue as long as a woman is in good health and is expected to live 10 more years or longer.

- All women should be familiar with the known benefits, limitations, and potential harms linked to breast cancer screening.

The U.S. Preventive Services Task Force (2016) recommends:

- Biennial screening mammography for women aged 50 to 74 years.
- Women 40 to 49 years: The decision to start screening mammography in women prior to age 50 years should be an individual one. Women who place a higher value on the potential benefit than the potential harms may choose to begin biennial screening between the ages of 40 and 49 years.

Clinical Breast Examinations

The American College of Obstetricians and Gynecologists (ACOG) recommends a clinical breast exam every year for women aged 19 or older (ACOG, 2015). Expert opinion suggests that the value of clinical breast examination and the ideal time to start such examinations is influenced by the patient's age and known risk factors for breast cancer (ACOG, 2012).

Routine Gynecological Examinations

ACOG (2015) recommends that the first visit to the obstetrician-gynecologist for screening and the provision of preventive healthcare services and guidance take place between the ages of 13 and 15 years. ACOG (2015) continues to recommend routine pelvic examinations as part of an annual well-woman visit starting at age 21.

Human Papillomavirus

The HPV is a group of more than 150 related viruses that can cause infection and genital warts and lead to cancer, especially cervical cancer. There are some HPV strains that do not cause symptoms. HPV is the most common sexually transmitted virus in the United States. Vaccination against HPV is the best method for preventing HPV-related diseases, including cervical cancers and genital warts (Sanslow, 2016). The current recommendation is for all females (and males) ages 9 to 26 to receive the HPV vaccine (Sanslow, 2016). Vaccination over the age of 26 is less effective in reducing HPV-related diseases and therefore not recommended (Sanslow, 2016).

Cervical Cancer Screening

The latest recommendations from ACS (2015b) for cervical cancer screenings are as follows:

- All women should begin cervical cancer screening at age 21.
- Women aged 21 to 29, should have a Pap test every 3 years. HPV testing should not be used for screening in this age group. (It may be used as part of follow-up for an abnormal Pap test.)
- Women between the ages of 30 and 65 should have both a Pap test and an HPV test every 5 years. This is the preferred approach, but it is also all right to have a Pap test alone every 3 years.
- Women over age 65 who have had regular screenings with normal results should not be screened for cervical cancer. Women who have been diagnosed with cervical pre-cancer should continue to be screened for at least 20 years.

Sexually Transmitted Infections

- The CDC (2015f) recommends that all sexually active women age 25 and younger be regularly screened for chlamydia and gonorrhea. Women over age 26 should be screened for chlamydia and gonorrhea annually if they have multiple sexual partners or if their partner has multiple sexual contacts.
- CDC (2015g) encourages HIV testing, at least once, as a routine part of medical care if the patient is an adolescent or adult between the ages of 13 and 64.
  - □ Educate patients on prevention of STIs.
  - □ Limit activity to one mutually monogamous uninfected partner.
  - □ Encourage use of condom or other barrier devices with oral, vaginal, and anal sexual activity.
  - □ Avoid sexual activity with multiple partners or with individuals with multiple partners.
- Avoid sexual activity with partners who use intravenous (IV) drugs.
- Have HIV test if you have had unprotect sex in the past or have used IV drugs or have intercourse with someone who is HIV positive, or they use IV drugs.

Hepatitis

Hepatitis viruses are the most common cause of hepatitis in the world, but other infections and autoimmune diseases, toxic substances (e.g., alcohol, certain drugs), contaminated food and water, infected blood, semen, and other body fluids can also cause hepatitis (WHO, 2015). There are five hepatitis viruses, A, B, C, D, and E. Patients should be educated about the causes and availability and benefits of vaccinations. Detailed information about hepatitis can be found on the WHO website (http://www.who.int/features/qa/76/en/).

Menopause

Menopause is a normal part of life, and women need to have accurate information about what to expect. Women who have the knowledge about this period of their life will know what to expect and understand related menopausal symptoms. Encourage women to:

- stay healthy and maintain a healthy weight
- exercise at least 150 minutes per week; weight-bearing exercises such as running and using weights are highly recommended
- eat a diet rich in calcium and vitamin D
- limit alcohol intake
- stop smoking
- discuss with the nurse or healthcare provider symptoms of concern.

TIP Women who smoke seem to go through menopause 1½ to 2 years earlier than women who do not smoke (National Institute on Aging, 2015).

INTRODUCTION

Reproductive and genitourinary health are sensitive topics to discuss and areas to examine. Men and women have their own unique perception of health, which is influenced by personal perception and receptivity of health assessment. There is strong evidence that on many health measures men are doing significantly worse than women, including lower life expectancy and increased cardiovascular mortality, rate of injury, depression, and suicide (Karoski, 2011). Women's health has been recognized as a nursing specialty, and the time has come to focus on the health needs of men. Men are less likely to visit a doctor, get regular preventative checkups, or live healthier lifestyles (Spar, 2014). Nurses can make a difference to help increase the awareness of men's health and health promotion. The male assessment requires essential assessment of the breasts and reproductive and genitourinary systems.

REVIEW OF ANATOMY AND PHYSIOLOGY

Male Breasts

- Extend from the second through sixth anterior ribs with the sternum as the medial border and the mid-axillary line being the endpoint laterally (Fig. 19-1)
- Consist of fibrous, glandular, and fatty tissue
- The male hormone, testosterone, inhibits the development and growth of breast tissue in males.
- Average diameter of a male areola is 1 inch.

Penis

- Composed of three parts (Fig. 19-2):
  - □ The root (radix) is attached to the abdominal wall and to the perineum.
  - □ The body, or shaft, is the middle portion; contains vascular erectile tissue; during an erection, the vascular tissue becomes engorged.
  - □ Glans penis is the cone-shaped head of the penis; the foreskin (prepuce) is loose skin that covers the glans penis; if a patient is circumcised, the foreskin is surgically removed (Fig. 19-3); this tip of the penis has nerve endings and is very sensitive; involved in sexual arousal.
- Urethral meatus is at the tip of the glans penis.

TIP Circumcision is one of the oldest and most controversial surgical procedures (Puri, Kumar, & Ramesh, 2010). Circumcision is performed for a variety of religious and cultural reasons. Male circumcision reduces the risk that a man will acquire HIV from a HIV-positive female partner, and also lowers the risk of other sexually transmitted infections (STIs), penile cancer, and urinary tract infections (CDC, 2012; WHO, 2016).

Scrotum

- Located at the base of the penis; covered with loose and wrinkled skin called rugae.
- The scrotum contains the following: a testicle on each side, epididymis, and parts of the spermatic cord.
- Cutaneous, fibromuscular sac containing the testes and lower parts of the spermatic cord has sebaceous glands, sweat glands, and nerve endings
- The scrotum acts as a climate control system, allowing the testicles to be slightly away from the rest of the body and keeping them slightly cooler than normal body temperature for optimal sperm development (Leslie, 2012).

Testes (Testicles)

- Right and left testes (testicles); each are oval shaped and feel soft and rubbery.
- Primary male reproductive organs responsible for sperm and testosterone production
- Spermatogenesis is the process of mature sperm development through cell divisions to produce spermatozoa.
- Left testis (testicle) lies lower than the right testis because the left spermatic cord is longer.

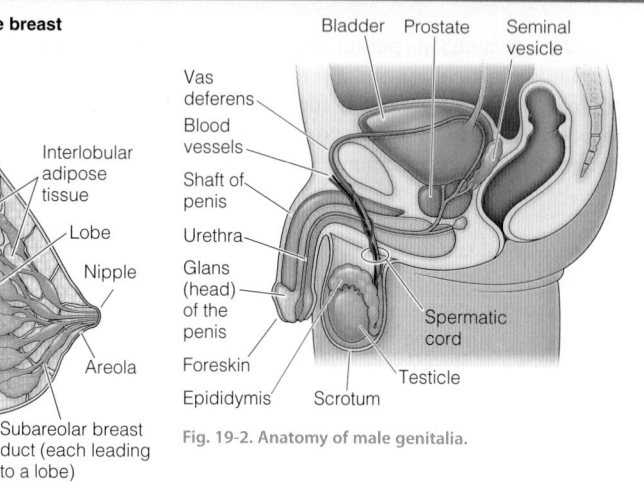

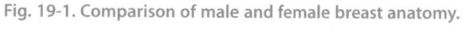

Fig. 19-1. Comparison of male and female breast anatomy.

Fig. 19-2. Anatomy of male genitalia.

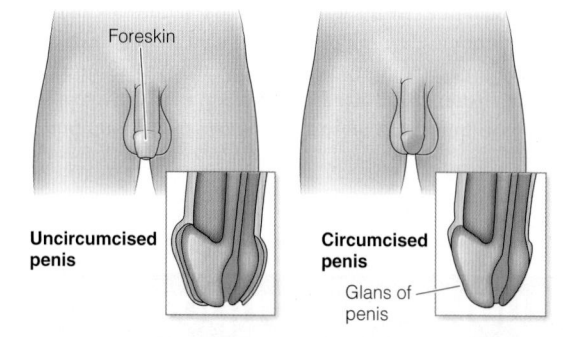

Fig. 19-3. Uncircumcised versus circumcised penis.

Epididymis
- Located on top and behind each testis
- Collection area for mature sperm

Spermatic Cord
- Suspends the testis in the scrotum
- Left cord is slightly longer than the right.
- Contains the vas deferens, testicular artery and veins

Vas Deferens
- Connects the testes with the urethra
- Stores and transports sperm through the epididymis
- Muscle contractions propel sperm into the ejaculatory duct and out through the urethra.

Seminal Vesicles
- Located behind the bladder and prostrate; approximately 5 cm long
- Transport sperm from the testes to the seminal vesicles
- Add fluid to semen during ejaculation

Urethra
- Passageway for urine to flow
- Transports semen during sexual intercourse

Prostate Gland
- Doughnut-shaped gland about the size of a walnut located between the bladder and the rectum
- Contains 15 to 20 branched, tubular glands which form lobules
- Secretes a viscid, alkaline fluid, which aids in sperm motility and in neutralizing the acidity of the vagina, thus enhancing fertilization (Bock, 2014).

DIAGNOSTICS
- **Prostate-specific antigen (PSA)** test is a blood test that measures the amount of PSA, a protein secreted by prostate epithelial cells; used as a biological marker for prostate cancer (Miller, 2013).
- **Prostate biopsy** procedure removes a sample of body tissue for examination under a microscope; a core needle biopsy is the main method used to diagnose prostate cancer; it is usually done by an urologist, a surgeon who treats cancers of the genital and urinary tract, which includes the prostate gland (ACS, 2015a).
- **Urethral specimens** are obtained in men with penile discharge; the specimen identifies the organisms causing the symptoms; commonly collected for sexually transmitted diseases such as gonorrhea or chlamydia.

HEALTH HISTORY

Review of Systems
Assessing the male reproductive and genitourinary system provides essential subjective data to identify risk factors, potential or actual health problems, and areas of health promotion. Using open-ended and direct, focused questions facilitates a thorough history. A gender-specific health history assesses sensitive topics that may be embarrassing or uncomfortable for the patient. Male patients may not feel comfortable discussing male symptoms or concerns with a female nurse and may request a male nurse (if available).

The history for the male assessment focuses on different types of cancers prevalent in men, healthcare practices, and symptoms. See Table 19-1 for risk factors for some of the more common types of cancers prevalent in males.

TABLE 19-1 Risk Factors for Male Cancers

Testicular Cancer	Family history
	Undescended testicle
	Men infected with HIV and AIDs
	Body size – tall men (ACS, 2016g)
Penile Cancer	Not being circumcised
	HPV infection
	Phimosis
	Smoking
	Advancing age
	Ultraviolet light treatment for psoriasis (ACS, 2016i)
Prostate Cancer	Men older than 50 years
	Family history (ACS, 2016f)
Male Breast Cancer	Advancing age
	Exposure to radiation prior to age 30
	High estrogen levels
	Family history of breast cancer
	Inherited gene mutation (*BRCA1, BRCA2*)
	Klinefelter syndrome
	Alcohol
	Testicular conditions
	(ACS, 2016h; Breastcancer.org, 2016)

Use the OLDCARTS (**O**nset, **L**ocation, **D**uration, **C**haracteristics, **A**ggravating/Alleviating factors, **R**elieving factors, **T**reatment, **S**everity) mnemonic to identify attributes of a symptom. Ask the patient the following questions.

Family History

■ Do you have any family history of the following cancers?

☐ **Bladder:** bladder cancer is the fourth most common cancer in men; the most common signs or symptoms include blood in the urine (hematuria), dysuria, and frequency of urination.

☐ **Breast:** male breast cancer is uncommon in men under the age of 35, but men do get breast cancer; men have breast tissue and low levels of the estrogen hormone: breast cancer is about 100 times less common among men than among women (ACS, 2016a).

☐ **Kidney:** kidney cancer is found about twice as often in men as in women; Caucasian men have double the risk of African-American men (Simon, 2011). Men are more likely to be smokers and are more likely to be exposed to cancer-causing chemicals at work, which may account for some of the difference (ACS, 2016b). The most common symptom is painless hematuria (blood in the urine).

☐ **Penis:** penile cancer is rare in North America and Europe; accounts for less than 1% percent of cancers in men living in the United States; more common in men living in parts of Asia, Africa, and South America (ACA, 2016c). The most common symptom is a change in the color or texture of the skin on the penis.

☐ **Prostate:** prostate cancer is one of the most common cancers among men (after skin cancer). Signs and symptoms include:
• difficulty or frequency urinating
• hematuria
• impotence (inability to have an erection)
• early prostate cancer may have no symptoms.

☐ **Testicular:** testicular cancer can develop in one or both testicles or scrotum. This cancer is more common in young and middle aged men; the average age at time of diagnosis is 33; Caucasian men have the highest risk. Worldwide, the risk of developing this disease is highest among men living in the United States and Europe and lowest among men living in Africa or Asia (ACS, 2016d). Signs and symptoms include:
• painless lump
• swelling
• pain.

Military History

In 2015, the U.S. Census Bureau reported 20.3 million male veterans in the United States (U.S. Census Bureau, 2015). Combat veterans experiencing traumatic events of the war are at higher risk for post-traumatic stress disorder (PTSD) (Gough & Robertson, 2010) or a new syndrome called post-deployment syndrome (PDS) (Cifu & Blake, 2015). These are illnesses of war that may have unexplained symptoms (Box 19-1, Box 19-2). The symptoms may be gradually present within months of returning home or may take years. These veterans may be at greater risk for substance abuse disorders or major depressive disorder. Symptoms of major depressive disorder may include:

- anorexia
- chronic fatigue
- chronic aches and pains
- insomnia
- inability to work
- loss of interest in activities, including sex
- being persistently sad, anxious, or irritable
- suicidal thoughts.

When assessing veterans, it is important for nurses to remember that each war comes with its own set of health risks.

SENC Safety Alert More men die by suicide than women. In high-income countries, three times as many men die by suicide than women. Men aged 50 years and over are particularly vulnerable (WHO, 2015).

Past Medical and Surgical History

- Do you have a past medical or surgical history of conditions related to the kidneys, bladder, rectum, or the genital area?
  - □ STIs are caused by bacteria and viruses; the six most common in men are:
    1. **Gonorrhea** is caused by gram-negative diplococcus *Neisseria gonorrhoeae* causing inflammation of the urethra, prostate, rectum, and/or pharynx in men; most common symptom in men is a yellow mucopurulent penile discharge.
    2. **Chlamydia** is an STI caused by a bacterium *Chlamydia trachomatis;* most common symptom in men is penile discharge and dysuria, pain with urination.

TIP One in four men with chlamydia has no symptoms; chlamydia is the most common STI.

BOX 19-1 Symptoms of Post-Traumatic Stress Disorder

- Pain
- Having nightmares, vivid memories, or flashbacks
- Feeling emotionally cut off from others
- Feeling numb or losing interest in things you used to care about
- Becoming depressed, anxious, jittery, or irritated
- Having difficulty sleeping
- Experiencing a sense of panic that something bad is about to happen
- Having difficulty concentrating/memory problems
- Having a hard time relating to and getting along with spouse, family, and friends

U.S. Department of Veteran Affairs, Make the Connection, PTSD, 2015.

BOX 19-2 Post-Deployment Syndrome

- Chronic unexplained symptoms
- Chronic pain
- Fatigue
- Traumatic brain injury
- Post-traumatic stress disorder symptoms
- General anxiety disorder

Data from Cifu, D. X., & Blake, C. (2011). *Overcoming post-deployment syndrome: A six-step mission to health.* New York: Demos Medical Publishing.

---

3. **Genital herpes** is an STI caused by herpes simplex viruses type 1 (HSV-1) or type 2 (HSV-2); painful fluid-filled blisters or vesicles form anywhere on the male genitalia or rectum.

4. **Human papillomavirus** (HPV) is an STI caused by the human papillomavirus; there are over 40 different types of HPV that are sexually transmitted (CDC, 2014); men may not have symptoms; some may cause genital warts.

5. **Human immunodeficiency virus** (HIV) is an STI viral infection caused by a retrovirus causing general flu-like symptoms in the early stages; the virus destroys the cells of the immune system and progresses and causes the acquired immunodeficiency syndrome (AIDS).

6. **Syphilis** is an STI caused by the spirochete *Treponema pallidum*; syphilis progresses through four different stages; the initial symptom is a sore called a "chancre" (Venes, 2013).

Medications

■ What prescriptive, herbal, and over-the-counter medications are you currently taking?
   □ Medications have side effects; certain medications can contribute to sexual dysfunction or impotence; testosterone, a steroid hormone, may be given to men with low testosterone levels.

Health Promotion

■ Do you perform testicular self-examinations? If so, how often?
   □ Most testicular cancers are found by the patient either unintentionally, through self-examination, or routine physical examination.

SENC Patient-Centered Care Therapeutic communication skills are needed to discuss sensitive health promotion recommendations.

SENC Evidence-Based Practice The sensitivity and specificity of routine screening of asymptomatic men for testicular cancer are not known; USPSTF (2011) recommends against screening for testicular cancer in adolescent or adult men.

□ The ACS recommends a testicular examination by a doctor as part of a routine cancer-related checkup; ACS does not have a recommendation about regular testicular self-examinations for all men (ACS, 2015a).
□ The most common symptom of testicular cancer is a painless testicular mass.
□ Young men may have the "Superman complex" where they feel nothing can hurt them and they do not need to go see a doctor (Cancer Survivor, Carl Olsen, 2012); men may also take the "it'll never happen to me" approach (Martinez, 2014).

■ **TIP** Testicular cancer is rare but the most common cancer in men younger than age 35.

■ Have you had prostate cancer screening?
   □ Many states have laws assuring that private health insurers cover procedures to detect prostate cancer, including the prostate-specific antigen (PSA) test and the digital rectal examination (DRE). Some of these states also assure that public employee benefit health plans provide coverage for prostate cancer screening procedures. Most state laws assure annual coverage for men ages 50 and over and for high-risk men, ages 40 and over (African-American men and/or men with a family history of prostate cancer) (ACS, 2015b).

Safety

■ Do you wear protective equipment when playing sports?
   □ Protection of the male genitalia during sports is important to prevent permanent damage or impotence.

Pain

- Are you experiencing any pain or burning during urination?
  - □ **Dysuria** is pain and difficulty with urination; usually described as a "burning" quality; may indicate infection or inflammation of the lower urinary tract.
  - □ **Bladder pain** may indicate cystitis, inflammation of the bladder due to infection.
- Do you have any back pain (costovertebral pain)?
  - □ **Back pain** elicited by costovertebral tenderness may indicate inflammation of the kidneys or possibly the presence of kidney stones.
- Do you experience any pain or discomfort in your scrotum?
  - □ **Testicular pain** may be related to trauma, infection, or cancer; testicular torsion occurs when the testicle twists inside the scrotum, decreasing the blood flow to the testicle and causing severe pain in the scrotum; this is a surgical emergency.
- Do you have any groin (inguinal) pain?
  - □ **Inguinal pain** may be related to an inguinal hernia; part of the intestine protrudes through the abdominal wall; more evident if the patient coughs, bends over, or lifts a heavy object exerting intra-abdominal pressure.

Urinary Symptoms

- Do you have difficulty starting the stream of urination?
- Do you experience hesitancy of urination?
- Do you feel that you do not completely empty your bladder (urinary retention)?
- Do you experience frequency of urination?
  - □ **Benign prostatic hypertrophy (BPH)** is a nonmalignant enlargement of the prostate gland as part of the aging process; BPH occurs only in men; approximately 8 percent of men aged 31 to 40 have BPH. In men over age 80, more than 80 percent have BPH (Cunningham & Kadmon, 2011).

Penile Lesions or Discharge

- Have you developed any sores or lesions on your penis?
  - □ Lesions or sores may be indicative of a bacterial or viral infection.
  - □ Have you had any discharge from your penis? When did it start? Ask about the:
    - color of discharge
    - amount of discharge
    - consistency of discharge
    - odor of discharge
  - □ A symptom of some STIs is penile discharge:
    - Gonorrhea: yellow, white, green
    - Chlamydia: a white or cloudy discharge from penis and rectum
    - Urethritis: clear and white

Scrotum

- Have you had any swelling or enlargement of the scrotum?
  - □ The scrotum may become swollen, filled with fluid, or enlarged; this may be caused by inflammation of internal structures, masses, and medical conditions such as congestive heart failure.
  - □ **Hydrocele** is an accumulation of fluid around the testes (Fig. 19-4).
  - □ **Epididymitis** is swelling and inflammation of the epididymis (Fig. 19-4); may be related to a STI.

Sexual Health

Healthy People 2020

Goal: Improve the health, safety, and well-being of lesbian, gay, bisexual, and transgender individuals (HHS, 2010). Sexual health is a fundamental part of our being. During healthcare encounters, patients often hide sexual problems, sometimes presenting to healthcare professionals with some "other" issue because that is more comfortable for them (French, 2010).

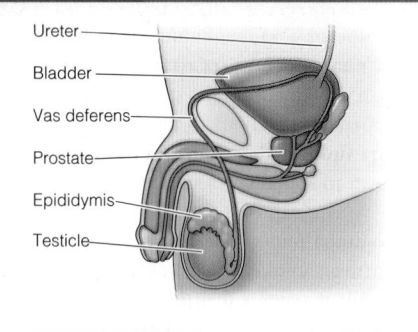

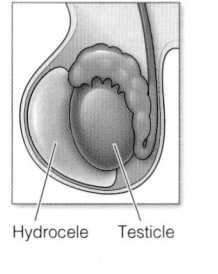 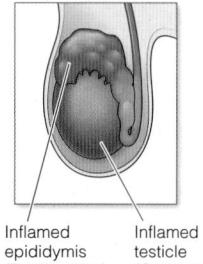

Fig. 19-4. Hydrocele and epididymitis.

The WHO (2014) has defined sexual health as:

- a state of physical, mental, and social well-being in relation to sexuality
- it requires a positive and respectful approach to sexuality and sexual relationships, as well as the possibility of having pleasurable and safe sexual experiences, free of coercion, discrimination, and violence.

SENC Safety Alert Unprotected sex places any patient at high risk for bacterial or viral STIs; do not miss this opportunity to educate the patient while performing the health history.

TIP The best time to discuss sexual health is toward the end of the assessment; this gives you and the patient time to build a relationship and rapport. Assure the patient that this information will remain confidential.

SENC Patient-Centered Care The topic of sexuality may create anxiety for both the patient and the nurse. A genuine presence is critical during this discussion. Patients sometimes hide sexual problems, and present other symptoms or concerns because it is more comfortable for them. Patients may not identify their sexual orientation until a trusting relationship has been established. Nurses must provide holistic patient care, establish a therapeutic relationship, and realize that sexual health is just another aspect of a patient's health and well-being (French, 2010).

Sexual history includes the four Ps (partners, practices, protection, past STIs) as a general guide.

- **Partners**
  - ☐ Are you in a relationship?
  - ☐ Are you satisfied with your sex life?
  - ☐ Do you have sexual relationships with women, men, or both?
    - Heterosexual is a person who has sexual orientation to a person of the opposite sex.
    - Homosexual is a person who has sexual orientation to a person of the same sex.
    - Bisexual is a person who has sexual orientation both to a person of the same and also of the opposite sex.

TIP Gender refers to the socially constructed roles, behaviors, activities, and attributes that a given society considers appropriate for boys and men, or girls and women. Gender identity refers to a person's internal sense of being male or female (APA, 2015).

- Transgender is a gender identity disorder (GID) and is used to describe someone who was assigned female or male at birth, but later realizes that label does not accurately reflect who the person feels he or she is inside (Lesbian and Gay Community Services Center, Inc., 2015).

□ Do you have several partners?

■ **Practices**

□ What types of sexual practices do you engage in?
  • Types of sexual practice include:
    • oral sex
    • penile-vaginal sex
    • penile-rectal sex

■ **Protection**

□ What types of precautions or protection do you use during sexual activity?
  • Latex condoms, when used consistently and correctly, are highly effective in preventing the sexual transmission of HIV and reduce the risk of other sexually transmitted diseases (STDs). Condom use may reduce the risk for genital HPV infection and HPV-associated diseases such as genital warts and cervical cancer in women (CDC, 2015a).

□ Have you had the hepatitis A or B immunizations?
  • Men who have sex with other men are at higher risk for contracting hepatitis A, hepatitis B, and although uncommon, hepatitis C (CDC, 2013a).

TIP There is no vaccine for hepatitis C, and testing for hepatitis C is not recommended for men who have sex with men (MSM) unless they were born from 1945 through 1965, have HIV, or are engaging in risky behaviors (CDC, 2015b).

■ **Past STIs**

□ Do you have a past history of STIs? If so, were you treated and when?

□ Do you have any concerns about having HIV?

■ **Erectile dysfunction (ED)**

□ Are you able to achieve or maintain an erection?

□ How long have these symptoms been present? Did they begin gradually or suddenly?
  • ED is when a man has trouble getting or keeping an erection.
  • ED becomes more common as men get older.
  • ED is not a natural part of aging.
  • Risk factors for ED include side effects of some medications.
  • ED is strongly linked to a number of other common diseases in men, such as diabetes, heart disease, high blood pressure, high cholesterol, vascular disease, neurologic conditions, chronic liver or kidney disease (Sexual Medicine Society of North America, 2016).

CULTURAL CONSIDERATIONS Cultural and racial considerations may place restrictions on discussing sexual issues. Certain cultures may only allow same-gender healthcare providers to perform their assessment. For example, Hispanics value modesty; the nurse should recognize that the area between the waist and knees is considered particularly private (Dayer-Berenson, 2011).

• The risk of testicular cancer among Caucasian men is about five times higher than that of African-American men and more than three times greater than that of Asian-American and American-Indian men (ACS, 2016d).

• Prostate cancer occurs more often in African-American men than in men of other races. African-American men are also more likely to be diagnosed at an advanced stage, and are more than twice as likely to die of prostate cancer as Caucasian men. Prostate cancer occurs less often in Asian-American and Hispanic/Latino men than in non-Hispanic whites (ACS, 2016e).

• Male breast cancer is more common among African-American men (American Society of Clinical Oncology, 2014).

• Renal cell carcinoma is the most frequently occurring kidney cancer in adults; risk factors include being a male and smoking (Story, 2012). Bladder cancer is more common in Caucasian men.

PREPARATION FOR ASSESSMENT

Equipment Needed
Gloves

Sequence of Assessment
1. Inspecting and palpating the male breasts
2. Inspecting the male genitalia

Preliminary Steps
- Reassure the patient that confidentiality will be maintained during the examination of the male genitalia.
- Ensure adequate lighting.
- Ensure privacy for the interview and examination.
- Provide a warm and comfortable room.
- Encourage the patient to empty his bladder.
- Expose only the area being assessed.
- Perform hand hygiene.

FOCUSED ASSESSMENT

TECHNIQUE 19-1: **Inspecting and Palpating the Male Breasts**

Purpose: To assess for lumps, nipple discharge or abnormalities

ASSESSMENT STEPS
1. Explain the technique to the patient.
2. With the patient lying in the supine position, inspect the male breasts for (Fig. 19-5A):
   - ☐ symmetry
   - ☐ color
   - ☐ contour (dimpling or retraction)
   - ☐ edema
   - ☐ lesions
   - ☐ ulcerations
   - ☐ texture of skin.
3. Inspect the areola for:
   - ☐ shape
   - ☐ color.

4. Inspect the nipples for:
- ☐ size
- ☐ position
- ☐ shape
- ☐ discharge
- ☐ scaling or crusting.

5. Ask the patient to raise his arms over his head and inspect the lateral aspect of the breasts toward the mid-axillary line for skin changes (Fig. 19-5B).

6. Gently palpate each breast and axillary area using the finger pads of your second, third, and fourth fingers using the vertical strip pattern assessment technique, assessing for lumps or masses (Fig. 19-6).

▧ **TIP** The most common presentation of male breast cancer is a painless, palpable, subareolar lump or mass (Block & Muradali, 2013).

- ☐ Palpate any lump or mass and note:
  - • Shape
  - • Size
  - • Consistency (hard, soft, or rubbery)
  - • Mobility (mobile or immobile)
  - • Location (document by using clock method)

7. Put on gloves and palpate each areola area.

8. Gently palpate and press each side of the nipple at the base noting any discharge; if discharge is present, assess (Fig. 19-7):
- ☐ color
- ☐ consistency
- ☐ odor.

9. Remove and discard gloves.

10. Document your findings.

NORMAL FINDINGS
- ▪ Breasts are symmetric.
- ▪ Skin has even color.

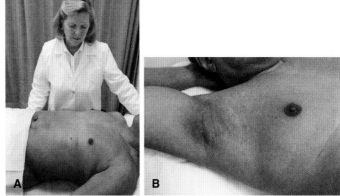

Fig. 19-5. (A) Inspecting the male breasts. (B) Inspecting the lateral aspect.

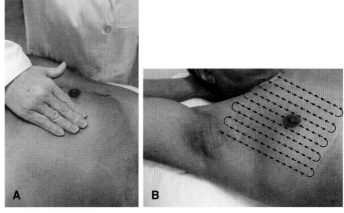

Fig. 19-6. (A) Palpating the male breasts. (B) Vertical strip pattern.

- There are no lesions, dimpling, or puckering.
- There are no lumps or masses.
- Axillary area has no lumps or masses.
- Areola is smooth, has uniform color, and is without skin changes.
- Nipple is everted, skin intact, and without drainage.

ABNORMAL FINDINGS

- Lump or mass is palpated.
- **Gynecomastia** is enlarged or overdeveloped fibroglandular breast tissue; term comes from the Greek words *gyne* meaning "woman" and *mastos* meaning "breast"; may be related to decreased testosterone levels in the aging male or a medication side effect; frequently associated with devastating social and emotional trauma; 60 percent of males worldwide have some degree of gynecomastia (http://www.gynecomastia.org/gynecomastia-men).
- Breast cancer may present as a hard painless lump, erythema of the skin, scaling of the nipple, or nipple discharge (Fig. 19-8).

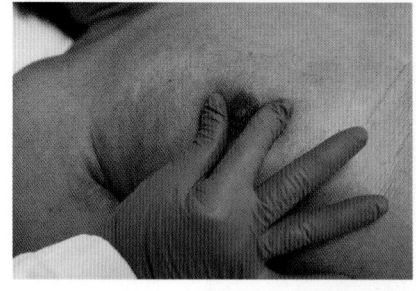

Fig. 19-7. Palpate nipple.

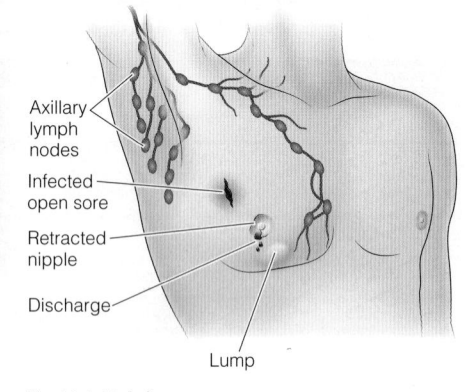

Fig. 19-8. Male breast cancer.

TECHNIQUE 19-2: **Inspecting the External Genitalia**

Purpose: To assess the external male genitalia for lesions, edema, and masses
Equipment: Gloves, tangential lighting

SENC Patient-Centered Care Inspecting the genitalia may be embarrassing for the patient; male patients are sensitive and very aware of nonverbal body language; always be professional and objective throughout the assessment.

ASSESSMENT STEPS

1. Explain to the patient that this technique requires two positions: lying supine and standing up.
2. Ask the patient to lie on the examination table in the supine position.
3. Put on gloves.
4. Drape the patient so that only the genital area being examined is exposed.

5. Inspect the skin of the male genitalia assessing for (Fig. 19-9):
- ☐ color
- ☐ lesions
- ☐ drainage
- ☐ edema
- ☐ hair distribution.

6. Assess the following structures:
- ☐ **Penis:** assess the ventral, lateral, and dorsal sides.
- ☐ **Prepuce:** note whether the patient is circumcised or not; if uncircumcised ask the patient to retract the foreskin.

▌**TIP** You may observe a white cheesy substance called smegma (Fig. 19-10); this is a clean substance that moisturizes the glans and keeps it smooth, soft, and supple; it has antibacterial and antiviral properties and is normal.

- ☐ **Urethral meatus:** note the location of the urethral opening (Fig. 19-11).
- ☐ **Pubic hair:** assess pattern of hair distribution.
- ☐ **Skin:** assess for irritation, erythema, or pubic lice (also known as Phthirus pubis), more commonly known as crabs, derive their name from the crab-shaped insects that sometimes take up residence in the pubic hair; itching is the most common symptom reported (Kennard, 2006).

7. Gently lift up the scrotum to assess the posterior side (Fig. 19-12).

8. Ask the patient to turn on his side with his upper leg slightly bent, and gently spread the buttocks apart to inspect the anus.

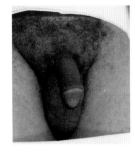

Fig. 19-9. Inspecting genitalia with draping.

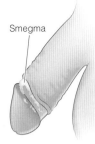

Fig. 19-10. Smegma moisturizes the glans.

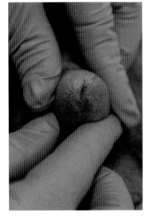

Fig. 19-11. Inspecting the urethral opening.

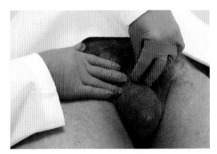

Fig. 19-12. Inspecting posterior side of scrotum.

9. Maintaining the patient's dignity, ask the patient to stand. Ask the patient to hold his penis up for this next part of the assessment. While sitting on a stool or squatting at eye level, compare right and left scrotal sacs (Fig. 19-13).

10. Assess the groin area for inguinal bulging; if suspected, ask the patient to cough for better visualization of any suspected bulging.

11. Remove and discard gloves.

12. Document your findings.

NORMAL FINDINGS

- **Penis:** Caucasians: pink to light brown; African Americans: light to dark brown; smooth, no hair; dorsal vein is visible; no lesions; no discharge
- **Prepuce:** circumcised foreskin is smooth and pink; uncircumcised foreskin easily retracts; smegma may or may not be present.
- **Urethra meatus:** pink, smooth, located at the center of the glans
- **Pubic hair:** at the base of the penis the hair distribution is in a triangular pattern consistent with age; coarse hair; no nits or lice.
- **Scrotum:** skin is a darker pigmentation; wrinkled surface, thin skin; left testis may hang lower than the right testis.
- **Epidermoid cysts:** sebaceous cysts that are yellow or white papules, nontender cutaneous lesions (Fig. 19-14)
- **Inguinal area:** skin is smooth, free from lumps or bumps, no signs of a hernia
- **Anus:** darker color skin, wrinkled around the orifice, no hemorrhoids

ABNORMAL FINDINGS

- **Penis:** skin has lesions or sores. Lesions indicative of common STIs include
  - ☐ **Syphilis chancre** lesion is a painless, firm, round, and open sore that forms during the primary stage of syphilis; commonly appears on the penis or anorectal area.
  - ☐ **Condyloma acuminatum** (genital warts) are soft, small, cauliflower-shaped growths on the skin; caused by HPV.
  - ☐ **Herpes lesions** typically develop on the penis; the painful lesions are vesicular small red bumps that change in appearance to blisters and ulcers as they progress through the four stages.
  - ☐ **Chancroid lesion** is a bacterial STI; painful open sore covered with gray or yellow gray material; has irregular borders
  - ☐ **Tinea cruris,** also known as "jock itch," is a fungal infection of the groin presenting as a bright red rash.
  - ☐ **Penile cancer** appears as a lump, ulcerative lesion, or redness and irritation of the skin; may or may not have drainage.

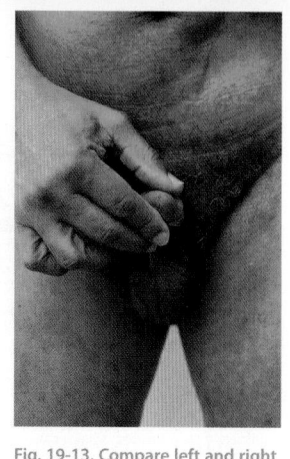

Fig. 19-13. Compare left and right scrotal sacs.

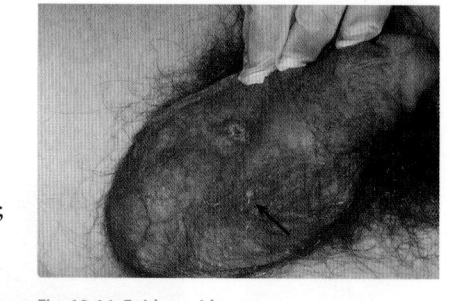

Fig. 19-14. Epidermoid cysts.

- ■ **Prepuce**
  - □ **Phimosis** is a stenosis of the preputial orifice so that the foreskin cannot be pushed back over the glans penis (Venes, 2013); may be a complication after recurrent infections; if it obstructs urinary flow, a circumcision may be needed.
  - □ **Paraphimosis** is an uncircumcised penis that may be covered with foreskin that once retracted, now cannot be returned to its original position; area becomes swollen; this requires immediate medical attention.
  - □ **Balanitis** is inflammation of the skin covering the glans penis (Venes, 2013).
- ■ **Pubic hair:** hair distribution is not consistent with age. Skin and pubic hair are infested with lice; when the hair is infested, the surrounding skin is inflamed secondary to scratching.
- ■ **Urethra:** opening has discharge; the opening to the urethra is not centrally located on the tip of the glans.
  - □ **Epispadias:** the urethral opening is located dorsally on the penis.
  - □ **Hypospadias:** urethral opening is located ventrally on the penis.
- ■ **Anus**
  - □ Hemorrhoids are swollen veins protruding from the anus.
  - □ Rectal bleeding
  - □ Protrusion of rectal mucosa related to rectal prolapse
- ■ **Scrotum**
  - □ Skin is swollen and stretched causing a decrease in the rugae; presence of scrotal swelling can be from several causes including edema, heart failure, renal failure, local inflammatory or infectious process.
  - □ Presence of any lesions on the scrotum is considered an abnormal finding.
  - □ Empty scrotal sac or scrotal sac with small testes
- ■ **Inguinal area**
  - □ Inguinal hernia is a weakening in the abdominal cavity wall with a protrusion of abdominal contents; any activity or medical problem that increases pressure on the abdominal wall tissue and muscles may cause an inguinal hernia (Fig. 19-15).

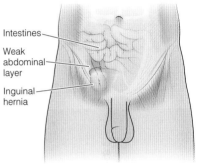

Intestines

Weak abdominal layer

Inguinal hernia

Fig. 19-15. Inguinal hernia.

ADVANCED ASSESSMENTS

The physician or midlevel practitioner will further assess the male patient during a comprehensive or focused examination using the technique of palpation. Nurses should be aware that these are common assessments that will be done on the male patient.

If a patient has urethral drainage, nurses may need to obtain a culture.

TECHNIQUE 19-3: **Obtaining a Urethral Culture**

Purpose: To identify the organism causing the infection
Equipment: Gloves, culturette tube, protective glasses
For accurate results, the patient should not have urinated for at least 1 hour prior to obtaining the culture. Read the institutional procedure prior to obtaining the culture.

ASSESSMENT STEPS

1. Gather your supplies.
2. Explain the technique to the patient.
3. Put on gloves.
4. Open up the culturette tube and remove the swab (Fig. 19-16).
5. Maintaining sterility of the swab tip, hold the shaft of the penis and gently insert the tip of the swab about 2 to 4 cm into the urethra.
6. Gently turn the swab clockwise for 2 to 3 seconds, maintaining contact with the mucosal surfaces.
7. Slowly withdraw the swab and insert into culturette tube and medium.
8. Break off the end of the swab at the score line.
9. Turn and recap tightly; document or attach preprinted label with the patient's name, date, and source of culture.
10. Remove and discard gloves.
11. Send specimen to the laboratory.

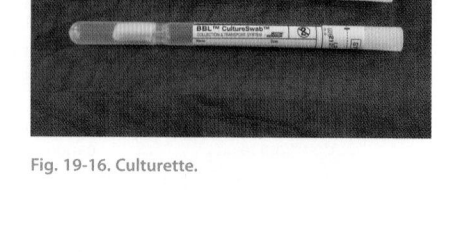

Fig. 19-16. Culturette.

PATIENT EDUCATION

Men should be educated on the risk factors and identification of signs and symptoms of breast, prostate, and testicular cancer. Offer general guidance to understand men's health and health promotion.

Male Breast Cancer

No screening guidelines exist for men in the general population (Block & Muradali, 2013). Male breast cancer is usually found in men 60 to 70 years of age (NIH, 2017). Screening is only recommended for men with a strong family history, genetic predisposition for, or strong family history of breast cancer or the history and physical assessment results suggest breast cancer (ACS, 2014). Recommendations include:

- Semiannual clinical breast examination (starting at age 35)
- Baseline mammography (at age 40) with further annual mammography if increased breast density is seen on a baseline mammogram
- Men should be taught about breast self-awareness and how to do breast self-examination (Box 19-3).

BOX 19-3 How to Perform a Male Breast Self-Examination

1. Make yourself soapy.
2. Place your left arm above and behind your head. With the three middle finger pads of your right hand, press your left breast against your chest wall.
3. In a circular motion, feel small portions of your left breast, going around until you have covered the entire breast and underarm. Make sure you do it slowly.
4. Repeat again on your opposite breast.

Remember: Look for changes, and if you find a lump or have discharge, or you think something may be wrong, make an appointment with your healthcare provider.

Testicular Cancer

- For men over the age of 14, a monthly self-examination of the testicles is an effective way of becoming familiar with this area of the body and thus enabling the detection of testicular cancer at an early and very curable stage (Testicular Cancer Resource Center, 2012).
- Males should be taught how to check their testicles for lumps; if one is found, it should be assessed by their healthcare provider. The best time to check the testicles is after a warm shower or bath (Box 19-4).

TIP The Testicular Cancer Society (2016) has developed an app for directions on doing a testicular self-examination and also to send monthly reminders. For a free mobile app, advise male patients to go to www.BallChecker.com.

BOX 19-4 How to Perform a Testicular Self-Examination

TIP Do not press hard during the examination; if you feel pain or pressure, you are pressing too hard.

1. Testicular assessment is easier to perform while in the shower or taking a warm bath, because the warmth will relax the scrotal area and the water will make it easier to smoothly move over the skin surface. The examination may also be performed after a shower or bath.

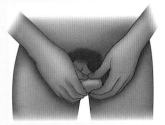

Testicular self-exam.

2. Feel each testicle with both hands by placing the index and middle fingers under the testicle with the thumbs placed on top.
3. Roll the testicle gently between the thumbs and fingers.
4. Feel for the epididymis, the soft, rope-like structure behind the testicle collects and carries sperm; palpate gently for any bumps.
5. If you find a lump on your testicle or any of the other signs of testicular cancer, see your healthcare provider as soon as possible for further evaluation.

Prostate Cancer

The ACS (2016) recommends that men should make an informed decision after getting information about the uncertainties, risks, and potential benefits of prostate cancer screening.

- A yearly screening be offered to all men over 50 who have a life expectancy of at least 10 years.
- For African-American men, or men with an affected first-degree family member, yearly screening is recommended beginning at age 45.
- For men who have multiple first-degree relatives affected with prostate cancer at an early age, a baseline screen is advocated at age 40. There are many experts who believe all men should initiate screening at age 40.

Healthy People 2020

Goal: Promote healthy sexual behaviors, strengthen community capacity, and increase access to quality services to prevent STIs and their complications (HHS, 2010).

Healthy People 2020 Corner—Men's Health Screenings

Compared to women, men are more likely to smoke and drink, make unhealthy or risky choices, and put off regular checkups and medical care.

Many men have the philosophy, "If it's not broken, don't fix it," not realizing part of maintaining a healthy body is preventive maintenance.

The two leading causes of death among men are heart disease and cancer. Advice from a healthcare provider about getting blood pressure, cholesterol, diabetes, and cancer screenings, as well as providing information on reducing controllable risk factors, such as smoking, physical inactivity, and obesity, can make a positive impact toward meeting Healthy People (HP) objectives (Health Net Federal Services, 2017).

Sexually Transmitted Infections

- Routine HIV screening for teens and adults between 15 and 65 years of age; younger adolescents and older adults who are at increased risk should also be screened (USPSTF, 2013).
- Advise protection through use of condoms:
  - □ Latex condoms, when used consistently and correctly, are highly effective in preventing and reducing the sexual transmission of HIV, the virus that causes AIDS, and other STIs (CDC, 2015a).
  - □ In addition, consistent and correct use of latex condoms reduces the risk of other STIs, including diseases transmitted by genital secretions, and to a lesser degree, genital ulcer diseases.

INTRODUCTION

The rectum and anus are intimate parts of the body that require the nurse to be professional and sensitive to the patient's feelings during this assessment. This assessment is the same for both the male and female patient. Healthcare providers may assess a woman's anus and rectum during their annual gynecological examination; men may have a digital rectal examination during a prostate assessment. Registered nurses perform rectal assessments for rectal symptoms such as rectal pain or bleeding, checking for fecal impactions, or giving suppository medications. Patients may fear having a rectal assessment; nurses should let patients know that rectal assessments are most often painless.

SENC Patient-Centered Care This assessment may be embarrassing for the patient and cause the patient to become anxious. Talking to the patient throughout the assessment may help to alleviate the anxiety.

REVIEW OF ANATOMY AND PHYSIOLOGY

Rectum

The rectum's primary function is to store processed fecal material. Fecal material accumulates in the rectum triggering the sensory nerves to tell the brain it is time to have a bowel movement (Ruggieri & Tolentino, 2011).

- Rectum is the lower part of the sigmoid colon, the large intestine; average length is approximately 12 to 14 cm in an adult (Mahadevan, 2014). The rectum is made up of transverse folds that propel waste materials into the anal canal; it contains arteries, veins, and visceral nerves; the main rectal artery is the superior rectal artery, and the main vein is the superior rectal vein (Fig. 20-1).
- Perirectal fat lines the entire length of the rectal walls; rectal lymph nodes are located in these walls (Mahadevan, 2014).

Anus

- The length of the anal canal is 4 to 5 cm in length in an adult (Mahadevan, 2014); located in the perineum.
- Anus is the terminal endpoint of the gastrointestinal tract and large intestine; lined with mucous-secreting anal glands and membranes arranged in longitudinal and curved folds (Fig. 20-1).
- These glands help to lubricate the anal canal to make it easier for feces to move through the canal and out of the body.
- The internal anal sphincter is composed of smooth, involuntary, ring-like muscle and supplied by parasympathetic nerve fibers; contributes to 60 to 75 percent of the anal resting tone (Mahadevan, 2014); relaxes in response to pressure from gas or fecal material.

- The external anal sphincter is composed of striated, voluntary, ring-like muscle and can be contracted voluntarily.

TIP During a rectal assessment, a nurse is able to feel both sphincters.

- The anorectal ring is the demarcation of the anal canal and the rectum.
- The dentate line is located at the junction of the rectum and the anus; mucus-secreting cells change to squamous cells.
- The perianal skin is composed of squamous cells and has hair, sweat, and sebaceous glands.

DIAGNOSTICS
See Chapter 14, Assessing the Abdomen.

CULTURAL CONSIDERATIONS Colorectal cancer is a leading cause of cancer-related deaths world-wide (Guda et al., 2015). Colorectal cancer rates are highest in African-American men and women and lowest in Asian/Pacific Islander (API) men and women (American Cancer Society, 2014). African-Americans have a higher incidence and higher mortality rates than Caucasian-Americans (Basa et al., 2016).

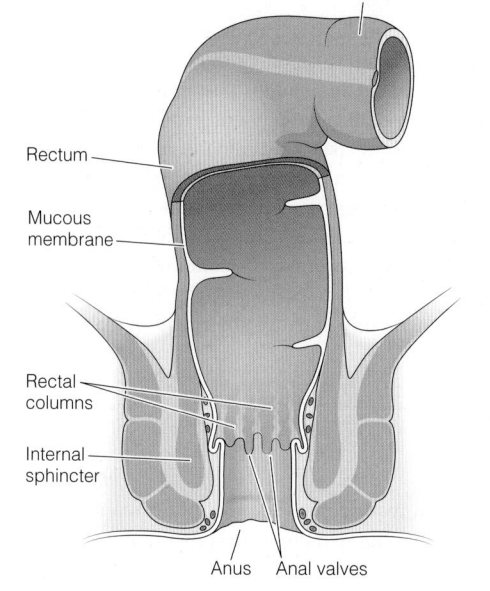

Fig. 20-1. Rectum and anus.

HEALTH HISTORY

Review of Systems
Ask the patient the following questions.

Rectum
- What is your normal bowel movement pattern? Have you noticed any change in the size and diameter of your stools? Are you constipated? Do you have any diarrhea?

☐ Constipation is when bowel movements are:
  - too hard or too small
  - become less frequent (less than 3 times per week)
  - difficulty having a bowel movement
  - a sense that bowels are not completely emptied (Wald, 2016).

The ROME III diagnostic criteria for functional constipation can be seen in Box 20-1.

BOX 20-1 ROME III: Diagnostic Criteria for Functional Constipation

1. Must include two or more of the following:
   a. Straining during at least 25 percent of defecations
   b. Lumpy or hard stools in at least 25 percent of defecations
   c. Sensation of incomplete evacuation for at least 25 percent of defecations
   d. Sensation of anorectal obstruction/blockage for at least 25 percent of defecations
   e. Manual maneuvers to facilitate at least 25 percent of defecations (e.g., digital evacuation, support of the pelvic floor)
   f. Fewer than three defecations per week
2. Loose stools are rarely present without the use of laxatives
3. Insufficient criteria for irritable bowel syndrome

*Criteria fulfilled for the last 3 months with symptom onset at least 6 months before diagnosis. From the ROME Foundation, Inc., 2015.

☐ Diarrhea is liquid stool; there are many causes including side effects of medications, viruses, food intolerances, and illness.
☐ Change in size and diameter of stools may indicate a partial obstruction or mass in the intestines.

SENC **Safety Alert** *Clostridium difficile* (*C. difficile*) is anaerobic toxin-producing gram-positive spore forming bacterium that is widely recognized as the leading cause of nosocomial diarrhea worldwide. Patients who have recently been on antibiotics may be at risk. Ask the patient to describe their diarrhea because three or more watery, nonbloody stools per 24-hr period is the hallmark of *C. difficile* illness (Ofosu, 2016). Patients experiencing watery, foul smelling diarrhea should have a specimen sent out for culture and sensitivity.

■ Do you have any rectal bleeding? If so, what is the color of the blood?
☐ Rectal bleeding (hematochezia) can present as bright red blood or cause the stool to have a black, tarry appearance. The color of blood can give clues to where the bleeding is occurring:
   • Bright red blood usually indicates bleeding low in the colon or rectum.
   • Dark red or maroon blood usually indicates bleeding higher in the colon or the small bowel.
   • Melena is black, tarry feces caused by digestion of blood in the gastrointestinal tract; commonly seen with gastrointestinal bleeding (Venes, 2013, p. 1483).
■ Some causes of rectal bleeding are as follows:
☐ An anal fissure is a tear in the opening of the anus that can cause pain, itching, and bleeding; the most common cause is constipation (Sugarman & Sugarman, 2014).
☐ Hemorrhoids are swollen, dilated veins that protrude from the lower rectum or anus; symptoms may include bleeding, irritation, and itching; hemorrhoids may be caused by increased rectal pressure such as chronic straining related to constipation. There are two locations of hemorrhoids (Fig. 20-2):

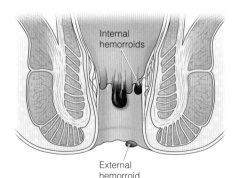

Fig. 20-2. Internal and external hemorrhoids.

- Internal hemorrhoids are located inside the rectum.
- External hemorrhoids protrude to the outside of the anus.
- Polyps are abnormal outgrowths of tissue in the lining of the colon; polyps may be precancerous.
- Inflammation of the gastrointestinal tract may cause rectal bleeding and need further evaluation.
■ Do you have any itching or pain in your anus? Any abnormal drainage?
  - Eighty percent of anal cancers are squamous cell in nature and arise in the anal canal, where the mucosa is made up of squamous cell epithelium; symptoms include anal pain, irritation, itching, and bleeding (Coakes & White, 2013).

- An anal fistula will drain pus and abnormal fluid from the anus. An anal fistula may increase the risk of developing anal cancer (ASCO, 2015).

CULTURAL CONSIDERATIONS Most squamous cell anal cancers seem to be linked to infection by the human papillomavirus (HPV). More Caucasian women get HPV-associated anal cancer than women of other races; more African-American men get HPV-associated anal cancer than men of other races (CDC, 2014). Overall, anal cancer is more common in women than men in most racial/ethnic groups. However, in African Americans it is more common in men than in women (CDC, 2015).

PREPARATION FOR ASSESSMENT

Equipment Needed
Gloves
Water-soluble lubricant
Stool for occult blood test kit

Sequence of the Examination
1. Inspecting
2. Digital rectal examination
3. Testing stool for occult blood

The anus and rectum are assessed at different times for the female and male assessment.
■ Female patient's rectum and anus are assessed after a gynecological assessment.
■ Male patient's rectum and anus are assessed after the male genital area assessment; the prostate gland is assessed at the same time.
This assessment may be performed with the patient in the Sims' (side-lying) or lithotomy position, for women. Inspection is a noninvasive assessment that is done by the nurse.

TECHNIQUE 20-1: **Inspecting the Anus**

Purpose: To assess for abnormalities of the anus
Equipment: Gloves

ASSESSMENT STEPS

1. Explain the technique to the patient.
2. Put on gloves.
3. Have the patient lie on his or her left side with the right knee slightly bent.
4. Gently spread the buttocks to expose the anus and perianal area (Fig. 20-3).
5. Assess the anus and the perianal area for:
  ☐ redness
  ☐ inflammation
  ☐ lesions or lumps
  ☐ wounds or excoriation
  ☐ hemorrhoids, fissures.
6. Remove and discard gloves.
7. Assist patient to sitting position.
8. Document your findings.

NORMAL FINDINGS

■ Anus is tightly closed.
■ Skin is moist and darkly pigmented; hair may be present.
■ No redness, inflammation, lesions, lumps, wounds, hemorrhoids, or fissures.

ABNORMAL FINDINGS

■ Patulous anus: open and distended
■ Redness, inflammation, lesions, wounds, or hemorrhoids
■ Rectal prolapse: rectum partially or fully intussuscepts and comes out through anus

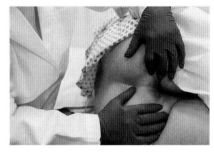

Fig. 20-3. Inspecting the anus.

ADVANCED ASSESSMENTS

A nurse may perform the digital rectal examination; this may be an uncomfortable assessment for the patient. Encourage the patient to let you know if he or she is experiencing any discomfort or pain. Encourage the patients to take some deep, relaxing breaths.

SENC Patient-Centered Care Talking to the patient throughout this assessment may help to alleviate some of the patient's anxiety.

TECHNIQUE 20-2: **Performing a Digital Rectal Examination**

Purpose: To assess for abnormalities of the rectum and prostate (in males)

Equipment: Gloves, water-soluable lubricant

SENC Patient-Centered Care Examining the rectum may be embarrassing for the patient. This examination may also cause the patient some discomfort. Give a careful explanation and be professional. Some patients are fearful of a rectal examination. Give your patient the choice of which position he or she would prefer. A rectal examination can be performed using any of the three positions:

- Lateral decubitus or side-lying position with the upper extremity slightly flexed (Fig. 20-4A)
- Lithotomy position is lying down on the examination table with feet in stirrups (Fig. 20-4B).
- Patient standing and bending over and holding onto the examination table (Fig. 20-4C)

SENC **Safety Alert** When the patient is standing for this assessment, instruct the patient to hold onto the examination table for support to prevent a fall.

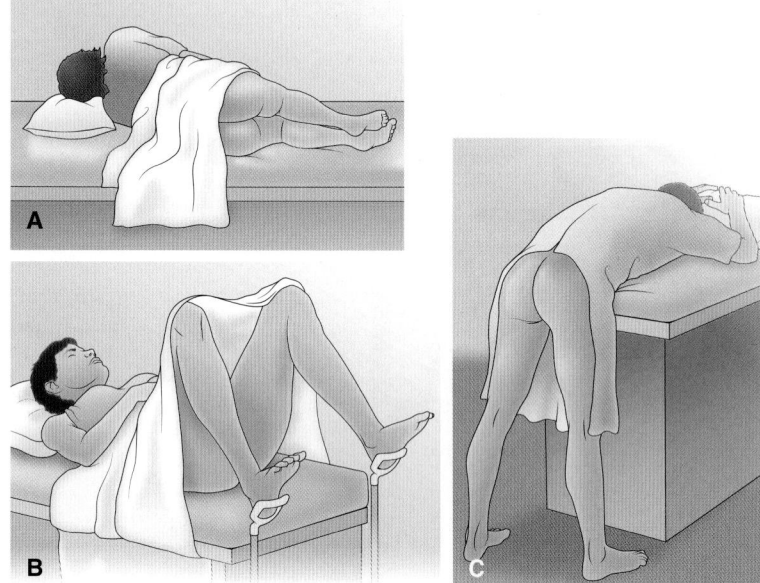

Fig. 20-4. Rectal exam positions. (A) Side-lying. (B) Lithotomy. (C) Standing and bending over the examination table.

ASSESSMENT STEPS

1. Explain the technique to the patient.

2. Assist your patient to the preferred position.

3. Put on gloves.

4. Apply a moderate to large amount of the water-soluble lubricant to your index finger of your dominant hand.

5. Gently touch the anus with your index finger and ask the patient to bear down on your finger as you gently insert your index finger into the lower rectum; assess the rectal sphincter muscle tone (Fig. 20-5).

6. Male patient only: Move your index finger so that it is positioned anteriorly pointing toward the umbilicus, and palpate the posterior surface of the prostate gland; assess the prostate gland for:

  ☐ size
  ☐ shape
  ☐ smoothness
  ☐ lumps
  ☐ tenderness.

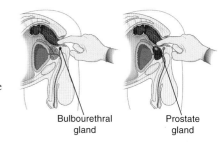

Bulbourethral gland   Prostate gland

Fig. 20-5. Digital rectal examination.

7. Using the pad of your index finger, gently palpate the inside of entire rectum assessing for tenderness, lumps, or masses.

8. If needed, a stool smear for occult blood may be taken to assess for hidden blood in the stool (see Technique 20-3).

9. After assessing the rectum and prostate (in the male), gently remove your index finger.

10. Remove and discard your glove.

11. Assist the patient to a comfortable position.

12. Document your findings.

SENC Patient-Centered Care Give your patient some tissues or wipes prior to getting dressed.

NORMAL FINDINGS

- Rectum is without masses or hemorrhoids.
- Male patient: Prostate gland has two smooth lobes within normal size, no hard nodules; nontender (Fig. 20-6).

ABNORMAL FINDINGS

- Rectum has a mass or nodule.
- Internal hemorrhoids, mass, or fissure is present.
- Prostate gland is enlarged, hard, or with nodules (Fig. 20-6).
- Benign prostatic hyperplasia is an enlargement of the prostate gland that occurs with advancing age; the exact cause is unknown, but declining testosterone and increasing estrogen levels are thought to cause enlargement of the prostate gland; does not increase risk for prostate cancer.

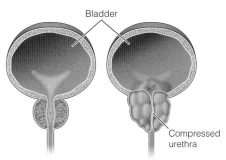

Bladder

Compressed urethra

Normal   **Enlarged prostate**

Fig. 20-6. Normal and enlarged prostate gland.

TECHNIQUE 20-3: **Assessing Stool for Fecal Occult Blood**

Purpose: To identify hidden blood in stool
Equipment: Gloves, Agency-specific Fecal Occult Blood Test (FOBT)
Sometimes the healthcare provider will want to test a stool specimen for hidden blood.

SENC Safety Alert Always read the directions of the FOBT testing kit. Check the expiration date of the FOBT developing solution.

ASSESSMENT STEPS

1. Set up the FOBT by opening up the side for the sample application.
2. Put on gloves.
3. Apply a sample specimen to both of the FOBT windows (Fig. 20-7).
4. Close the specimen-side FOBT slide.
5. Open the opposite side of the FOBT slide and follow the directions for dropping one or two drops on each window.
6. Observe the specimen sites color.
7. Remove and discard gloves.
8. Document your findings.

NORMAL FINDINGS

■ Window remains brown in color
■ Negative for occult blood

ABNORMAL FINDINGS

■ Window turns a bluish hue
■ Positive for occult blood

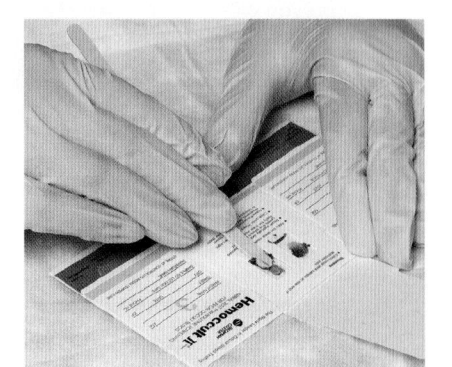

Fig. 20-7. Fecal occult blood test.

PATIENT EDUCATION

Patient education should include discussing the signs and symptoms of rectal cancer.

- A change in bowel habits (constipation or diarrhea)
- Feeling that the bowel does not empty completely
- Stools that are narrower, pencil-like, or change from their usual shape
- Blood in the stool
- General abdominal discomfort (frequent gas pains, fullness, bloating, or cramps)
- Change in appetite
- Weight loss for no known reason
- Fatigue (National Cancer Institute at the National Institute of Health, 2013)

INTRODUCTION

Newborns are a specialized population to be assessed. Newborns make multiple adjustments to their respiratory and circulatory systems as they adjust to extrauterine life. Unlike adults, newborns are not able to communicate verbally, and therefore communicate primarily by behavior. The nurse must assess and interpret the newborn's behavior in order to form an accurate picture of the newborn's health. Accurate assessment of the newborn includes a history, estimation of gestational age, physical examination, and neurological examination.

REVIEW OF ANATOMY AND PHYSIOLOGY

Newborn is the term used for a child from birth through 28 days old. Newborns grow rapidly and at different rates.

Head

A newborn's head is large in proportion to the infant's body.
- The newborn head is composed of five major bones:
  - One occipital bone
  - Two frontal bones
  - Two parietal bones
- The skull of a newborn is soft and flexible with two open areas:
  - Anterior fontanel (called "soft spot") is a diamond shaped space; measures about 4 to 5 cm at birth; this area remains soft to about age 2
  - Posterior fontanel is triangular in shape; measures about 1 cm at birth; closes up to 2 months after birth
- The skull's bones are connected by fibrous cranial sutures; these sutures permit the skull to expand as the brain grows (Fig. 21-1).

- During a vaginal delivery, pressure from the vagina and pelvic bones on the newborn's head may cause molding of the head; molding is an overriding of the cranial bones; this causes the head to become asymmetric (plagiocephaly).
- Changes in the head circumference may occur during the first postnatal days as the

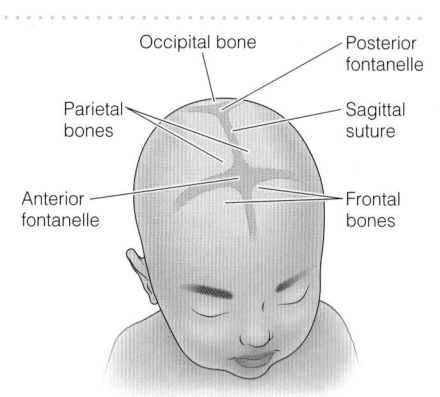

Fig. 21-1. The newborn head.

result of scalp edema and molding resolution (Klarić, Rajić, & Crnković, 2014).

- If the infant is delivered by caesarean section, the head is usually round.
- Average head circumference is 34 cm and is about 2 cm larger in diameter than the chest circumference.

Skin

- Skin is critical to the newborn's transition from the intrauterine environment to the extrauterine environment; adaptation of the newborn's skin to the extrauterine environment is an ongoing process during the first year of life (Dyer, 2013).
- The newborn's skin performs many functions, including:
  - □ barrier to water loss, light, and irritants
  - □ protects against bacteria, viruses, and infection
  - □ provides resilience to mechanical trauma
  - □ provides sensation and tactile discrimination
  - □ maintains thermal regulation (Visscher, Brink, & Odio, 2015).
- The newborn's skin is not fully developed at birth and matures with age; the skin will vary depending on the length of pregnancy.
  - □ Premature infants will have thin, transparent skin.
  - □ Postmature infants will have thicker skin.
- The newborn's skin is smooth and thin and drier than the skin of older (1-, 2-, and 6-month-old) infants (Dyer, 2013).

SENC Safety Alert The infant has a thin layer of subcutaneous fat resulting in an ineffective thermoregulatory system; thereby, infants need to be kept in a warm environment because of their inability to contract and shiver. Assess for changes in color of skin and decreased activity.

- Color of the skin can vary; mottling (spotting) is commonly seen on the trunk and extremities.

- At birth, a thick, cheesy, waxy substance called *vernix caseosa* covers the skin; this covering is made of a mixture of a variety of substances including protein (10 percent), lipid (10 percent), and water (80 percent) (Dyer, 2013).
- Fingernails and toenails are present at birth.

Hair

- Lanugo is the fine, soft hair that will cover most of the newborn's body; disappears within a month; this hair is now replaced by fine, light-colored vellus hair.

Nose

- Newborns are obligate nose breathers—that is, they prefer to breathe through their noses, although they can, if needed, breathe through their mouths.

Neck

- A newborn's neck muscles are weak and cannot support the head.
- The neck is short during the newborn period.

TIP The newborn should be able to hold his or her head up at a 45-degree angle around 4 months of age.

Eyes

- The macula is absent at birth and develops fully around 8 months of life; therefore, the infant does not have central vision.
- Peripheral vision is developed at birth.
- Iris eye color depends on a protein melanin; it will take up to one year before the melanocytes mature and present with a permanent eye color.
- Newborns have the ability to see objects and colors.
- Newborns are nearsighted.

Ears
- The inner ear develops during the first weeks of gestation.
- Ears are soft because the cartilage is not fully developed.
- The eustachian tube is shorter and wider and more horizontal.
- The outer ear canal is shorter.
- Newborns respond better to high-pitched sounds because the inner ear is not fully developed.

■ **TIP** The position of the eustachian tube and its close proximity to the nasopharynx place the newborn at higher risk for developing ear infections.

Thorax
- The thorax in a newborn is round.
- Anteroposterior and transverse chest diameters are equal.
- The average chest circumference is 32 cm.
- Thin chest walls with increased cartilage make the thoracic cage more flexible.

Breasts
- A newborn's breasts may be temporarily enlarged due to retention of the maternal hormone, estrogen, which crosses the placenta during pregnancy.
- "Witch's milk" is neonatal milk that may be seen coming from the newborn's nipple as a result of maternal hormones; more commonly seen in full-term infants.

Heart
- The heart lies more horizontal in the chest of a newborn.
- The apex is at the left fourth intercostal space.

Abdomen
- The umbilical cord has two arteries and one vein.

Urinary System
- The urinary bladder is located between the symphysis pubis and the umbilicus.
- Bladder capacity increases with age.

Neurological System
- The neurological system of a newborn is not fully developed at birth.
- Newborns are all born with the same primitive reflexes that originate in the central nervous system; reflexes are instinctual and protect the newborn.
- Newborns have rudimentary sensation; this means that only a strong sensation will cause a reaction in the newborn.

DIAGNOSTICS
Laboratory samples may be drawn from the newborn to identify disorders that may affect the health of the newborn. Each state varies on the amount and type of disorders screened.

- **Metabolic profile** is the most common laboratory test performed after the infant is 24 hours old; this is drawn via heel stick. The metabolic screen checks for inborn errors of metabolism and blood disorders.
- **Phenylketonuria (PKU) test** is a blood test to check for phenylalanine, an amino acid that is required for normal growth and development. It is a state requirement in the United States and Canada.
  - □ Infants with PKU are deficient in an enzyme called phenylalanine hydroxylase; this enzyme is needed to break down the essential amino acid called phenylalanine.
  - □ Deficiency of this enzyme could cause serious neurological and intellectual disabilities.
  - □ The test is conducted 24 to 48 hours after the infant is born.

CULTURAL CONSIDERATIONS PKU is inherited from both parents; it occurs more in Caucasians and American Indians and is less common in blacks, Hispanics, and Asians.

■ **Serum bilirubin level** is a blood test measuring the amount of bilirubin in the blood.
  □ Bilirubin is a by-product of heme catabolism from old red blood cells (RBCs).
  □ Bilirubin is a yellow-brown substance found in bile; bile is produced by the liver.
  □ When bilirubin levels are high, the yellowish pigment deposits under the skin and sclera of the infant's eyes may turn yellow; this is called jaundice.

■ **Glucose screening** differs by institution; certain infants are at higher risk for developing hypoglycemia; these include infants who are:
  □ small for gestational age (SGA): infant who is smaller in size than normal for age and gender
  □ large for gestational age (LGA): infant who is larger in size than normal for age and gender
  □ premature infants with low Apgar scores at 5 minutes
  □ infants of diabetic mothers
  □ infants with thermoregulation issues.

Healthy People 2020
Goal: Increase appropriate newborn blood-spot screening and follow-up testing (HHS, 2010).

HEALTH HISTORY

Review of Systems
It is important to include the parent(s) in the assessment process from the moment of the newborn's birth. The mother, parents, or primary caretaker are the primary sources for gathering information about the newborn. During the review of systems (ROS), the nurse should:
■ be nonjudgmental
■ demonstrate caring and genuineness
■ understand there may be cultural variations among families
■ encourage open communication
■ encourage the mother, parent, or primary caretaker to ask questions
■ provide teaching when appropriate.
Begin by reviewing the perinatal history. Use the OLDCARTS mnemonic (**O**nset, **L**ocation, **D**uration, **C**haracteristics, **A**ggravating/Alleviating factors, **R**elieving factors, **T**reatment, **S**everity) to identify attributes of a symptom. Ask the mother or caretaker the following questions.

Past Medical History of Mother
The past history is important to identify risk factors or past medical complications experienced by the mother during her pregnancy that may have had an effect on the newborn.
■ Have you ever had any diseases during pregnancy, including hypertension, anemia, or diabetes?
  □ Hypertension can decrease placental perfusion causing intrauterine growth restriction (IUGR) or small for gestational age (SGA) and preterm birth.
  □ Anemia can increase the risk for preterm delivery and low birth weight in the newborn.
  □ Diabetes can cause large for gestational age (LGA), or macrosomia, in the newborn, which can lead to birth trauma and newborn hypoglycemia.
    • **Macrosomia** is an infant that weighs greater than 4000 grams or 8 lb. 13 oz.

- Did you ever have a preterm labor (labor weeks' gestation) and antepartum bleeding?
  - ☐ Preterm labor is labor that occurs before 37 weeks' gestation.
  - ☐ Antepartum bleeding is abnormal bleeding occurring from 24 weeks' gestation.

SENC Safety Alert Bleeding such as placental abruption can decrease the placental perfusion, cutting down the fetal oxygen supply. It can also become a medical emergency leading to preterm delivery.

- What is your blood type?
  - ☐ Infants born to mothers with any negative blood type or O blood type are at increased risk for jaundice.
- Did you have an illnesses or infectious disease during your pregnancy?
  - ☐ TORCH infections can cross the placenta and have teratogenic effects on the fetus. TORCH infections are major contributors to prenatal, perinatal, and postnatal morbidity and mortality (Neu, Duchon, & Zachariah, 2015). Focus on TORCH infections that include the following:
    - Toxoplasmosis is a parasitic disease.
    - Treponema pallidum is a spirochete bacterium causing syphilis.
    - Rubella is caused by the rubella virus causing German Measles.
    - Cytomegalovirus (CMV) is a common virus and related to the virus that causes chicken pox and mononucleosis (National Library of Medicine [NLM], 2017).
    - Herpes viruses
  - ☐ In addition, review human immunodeficiency virus (HIV) and hepatitis status; these diseases can be passed through the placenta to the newborn.
  - ☐ Infections such as Group B strep, gonorrhea, and chlamydia can be passed to the infant during labor and delivery.
    - Group B strep can cause pneumonia and sepsis.
    - Gonorrhea and chlamydia can cause blindness in the newborn.

Medication History

- What type of medications, if any, did you take while you were pregnant (prescription medications, herbal therapies, over-the-counter drugs)?
- What medications did you take during the birth of your baby (prescription medications, herbal therapies, over-the-counter drugs)?

Psychosocial History of the Mother

- Do you smoke? If so, did you smoke during your pregnancy?
  - ☐ Smoking can lead to prematurity, low birth weight, increased risk of sudden infant death syndrome (SIDS), as well as an increased risk for bronchitis and pneumonia.
- Do you drink alcohol? If so, how much and how often? Did you drink during your pregnancy?
  - ☐ Drinking alcohol during pregnancy can cause fetal alcohol syndrome (FAS), which can cause facial anomalies, deafness, heart defects, developmental delays, and neurological abnormalities.
- Are you a substance user? If so, prescription or "street" drugs? Did you use drugs during your pregnancy?
  - ☐ Substance use, whether prescription or "street" drugs, can lead to newborn prematurity, low birth weight, and drug withdrawal.

Family History

- Do you and your family have any of the following?
  - ☐ History of birth defects such as spina bifida or congenital heart defects
    - Spina bifida is a congenital neural tube defect that can affect the spine, spinal cord, brain, and meninges; the vertebrae do not form normally, and the spinal cord may be exposed. The infant may have motor and sensory loss, bowel and bladder dysfunction.
  - ☐ History of congenital anomalies

□ History of cardiac abnormalities
□ History of blood disorders

Birth History

■ Tell me about the following aspects of your infant's birth:
  □ Estimated due date (preterm or post term delivery)
  □ Length of rupture of membranes
    • Once the membranes have ruptured, the mother and infant are at risk for infection.
  □ Length of labor
  □ Medications used during labor and birth
  □ Type of delivery
    • Vaginal delivery
      • Forceps assisted
      • Vacuum assisted
    • Operative delivery
      • Cesarean section

■ The **Apgar score** provides a quick assessment of the newborn's transition to extrauterine life. The Apgar score is evaluated at 1 and 5 minutes after birth. The score is based on five categories:
  □ Heart rate
  □ Respiratory rate
  □ Muscle tone
  □ Reflex irritability
  □ Skin color

The interpretation of each of the above areas is scored 0, 1, or 2. The maximum total score is 10 and low score at 1 minute is a sign of perinatal asphyxia and the need for immediate assisted ventilation.
  □ 7 to 10 is good to excellent
  □ 4 to 6 is fair
  □ Less than 4 is poor condition (Venes, 2013, p. 167).

PREPARATION FOR ASSESSMENT

Equipment Needed

■ Stethoscope: neonatal stethoscope preferred
■ Measuring tape
■ Digital thermometer
■ Newborn blood pressure machine
■ Gloves
■ Scale

SENC Safety Alert Clean gloves must always be worn during the assessment if the newborn has not had his or her initial bath.

Preliminary Steps

The newborn assessment should take place in an area that is well lit, warm, and draft free.

■ The best place to assess a newborn is on a radiant warmer bed.
■ The radiant warmer should be prewarmed before the infant is placed on the surface to avoid heat loss.
■ The infant should be undressed.

FOCUSED ASSESSMENT

TECHNIQUE 21-1: **Gestational Age Assessment**

Purpose: To determine the infant's gestational age based on physical and neuromuscular examination
Equipment: Radiant warmer, gloves, Ballard Assessment Tool, pen, or pencil
- Estimated gestational age is calculated by an early first trimester ultrasound or last menstrual period (LMP).
- The Ballard Gestational Age Assessment Tool determines gestational age through neuromuscular and physical assessment of the newborn. Scores range from −1 to 4 or 5 for each criterion (Fig. 21-2) (Ballard et al, 1991).
- Assessment of the newborn should be completed within 2 hours of birth. It is important to identify any potential complications early in the infant's life in order to intervene quickly.

> **SENC Safety Alert** Always check the infant's identification band prior to beginning an assessment. It is important to be sure that you are assessing the correct infant.

ASSESSMENT STEPS

While assessing the infant, mark the appropriate box on the Ballard Assessment Tool for each of the following assessments:
1. Place the naked infant supine on radiant warmer.
2. **Posture:** observe resting posture and score the infant (0–4) based on resting posture. Choose the illustration that best represents the infant's posture. Mark the appropriate box.
3. **Square window:** apply gentle pressure to the dorsum of the infant's hand, bending the hand toward the forearm. Continue applying pressure until resistance is noted. Note the angle that is made between the hand and wrist. Mark the appropriate box.
4. **Arm recoil:** place one hand below the infant's elbow. Holding the infant's hand, briefly hold the infant's arms, set in flexion and then extension. Release the infant's hand. Note the angle of recoil the forearm returns to. Mark the appropriate box.
5. **Popliteal angle:** with the infant's knee flexed, place the infant's thigh onto the infant's abdomen. Once the infant is relaxed in this position, grasp the infant's foot with one hand while supporting the thigh with the other hand. Apply gentle pressure as you straighten the infant's leg until initial resistance is met. Measure the angle formed by the upper and lower leg. Mark the appropriate box.
6. **Scarf sign:** place the infant's head midline and support the infant's hand across the upper chest. Place the thumb of your other hand on the infant's elbow. With gentle pressure, move the infant's elbow across his or her chest. When resistance is noted, note the position of the infant's elbow on the chest. Mark the appropriate box.
7. **Heel to ear:** with the infant in a resting position, grasp the infant's foot and bring it toward the ear using gentle pressure. When resistance is felt, note the position of the infant's foot in relation to the ear. Mark the appropriate box.

MATURATIONAL ASSESSMENT OF GESTATIONAL AGE (New Ballard Score)

NAME _____ SEX _____
HOSPITAL NO. _____ BIRTH WEIGHT _____
RACE _____ LENGTH _____
DATE/TIME OF BIRTH _____ HEAD CIRC. _____
DATE/TIME OF EXAM _____ EXAMINER _____
AGE WHEN EXAMINED _____
APGAR SCORE: 1 MINUTE _____ 5 MINUTES _____ 10 MINUTES _____

NEUROMUSCULAR MATURITY

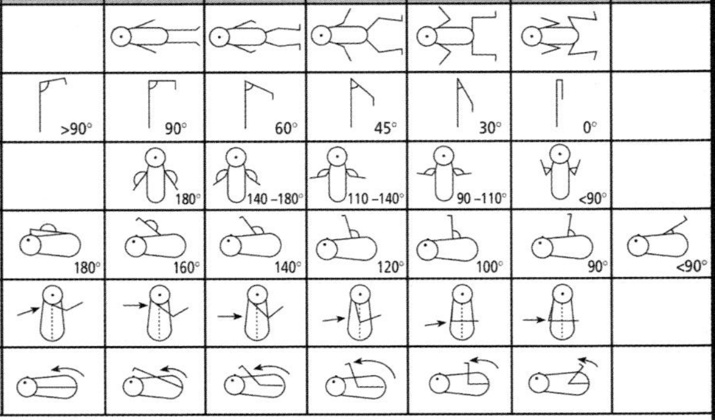

NEUROMUSCULAR MATURITY SIGN	SCORE							RECORD SCORE HERE
	-1	0	1	2	3	4	5	
POSTURE								
SQUARE WINDOW (Wrist)	>90°	90°	60°	45°	30°	0°		
ARM RECOIL		180°	140°–180°	110°–140°	90°–110°	<90°		
POPLITEAL ANGLE	180°	160°	140°	120°	100°	90°	<90°	
SCARF SIGN								
HEEL TO EAR								

TOTAL NEUROMUSCULAR MATURITY SCORE

PHYSICAL MATURITY

PHYSICAL MATURITY SIGN	SCORE							RECORD SCORE HERE
	-1	0	1	2	3	4	5	
SKIN	sticky friable transparent	gelatinous red translucent	smooth pink visible veins	superficial peeling &/or rash, few veins	cracking pale areas rare veins	parchment deep cracking no vessels	leathery cracked wrinkled	
LANUGO	none	sparse	abundant	thinning	bald areas	mostly bald		
PLANTAR SURFACE	heel-toe 40–50 mm: -1 < 40 mm: -2	>50 mm no crease	faint red marks	anterior transverse crease only	creases ant. 2/3	creases over entire sole		
BREAST	imperceptible	barely perceptible	flat areola no bud	stippled areola 1–2 mm bud	raised areola 3–4 mm bud	full areola 5–10 mm bud		
EYE / EAR	lids fused loosely: -1 tightly: -2	lids open pinna flat stays folded	sl. curved pinna; soft; slow recoil	well-curved pinna; soft but ready recoil	formed & firm instant recoil	thick cartilage ear stiff		
GENITALS (Male)	scrotum flat, smooth	scrotum empty faint rugae	testes in upper canal rare rugae	testes descending few rugae	testes down good rugae	testes pendulous deep rugae		
GENITALS (Female)	clitoris prominent & labia flat	prominent clitoris & small labia minora	prominent clitoris & enlarging minora	majora & minora equally prominent	majora large minora small	majora cover clitoris & minora		

TOTAL PHYSICAL MATURITY SCORE

SCORE

Neuromuscular _____
Physical _____
Total _____

MATURITY RATING

SCORE	WEEKS
-10	20
-5	22
0	24
5	26
10	28
15	30
20	32
25	34
30	36
35	38
40	40
45	42
50	44

GESTATIONAL AGE (weeks)
By dates _____
By ultrasound _____
By exam _____

Reference
Ballard JL, Khoury JC, Wedig K, et al: New Ballard Score, expanded to include extremely premature infants. J Pediatr 1991; 119:417–423. Reprinted by permission of Dr Ballard and Mosby—Year Book, Inc.

Fig. 21-2. Ballard Gestational Assessment tool.

8. **Skin:** note skin turgor, color, texture, and predominance of vessels throughout the infant's body.

   ▦ **TIP** the easiest place to assess the infant's skin for the Gestational Age Assessment is on the abdomen. Mark the appropriate box.

9. **Lanugo:** note the distribution of lanugo; fine downy hair. Begin with the face and trunk, followed by the rest of the body. Mark the appropriate box.

10. **Plantar surface:** note the presence and location of creases on the soles of the infant's feet. Mark the appropriate box.

11. **Breast:** note the size of the breast bud. Palpate the nodule to determine its size. Mark the appropriate box.

12. **Eye/ear:** place your index finger on the infant's upper eyelid, with the thumb on the lower lid. Gently try to open the infant's eye. Note the degree to which you can open the eye. Palpate the infant's ear. Note the amount of cartilage. Fold the pinna of the ear toward the face and release it. Note the recoil. Mark the appropriate box.

13. **Genitals, male:** note the size of the scrotum and presence or absence of rugae. Gently palpate for descended testes. Place your fingers over the inguinal canal to prevent the testes from ascending into the abdominal cavity. Mark the appropriate box.

14. **Genitals, female:** note the prominence of the labia majora, and whether it covers the clitoris and labia minora. Mark the appropriate box.

15. Add up the scores from both the neuromuscular and physical maturity sections of the Ballard Assessment Tool. Determine the weeks that most closely match your score. This is your estimated gestational age.

NORMAL FINDINGS

- Appropriate for Gestational Age (AGA): weight is between 10th and 90th percentile.
- Full term: birth occurred between 39 0/7 weeks' gestation and 40 6/7 weeks' gestation (ACOG, 2013).

   ▦ **TIP** Weeks' gestation 40 6/7 means 40 weeks and 6 out of a 7 day week.

ABNORMAL FINDINGS

- Small for gestational age (SGA): weight is below 10th percentile.
- Large for gestational age (LGA): weight is above 90th percentile.
- Late preterm: birth occurred 34 0/7 weeks' gestation to 36 6/7 weeks' gestation.
- Early term: birth occurred prior to the completion of 37 0/7 weeks' gestation through 38 6/7 weeks' gestation.
- Late term: birth occurred 41 0/7 weeks' gestation through 41 6/7 weeks' gestation
- Post-term: birth occurred after the completion of 42 0/7 weeks' gestation or later (ACOG, 2013).

SENC Safety Alert Infants born just three to six weeks early are at greater risk for potentially serious health problems related to: hypoglycemia, poor feeding, respiratory compromise, lower temperature, jaundice, and infections (Forsythe, & Allen, 2013).

TECHNIQUE 21-2: **Assessing Newborn Measurements**

Purpose: To obtain accurate initial measurements of newborn height, weight, head and chest circumference

Technique 21-2A: **Assessing Weight**

Purpose: To obtain accurate initial weight of newborn

Equipment: Digital scale, gloves (optional)

> **SENC Safety Alert** Never leave an infant alone on the scale.

ASSESSMENT STEPS

1. Place a receiving blanket on the scale, and zero out the scale.
   ▪ **TIP** Procedure for zeroing the scale differs on the make and model of each scale. Refer to manufacturer's guidelines.
2. Ensure that the infant is completely naked.
3. Gently place the infant on the scale, placing a hand above the infant to ensure safety (Fig. 21-3).
4. Read and record the weight in both grams and pounds.
5. Gently place the infant back in the bassinet.
6. Plot the weight on a growth curve for gender (Fig. 21-4).
7. Document your findings.

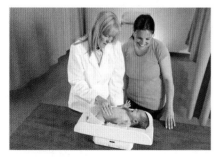

Fig. 21-3. Weighing an infant.

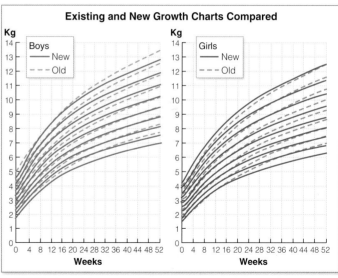

Fig. 21-4. Plotting weight on a growth curve.

▣ **TIP** About 10 percent weight loss related to decreased fluid intake and fluid loss is expected over the first 3 to 4 days after the infant is delivered.

NORMAL FINDINGS

■ Weight range for full-term infant is 2500 to 4000 g (5 lb. 8 oz. to 8 lb. 13 oz.) (Durham & Chapman, 2014).
■ Weight: average for full-term infant is 3400 g (7 lb. 8 oz.)

▣ **TIP** Weight must be related to gestational age. Weights above 90th percentile for gestational age are considered to be LGA. Weights below 10th percentile are considered to be SGA. Both of these categories increase an infant's risk for complications such as hypoglycemia and hypothermia.

ABNORMAL FINDINGS

■ Weight loss of more than 10 percent in the first 3 to 5 days of life

Technique 21-2B: Assessing Length

Purpose: To obtain an initial length of newborn
Equipment: Measuring tape, gloves (optional)

SENC Safety Alert If the infant has not had an initial bath, standard precautions should be taken and gloves should be put on to prevent the acquisition of infection.

ASSESSMENT STEPS

1. Gently place infant supine on a flat surface (i.e., examining table with disposable paper).
2. Place a mark at the top of the infant's head (Fig. 21-5A).
3. Gently extend the infant's leg and make a mark at the bottom of the infant's heel (Fig. 21-5B).
4. Gently place the infant back in the bassinet.
5. Measure the length from the head marking (lining the "0" of the tape measure at this mark) to the heel marking (Fig. 21-5C).

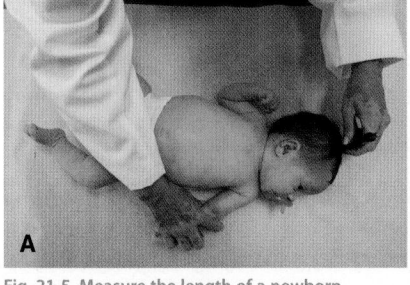
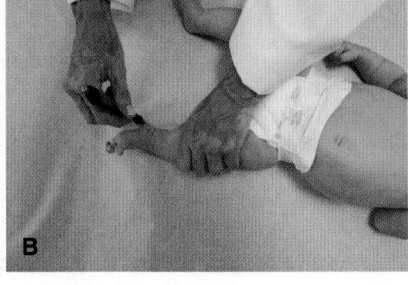
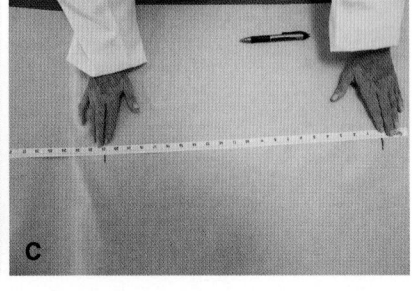

Fig. 21-5. Measure the length of a newborn.

6. Record the length in inches and centimeters.

7. Plot the length on a growth curve for gender.

NORMAL FINDINGS

■ Length range for term infant is 48 to 52 cm (18 to 22 inches).

    ▓ **TIP** The average length of a healthy term newborn is 50 cm (20 inches).

ABNORMAL FINDINGS

■ Length of less than 45 cm (17.7 inches) or greater than 55 cm (21.7 inches) may be indicative of a chromosomal abnormality.

    ▓ **TIP** Measuring can be difficult in the term infant because of molding of the head, or in breech delivery. In this case, use the initial measurement but know that the measurement might be different after the molding has resolved.

Technique 21-2C: **Measuring Chest Circumference**

Purpose: To obtain initial measurement of infant's chest circumference

Equipment: Paper measuring tape, gloves (optional)

ASSESSMENT STEPS

1. Place tape measure across infant's nipple line (Fig. 21-6).

2. Pull snugly upon infant's expiratory breath.

3. Note the measurement in inches and centimeters.

4. Discard tape measure.

5. Document your findings.

NORMAL FINDINGS

■ Ranges 30 to 35 cm (11.8 to 13.8 inches)

ABNORMAL FINDINGS

■ Chest circumference is greater than head circumference.

    ▓ **TIP** The average chest circumference is 32 cm (12.6 inches).

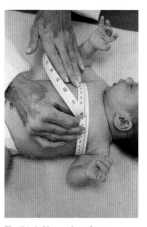

Fig. 21-6. Measuring chest circumference of an infant.

Technique 21-2D: **Measuring Head Circumference**

Purpose: To assess the infant's head circumference
Equipment: Measuring tape, gloves (optional)
ASSESSMENT STEPS

1. Find the greatest diameter of head-occipital frontal area (Fig. 21-7).
2. Gently place the measuring tape securely around the infant's head.
3. Place the center of the measuring tape at the back of the infant's head while the infant is laying supine. This prevents slippage.
4. Gently pull the measuring tape snugly and note the size of the head circumference.
5. Discard the tape measure.
6. Document the head circumference in centimeters or inches, per institutional policy.

NORMAL FINDINGS

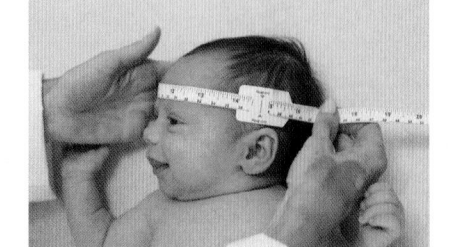

Fig. 21-7. Measuring head circumference of an infant.

■ Head circumference is 32 to 37 cm (12.6 to 14.6 inches)

ABNORMAL FINDINGS

■ Head circumference less than 32 cm (12.6 in), or 4 cm (1.6 in) greater than the chest circumference.
■ **Macrocephalic** is an enlarged head greater than two standard deviations above the mean for a given age, sex and gestation; abnormally large head.
■ **Microcephalic** is a head circumference greater than two standard deviations below the mean for a given age, sex, and gestation; abnormally small head.

　TIP A newborn's head circumference should be about 2 cm greater than chest circumference.

TECHNIQUE 21-3: **Assessing Vital Signs**

Purpose: To assess the general health of the infant

Technique 21-3A: **Assessing Temperature**

Purpose: To assess the body's core temperature
Equipment: Digital thermometer, gloves
ASSESSMENT STEPS

1. Remove any clothing from the infant's torso.
2. Visualize the infant's axilla.

3. Gently place the thermometer probe in the deepest part of the axilla (Fig. 21-8).

4. Gently hold the infant's arm in place snugly against the torso.

5. When thermometer registers and beeps, note the temperature.

6. Document your findings.

NORMAL FINDINGS

■ Normal range is 36.5 to 37.4°C (97.7°F to 99.3°F)

ABNORMAL FINDINGS

■ Below 36.5°C (97.7°F) or above 38°C (100.4°F)

SENC Safety Alert Rectal temperature is assumed to be the most accurate representation of the newborn's core temperature. However, this method is not recommended as a routine method because it may cause health risks (Yi-Chien, Chieh-Yu, Chia-Chi, & Wei-Wen, 2013).

SENC Safety Alert Notify the healthcare provider for temperatures below 36.5°C (97.7°F) or above 38°C (100.4°F) or 36.4°C (97.5°F); Rather than becoming hyperthermic, septic infants tend to become hypothermic.

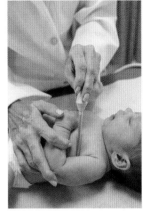

Fig. 21-8. Taking axillary temperature.

Technique 21-3B: Assessing the Heart Rate

Purpose: To assess the heart rate of the newborn

Equipment: Neonatal stethoscope, watch or clock with a second hand, gloves (optional)

TIP If infant is quiet or sleeping, obtain heart rate before any other part of your assessment. Heart rate will be easiest to assess on a quiet infant.

Healthy People 2020

Goal: To decrease the rate of infant deaths related to congenital heart birth defects (HHS, 2010).

ASSESSMENT STEPS

1. Wipe off the stethoscope with an alcohol swab.

2. Warm the stethoscope between the palms of your hands.

3. Place stethoscope on infant's chest, near the left nipple, at the fourth intercostal space (Fig. 21-9).

4. Auscultate the heart rate.

5. Listen for the crisp S1 and S2 sounds and for heart murmurs.

6. Determine whether rhythm is regular or irregular.

7. Count the apical heart rate for 1 full minute.

8. Document your findings.

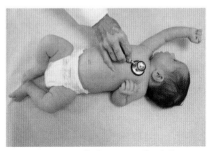

Fig. 21-9. Assessing the heart rate of an infant.

■ **TIP** Any deviation from the crisp sounds qualifies as a murmur.

NORMAL FINDINGS

■ Heart rate ranges from 120 to 160 beats per minute (bpm).

ABNORMAL FINDINGS

■ Heart rate greater than 160 bpm (**tachycardia**)
■ Heart rate less than 100 bpm (**bradycardia**)
■ **Heart murmur** is an abnormal sound during the heartbeat cycle such as a whooshing or swishing sound made by turbulent blood in or near the heart.
■ **Cardiac arrhythmia** is an abnormal heart rhythm.

SENC Safety Alert Notify the healthcare provider upon auscultation of an irregular heart rate, or a heart murmur.

■ **TIP** Be sure to note the activity level of the infant when interpreting the results. An infant who is in a deep sleep may have a heart rate of as low as 100, while a crying infant may have a heart rate above 160.

Technique 21-3C: **Assessing the Respiratory Rate**

Purpose: To assess pulmonary ventilation
Equipment: Neonatal stethoscope, watch or clock with a second hand
■ **TIP** If the infant is quiet and/or sleeping, obtain respiratory rate before any other vital sign.

Infants are abdominal breathers. It is easiest to assess the respiratory rate by viewing the infant's abdomen. The respiratory rate can be obtained by direct observation or auscultation with a stethoscope.

ASSESSMENT STEPS

1. Carefully observe the rise and fall (one breath) of the infant's abdomen.
2. Count respirations for 1 full minute.
3. Document your findings.

NORMAL FINDINGS

■ Respiratory rate will be irregular in depth, rate, and rhythm; short pauses between 5 to 10 seconds are normal.
■ Ranges from 30 to 60 breaths/minute

ABNORMAL FINDINGS

■ Apneic period of 20 seconds or longer
■ Respiratory rate of greater than 60 breaths/minute
■ Seesaw or paradoxical respirations instead of abdominal respirations. In normal respirations, the newborn's chest and abdomen rise simultaneously. With seesaw respirations, the newborn's chest wall retracts and the abdomen rises with inspirations (Davidson, LonPut on, & Ladewig, 2012).

SENC Safety Alert Notify the healthcare provider if the infant has prolonged apnea with a noted color change or more than one apneic period, or prolonged tachypnea.

■ **TIP** If you cannot clearly see the rise and fall of the newborn's abdomen, auscultate both the anterior and posterior chest. It can be difficult to distinguish between heart rate, respiratory rate, and bowel sounds in an infant. It is helpful to close your eyes and focus in on the respiratory rate alone. This can be done most easily by auscultating breath sounds on the right side of the infant's chest (anterior). Attempt to correlate the respirations heard upon auscultation with the infant's abdominal respirations.

Technique 21-3D: Assessing Blood Pressure

Purpose: To assess circulatory blood volume as the heart contracts and relaxes
Equipment: Noninvasive electronic BP device, BP cuff (appropriately sized for the newborn)

Healthy People 2020

Goal: To obtain accurate blood pressure (BP) measurement and screen for congenital heart defects (HHS, 2010).

■ **TIP** The preferred time to obtain the BP reading is while the infant is asleep.

BP is not routinely measured on healthy newborns. However, BP monitoring is an essential measurement in newborns who are premature or have cardiac or renal disease (Davidson et al., 2012).

■ **TIP** Swaddling the infant or giving the infant a pacifier can help soothe and calm the infant.

ASSESSMENT STEPS

1. Determine appropriate BP cuff size for the newborn: the cuff should cover two thirds of the upper arm or upper leg.
2. Gently restrain the limb that you are going to use for the BP by gently holding the corresponding hand or foot with your hand.
3. Position the BP cuff on the infant's extremity and wait until the infant becomes calm (Fig. 21-10).
4. Press the button on the digital BP monitor to allow the BP measurement to begin.
5. Continue to gently restrain the limb until the BP measurement appears on the screen.
6. Document your findings.

NORMAL FINDINGS

■ The normal BP range for a newborn is 50–75/30–45 mm Hg at birth.
■ Normal BP for a full-term infant at birth is 72/42.

ABNORMAL FINDINGS

■ BP exceeding 95 mm Hg systolic or 75 mm Hg diastolic in a term newborn is considered to be hypertensive; may be related to kidney or congenital heart conditions.

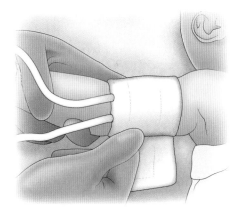

Fig. 21-10. Taking an infant's blood pressure.

- To determine hypertension in the newborn, BP readings must meet this criterion for at least three consecutive days (Merenstein & Gardner, 2010).
- Coarctation of the aorta is a common congenital heart defect, an abnormality in the structure of the aorta that is present at birth or shortly after birth; the blood pressure in the upper body is high and in the lower body is very low; the quality of pulses of the upper and lower extremities is different (O'Brien & Marshall, 2015).

  SENC Safety Alert If a cardiac anomaly is suspected, BP readings and pulses in all four extremities must be assessed.

  TIP Movement, crying, and using a too-small BP cuff can falsely increase the BP reading.

TECHNIQUE 21-4: **General Assessment**

Purpose: To assess the newborn's systems and observe for any abnormalities
A portion of this assessment can be completed without rousing the infant.

  SENC Safety Alert The infant can become cold quickly. Be sure to perform the examination quickly and in a heated environment.

  TIP A newborn assessment should be completed in a head-to-toe fashion.

ASSESSMENT STEPS

1. Stand at the infant's side and inspect and observe the infant's

  ☐ Activity level
  • Deep sleep
  • Light sleep
  • Drowsy
  • Quiet alert
  • Active alert
  • Crying

  TIP A newborn in the quiet alert phase may smile, vocalize, and respond to people talking to her or him. The infant's respiratory rate is regular, and the infant will lay still and focus on objects in front of him or her. In the active alert phase, the infant appears restless and may move his or her head from side to side. Respirations may be irregular, and the infant may not be interested in stimulation.

  ☐ Resting posture
  ☐ Muscle tone

  TIP A normal newborn muscle tone includes flexed upper and lower extremities.

2. Assess the skin throughout the assessment. Skin deviations can be found anywhere on the infant's body.
- ☐ Color
  - Pink
  - Jaundiced (yellow) is a symptom of hyperbilirubinemia; increased bilirubin levels

    TIP You can assess if an infant is jaundiced by pressing one finger on the infant's forehead, nose, or sternum; if the skin is jaundiced, it will appear yellow when you release pressure from the skin; jaundice commonly is seen in the face and then progresses to the lower extremities.

  - Pale
  - **Acrocyanosis:** blue hands and feet related to peripheral vasoconstriction; more common when exposed to low temperatures and the infant is cold (Fig. 21-11A)

    TIP Acrocyanosis is normal in the first 24 to 48 hours of life.

  - Mottled-lacy pattern of dilated blood vessels under the skin (Fig. 21-11B)

NORMAL FINDINGS
- ■ Depends on gestational age and ethnicity
  - ☐ Preterm infants will have lanugo and vernix caseosa present.
    - **Lanugo** is fine hair covering the body, present on the upper head, back, shoulders; decreases with advancing gestation (Fig. 21-12).
    - **Vernix caseosa** is a thick, white, cheese-like coating made up of oil on the skin and dead skin cells; may be present at birth especially in the folds of the skin (Fig. 21-13).

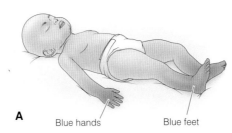
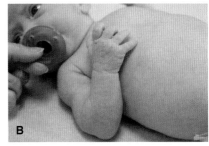

A Blue hands   Blue feet

Fig. 21-11. (A) Acrocyanosis. (B) Mottling.

B

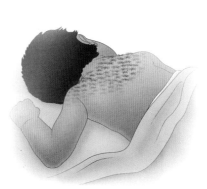

Fig. 21-12. Lanugo.

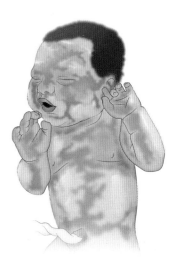

Fig. 21-13. Vernix caseosa.

- ☐ Postterm infants will have peeling, dry, cracked skin.
- ☐ **Milia** are pearly white cysts on the skin formed from the sebaceous glands; often found on the nose (Fig. 21-14).
- ■ Birthmarks can include:
  - ☐ **Nevus simplex (stork bites)** are capillaries close to the surface of the skin; flat and red in color, and become more saturated with color when the infant cries; commonly seen on the nape of the neck and between the eyebrows (Fig. 21-15).
  - ☐ **Mongolian spots:** bluish-black pigmented areas common in infants of African, Asian, and Mediterranean descent; commonly found on the sacral area (Fig. 21-16).

CULTURAL CONSIDERATIONS Mongolian spots are commonly found on African-American, Filipino-American, Navajo Native-American, and Chinese-American newborns; reassure the family that most Mongolian spots will disappear over time (Purnell, 2014).

  - ☐ **Hemangioma** is a harmless growth or tumor made up of tiny blood vessels; also called a "strawberry mark." Most commonly found on the head and trunk (Fig. 21-17).

    ■ **TIP** Hemangiomas affect about 10 percent of infants, and the risk is about five times higher in females than males. Caucasian infants and premature infants are at an increased risk for hemangioma, as are infants born to mothers with an abnormal placenta (Skinsight, 2008).
  - ☐ **Café au lait spots** are permanent flat patches that can be found anywhere on the body; tan to light brown in color (Fig. 21-18).

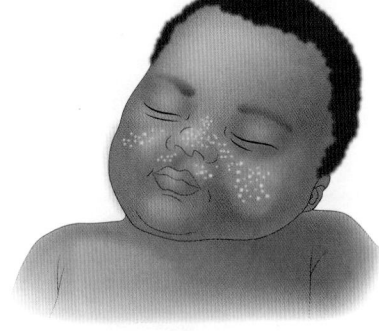

Fig. 21-14. Milia.

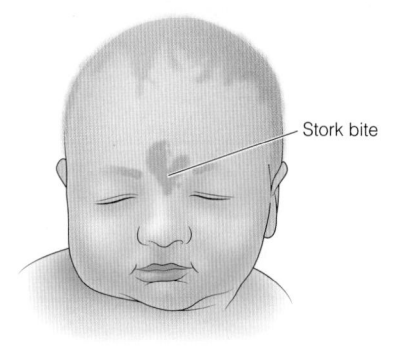

Stork bite

Fig. 21-15. Stork bites.

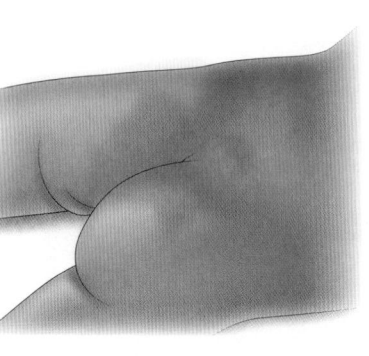

Fig. 21-16. Mongolian spots.

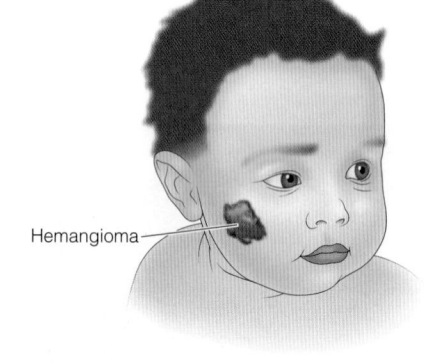

Hemangioma

Fig. 21-17. Hemangioma.

- □ **Nevus flammeus (port-wine stain)** is a capillary malformation of superficial dermal blood vessels just below the surface of the skin; red or purple in color; does not blanche; this is a permanent malformation (Fig. 21-19).
- □ **Erythema toxicum** is a benign newborn rash; presents as firm yellow-white papules or pustules with a red base (Venes, 2013); often found on the face and trunk (Fig. 21-20).

ABNORMAL FINDINGS

- ■ **Pathological jaundice** (jaundice that appears before 24 hours of age) is associated with anemia and hepatosplenomegaly (enlarged liver and spleen). It is usually caused by a blood group incompatibility but can also be caused by infection or blood disorders.
- ■ **Pale color and mottled skin** may indicate poor perfusion or poor thermoregulation.
- ■ **Central cyanosis** is a bluish hue to the skin and mucus membranes indicative of hypoxia, signs of pulmonary disease, or congenital heart malformations.
- ■ **Petechiae** are small, flat, red or purplish spots below the surface of the skin caused by broken capillaries and can be a result of birth injury, infection, or blood disorder.

▋**TIP** Skin color is most easily assessed by blanching the skin. Regardless of the ethnicity of the infant, the underlying color when blanched should be pink. Color is best assessed along with capillary refill on the infant's sternum.

SENC Safety Alert If the infant has multiple café au lait spots or a hemangioma on the face or neck, notify the healthcare provider. Multiple café au lait spots may indicate neurofibromatosis type 1, a genetic disorder (James & Sheth, 2011).

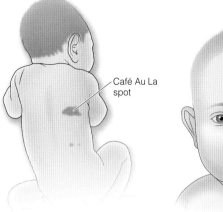

Café Au La spot

Fig. 21-18. Café au lait spots.

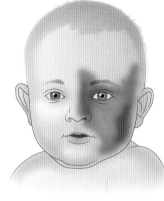

Fig. 21-19. Nevus flammeus.

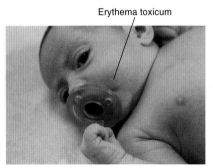

Erythema toxicum

Fig. 21-20. Erythema toxicum.

Technique 21-4A: Inspecting and Palpating the Head

Purpose: To assess abnormalities of the head

Equipment: Gloves (optional)

ASSESSMENT STEPS

1. Carefully inspect the parts of the infant's head:
- ☐ Anterior fontanel
- ☐ Posterior fontanel

2. Standing on the side of the infant, inspect the shape of the infant's head for abnormal deviations.

3. Gently palpate the anterior fontanel (Fig. 21-21).

4. Gently palpate the cranial suture line from the anterior fontanel to the posterior fontanel; may be separated, approximated, or overriding.

5. Gently palpate for the posterior fontanel.

6. Document your findings.

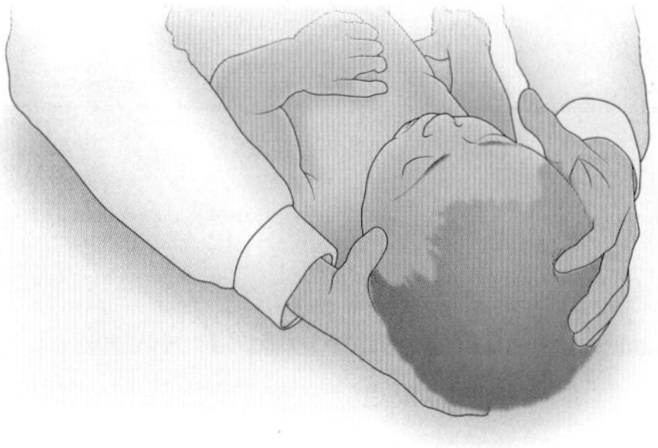

Fig. 21-21. Palpating the anterior fontanel.

NORMAL FINDINGS

- Anterior fontanel: diamond shaped, should feel soft and flat
- Posterior fontanel: may be nonpalpable; triangular in shape and smaller than the anterior fontanel
- Sutures may be separated, approximated, or overriding
- Shape of head: round or molding
- Common deviations include
  - ☐ Molding of head
  - ☐ Lacerations may be present on the scalp from amniohook or fetal scalp electrode that was needed during labor.
  - ☐ Bruising and swelling may be evident if the pushing stage of labor was prolonged.

ABNORMAL FINDINGS

- Bulging or depressed fontanels
- **Caput succedaneum** is diffuse edema of the fetal scalp that crosses the suture lines (Venes, 2013); often caused by pressure on the head during a head-first delivery (Fig. 21-22A).
- **Cephalohematoma** is a unilateral collection of blood between the skull and the periosteum; does not cross the suture line; often caused by birth trauma (Fig. 21-22B).
- Bruising may or may not be evident.

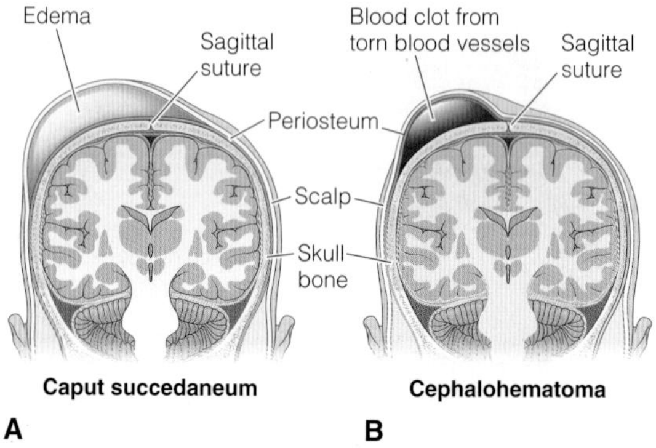

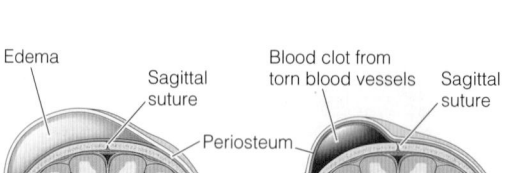

Caput succedaneum   **Cephalohematoma**

A   **B**

Fig. 21-22. (A) Caput succedaneum. (B) Cephalohematoma.

Technique 21-4B: **Inspecting the Face**

Purpose: To assess deviations and abnormalities of the eyes, ears, nose, and mouth
Equipment: Gloves (optional), penlight

SENC Safety Alert Infants are obligate nose breathers but do not develop the response of opening the mouth due to a nasal obstruction for several weeks after birth. If an infant has complete nasal obstruction of both nares, the newborn will go into respiratory distress; flaring of nostrils is a sign of respiratory distress. Before notifying the healthcare provider, assess for other signs of respiratory distress such as tachypnea (RR greater than 60 breaths per minute), grunting, retractions, or see-saw breathing.

ASSESSMENT STEPS

1. Inspect the face for symmetry; compare both sides.
2. Inspect the following parts of the eyes:
   □ Color of the eye
   □ Sclera for color
   □ Conjunctiva
   □ Eyelid edema may be present due to prolonged pushing during delivery.
   □ Presence of yellow or white discharge may indicate a clogged tear duct or conjunctivitis.
   ▓ **TIP** A jaundiced infant will often have yellow sclera. Jaundice begins at the head and moves to the toes and recedes in the reverse order. Therefore, yellow sclera is often the first sign of jaundice, as well as the last part of the body to remain jaundiced when it is resolving. Treatment for jaundice includes hydration and phototherapy.
3. Inspect the nose for patency.
4. Occlude the left naris (nostril) with one finger.
5. Observe for flaring of the right naris for cyanosis or asphyxia (decreased oxygen to the body).
6. Occlude the right naris with one finger.
7. Observe for flaring of the left naris for cyanosis or asphyxia.
   ▓ **TIP** Some mucous discharge may be present, but there should be no drainage
8. Inspect the ears for:
   □ Size
   □ Position in relation to the eyes
9. Determine the position of the ears in relation to the eyes; draw an imaginary line from the inner canthus of the eye outward. The eye should be even with the upper tip of the pinna of the ear (Fig. 21-23).
10. Clap next to the infant's right ear; observe to see if the infant turns his or her head toward the direction of the sound.
11. Clap next to the infant's left ear; observe to see if the infant turns his or her head toward the direction of the sound.

TIP Most states mandate hearing testing of the newborns prior to discharge from the hospital so early intervention can be initiated if hearing impairment is found.

12. Using a penlight, inspect the inside of the infant's mouth. If the infant does not open his or her mouth, place your finger on the infant's chin and apply gentle pressure to open the mouth. Inspect the color and mucous membranes.

13. Put on gloves, gently insert an index finger into the infant's mouth with the pad of the index finger touching the infant's palate. Palpate for a smooth, uninterrupted palate (Fig. 21-24).

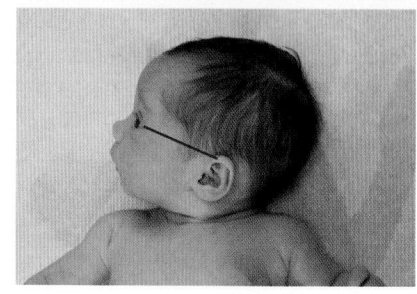

Fig. 21-23. Determining position of the ears.

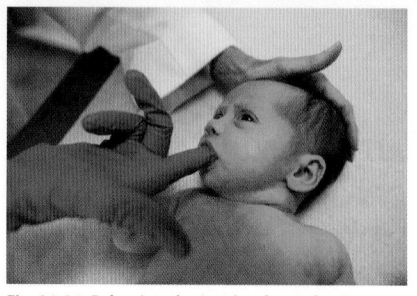

Fig. 21-24. Palpating the inside of an infant's mouth.

TIP It is easier to assess the infant's mouth when the infant is crying. If the infant is not crying, gently apply pressure on the infant's chin with your index finger to open the mouth.

14. Gently palpate the hard and soft palates to determine whether they are intact.

15. Assess the positive **sucking reflex** by inserting a gloved index finger into the infant's mouth with the pad of your finger touching the roof of the infant's mouth. The infant should begin to suck on your finger (Fig. 21-25).

16. Assess the **gag reflex.** After assessing the suck, move your index finger back toward the infant's uvula. This will elicit the gag reflex, and the infant will attempt to push your finger out of the mouth using his or her tongue.

17. Assess the **rooting reflex** by gently stroking the infant's cheek, moving from the mouth outward. The infant should turn his or her head toward the direction of your finger (Fig. 21-26).

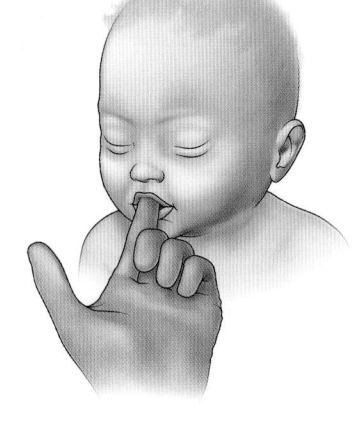

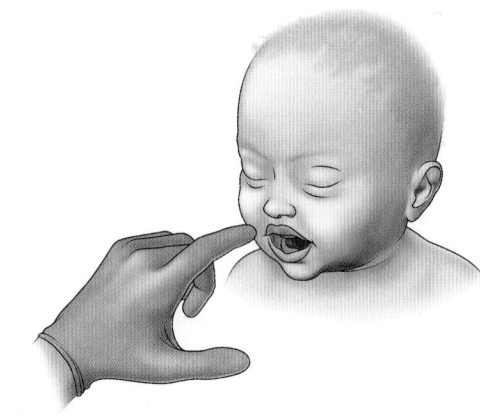

Fig. 21-25. Assessing the sucking reflex.

Fig. 21-26. Assessing the rooting reflex.

18. Remove and discard gloves.

19. Document your findings.

NORMAL FINDINGS

- Face is symmetrical.
- Eyes are symmetrical, no discharge, sclera white, conjunctiva pink.
- Nose is patent bilaterally; no nasal flaring or discharge.
- Ears: normally placed, no pits or tags
- Mouth: mucous membranes pink and moist. Hard and soft palates intact. Epstein pearls may be present. Epstein pearls are small cysts on the roof of the mouth formed when the palate fused (Fig. 21-27).
- Infant will turn his/her head toward the clapping sound.
- Suck, gag, and rooting reflex are present.

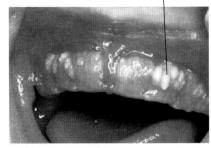

Epstein's pearls

Fig. 21-27. Epstein's pearls.

ABNORMAL FINDINGS

- Face is asymmetrical, often due to position in utero.
- Eyes: eyelid edema can be expected when there is an extended pushing phase of labor; subconjunctival hemorrhage is a ruptured blood vessel(s) are seen in the white of the eye.
- Nose: nasal flaring, nasal discharge, asymmetry of the nose
- Ears: preauricular pits appear to be dimples resembling pin pricks near the ear.
  - □ Preauricular skin tags can occasionally be found near the ear. They do not contain cartilage or bone. Infants with preauricular pits or tags should be closely evaluated for additional congenital malformations.
  - □ Low-set ears can be a sign of a chromosomal abnormality or a renal disorder.
- Mouth: mucous membranes dry, cyanotic, cleft hard or soft palate, natal teeth are present
  - □ Absent suck, rooting, or gag reflex

SENC Safety Alert Be alert to the infant's mouth when crying. Facial paralysis is evident when the mouth is asymmetric with crying. This can occur from the pressure on the facial nerve caused by pressure of the maternal pelvis or forceps during deliver (Nagtalon-Ramos, 2013).

Technique 21-4C: **Assessing the Neck**

Purpose: To assess range of motion (ROM) of the neck

ASSESSMENT STEPS

1. Inspect the skin folds of the neck.

2. Assess ROM.
  - □ If infant is active, observe infant's ability to turn head to the right and left, up and down.
  - □ If infant is sleeping or not actively moving, gently manipulate head to the left and right, up and down to observe passive ROM.

3. Document your findings.

NORMAL FINDINGS

■ Neck short, thick, no webbing

■ ROM: full, neck moves freely from side to side and up and down

ABNORMAL FINDINGS

■ Webbing of the neck is when the skin folds appear as loose folds of skin (may indicate Down's syndrome or Turner's syndrome)

  □ **Down's syndrome** is a genetic disorder caused by an error in cell division. The newborn has a pair or extra copy of chromosome 21.

  □ **Turner's syndrome** is a genetic disorder that is related to the females having only one X chromosome; the second X chromosome is missing.

■ ROM: limited (may indicate nerve damage)

TECHNIQUE 21-5: **Assessing the Peripheral Vascular System**

Purpose: To assess cardiovascular perfusion

Technique 21-5A: **Assessing Capillary Refill**
Purpose: To assess peripheral perfusion
Equipment: Watch with a second hand, gloves (optional)

ASSESSMENT STEPS

1. Position the infant in the supine position.

2. Using the finger pad of the index finger, gently press down and blanche the skin on the infant's sternum (Fig. 21-28).

  SENC Safety Alert Be sure to position your finger on the sternum, not the xiphoid process. Pressing too hard on the xiphoid process can cause a fracture.

3. Note the time in seconds that it takes for the blanched skin to return to a normal color.

4. Document your findings.

NORMAL FINDINGS

■ Capillary refill less than 3 seconds

ABNORMAL FINDINGS

■ Poor perfusion if capillary refill is greater than 3 seconds

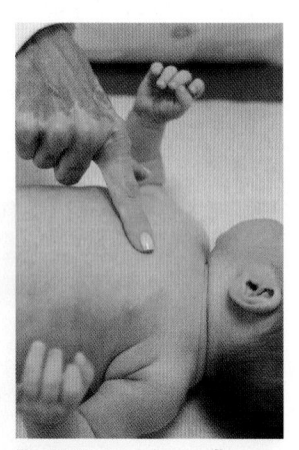

Fig. 21-28. Assessing capillary refill on the sternum.

Technique 21-5B: **Palpating Peripheral Pulses**

Purpose: To assess peripheral perfusion

Equipment: Gloves (optional)

ASSESSMENT STEPS

1. Position the infant in supine position.

2. Using the finger pads of your index finger of both your hands, gently palpate both the right and left brachial pulses between the triceps and the biceps muscles.

☐ Assess both the right and left brachial pulses simultaneously makes it easier to determine whether they are equal (Fig. 21-29A).

3. Note the rhythm and equality.

TIP If you are certain that you are feeling for the pulse in the correct location but cannot seem to find it, ease up on the pressure exerted by your finger; an infant's brachial pulse is easily occluded by moderate pressure of a finger pad.

4. Using the finger pad of your index finger of both your hands, gently palpate both the right and left femoral pulses in the infant's inguinal area (groin area) (Fig. 21-29B).

☐ Assessing both the right and left femoral pulses simultaneously makes it easier to determine whether the pulses are equal.

5. Document your findings.

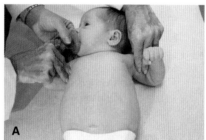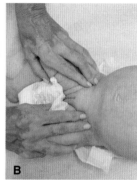

Fig. 21-29. (A) Assessing brachial pulses. (B) Assessing femoral pulses.

NORMAL FINDINGS

■ Brachial and femoral pulsations are present and equal.

ABNORMAL FINDINGS

■ Peripheral pulses are nonpalpable.

SENC Safety Alert If the pulses are nonpalpable, note the color and temperature of the extremity as well as the ROM. If there is a nonpalpable pulse along with a cool, pale extremity, or limited ROM, notify the healthcare provider immediately.

TECHNIQUE 21-6: **Assessing the Respiratory System**

Purpose: To assess pulmonary perfusion
Equipment: Neonatal stethoscope, gloves (optional)

ASSESSMENT STEPS

1. Place infant in supine position.
2. Observe the clavicular, substernal, and intercostal areas of the chest.
3. Closely observe the rise and fall of the infant's chest while breathing and count the number of breaths for one minute.

    ■ **TIP** One inspiration and one expiration equals one breath.

4. Using the bell of the neonatal stethoscope, auscultate the anterior and posterior lungs.
5. Place stethoscope on infant's anterior chest bilaterally and listen for equality of bilateral breath sounds in a systematic pattern from the apex to the base of the lungs.
6. Gently roll the infant to his or her side, place the stethoscope on the infant's posterior chest bilaterally and listen for equality of bilateral breath sounds in a systematic pattern from the apex to the base of the lungs (Fig. 21-30).

    ■ **TIP** There is no need to reposition the infant to the prone position to listen to the posterior portion of the chest. Simply roll the infant to his or her side to auscultate the lungs. This will cause less manipulation of the infant, and will make it less likely that the infant will cry.

7. Document your findings.

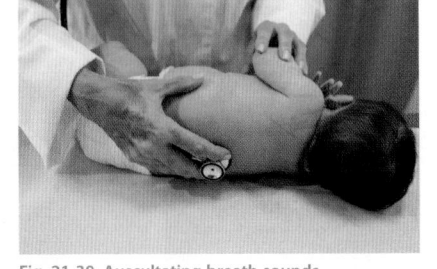

Fig. 21-30. Auscultating breath sounds.

NORMAL FINDINGS

■ Thoracic area: no retractions observed
■ Diaphragmatic respirations are present; rate between 30 and 60 bpm
■ Breath sounds are clear and equal bilaterally.

ABNORMAL FINDINGS

■ Substernal, intercostal, or suprasternal retractions are present; may indicate respiratory distress.
■ Breath sounds are decreased on one side (may indicate a pneumothorax, a collapsed lung), crackles are heard (may indicate retained fluid in the lungs).

TECHNIQUE 21-7: **Inspecting and Palpating the Chest**

Purpose: To assess and screen for fractured clavicles
Equipment: Gloves (optional)

ASSESSMENT STEPS

1. Place the infant in the supine position.
2. Standing on the side of the infant, inspect the shape of the infant's chest.
3. Draw an imaginary line down the center of the infant's chest and observe for symmetry of both sides (Fig. 21-31).
4. Using your index finger pads, gently palpate each clavicle from the shoulder to the sternum; listen and feel for crepitus, edema, or a noticeable step-off.

   ▌**TIP Crepitus** is a crackling, grating, or crinkly feeling or sound under the skin; it is heard when two ends of a broken bone grate together (Venes, 2013).

5. Inspect breasts for symmetry.
6. Inspect the number of nipples; observe for number of nipples along the nipple line.

   ▌**TIP** Occasionally infants will have **supernumerary nipples** (extra nipples) that are smaller and located in line with the nipple line (Fig. 21-32).

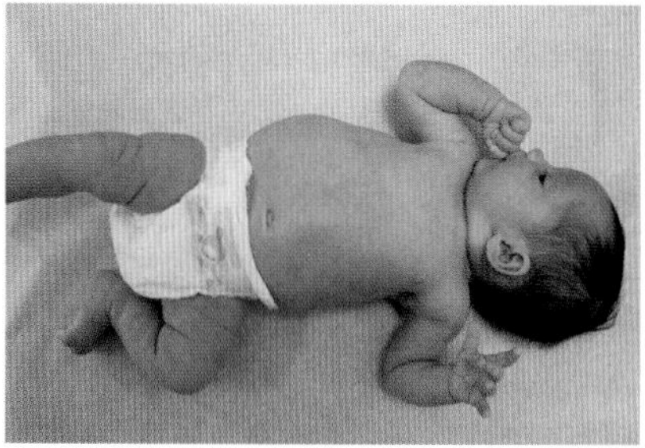

CULTURAL CONSIDERATIONS Supernumerary nipples are commonly found in dark-skinned infants (Nagtalon-Ramos, 2013).

7. Using the finger pads of the second and third fingers, gently palpate the breasts for size of breast buds.
8. Put on gloves, gently squeeze each breast bud with the finger pads of your fingertips to assess for galactorrhea (witch's milk) (Fig. 21-33).

   ▌**TIP Galactorrhea** is milky white discharge from the nipple. It is caused by high maternal estrogen hormonal levels and is considered a normal deviation.

SENC Safety Alert In some healthcare institutions, massage or manipulation of the breast tissue may not be done because it may force bacteria into the milk glands, which can lead to mastitis (Wammanda, 2004).

9. Remove and discard gloves.
10. Document your findings.

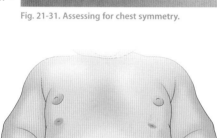

Fig. 21-31. Assessing for chest symmetry.

Fig. 21-32. Supernumerary nipples.

NORMAL FINDINGS
- Chest is symmetrical, barrel shaped.
- Clavicles are intact, feel straight and smooth.
- Breasts have two well-formed, symmetrical breast buds.
- Breast nodule is approximately 6 mm in diameter.
- Galactorrhea may be present.

ABNORMAL FINDINGS
- Symmetry: asymmetrical chest
- Clavicles: crepitus on one or more clavicles (may indicate a fractured clavicle)
- Breasts: supernumerary nipples present
- Engorged breast nodule (greater than 6 mm in diameter)

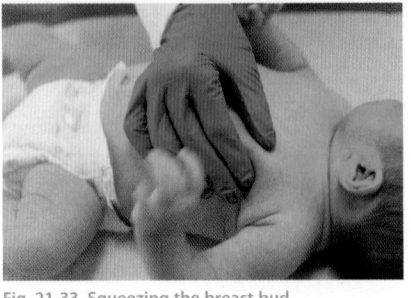

Fig. 21-33. Squeezing the breast bud.

TECHNIQUE 21-8: **Assessing the Abdomen**

Purpose: To assess the gastrointestinal system
Equipment: Neonatal stethoscope, gloves (optional)

Technique 21-8A: **Inspecting the Abdomen**
Purpose: To assess symmetry of the abdomen

ASSESSMENT STEPS
1. Place the infant in the supine position.
2. Standing on the side of the infant, assess the infant's abdomen for symmetry.
3. Draw an imaginary line down the center of the infant's abdomen, and assess whether both sides are equal (Fig. 21-34).
4. Inspect the infant's abdomen from the side, noting the shape.
5. Inspect the umbilical cord for number of vessels, color, consistency, drainage, odor, and signs of infection.
6. Document your findings.

NORMAL FINDINGS
- Abdomen is symmetrical.
- Shape: round, dome shaped, nondistended

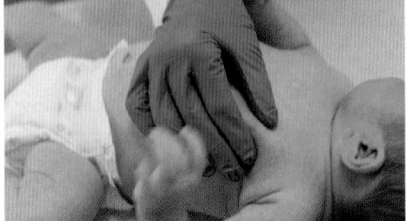

Fig. 21-34. Assessing the newborn abdomen for symmetry.

- Umbilical cord has two arteries and one vein present; no odor, no drainage, no signs of redness or inflammation around the base of the umbilical cord (Fig. 21-35).

   ▓ **TIP** If the assessment is within the first 24 hours after birth, the cord will appear moist and jelly-like. After 24 hours, the cord will begin to shrivel up and dry.

ABNORMAL FINDINGS
- Asymmetrical
- Shape: scaphoid may indicate diaphragmatic hernia (where the intestines are herniated into the chest cavity), distended abdomen (may indicate intestinal obstruction)
- Umbilical cord: one artery and one vein present (known as a two-vessel cord); these infants have an increased risk of cardiac, renal, and gastrointestinal anomalies.
- Signs of infection may be present; redness, foul odor, discharge.

CULTURAL CONSIDERATIONS People of European-American heritage believe the infant should wear a band around the abdomen to prevent the umbilicus from protruding and becoming herniated (Purnell, 2014).

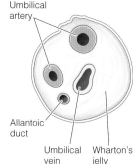
Fig. 21-35. Umbilical cord: two arteries, one vein.

Technique 21-8B: Auscultating Bowel Sounds

Purpose: To assess peristalsis
Equipment: Neonatal stethoscope
▓ **TIP** Always auscultate bowel sounds before you palpate the abdomen. Palpation can trigger increased bowel sounds.
The environment should be quiet to accurately auscultate bowel sounds.

ASSESSMENT STEPS
1. Place the infant in the supine position.
2. Using the bell of the neonatal stethoscope, auscultate for bowel sounds in all four quadrants (right lower, right upper, left upper, and left lower) of the infant's abdomen (Fig. 21-36).
3. Listen for up to one full minute before stating that there are no bowel sounds.
4. Document your findings.

   ▓ **TIP** Infant bowel sounds often sound quieter and have a lower frequency than those of the adult due to the smaller size of the infant's intestines.

NORMAL FINDINGS
- Bowel sounds are present in all four quadrants within 1 to 2 hours after birth.

ABNORMAL FINDINGS
- Absent or hypoactive bowel sounds may indicate an intestinal obstruction.

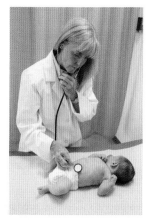
Fig. 21-36. Auscultating bowel sounds using the bell of the stethoscope.

Technique 21-8C: **Palpating the Abdomen**

Purpose: To assess for abdominal distention and masses
Equipment: Bulb syringe, gloves (optional), pediatric stethoscope

■ **TIP** Palpating the infant's abdomen may cause the infant to spit up some of his or her last feeding. The best time to palpate the infant's abdomen is prior to a feeding or 2 to 3 hours after a feeding.

SENC Safety Alert Always have a bulb syringe in the infant's crib in case of spitting up or choking.

ASSESSMENT STEPS

1. Note the time of the infant's last feeding.
2. Place the infant in the supine position.
3. Using the finger pads of the second and third fingers, gently palpate all four quadrants of the infant's abdomen (Fig. 21-37).
4. Document your findings.

NORMAL FINDINGS

■ Abdomen is soft, nontender to touch, no masses palpated.

ABNORMAL FINDINGS

■ Abdomen tense and firm (may indicate abdominal mass or intestinal obstruction), mass

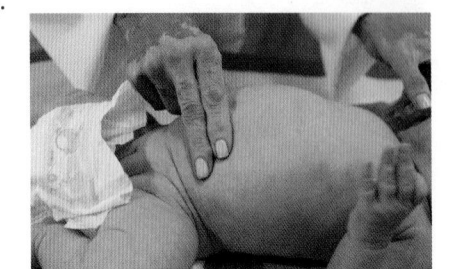

Fig. 21-37. Palpating the abdomen.

TECHNIQUE 21-9: **Assessing the Musculoskeletal System**

Purpose: To assess ROM and neurological integrity of the extremities
Equipment: Gloves (optional)

ASSESSMENT STEPS

1. Place the infant in the supine position.
2. Standing on the side of the infant, assess both the upper and lower extremities for
  □ Full ROM of all four extremities
  □ Active ROM of all four extremities
  □ Symmetrical ROM of all four extremities
3. Assess the degree of flexion of the infant's upper and lower extremities.
4. Document your findings.

NORMAL FINDINGS

■ Infant has full, active, symmetrical ROM and flexion of all four extremities.

■ Asymmetrical, absent, stiff, or incomplete ROM of any of the four extremities.

Technique 21-9A: **Assessing the Hands**

Purpose: To assess the number of digits on the hands and screen for potential abnormalities

Equipment: Gloves (optional)

ASSESSMENT STEPS

1. Place infant in the supine position.

2. Using your thumb, gently unfurl (uncurl) the infant's fingers.

▨ **TIP** Infants like to maintain their hands balled into a fist. Gently unfurl the fingers to count the digits. Often when there is an extra digit, the infant is grasping it in the other fingers.

3. Count the number of digits on the infant's hand.

4. Inspect the infant's right palmar creases while gently holding the infant's hand open.

5. Inspect the infant's left palmar creases while gently holding the infant's hand open.

6. Assess the **palmar grasp reflex.** Gently insert your thumbs into the palms of the infant's hands and observe the infant curling his or her fingers around your thumb (Fig. 21-38).

▨ **TIP** You can easily test for the Moro reflex along with the palmar grasp.

7. Before releasing the infant's hands from the palmar grasp, allow the infant to lay his or her head and trunk back onto a flat surface; abruptly let go of the hands, thereby eliciting a startle reflex (**Moro reflex**).With the Moro reflex, the newborn's arms and legs will symmetrically extend and then abduct while its fingers spread to form a *C* (Fig. 21-39).

8. Document your findings.

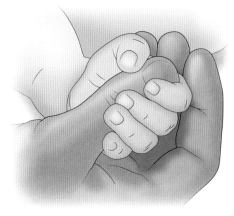

Fig. 21-38. Assessing the palmar grasp reflex.

NORMAL FINDINGS

■ Full ROM of all extremities

■ Flexion-flexed extremities

■ Each hand has five fingers with normal palmar creasing and positive grasp reflex

■ Moro reflex is positive

ABNORMAL FINDINGS

■ Restricted ROM of the legs can indicate possible hip dislocation; restricted ROM of the arms can indicate a fractured clavicle.

■ Infant's flexion is limp with arm(s) and/or leg(s) fully extended.

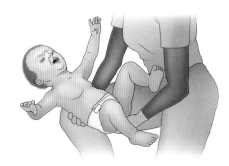

Fig. 21-39. Assessing the Moro reflex.

■ Extra hand digits noted; **Simian crease** (one single crease across the infant's palm may indicate Down syndrome); poor or absent grasp reflex (may indicate neurological or musculoskeletal concern).

■ Moro reflex is absent, decreased, or unilateral; Moro reflex can indicate nerve damage or a neurological deficit.

Technique 21-9B: **Assessing the Hips**

Purpose: To assess for newborn hip stability

The hip joint is a ball and socket joint. Newborns may have hips that are not in their socket (dislocated) or hips that are improperly formed (dysplasia) (Shorter, Hong, & Osborn, 2013). The American Academy of Pediatrics (AAP, 2000) recommends that all newborns be screened for hip dysplasia. Hip dysplasia is partial or total dislocation of the hip. There is no evidence of the cause of hip dysplasia. One theory is the baby is exposed to maternal hormones before birth; these maternal hormones relax muscles in the pregnant mother's body and may cause a baby's joints to become too relaxed and prone to dislocation (AAP, 2016).

> **SENC Safety Alert** The Barlow Ortolani maneuvers (Fig. 21-40) should be done by a healthcare provider who has experience and training to prevent a further hip complication if dysplasia of the hip is present.

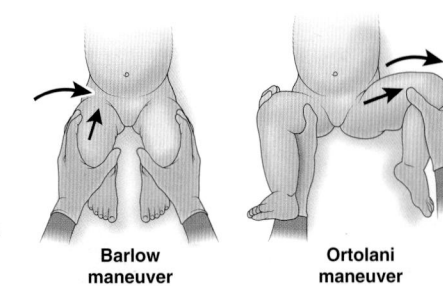

Barlow maneuver   Ortolani maneuver

Fig. 21-40. (A) Barlow maneuver. (B) Ortolani maneuver.

ASSESSMENT STEPS

1. Place the infant in the supine position.
2. Place your index and middle fingers along the greater trochanter of the infant's femur with your thumb along the inner thigh.
   > **TIP** Be sure to keep your index and middle fingers on the greater trochanter through step #6 so that you can palpate for any hip clicks or clunks.
3. Ensure that the infant's legs are in a neutral position.
4. Flex and adduct the infant's hips 90 degrees (Barlow maneuver).
5. Feel for a "click" or a "clunk."
   > **TIP** If the hip is unstable, the femoral head will slip over the posterior rim of the acetabulum and you will feel a "click or a clunk."
6. Gently abduct the hips while lifting forward on the femur (Fig. 21-41A, Ortolani maneuver).
7. Feel for a "click" or a "clunk."
8. Release the infant's hips.
9. Gently straighten the infant's legs by putting gentle downward pressure on the infant's feet (Fig. 21-41B).
10. Observe the thigh folds for leg symmetry.
11. Place infant in prone position.
12. Gently straighten infant's legs by applying gentle downward pressure (Fig. 21-41C).

13. Observe the gluteal folds for symmetry.

14. Document your findings.

NORMAL FINDINGS

- Hips: no "click" or "clunk" is felt upon adduction or abduction of the hips.
- Symmetrical thigh and gluteal folds are found in supine and prone positions.

ABNORMAL FINDINGS

- Positive **Barlow's maneuver** is when a "click" or "clunk" is felt and the hip subluxates or pops out of the socket during adduction of the hips.
- A positive **Ortolani's sign** is noted if the hip is dislocated, by a characteristic "click" or "clunk" that is felt as the femoral head slides over the posterior rim of the acetabulum.
- Asymmetrical gluteal folds and uneven limb length are all signs of possible hip dislocation.

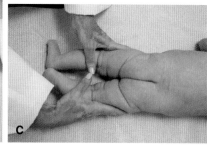

Fig. 21-41. Assessing for hip dysplasia. (A) Abducting hips. (B) Straightening legs. (C) Gluteal folds.

SENC **Safety Alert** Notify the healthcare provider if a hip dislocation is suspected.

Technique 21-9C: **Assessing the Feet**

Purpose: To assess foot position, digits, and physical maturity

ASSESSMENT STEPS

1. Place infant in a supine position.

2. Observe the infant's feet in relation to the leg while the infant is at rest.

3. Count the number of toes on each foot.

4. Observe the creasing along the bottom of the infant's feet.

5. Gently press the sole of the infant's left foot with your thumb near the toes and observe for the plantar reflex (Fig. 21-42); repeat on the right foot and observe the plantar reflex.

6. Assess the **Babinski's reflex** by stroking the outer edge of the sole of the left foot, moving from the heel up toward the pinkie toe and across the the ball of the foot (Fig. 21-43). Observe the Babinski sign; repeat on the right foot.

7. Document your findings.

NORMAL FINDINGS
- Foot position has five toes on each foot.
- Positive plantar reflex (infant will curl his or her toes around your finger)
- Positive Babinski (infant will extend the big toe and the rest of the toes will fan upward and out)
- Creasing present on two thirds of foot

ABNORMAL FINDINGS
- Smooth plantar surfaces may indicate prematurity.
- If the infant's foot can be returned to a neutral position, this is just called abnormal foot position. If it is unable to be returned to a neutral position, it is considered to be a **club foot.**
- **Polydactyly** is more than five toes on the foot.
- Negative plantar reflex (infant will not curl his or her toes around your finger); may indicate neurological disorder.
- Negative Babinski reflex (infant will not extend the bit toe and toes will not fan out); may indicate neurological disorder.

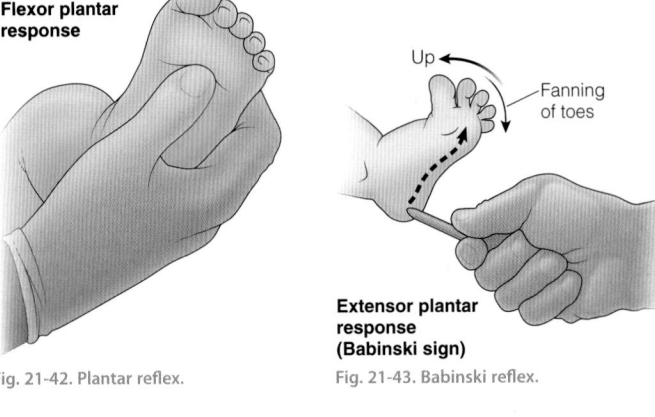

Flexor plantar response

Up

Fanning of toes

Extensor plantar response (Babinski sign)

Fig. 21-42. Plantar reflex.

Fig. 21-43. Babinski reflex.

TIP Extra digits tend to be familial. If there is no bone in the digit, it is often tied off with a suture by the healthcare provider.

SENC Safety Alert If a bone is palpated in the extra digit, or if a nailbed is noted, the infant should be referred to an orthopedist or plastic surgeon for further evaluation.

TECHNIQUE 21-10: **Assessing the Genitalia and Rectum**

Purpose: To assess gender and maturity of newborn
Equipment: Gloves, extra diaper and wipes
TIP Have an extra diaper and baby wipes available in case the infant has soiled the diaper.

SENC Safety Alert Always wear clean gloves when changing an infant's diaper, and always wash your hands after changing the infant's diaper.

Technique 21-10A: **Inspecting and Palpating the Male Genitalia**

Purpose: To assess physical maturity and testicular descent

ASSESSMENT STEPS

1. Put on gloves.
2. Place the infant in the supine position.
3. Remove the infant's diaper.
4. Inspect the scrotum for rugae (grooves or wrinkling of the skin).
5. Inspect the penis for the presence of the foreskin.
6. Inspect the location of the urinary meatus.
7. Place the index finger of the nondominant hand over the infant's inguinal canal. This prevents the testicle from traveling up the inguinal canal.
8. Gently palpate the scrotum using the index finger and thumb to determine whether the testicles have descended (Fig. 21-44).
   ■ **TIP** The testicle will feel like a small rubber ball, roughly the size of a pea.
9. Remove and discard gloves.
10. Document your findings.

NORMAL FINDINGS

■ Male genitalia: scrotum show rugae.
■ The urinary meatus is located on the tip of the penis.
■ Testicles are descended.
■ Foreskin is intact.

ABNORMAL FINDINGS

■ Male genitalia: scrotum with little or no rugae (indicative of prematurity)
■ Presence of a **hydrocele** (fluid surrounding the testicle; will spontaneously resorb)
■ **Hypospadias:** urinary meatus is located on the underside of the glans of the penis.
■ **Epispadias:** urinary meatus is located on the dorsal side of the glans of the penis.

  SENC Safety Alert Notify healthcare provider if hypospadias or epispadias are present; these infants cannot be circumcised.

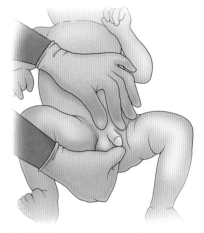

Fig. 21-44. Palpating the scrotum for descended testicles.

Technique 21-10B: **Inspecting Female Genitalia**

Purpose: To assess physical maturity

Equipment: Gloves

ASSESSMENT STEPS

1. Put on gloves.

2. Place infant in the supine position.

3. Remove the infant's diaper.

4. Inspect the labia majora, labia minora, and clitoris (Fig. 21-45).

5. Inspect for any noticeable discharge.

6. Remove and discard gloves.

7. Document your findings.

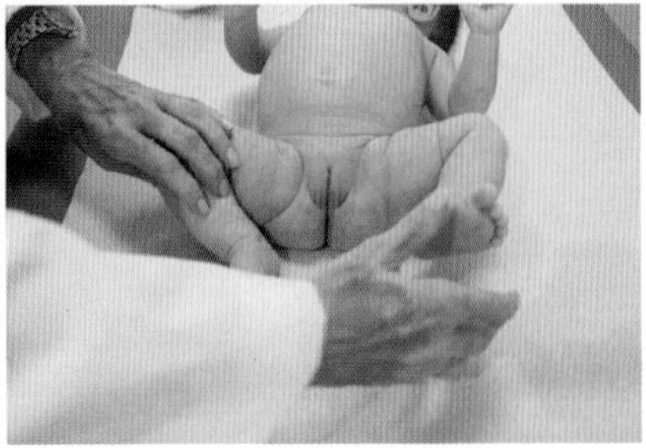

NORMAL FINDINGS

Fig. 21-45. Inspecting the female genitalia.

■ Female genitalia: labia majora cover labia minora and clitoris.

■ Labia may be edematous.

■ White or clear mucous-like discharge may be present; blood-tinged discharge may occur and is caused by maternal hormones.

ABNORMAL FINDINGS

■ Female genitalia: labia majora that does not cover labia minora is indicative of prematurity; vaginal skin tag is present.

> **SENC Safety Alert** Ambiguous genitalia are suspected when the clitoris is excessively prominent and a vaginal orifice is not clearly patent (Nagtalon-Ramos, 2013); this is related to a sexual development disorder.

Technique 21-10C: **Inspecting the Anus and Urine**

Purpose: To assess urine elimination and anal patency

Equipment: Gloves

ASSESSMENT STEPS

1. Put on gloves

2. Place the infant in supine position.

3. Remove the infant's diaper.

4. Inspect the infant's diaper for the presence of urine or stool.

5. Place the infant in the prone position.

6. Inspect the anus and assess whether stool is visible.

7. If stool is available, assess the color, amount, and consistency.

8. Remove and discard gloves.

9. Document your findings.

NORMAL FINDINGS

- Anus appears patent.
- Urine present within first 24 hours; clear or light yellow in color.
- Stool: meconium present within first 24 hours.
- Meconium is black, thick, and tar-like and then transitions to become looser; color changes from a black to green.

ABNORMAL FINDINGS

- No urine present within 6 to 8 hours (sign of dehydration) or foul smelling urine.
- No meconium present within 24 hours may indicate an intestinal obstruction.

    SENC Safety Alert Notify a healthcare provider immediately if the anus is not patent. Never try to perforate a nonpatent anus.

TECHNIQUE 21-11: **Inspecting and Palpating the Spine**

Purpose: To assess for an intact spine

   SENC Safety Alert Spina bifida is an opening in the spinal column. Depending on the severity of the opening, it may be palpated or visualized.

Equipment: Gloves (optional)

ASSESSMENT STEPS

1. Place infant in the prone position.

2. Inspect the entire length of the spine, including the base, where the spine meets the anus.

3. Using the finger pad of your index finger, gently palpate the entire length of the spine feeling the vertebrae (Fig. 21-46).

4. Document your findings.

NORMAL FINDINGS

- Spine appears straight and midline.
- Vertebrae are straight, flat, midline, and easily flexed.
- **Pilonidal dimple** is a small depression at the base of the sacrum without any clinical significance.

ABNORMAL FINDINGS

- Tuft of hair present at base of spine with a sacral dimple (may indicate spina bifida)
- A void (depression) in spinal column (may indicate spina bifida)

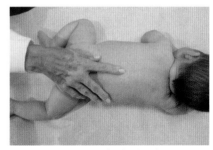

Fig. 21-46. Inspecting and palpating the spine.

TECHNIQUE 21-12: **Neurological Assessment**

Purpose: To assess for neurological deficits
Equipment: Gloves (optional)
The neurological examination consists of a series of observations as well as eliciting various reflexes. The neurological examination can be easily integrated throughout the physical examination of the newborn.

ASSESSMENT STEPS

1. Place the infant in the supine position.
2. Assess the sound of the infant's cry.
　■ **TIP** The newborn's cry can be assessed throughout your assessment.
3. Assess the infant's resting posture.
　■ **TIP** Resting posture should be assessed at the beginning of the examination, before touching the infant.
4. Assess the infant's muscle tone.
5. Assess the infant's state of alertness.
　□ Level 1 is quiet sleep
　□ Level 2 is active sleep
　□ Level 3 is quiet awake (best time for an assessment)
　□ Level 4 is active and alert
　□ Level 5 is crying
　■ **TIP** The level of alertness is one of the most sensitive indicators of neurologic injury in newborns (Gooding & McClead, 2015).
6. Elicit the sucking reflex (see Technique 21-4B).
7. Elicit the rooting reflex (see Technique 21-4B).
8. Elicit the grasping reflex (see Technique 21-9A).
9. Elicit the Moro reflex (see Technique 21-9A).
10. Elicit the Plantar reflex (see Technique 21-9C).
11. Elicit the Babinski's reflex (see Technique 21-9C).
12. Document your findings.

NORMAL FINDINGS

■ Cry: strong, lusty, medium pitch
■ Resting posture: partially flexed extremities with the legs abducted to the abdomen, bilateral movement of the extremities noted
■ Muscle tone: symmetrical, slightly hypertonic
■ State of alertness: alert, quiet, or sleeping

- Sucking reflex is present
- Rooting reflex is present.
- Grasping reflex is present.
- Moro reflex is present.
- Plantar reflex is present.
- Babinski's reflex is present.

ABNORMAL FINDINGS
- Cry: high-pitched or cat-like cry (may indicate a neurological disorder)
- Resting posture: extended extremities, absent or asymmetric movements (may indicate a neurological disorder)
- Muscle tone: decreased muscle tone (flaccid), jitteriness (may indicate hypoglycemia, hypocalcemia, or substance withdrawal), seizure activity (may indicate neurological disorder)

> **SENC Safety Alert** Jitteriness can be differentiated from seizure activity by gently placing a hand on the affected limb; if the movement stops, it is jitteriness.

- State of alertness: infant unable to be aroused
- Reflexes: absent or only are unilateral

TECHNIQUE 21-13: **Pain Assessment**

Purpose: To assess pain level
Equipment: Neonatal stethoscope, watch or clock with a second hand
Pain assessment in the newborn presents a challenge, because the newborn cannot communicate pain verbally. Instead, pain is identified by observing physiological and behavioral changes in the newborn (Merenstein & Gardner, 2010).

ASSESSMENT STEPS
1. Place the infant in the supine position.
2. Assess the infant's body for skin color.
3. Assess the infant for the presence of crying.
4. Assess the infant's facial expressions.
5. Assess the infant's muscle tone.
6. Assess the infant's activity level.
7. Assess the infant's state of arousal.
8. Document your findings.

NORMAL FINDINGS
- Infant's color is pink.
- Behavioral cues include the following:
  - ☐ Cry: absent or not continuous, able to be soothed
  - ☐ Facial expressions: nonfurrowed brow, face appears relaxed
  - ☐ Body movements: normal tone and posture
  - ☐ State of arousal: quiet, sleeping, calm

ABNORMAL FINDINGS

▇ **TIP** Physiological manifestations of pain may include bradycardia or tachycardia, tachypnea or apnea, cyanosis, mottling, duskiness, or pallor that all indicate that the newborn may be experiencing pain.

- Behavioral cues include:
  - ☐ Cry: whining, intense, urgent cry, high pitched, unable to be soothed
  - ☐ Facial expressions: frowning, gaze aversion
  - ☐ Body movements: rigid, hyperextended neck, flailing, thrashing, frantic behavior
  - ☐ State of arousal: hyperalert (infant's eyes are continually open wide, with little blinking)

TECHNIQUE 21-14: **Assessing Hydration**

Purpose: To assess newborn's hydration status

Hydration is assessed by reviewing the infant's record and obtaining information from the parent(s) or caregiver.

ASSESSMENT STEPS

1. Assess whether the infant is breast fed or formula fed.

2. Assess the amount of milk taken.

   ▇ **TIP** The time for breastfeeding is measured from the beginning of one feeding to the beginning of the next feeding.

   ☐ Breastfeeding: number of minutes per feeding

   ☐ Formula fed: number of ounces per feeding

3. Assess the frequency of feeding.

4. Assess the toleration of feeding (does the infant spit up any of the feeding?).

5. Assess the voiding amount and pattern by

   ☐ The number of wet diapers an infant has in a 24-hour period

   ☐ The number of stools an infant has in a 24-hour period

6. Document your findings.

SENC Safety Alert For initial feeds, the newborn generally receives no more than 15 mL or else the newborn will end up throwing up or pooping out excess; may become irritable from overfeeding.

- The breastfed infant will nurse well on at least one breast every 1.5 to 3 hours; appears satiated at the end of the feeding.
- The formula-fed infant will feed approximately 2 oz of formula every 3 to 4 hours by day 7.
  - **TIP** Initial formula feedings are much smaller due to the size of the infant's stomach, which eventually stretches from the size of a marble to the size of a golf ball, to allow the newborn to feed larger amounts.
- Presence of six to eight wet diapers a day
- The breastfed infant will have at least two to three stools/day but may have more; the stool will be loose, yellow, and seedy, with a slight sour-milk odor.
- The formula-fed infant will have at least two to three stools/day; the stool will be brown, soft, and may have an odor.

ABNORMAL FINDINGS
- Infant feeding is less than six times/day; vomits large amounts after feedings
- Less than six wet diapers in a 24-hour period (a week after birth); presence of uric acid crystals (indicates dehydration)
  - **TIP** Uric acid crystals will appear as a pink to dark pink staining in the diaper; related to concentrated urine.
- Zero to one stool/day may indicate constipation; blood or mucous in the stool may indicate digestive problems.

PATIENT EDUCATION

Patient education is one of the greatest responsibilities of a nurse. The parent or caregiver of the newborn will need education. Ideally, teaching about the newborn should begin before the baby is born through education during prenatal classes. However, not every parent is able to attend such classes. This is why teaching in the hospital setting is so important. Because of the large amount of information that new parents must learn, teaching is best spread out throughout the hospital stay. The nurse is responsible for arming the new parent(s) with the basic skills needed to care for the newborn, including information relating to temperature regulation, feeding, voiding, infant behaviors, safety, and signs and symptoms of illness. Because this can be overwhelming for the new parent(s), it can be helpful to reinforce verbal teaching with handouts, and to review the information before discharge.

- Give parents instructions for and explain the importance of follow-up testing if necessary.
- Infants are not as effective at keeping warm as adults. At most, place one additional layer of clothing on the infant (that layer can be a swaddling blanket).
- Take your infant's temperature only when the infant feels hot or cold, or if the infant appears to be sick.
- Infant temperatures should be taken using a digital thermometer in the infant's armpit.
- After day 6, your infant should have at least six to eight wet diapers a day, and two to three stools a day.
- When changing a baby girl's diaper, always wipe from front to back, never using the same part of the wipe twice.

- Call the pediatrician if the infant
  - ☐ Is vomiting or has diarrhea
  - ☐ Has blood in the stool
  - ☐ Is difficult to rouse
  - ☐ Has signs/symptoms of infection in the umbilical cord (redness, drainage, odor)
  - ☐ Has less than six wet diapers/day
  - ☐ Has less than one stool/day
  - ☐ Has a temperature 100.4°F or above
  - ☐ Does not respond to loud sounds with a startle reaction; this may be a sign of hearing loss

Healthy People 2020

Goal: Increase the proportion of infants who are put on their backs to sleep (HHS, 2010).

- Always place your infant flat on the back to sleep in the crib. Do not have anything other than the baby in the crib; no crib bumpers, loose blankets, toys etc. (American Academy of Pediatrics, 2011; Esposito, Hegyi, & Ostfeld, 2007).
- Infant sleep clothing that is designed to keep the infant warm without the possible hazard of head covering or entrapment can be used in place of blankets; however, care must be taken to select appropriately sized clothing and to avoid overheating. If a blanket is used, it should be thin and tucked under the mattress so as to avoid head or face covering. These practices should also be modeled in hospital settings (Moon & Task Force on Sudden Infant Death Syndrome, 2011).
- Feed your infant at least every 4 hours.
- Your infant's umbilical cord will fall off between 7 and 10 days after birth. Until then, keep it clean and dry.
- Until your infant's umbilical cord has fallen off, just give the infant a sponge bath; not a tub bath.

- When traveling in the car, the infant should always be secured in a rear-facing car seat in the back seat. Infants must stay rear-facing until they are at least 2 years old and 20 lbs. (Governors Highway Safety Association, 2013). "The American Academy of Pediatrics (AAP) recommends that all infants should ride rear-facing starting with their first ride home from the hospital. All infants and toddlers should ride in a Rear-Facing Car Seat until they are 2 years of age or until they reach the highest weight or height allowed by their car seat's manufacturer" (American Academy of Pediatrics, 2013).

CULTURAL CONSIDERATIONS American Indian and Alaska Native infants are 2 to 4 times more likely to die of Sudden Infant Death Syndrome (SIDS) as Caucasian infants, making it the leading cause of post-neonatal deaths for Native babies (Pierce-Bulger, 2013).

Healthy People 2020

Goal: Increase the proportion of infants who are breastfed (HHS, 2010)

Breastfeeding is the normal way of providing young infants with the nutrients they need for healthy growth and development.

- The World Health Organization (WHO, 2015) supports breastfeeding and encourages mothers to breastfeed within the first hour after birth.
- The American Academy of Pediatrics (AAP, 2012) recommends exclusive breastfeeding for about the first six months of a baby's life, followed by breastfeeding in combination with the introduction of complementary foods until at least 12 months of age, and continuation of breastfeeding for as long as mutually desired by mother and baby.
- There are physical, emotional, and health advantages for both mother and child. Breastfeeding has a protective effect for the infant, giving increased immunity for the baby against getting:
  - ☐ respiratory infections

□ ear infections
□ gastrointestinal disease
□ allergies.

CULTURAL CONSIDERATIONS Some people of the Hindu Heritage believe that colostrum is unsuited for infants; most women think that the milk does not "descend from the breast" until the ritual bath on the third day, and as a result, newborns are fed sugar water or milk expressed from lactating women (Purnell, 2014).

■ **Postpartum depression** is one of the most common complications in the postpartum period and has potentially significant negative consequences for mothers and their families (Guille, Newman, Fryml, Lifton, & Epperson, 2013).

　□ Postpartum depression may have a genetic predisposition; it may also be caused by hormonal changes following delivery and the many physical, emotional, and social stressors of being a new parent.

　□ Nurses should be alert to some of the signs and symptoms of postpartum depression, including but not limited to:
　　• fatigue
　　• insomnia
　　• mood changes
　　• depression
　　• lack of interest or feelings toward the newborn
　　• diminished ability to think or concentrate.

□ Nurses should also be alert to signs of postpartum depression that may cause physical or emotional abuse of an infant. Nurses must be attentive to signs of potential child abuse that may include:
• Mother is unable to care for herself or her baby.
• Mother is afraid to be alone with her baby.
• Mother has negative feelings toward the baby or even thinks about harming the baby.
• Unexplained bruises are found on the baby.
• Repeated hospitalizations related to unexplained injuries are noted.

SENC Evidence-Based Practice The Agency for Research, Healthcare and Quality (Myers et al., 2013) searched PubMed, Embase, PsycINFO, and the Cochrane Database of Systematic Reviews for relevant English-language studies published from January 1, 2004, to July 24, 2012, that evaluated the performance of screening instruments for postpartum depression, potential benefits and harms of screening, and impact on appropriate post-screening actions. The potential effectiveness of screening for postpartum depression appears to be related to the availability of systems to ensure adequate follow-up of women with positive results. The ideal characteristics of a screening test for postpartum depression, including sensitivity, specificity, timing, and frequency, have not been defined.

INTRODUCTION

Assessing the child and adolescent entails collecting data in a variety of ways. The health history and physical examination provide important information, but it is equally important to observe the child's behavior and the parent-child interaction during the visit. Even when the child and the parent are on their best behavior, their interactions can serve as a springboard for discussion. Careful observation may reveal behavioral problems, developmental delays, social or environmental problems, and neurological problems.

SENC Child-Centered Care A family-centered approach to a child's health is essential because there is a strong correlation between the health of parents and the health of their children. From the moment you enter the room, you are developing a relationship with the child and parent. The rapport you develop helps to set the tone for the entire visit and future visits. A white lab coat can be threatening to a child and intimidating to a parent, and is not necessary to maintain a professional demeanor. The slightest hint of irritability, boredom, or a feeling of being rushed can also compromise your relationship with the child and parent.

DEVELOPMENTAL PRINCIPLES

The following are the pediatric stages of development, according to the American Academy of Pediatrics (2017a):

- Baby: 0 to 12 months
- Toddler: 1 to 3 years
- Preschool child: 3 to 5 years
- Grade school child: 5 to 12 years
- Adolescent/Teen: 12 to 18 years

Keep in mind the following developmental principles:

- Many events in a child's life, including illness, may hinder a child's development; some events may move the child to maturity more quickly.

- Development may not advance steadily in all the domains, but growth and development proceed in an orderly, sequential process along a predicable path that is governed by the maturing brain.
- Development is directional.
  - Development occurs in a cephalocaudal (head to toe) and proximodistal direction (midline to the periphery).
  - Children develop gross motor skills, such as crawling, walking, and running, before fine motor skills, such as using a pincer grasp (uses pointer finger and thumb) to pick up food, drawing with crayons, or writing with a pencil.

- As the child matures, developmental abilities become increasingly integrated, organized, and differentiated.
- The pace of one child's growth and development is specific to the child.

TIP Parent teaching and anticipatory guidance should be specific to the individual child.

- Increases in reproductive hormones leading to pubertal maturation are manifested in a sequence of predictable changes in secondary sexual characteristics.
  - Tanner staging (Marshall, 1969, 1970) ranks maturity level from stage 1 (immature) to stage 5 (mature) for both males and females (Table 22-1).
  - In females, staging is based on breast size and shape and the distribution of pubic hair.
  - In males, staging is based on the size and shape of the penis and scrotum and the shape and distribution of pubic hair.

- The physical assessment should be tailored to the developmental level of the child.

DIAGNOSTICS

The American Academy of Pediatrics recommends regular evaluations and periodic laboratory tests even if the child does not appear ill. These evaluations function to screen for general health (mental and physical) and to test for specific disorders.

- **Kidney disease:** Urinalysis at age 5 years and at least once in adolescence
- **Iron deficiency anemia:** Annual testing (hematocrit) is recommended for at-risk children ages 2 to 5 who
  - Consume a diet low in iron
  - Have limited access to food because of poverty or neglect
  - Have special healthcare needs
- **Blood lead levels:** Periodic screening for infants and children ages 6 months to 6 years for a history of *possible* lead exposure

TABLE 22-1 Tanner Stages

Sexual Maturity Rating (Tanner Stage)	Pubic Hair	Female Breast Development	Testicular Length (cm)	Testicular Volume (mL)
I	None	No development	<2.5	<4
II	Sparse	Bud	≥2.5	4–6
III	Coarse, easily visible	Breast tissue beyond areola	≥3.0	6–10
IV	Confined to suprapubic area	Secondary mound	≥4.0	10–15
V	Adult type on medial thighs	Adult	≥5.0	>15

From Marshall, 1969, 1970, with permission.

☐ Infants at risk should be tested beginning at 9 to 12 months, and retested at 24 months.

☐ Testing of abused or neglected children and for children who have conditions associated with increased lead exposure, including:
  • using pottery or dishes containing lead
  • using some cosmetics and some folklore remedies
  • living in poverty
  • living in urban areas or older homes where lead decontamination has not occurred
  • inhaling lead-based paint dust or eating lead-based paint chips.

■ **Cardiovascular health:** Depending on family history, children at risk for hyperlipidemia should be selectively tested after age 2 and no later than 10 years old (AAP, 2017b).

TIP Evidence suggests that atherosclerosis and coronary heart disease (CHD) involve processes that begin in childhood or adolescence (Kwiterovich, 2012).

■ **Infectious Diseases**
  ☐ **Purified protein derivative (PPD) skin test for tuberculosis** is done if the child is at risk for having the illness.
  ☐ **Testing for sexually transmitted infections (STIs)** should be performed for sexually active male and female adolescents.
  ☐ **Testing for human immunodeficiency virus (HIV)** is done for all adolescents beginning at age 15 years; testing is also indicated for adolescents younger than 15 years who are sexually active.

SENC Safety Alert Always maintain the "three Cs" when screening or testing for HIV: (1) obtain an informed *consent,* (2) provide *counseling,* and (3) maintain *confidentiality.*

■ **Tympanometry** is used to identify the presence of fluid in the middle ear, mobility and patency of the eardrum and tympanostomy tubes; used to diagnose otitis media or fluid in the middle ear.

CULTURAL CONSIDERATIONS Trusting relationships take time to develop under the best of circumstances. When the belief systems of the healthcare provider and the child and family differ, there is an additional layer of complexity when forging a relationship between the healthcare provider, the healthcare system, and the child and family. Some members of diverse populations can find it difficult to communicate with healthcare providers not only because of language barriers, but because healthcare providers are often seen as having greater power or prestige. If communication barriers are anticipated:

• Seek individuals trained in medical translation to assist.
• Learn basic words and phrases and avoid technical terms.
• Speak slowly and carefully, but not loudly, in your conversations with the child and parent.
• Allow time for the child and parents to process your questions. The parents may be translating your question into their native language, formulating an answer, translating the answer back into English, and then responding.

Demonstrating respect for cultural differences is essential because families may be reluctant to disclose personal or health-related information if they anticipate receiving discriminatory treatment or negative reactions. Therefore, careful monitoring of one's own reactions or assumptions is foundational for developing positive working relationships (Victorson et al, 2013).

It is helpful to explain to the parent and child/adolescent that the review of systems will require many questions to determine how the child has been since the last visit.

Review of Systems

The parent generally answers the questions in the health history. Children as young as 3 years of age can effectively participate in the health interview; however, the child (age appropriate) or adolescent should be encouraged to participate in the interview. During this period of the assessment, observe the interaction and communication between the parent/caregiver and child. Children will respond better when the nurse is able to build a trusting relationship with parent and child. As a nurse, you will be able to gather the data, teach, and answer questions throughout this part of the assessment.

Use the OLDCARTS mnemonic (**O**nset, **L**ocation, **D**uration, **C**haracteristics, **A**ggravating/Alleviating factors, **R**elieving factors, **T**reatment, **S**everity) to identify attributes of a symptom.

SENC Child-Centered Care Always take a few moments to warmly greet the child and parent, sit on a stool or chair to maintain eye level with the child, and be attentive to what both the child and the parent are saying (Fig. 22-1). You may ask the child if he or she has a nickname.

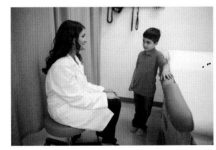

TIP Use toys, books, or other items that do not produce sound for developing rapport with

Fig. 22-1. Greeting the child.

a child, for distraction, or to occupy the child while interviewing the parent.

Reason for Visit
■ What brought you in today?
   □ The reason for the visit can be any number of reasons, such as a well-child visit with a routine physical examination and screening, an examination for clearance to play sports in school, a preoperative physical examination, a sick visit, or an emergency.
   □ Asking the parent/caregiver if he or she has any additional worries can reveal further information that may be helpful while assessing the child.
   □ Most parents are acutely sensitive to their child's physical, social, and emotional well-being and have very good sense of when something is wrong. Their concerns should be taken seriously.

TIP The child's position of comfort is an important clue about the overall health of the child. Observe the child's nonverbal body language and level of comfort. Some signs of pain may be facial grimacing, restlessness, rigid posture, or irritability.

Birth History
Prenatal and birth history will provide information about factors that may affect the physical and cognitive development of the child. Ask the parent/caregiver of the child the following:
■ Describe the pregnancy and delivery.
■ Did you take any medications during the pregnancy?
■ Did you smoke or drink alcohol during the pregnancy?

Past Medical History
The following should be carefully reviewed with parent/caregiver for all stages of development:

- Has your child had any major illnesses or injuries?
- Has your child had any hospitalizations or surgeries?
- Is your child up to date with his or her immunizations?
  - □ Immunizations are the most effective intervention to prevent and control infectious diseases. Parents have the right to decide whether their child is vaccinated or not. Nurses should educate parents about the benefits of immunizations but respect their decision. You can encourage parents to educate themselves about the immunization. Increased knowledge helps the parent to make the best decision for the child. You can refer the parent to read more about immunizations. You can give handouts or encourage the parent to review the American Academy of Pediatrics website at http://www2.aap.org/immunization/izschedule.html.

▬ **TIP** Some parents refuse to have their child immunized because of religious, medical, or philosophical reasons. State law determines exemptions. There are some states that have religious and philosophical exemptions. All 50 states allow medical exemptions for persons who have medical contraindication to vaccination(s) (CDC, 2017c). A nurse should be nonjudgmental.

- Has your child had any reactions to the immunizations?
- Do you have a record of your child's immunizations?
  - □ All immunizations are recorded in the child's chart and in the record immunization booklet kept by the parent.
  - □ The immunization history should include the most recent PPD test for tuberculosis and the response.
- What medications are your child taking, including over-the-counter medications or supplements?
- What allergies does your child have? What are the types of reactions?

Family History

Family history is similar to the adult family history. (See Chapter 3.) Family histories may be unknown if the child is adopted or in foster care.

Psychosocial History

Psychosocial questions are mostly directed to the parent or age appropriate child or adolescent.

Living Arrangements

- □ Describe the child's living arrangements.
- □ What type of neighborhood do you live in?
- □ Are both parents living in the home?
- □ How many people live in the house? How many other children live in the home?
- □ If a single parent, is the mother or father involved?
- □ Do one or both parents work? What are the day care or after-school care arrangements?
- □ Do you receive any social services support?

School

- □ Does your child attend school, or is she or he home-schooled?
- □ Does your child struggle with school? Does your child avoid reading out loud or have trouble completing homework assignments on time?
  - • **Learning disabilities** is an umbrella term for a wide variety of specific learning differences. Children with learning differences are often misunderstood as having a problem with motivation or intelligence, placing them at risk for difficulties with adjustment in the home or at school. Early identification of learning differences is key for providing appropriate intervention and support services to maximize the child's potential and maintain self-esteem (Harrison, 2009).
- □ How often does he or she miss school? If so, why?
- □ Does your child like school? Does your child like his or her teacher? Classmates?
- □ Does your child participate in extracurricular activities?
- □ Do you have any concerns about **attention deficit-hyperactivity disorder (ADHD)**?

- ADHD is a neurobehavioral disorder characterized by symptoms of a persistent pattern of inattention, hyperactivity, or impulsivity (Venes, 2013, p. 229).
- ☐ Does your child have friends with whom he or she plays or socializes?
  - Asking questions about what an adolescent's peer group is doing may better serve to engage the adolescent child in conversation while providing valuable insights.

Sports
- ☐ Does your child play sports? If so, which ones? Does he or she wear protective equipment?
- ☐ Does your child wear a helmet when riding his or her bicycle?
  - Bicycle helmets are a proven intervention that reduce the risk of bicycle-related head injury by about 80 percent; only 15 percent of children use helmets all or most of the time while cycling (CDC, 2011).

Smoking or Alcohol
Ask the parent:
- ☐ Do you smoke? If so, do you smoke in the presence of your child?
  - A significant number of parents are unaware or unconvinced of the health consequences of passive smoking (second-hand smoke) in children. Passive smoking contributes significantly to morbidity and mortality; these children are at higher risk for respiratory infections, wheezing, and asthma (Hutchinson et al, 2014).

■ **TIP** Nurses should increase parental awareness to the effects of passive smoking for their children.

Ask the school-age or adolescent child:
- ☐ Do you smoke or chew tobacco?
  - Each day in the United States, more than 3,200 children under 18 years of age smoke their first cigarette, and an estimated 700

become daily cigarette smokers (U.S. Food and Drug Administration [FDA], 2014).
- The majority of children in elementary school and the early part of middle school have never tried a cigarette. If they do try their first cigarette, it is around the age of 11, and many are addicted by the time they turn 14 (American Lung Association, 2014).

■ **TIP** The Family Smoking Prevention and Tobacco Control Act, signed into law by President Barack Obama on June 22, 2009, contains several provisions aimed at preventing young people from starting to smoke by restricting marketing and sales to youth.
- ☐ Do you drink alcohol?
- ☐ Do you use recreational drugs?

■ **TIP** Adolescents are less likely to truthfully share information about smoking, drugs, and drinking while the parent is present; you may wait until you are alone with the adolescent and ask these questions when other sensitive topics are discussed.

Behavioral Issues
Ask the parent of a young child:
- ☐ Does your child have tantrums?
- ☐ How do you handle tantrums or disobedience? What method of discipline do you use?
  - Spanking is shown to increase aggression and decrease language skills (Gershoff, 2013; MacKenzie, 2013).

Ask the parent of an older child (preferably without the child being present):
- ☐ Does your child have any behaviors that concern you?

Sleep History
Ask the parent or child (age-appropriate):
- ■ What are the sleeping arrangements?
- ■ How many hours does your child sleep?
- ■ Describe the bedtime routine?

- Does your child have difficulty falling asleep?
- Does your child experience any night terrors or nightmares?
  - □ **Night terrors** is a form of nightmare experienced by children in which a frightening hallucination is accompanied by an inability to awaken from sleep; the fear continues for a period after the child awakens (Venes, 2013, p. 1624).

■ **TIP** The American Academy of Pediatrics recommends that a child's bedroom be an internet- and television-free zone because studies have demonstrated an increased association with obesity and sleep problems (American Academy of Pediatrics Council on Communications and the Media, 2013; Chahal, H., Fung, C., Kuhle, S., & Veugelers, 2013; Foley et al, 2013).

Nutrition

In the last 30 years, the prevalence of overweight children and adolescents has tripled. The greatest numbers of overweight children and adolescents are among populations with the highest rates of poverty and lowest education levels.

- Intervention at the primary care level is foundational for prevention.
- Parents and children must be made aware of the significant health risks such as type 2 diabetes, hyperlipidemia, and heart disease, and taught how to modify their behaviors to prevent future health problems.

Ask the mother, if breastfeeding:

- How long do you plan to breastfeed?
  - □ Exclusive breastfeeding for 6 months is associated with a reduced incidence of eczema and food allergies, and provides a long-term protective effect against respiratory allergies. Breastfeeding also reduces the incidence and severity of colds (American Academy of Pediatrics, 2012).

Ask the parent or child (age-appropriate):

- How many meals each day does your child consume?
- What does his/her usual breakfast, lunch, and dinner consist of?

- How many snacks per day? Food choices?
- Does the family eat together?
- Where does the child eat most of his or her meals?
- Does the child feed self? Use a cup? Use eating utensils?
  - □ **Pica** is an eating disorder defined as the persistent ingestion of nonnutritive substances for a period of at least 1 month at an age for which this behavior is developmentally inappropriate. Pica may be benign, or it may have life-threatening consequences. A wide variety of nonfood substances may be ingested including, but not limited to, clay, dirt, sand, stones, pebbles, hair, feces, lead, laundry starch, vinyl gloves, plastic, pencil erasers, ice, fingernails, paper, paint chips, coal, chalk, wood, plaster, light bulbs, needles, string, cigarette butts, wire, and burnt matches.

■ **TIP** Pica is the most common eating disorder in individuals with developmental disabilities. In some societies, pica is a culturally sanctioned practice and is not considered to be pathologic.

Ask the adolescent:

- Do you drink caffeinated beverages such as coffee or cola beverages? If so, how much per day?
- Do you take any nutrition supplements? If yes, which ones?
- How do you feel about how much you eat and your current weight?
  - □ Self-image is important during the adolescent stage. Some adolescents may refuse to maintain body weight at or above a minimal normal weight for age and height. The weight loss is usually self-imposed and is usually less than 85 percent of expected weight (American Academy of Adolescent and Child Psychiatry, 2014).

■ **TIP** The most common and easiest method to assess daily intake is a 24-hour recall; however, many children, adolescents, and even adults have limited and inaccurate recall of their diets. To improve reliability of the daily recall, the family should document a food diary that includes two weekdays and one weekend day in the diary.

Elimination

Ask the parent of an infant or toddler:

■ Is your child being toilet trained? If so, how are you training her or him?

■ If not, when do you plan to begin toilet training?

☐ Toilet training is a significant milestone that hinges on the physical and emotional development of the child and not necessarily the age of the child.

☐ The American Academy of Pediatrics recommends a child-centered approach in which the child demonstrates an interest and ability for toilet training.

☐ Readiness behaviors include the ability to understand and follow directions, to sit on and rise from a potty chair, to pull down his or her pants and pull them up again, to imitate and identify with mentors, and to express the need to eliminate or complain about wet or dirty diapers (Choby & George, 2008).

■ Does your child remain dry through the night? Have accidents in the daytime?

☐ **Enuresis (bedwetting)** is a condition that is not diagnosed unless the child is 5 years or older, may or may not be purposeful behavior, and occurs more often in boys than girls.

• Nocturnal enuresis is the most common type of elimination disorder. Daytime wetting is called diurnal enuresis. Some children experience both.

• Main symptoms of enuresis include repeated nocturnal enuresis, repeated diurnal enuresis, and wetting at least twice a week for approximately three months.

• There are many causes of enuresis, such as a small bladder, persistent urinary tract infections, severe stress, or developmental delays that interfere with toilet training.

General Health

Ask the parent or child (age-appropriate):

■ How would you describe the child's usual state of health?

Skin

Ask the parent or child (age-appropriate):

■ Do you help your child avoid the sun and apply sunscreen?

☐ UV-induced skin changes may begin as early as the first summer of life. Infants younger than 6 months should avoid sun exposure. Sunscreen should be applied to children older than 6 months for uncovered areas of the skin (Paller, 2011).

Ask the school-age or adolescent child:

■ Do you have any problems with oily skin or skin blemishes?

☐ Acne, a condition that affects almost all teenagers, results from the action of androgen on the skin's sebaceous glands, causing them to get larger and produce more sebum.

SENC Child-Centered Care Acne can have significant physical and psychological consequences, such as causing a poor self-image, social inhibition, and anxiety. The nurse can educate the child about care that may help to control acne:

■ Perform two gentle skin care washings twice a day. Acne is not caused by dirt, so over-washing or using harsh scrubs on skin can dry or irritate the skin triggering the sebaceous glands to produce more oil and increasing the likelihood of pimples.

■ Use oil-free or noncomedogenic products for washing the face. These products help to prevent clogged pores.

■ Do not squeeze or pick blemishes. Doing so allows bacteria to penetrate deeper into the skin, causing more inflammation and the possibility of permanent scarring.

■ Do you have any tattoos or piercings? If so, where?

☐ Tattooing is a common practice, especially among young people, and we are witnessing a gradual increase of numerous potential complications to tattoo placement: the most common skin reactions to tattooing include a transient acute inflammatory reaction due to trauma of the skin with needles and medical complications (Bassi et al, 2014)

- Do you go to the tanning salons? If so, how often?
  - □ The FDA announced a reclassification of sunlamp products such as tanning beds from low to moderate risk, and ordered that these machines have a black-box warning against their use by children under 18 (FDA, 2014).

SENC Evidence-Based Practice Melanoma is the most common form of cancer for young adults, 25 to 29 years old, and the second most common form of cancer for adolescents and young adults, 15 to 29 years old. Studies have found a 75 percent increase in the risk of melanoma in those who have been exposed to UV radiation from indoor tanning. A recent review of 27 studies demonstrated that one in 20 cases of melanoma can be attributed to use of indoor tanning salons (Severs, 2012).

Hair and Nails

Ask the parent or child (age-appropriate):

- Does your child bite his or her nails?
  - □ Nail biting is of the most common habits of children and teens.
  - □ It is a behavior associated with the infant reflex of putting hands in the mouth for comfort. Children who bite their nails or suck their thumbs are usually seeking comfort, relief from stress, anxiety, loneliness, or boredom.
  - □ Children may also be imitating a family member. Children most often bite their nails when their hands are not engaged, such as while watching television, reading, sitting in class, or riding in the car.
  - □ The incidence of nail biting is greater between the ages of 4 and 6 years than in younger years and then increases during adolescence.

The rate of nail biting decreases following adolescence (Tanaka et al, 2008).

Eyes and Vision

Ask the parent of an infant or toddler:

- Does your child squint, tilt his or her head, close one eye, or peek around corners with one eye trying to see?
  - □ These are classic signs of double vision in children that few parents associate with visual impairments.
  - □ Strabismus is a misalignment of the eye; can be present with or without eye-crossing. Failing to treat strabismus can lead to vision loss (Miller, 2012).

Ask the older child:

- Are you able to see the blackboard? Any headaches or eye pain during or after reading? (If applicable: Do you wear your glasses or contacts all the time?)

TIP Visual acuity should be tested regularly beginning at age 3 (Miller, 2012). If a child older than 4 years is uncooperative on two separate visits, refer to an ophthalmologist experienced with children.

Ears

Ask the parent or child (age-appropriate):

- Does your child have recurrent ear infections?
- Does your child get infections after swimming?
- Does your child have ear pain? Have you observed any ear drainage?
  - □ Children experiencing prolonged middle ear infections can develop hearing loss and are at risk for altered development of speech and language.
  - □ Tympanostomy is a procedure in which a tube is placed through the tympanic membrane of the ear to allow ventilation of the middle ear as part of the treatment for otitis media with effusion (Fig. 22-2).

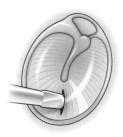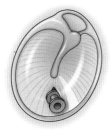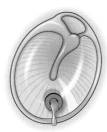

Fig. 22-2. Tympanostomy.

Ask the parent or child (age appropriate):

■ Does your child have any difficulty hearing?
  □ Screenings for hearing loss are recommended throughout a child's life span.
  □ Hearing loss in infants and children has been associated with deficits in language and speech acquisition, poor academic performance, emotional difficulties, and personal-social maladjustments (Harlor & Bower, 2009).
■ Has your child had a hearing test? If so, what were the results?
■ Does your child listen to loud music or is your child exposed to loud noises?
  □ Concern about hearing loss from a parent or caregiver is sufficient reason for a referral to a specialist (AAP 2009).

Nose and Sinuses

Ask the parent or child (age appropriate):

■ How often does your child seem to have a cold?
■ Does your child rub his or her nose often? Complain of itchy nose or eyes?

□ Allergy-related disorders, such as food allergies, asthma, and allergic rhinitis, are among the leading chronic diseases diagnosed in children.
□ Children with allergies account for hundreds of thousands of missed school days every year.
□ The most commonly diagnosed allergy is to milk, accounting for one fifth of all diagnosed allergies.

CULTURAL CONSIDERATIONS Milk allergy is more prevalent in Caucasians than other ethnicities (Warren, Jhaveri, Warrier, Smith, & Gupta, 2013).

□ Allergic reactions to food, insect stings, or medications should be evaluated by an allergist. Other common allergens are peanuts, tree nuts, dust mites, mold, pet dander, and pollen.

SENC Safety Alert Peanut allergy is one of the most common causes of severe allergic responses, especially in children. Peanut allergy symptoms can range from a minor irritation to a life-threatening anaphylactic reaction, so parents should be encouraged to have their children seen by a specialist even if a child has only experienced a minor reaction to peanuts. The proteins in peanuts are similar in structure to those in tree nuts; therefore, children who are allergic to peanuts may also be allergic to tree nuts, such as almonds, Brazil nuts, walnuts, hazelnuts, macadamias, pistachios, pecans, and cashews. High-risk foods for children with peanut or tree nut allergy include cookies, baked goods, candy, ice cream, and Asian and African cuisine. Peanuts or peanut butter can be used to thicken sauces and chili.

Mouth, Teeth, and Throat

Ask the parent or child (age appropriate):

■ Does your child drool?
■ Have pain with teething? Have tooth pain? (For the older child.)
■ Use a pacifier or suck his or her thumb?

- Has your child been to the dentist for an oral examination?
  - □ The Department of Health and Human Services (DHHS) recognizes that oral health can have a significant impact on overall health and well-being (American Academy of Pediatric Dentistry, 2014).

SENC Child-Centered Care An oral risk assessment should be performed on all infants by age 12 months (American Academy of Pediatrics, 2004). Risk factors for caries include:

- children with special healthcare needs
- mother with significant history of caries
- low socioeconomic status
- breastfeeding throughout the night or sleeping with bottle
- visible plaque, stains
- later-order offspring.

Ask the older child:

- How often do you brush your teeth? Do you use floss?
  - □ Children should brush their teeth twice a day with fluoridated toothpaste and floss once a day (Bright Futures/American Academy of Pediatrics, 2008).

Ask the parent:

- How often does your child see the dentist?
  - □ Toddlers should have visited a dentist by their first birthday (American Academy of Pediatric Section on Pediatric Dentistry and Oral Health, 2008). Older children should visit the dentist twice a year (Bright Futures/American Academy of Pediatrics, 2008).

TIP There is no evidence for or against primary care providers screening for children at risk for caries, but the American Academy of Pediatrics suggests that each child should receive a risk assessment before the age of 12 months so that preventive measures can be instituted by a dentist (Prevention of Dental Caries in Preschool Aged Children, 2013).

Ask the parent or child (age-appropriate):

- How much juice or soda does your child drink?
  - □ Juice, including 100 percent fruit juice, is associated with caries and obesity. Children should avoid carbonated beverages and fruit juices particularly between meals. One hundred percent fruit juices should be limited to 4 oz per day (American Academy of Pediatric Section on Pediatric Dentistry and Oral Health, 2008).

Respiratory

Ask the parent:

- Has your child ever had croup? If so, how often?
  - □ Recurrent **croup,** a respiratory condition that is usually triggered by an acute viral infection of the upper airway and characterized by a harsh, barking cough, may indicate upper respiratory abnormalities. Referral to a specialist may be indicated (Rankin, Wang, Waters, Clement, & Kubba, 2013).

Ask the parent of a child diagnosed with asthma:

- How often has your child visited the emergency room in the past 12 months?
- How often does your child use short-acting bronchodilators?
  - □ Emergency room visits and the use of short-acting bronchodilators (more than twice a week) indicate uncontrolled asthma. A review of the diagnosis and treatment plan is indicated.

Ask the parent or child if a nebulizer is available:

- Show me how you use the nebulizer/inhaler.
  - □ Commonly, asthma inhalers and nebulizers are used incorrectly even with appropriate education.
  - □ Incorrect delivery of inhaled medication leads to unnecessary exacerbations and hospitalizations.
  - □ Any child who uses an inhaler and any parent who administers nebulizer treatments should receive education on inhaler/nebulizer technique at each visit (Sleath et al, 2012; Inhaler Error Steering Committee et al, 2013).

Female Breasts

Ask the parent or age-appropriate female child/adolescent:

- Have your child's breasts (or your breasts, if this is being asked of a child) started to develop? If so, at what age did breast development begin?
- When did you start wearing a bra (if this is being asked of a child)?
- Do you have any tenderness or pain in your breasts (if this is being asked of a child)?
  - ☐ Thelarche is the beginning of breast development.
  - ☐ Changes in breasts of females that are not age appropriate may indicate precocious puberty.
  - ☐ Breast cancer is very rare in children and most causes of breast swelling in children are not serious.

▌TIP Adolescents will discuss sensitive topics with their healthcare provider only when they trust the confidentiality of their revelations. Typically a healthcare provider will talk with children without parents present for part of the visit starting around age 11.

Male Breasts

Ask the parent or age-appropriate male child/adolescent:
- Have you noticed any enlargement of breast tissue?
  - ☐ **Gynecomastia** is enlargement of breast tissue in the male. Nearly one half of adolescent males, ages 13 to 14 years, will develop physiologic gynecomastia, a self-limiting, benign proliferation of breast tissue in males (Dickson, 2012).

SENC Child-Centered Care Remind late school-age children and adolescents, in a matter-of-fact way, that the changes they are experiencing related to developing secondary sex characteristics are a normal part of growth and development. Many boys during early to middle puberty may experience gynecomastia or an overdevelopment of the male breast. Young boys experiencing emotional distress from having developed gynecomastia should be assured that it usually goes away within 6 months to 2 years and can seek treatment to reduce the symptoms if warranted (Dickson, 2012).

Cardiovascular

Ask the parent:
- Was your child born with any congenital heart problems? If so, how was he or she treated?
- Does your child see a cardiologist?
  - ☐ Although a rare event, **congenital cardiovascular disease** is the leading cause of nontraumatic sudden death in young athletes, with hypertrophic cardiomyopathy being the most common cause. Pulmonary causes of sudden death, such as asthma and anaphylaxis, or neurovascular congenital abnormalities such as aneurysms, are second to sudden cardiac death in young athletes (National Institutes of Health, National Heart, Lung, and Blood Institutes, 2006).
- Does your child fatigue easily?
  - ☐ Fatigue may be sign of decreased cardiac output. Children may get tired easily when playing or with increased activity.
- Have you noticed that your child's skin color becomes pale or has a bluish hue with increased activity?
  - ☐ **Cyanosis** is a sign of decreased oxygen or hemoglobin in the blood.

Abdominal

Ask the parent or child (age-appropriate):
- Does your child complain of abdominal pain? If so when and how often?
- Does your child complain of nausea or vomiting?
- Does your child have regular bowel movements? Bowel accidents?
  - ☐ **Encopresis** occurs when a child beyond the age of toilet teaching resists having bowel movements, causing impacted stool to collect

in the colon and rectum. When the colon is full of impacted stool, liquid stool can leak around the impacted stool and out of the anus, staining the child's underwear. Encopresis may also be called "stool holding."

SENC Child-Centered Care Recurrent abdominal pain is a common pediatric complaint. Children who internalize stress may experience abdominal pain. Typically, laboratory work-ups do not yield positive results when abdominal pain is the only symptom. (Dhroove, 2010). Administering a validated screening instrument to the child/family may identify a need for a referral to a mental health provider (American Academy of Pediatrics, 2010).

Female Genitalia/Genitourinary

Ask the parent:

- How often do you change a wet diaper?

Ask the parent or child (age-appropriate):

- Does your child complain of pain with urination?
- Do you have any pain in your private area?
- Have you noticed any colored drainage on toilet paper or your underpants when you wipe yourself?

In adolescent females, assess for the following:

- Have you started menstruating? If so, at what age did you start to have your periods? How long do your periods last?
- Do you have any pain with your periods? If so, what medications do you take to help the pain?
- Do you miss any school when you have your period? Do you use sanitary napkins or tampons?
- Are you sexually active?
- Are you on birth control or do you use safe sex practices? If so, what do you use for protection?

☐ Risky sexual behaviors (early sexual onset, unprotected sex, multiple partners) during adolescence are associated with unintended pregnancies and sexually transmitted infections (STIs) (Kao & Salerno, 2014).

☐ Fewer than 2 percent of adolescents have had sex by the time they reach their 12th birthday; on average, young people have sex for the first time at about age 17 (Planned Parenthood Federation of America, 2016).

SENC Evidence-Based Practice Evidence shows that male latex condoms have an 85 percent or greater protective effect against the sexual transmission of HIV and other sexually transmitted infections (STIs) (World Health Organization, 2016).

■ **TIP** Media coverage of vaccines can influence social norms, parental attitudes, and vaccine acceptance or refusal.

- Have you received the human papillomavirus (HPV) vaccine?

■ **TIP** Parental permission is required for vaccines to be administered to a child or adolescent younger than 18 years of age.

☐ The American College of Obstetricians and Gynecologists (2017) makes the following recommendations: routine HPV vaccination for girls and boys at the target age of 11–12 years (but it may be given from the age of 9 years) as part of the adolescent immunization platform.

■ **TIP** Sexualized behaviors are a normal part of child development. In children younger than age 5 years, these behaviors are more common in a child who has been physically abused, neglected, or sexually abused.

■ **TIP** Healthcare providers should carefully gather and document data collected when a child is a suspected victim of physical or sexual abuse. Asking children or adolescents specific questions about physical or sexual abuse, especially when the parent or legal guardian is not present, should be conducted by persons who are explicitly trained to work with suspected victims or victims of abuse.

TIP A child needs to understand that confidentiality may be breached if you suspect that he/she may be a danger to him/herself or a danger to others, or if you suspect that the child has been abused or is in danger of being abused (McConaughy, 2013).

Ask the appropriate questions of an older child:

- How did you first learn about sex?
- Do you have any concerns about your body?
- Do you know of anyone who has experienced sexual abuse?
- Has anyone touched you in a way that made you feel uncomfortable
  - Children are more likely to confide in a teacher or trusted relative or friend (McElvaney, 2015). Nurses should be alert to the nonspecific symptoms of child sexual abuse (Table 22-2).

SENC Child-Centered Care Lesbian, gay, bisexual, transgender and queer (LGBTQ) youth have to deal with harassment, intimidation, and bullying on a regular basis (Perron, Kartoz, & Himelfarb, 2017).

TABLE 22-2 Signs of Sexual Abuse

Physical Symptoms	Behavior Symptoms
Pregnancy	Withdrawal
Genital lacerations	Anxiety, fearlessness
Rectal tears	Sleep disturbance, nightmares
Pain or discoloration in in the mouth, anus, or genital area	Somatic complaints
Bruising near genitals	Eroticization, increased sex play
Stomachaches	Self-destructive behaviors
Blood in stool	Acting-out behaviors, self-harm such as cutting him- or herself
Discharge	School problems
	Depression, low self-esteem
	Regressing to younger behaviors

These youth experience higher rates of depression and suicidal ideation, higher rates of substance abuse, and STIs. A confidential, comprehensive socio-emotional history can identify those adolescents who may benefit from mental health services (American Academy of Pediatric Committee on Adolescence, 2013).

Male Genitalia

Ask the parent or child (age-appropriate):

- Does your child complain of pain with urination?
- Do you have any pain in your private area?
- Do you have any drainage from your penis?

Ask the adolescent boy (if age-appropriate):

- Do you do a testicular self-examination?
- Do you know why it is important to do testicular self-examination?
- Do you know how to perform a testicular self-examination?
  - Adolescent boys over the age of 14 should start performing testicular self-examinations to become familiar with this area of the body and to learn what normal testicles feel like and to check every month that there have been no changes. (See Chapter 19, Box 19-3, for directions to perform testicular self-examination.)

Musculoskeletal

Ask the parent or child (age-appropriate):

- Do you have any difficulty walking or moving your arms or legs?
- Are you able to run, jump, and climb during playtime?
- Do you have any pain or stiffness in your arms, legs, or back?
- Have you had any bone deformities and had to wear corrective devices?

Neurological

Ask the parent or child (age-appropriate):

- Does your child have any headaches?

TIP Headaches are very common in children. About 50 to 75 percent of children report having a headache each month. Serious causes of headaches in children and adolescents are rare. Among children and adolescents, headaches are most often a symptom of other medical or emotional problems (Moreno, Furtner, & Rivara, 2013).

■ Does your child complain of dizziness or feeling faint?
■ How is your child's muscle strength?
■ Has your child had any difficulty walking or with muscle coordination?
■ Has your child had any changes in her or his speech or articulation of words?
■ Has your child had a sport-related concussion?

SENC Evidence-Based Practice An evidence-based definition of concussion is:
■ change in brain function
■ following a force to the head, which
■ may be accompanied by temporary loss of consciousness, but is identified in awake individuals, with measures of neurologic and cognitive dysfunction (National Collegiate Athletic Association, 2014).

SENC Safety Alert Concussion is a common brain injury among children and adolescents participating in organized sports and recreational activities. A Safety in College Football Summit was held January 2014 and 2016, to bring together a multifaceted group of experts who share a common interest in improving the culture of safety in intercollegiate sports in general, and football in particular.

Student athletes are to be knowledgeable about the signs of a concussion. (See Box 22-1.) Parents should be educated that symptoms may occur immediately following the injury or hours to days after the injury. Any child or youth who sustains a concussion should be removed from

---

> **BOX 22-1 Signs and Symptoms of a Concussion**
>
> • Loss of consciousness
> • Headache
> • Changes in vision
> • Dizziness
> • Nausea/vomiting
> • Feeling faint
> • Agitation
> • Irritability
> • Memory loss
> • Insomnia
> • Problems with balance and coordination

play immediately and medically evaluated as soon as possible (Purcell, 2014). Medical clearance for the student-athlete is required prior to returning to the sport.

Endocrine
Ask the older child:
■ How often do you urinate?
■ Are you unusually hungry?
■ Are you unusually tired?
  □ The symptoms of type 1 diabetes include urinating often (polyuria), feeling very thirsty (polydipsia), feeling very hungry even though eating normally (polyphagia), extreme fatigue, blurry vision, cuts and bruises that are slow to heal, and weight loss despite eating normally.
  • Growth pattern changes, delayed sexual maturation, or precocious puberty may indicate pituitary gland issues.

PREPARATION FOR ASSESSMENT

Equipment Needed

Gloves
Age-appropriate scale
Age-appropriate: stadiometer or length board
Paper measuring tape
Stethoscope
Thermometer

Sequence of Assessment

- Inspection
- Auscultation
- Palpation

TIP For younger children, begin with the least invasive assessment. For example, consider auscultating heart and breath sounds first, saving inspection of the ears, eyes, nose, and mouth for last.

Preliminary Steps

- Maintain privacy throughout the assessment. Respect for the child/adolescent's privacy must be maintained, including removing one's clothing, providing gowns that fit appropriately, and obtaining measurements in a location that offers privacy. Even young children are aware of their feelings of vulnerability when exposed.
- Approach the child according to his or her developmental age (Table 22-3).

- Be attentive to your initial impressions, recognizing that a child's chronological age is not always an indicator of the child's developmental stage.
- Ask the parents of an older school-age child or adolescent to leave the room during the physical examination unless the child/adolescent prefers the parent to remain in the room.
- Explain the steps of the assessment as you proceed using age-appropriate explanations.
- Ask permission to assess private areas.
- Answer the child's questions, using age-appropriate explanations.
- Keep the room warm and free of drafts.
- Perform hand hygiene and warm hands before touching the child in all of the following assessments.
- Engage the child in an age-appropriate conversation by asking simple questions about themselves, toys, or favorite activities.

SENC Child-Centered Care Establishing a calm, relaxed, yet professional approach that demonstrates understanding of child development builds parental confidence and is essential for best meeting the needs of the child.

TIP Compliment the child's cooperation during the physical assessment and use the temperament of the child as the guide in your approach.

TABLE 22-3 Developmental Approaches for Pediatric Examination

Developmental Age Group	Toddler	Preschooler	School-age	Adolescents
Place to perform the examination	If possible, perform the examination on an examining table with the parent by the child's side. Otherwise, allow the child to either sit on the parent's lap or stand by the parent. Toddlers will attempt to stay in the upright position so examination in a prone or supine position is best accomplished in the parent's lap.	Prefers standing or sitting with the parent close by. Is likely to be cooperative in the prone or supine position.	Sitting on the examination table and is generally cooperative in most positions. Younger school-agers prefer the parent within their line of sight; an older school-aged child may prefer privacy.	Same as the school-age child. Older teens may prefer that the parent leave the room during the examination and return afterward. Offer the option of parent's presence.
Approach	Expect that a toddler will start to scream soon after you enter the room. Remain calm, and speak to the parent in an assuring manner. If the parent feels comfortable, this feeling will be conveyed to the child. Make sure the child remains safely in the parent's lap through most of the examination. Provide a simple explanation of the steps of the examination to the child and a more detailed explanation to the parent. Perform the least invasive parts of the examination first. Allow the child to touch and explore your stethoscope. Attaching a small toy to the tubing will increase the child's curiosity.	Encourage the child to be an active participant in the examination. Using a hand-over-hand technique while listening with a stethoscope (allow the child to hold the diaphragm of the stethoscope and place your hand over the child's) will engage the child. Making a game of the examination is helpful because the child is both curious and worried about what you are doing. Use a slow, deliberate approach.	Use a head-to-toe approach with the examination of the genitals last. Speak with the parent before and after the examination. Ask the child direct questions, and explain what you are doing in simple terms. Tell the child when something you are going to do will be uncomfortable or hurt. Include the child in the conversation when appropriate.	Use a head-to-toe approach with the examination of the genitals last. Adolescents prefer to be treated more as adults. Speak to the adolescent using appropriate terminology and explanations. Use open-ended questions to encourage conversation. Limiting direct eye contact and asking questions in a casual, matter-of-fact way creates a more comfortable tone. Questions about the behaviors of the adolescent's peer group may offer additional insights. Explain confidentiality to the parent and teen; speak to the parent and teen together and separately.

TABLE 22-3 Developmental Approaches for Pediatric Examination—cont'd

Developmental Age Group	Toddler	Preschooler	School-age	Adolescents
Preparation	Have the parent remove the child's clothing except underwear which should be removed as the body part is being examined. Allow the child to see and/or touch the equipment. Move quickly if the child is uncooperative. Request parent's assistance during restraining, positioning the parent near the head of the child.	Request the child undress except for underpants. Allow the child to see the equipment, offering a brief demonstration. Expect cooperation and give choice when possible. Make up stories about procedures ("I am giving you a hands-free hug" for BP).	Request the child to undress, providing a gown to wear in place of clothing. Allow the child to wear underpants. Explain the purpose of the equipment and provide a simple explanation for what the procedure will accomplish. Teach about body function and care.	Allow to undress in private, providing a gown. Maintain privacy, exposing only the parts being examined. Explain findings as you go through the examination using an "a-matter-of-fact" approach about sexual development. Examine genitalia last. Reinforce normalcy of development when examining each body area.
Sequence	Use minimum physical contact initially using play to inspect each body area. Introduce equipment slowly. Auscultate, percuss, and palpate when the child is quiet; perform the most invasive or traumatic procedures last.	If cooperative, proceed in head-to-toe fashion; otherwise, proceed as with toddler.	Proceed in head-to-toe fashion, examining genitalia last in older child.	Proceed in head-to-toe fashion, examining genitalia last.

From Hockenberry, 2011; Ricci, 2009.

FOCUSED ASSESSMENT

TECHNIQUE 22-1: **Performing a General Survey**

Purpose: To assess the child's physical appearance, state of nutrition, personality, interaction with the parent(s), siblings (if present), nurse, and healthcare provider.

ASSESSMENT STEPS

1. Assess hygiene, cleanliness, unusual body odor, and condition of clothing.

■ **TIP** The hygiene of a child can be an important clue to possible instances of neglect, limited financial resources, housing difficulties such as no heat or running water, or a lack of knowledge concerning the basic needs of the child. For the older child it may indicate difficulties with changing body image.

2. Assess posture, overall development, and speech.

3. Assess the child's behavior: activity level, reaction to stress, interactions with others, attention span, ability to follow directions, use of eye contact, and the child's overall personality.

4. Document overall assessment of child's speech development, motor skills, coordination, and recent area of achievement.

NORMAL FINDINGS

■ Good hygiene, no body odor
■ Clothed appropriately for season
■ Straight posture, within normal parameters for growth and development
■ Makes eye contact
■ Alert and cooperative (age appropriate)
■ Motor skills and coordination (age appropriate)
■ Positive interactions with parent/caregiver, nurse, and healthcare provider

ABNORMAL FINDINGS

■ Poor hygiene, body odor
■ Clothed inappropriately for the season
■ Poor posture, not within normal parameters for growth and development
■ No eye contact, aggressive or uncooperative (age appropriate)
■ Decreased motor skills and coordination (age appropriate)
■ Negative interactions with parent/caregiver, nurse, or healthcare provider

TECHNIQUE 22-2: **Assessing Weight**

Purpose: To assess normal somatic growth specific to weight
Equipment: Age-appropriate scale
- The child or adolescent should be weighed wearing only lightweight underclothing or a hospital gown.
- A toddler should be weighed nude; otherwise, the weight should be documented including a notation of the additional clothing or shoes the child was wearing. If a diaper is worn then it should be clean and dry.
- A child must be able to stand independently to obtain an accurate weight on a standing scale.
- Generally, children older than 36 months can be weighed on a standing scale.

   ■ **TIP** For toddlers weighing less than 40 pounds and who are unable to stand long enough to obtain an accurate weight, use an infant scale (Fig. 22-3A).

   ■ **TIP** When a child is too active or distressed to obtain an accurate weight measurement, an alternative, but less accurate, weighing technique is to have the parent stand on an adult standing scale, document the weight, reset the scale to zero, and then have the parent hold the child and weigh the child and parent together. The difference between the two values will provide an approximate weight of the child.

ASSESSMENT STEPS
1. Move the large and small weights to zero or make the balance beam level and steady by adjusting the calibrating knob.
2. Once calibrated, have the child/adolescent stand on the scale with feet a comfortable distance apart, arms and hands at his or her side, and head up and facing forward (Fig. 22-3B).
3. Move the largest weight to the increment just under the child's weight.
4. Adjust the smaller weight to balance the scale to the nearest quarter pound or 0.1 kg.
5. Note the weight.
6. Have the child step off the scale.
7. Document the weight in pounds and kilograms.

NORMAL FINDINGS
- Normal weight for age

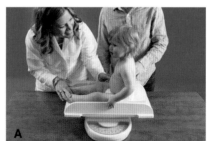
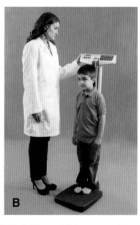

Fig. 22-3. (A) Weighing a toddler on an infant scale. (B) Weighing a child on a stand up scale.

ABNORMAL FINDINGS
■ **Growth failure** is failure to grow, gain weight, or both (Nofal & Schwenk, 2013). It is reflected as weight lower than the fifth percentile for the child's age on standard growth charts or a weight curve that falls more than two percentile lines on the National Center for Health Statistics (Center for Disease Control and Prevention, 2015).

TECHNIQUE 22-3: ASSESSING LENGTH OR HEIGHT

Purpose: To assess for somatic growth specific to length or height
Equipment: Age-appropriate: stadiometer, or length board

Length
ASSESSMENT STEPS
1. Two measurers are required for an accurate measurement. One measurer holds the infant's head, and the second aligns the infant's trunk and legs.
2. To measure a child using a length board, gently position the child on his or her back in the center of the board so that the shoulders and buttocks are flat against the board (Fig. 22-4A).
   □ Length boards are used for measuring children younger than 24 months of age or for children 24 to 36 months who cannot stand unassisted.
   ■ **TIP** The child's eyes should be looking straight up, both legs fully extended, and feet flat against the footboard so the toes are pointing upward.
3. Gently hold the head in midline, firmly press on both knees to fully extend both legs while bringing the footboard firmly against the heels, toes pointing upward. Both legs should be fully extended for an accurate measurement.
4. Note the length in centimeters.
5. Document your findings.

Height
ASSESSMENT STEPS
1. Ask the patient to remove shoes and place feet together before measuring height.
2. Measure the patient's height by standing upright under a stadiometer (Fig. 22-4B).

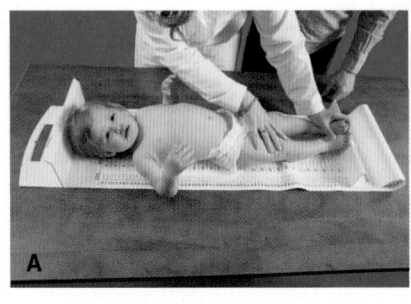
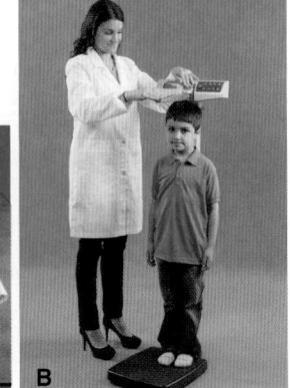

Fig. 22-4. (A) Measuring height of toddler using a length board. (B) Measuring height of school-aged child using a stadiometer.

3. Carefully lower the horizontal bar until it touches the top of the patient's head.

4. Record the measurement.

NORMAL FINDINGS

- Normal height for age
- Familial short stature or temporary delay in skeletal growth can lead to a normal variant. Delayed skeletal growth may also be related to endocrine or other diseases such as growth hormone deficiency, inflammatory bowel disease, celiac disease, renal disease, or genetic syndromes.

ABNORMAL FINDINGS

- Short stature, subnormal height for age

TECHNIQUE 22-4: **Assessing Temperature**

Purpose: To assess the body's core temperature

Technique 22-4A: **Assessing Rectal Temperature**

Purpose: To assess core body temperature

Equipment: Digital thermometer, gloves, lubricant

- Rectal temperature is considered an accurate route for assessing body core temperature because it is an indication of deep visceral temperature.
- Rectal temperatures taken with digital thermometers are recommended by the American Academy of Pediatrics (American Academy of Pediatrics, 2015) for children 3 years of age or younger.

   TIP In some institutions, rectal temperatures require a healthcare provider's order.

ASSESSMENT STEPS

1. Explain the procedure to the parent or caregiver.
2. Put on clean gloves.
3. Position the child in the prone position on a firm surface or prone on the parent's or caregiver's lap; the smaller child may be supine holding the legs up.
4. Remove the temperature probe from the electronic thermometer base.
5. Insert probe into the disposable probe cover.
6. Lubricate the tip of the probe with lubricant.
7. Gently insert the tip of the thermometer into the rectum about 1/2 inch in the younger child and 1 inch in an older child.
8. Hold the probe in place until the temperature reading registers.
9. Slowly remove the probe from the rectum and discard the disposable plastic cover and gloves in the garbage.
10. Assist or place the child in a comfortable position.

11. Return the thermometer back to the charger stand.

12. Document the site and temperature reading.

NORMAL FINDINGS

■ 98.7°F to 100.5°F or 37.1°C to 38.1°C

ABNORMAL FINDINGS

■ <98.7°F to >100.5°F or <37.1°C to >38.1°C

Technique 22-4B: **Assessing Oral Temperature**

Purpose: To assess the core body temperature

Equipment: Electronic thermometer

■ A digital oral thermometer can be used when children reach the age of 4 to 5 years and are able to keep their mouths closed with the probe correctly positioned under the tongue long enough to obtain a temperature reading.

  ■ **TIP** Always make sure your thermometer is fully charged and calibrated.

ASSESSMENT STEPS

1. Take the thermometer off the charger prior to assessing the child.

2. Explain the procedure to the child.

3. Ask the child or adolescent if he or she has smoked, or consumed any hot or cold foods or beverages in the last 30 minutes; if so, wait until 30 minutes has passed to maintain the accuracy of the reading.

4. Take the thermometer probe out of the holder and attach a plastic disposable probe cover.

5. Ask the child to open his or her mouth and lift up the tongue.

6. Gently place the thermometer probe underneath the tongue (sublingually).

7. Ask the child to gently but firmly close her or his mouth.

8. Observe the calculation of the thermometer; a sound or blinking will occur as the temperature reading registers.

9. Dispose of the dispensable thermometer probe cover.

10. Return the thermometer to the charger.

11. Document the site and temperature reading.

NORMAL FINDINGS

■ 97.5°F to 99.5°F or 36°C to 38°C

ABNORMAL FINDINGS

■ Less than 97.7°F to greater than 100°F or less than 36.5°C to greater than 37.8°C

  □ Hypothermia is a core body temperature below 35°C (95°F) (Venes, 2013).

  □ Hyperthermia (pyrexia) is an elevated body temperature greater than 37.8°C (greater than 100°F).

SENC Safety Alert Hypothermia should be confirmed by temperature readings at two different core locations (Venes, 2013).

Technique 22-4C: **Assessing Tympanic Temperature**

Purpose: To assess the core body temperature for children 6 months and older.

Equipment: Tympanic thermometer

■ Tympanic thermometers may be used in infants 6 months or older but must be placed in the ear canal correctly to obtain an accurate reading.

ASSESSMENT STEPS

1. Explain the procedure to the child (age-appropriate).

2. Take the tympanic thermometer off the charging stand.

3. Attach a clear dispensable plastic ear probe.

4. Gently pull the upper earlobe up and back.

5. Insert the ear probe snugly pointing it toward the tympanic membrane.

6. Push the button to register the temperature reading.

7. Once the temperature reading registers, dispose of the dispensable thermometer probe cover.

8. Return the thermometer to the charger.

9. Document the site and temperature reading.

NORMAL FINDINGS

■ 98.2°F to 100°F or 36.8°C to 37.8°C

ABNORMAL FINDINGS

■ Less than 98.2°F to greater than 100°F or less than 36.8°C to greater than 37.8°C

Technique 22-4D: **Assessing Temporal Temperature**

Purpose: To assess core body temperature

Equipment: Temporal artery thermometer

■ Axillary temperatures and temporal artery thermometry (TAT) (Carr, 2011; Penning, 2011) are not considered reliable but can be helpful in screening for fever in a less invasive manner.

ASSESSMENT STEPS

1. Explain the procedure to the child (age-appropriate).

2. Place the sensor head of the temporal artery thermometer at the center of the forehead midway between the eyebrow and the hairline.

3. Press the button down to start the scan.

4. Slowly slide the thermometer straight across the forehead toward the top of the ear maintaining direct contact with the skin.

SENC Safety Alert Lifting the temporal artery thermometer off the skin will affect the reliability of the temperature.

5. Stop when you reach the hairline and release the button.

6. Lift up the thermometer from the skin and read the temperature on the display screen.

7. Wipe the probe with an alcohol wipe.

8. Return the thermometer back to the charger.

9. Document the site and temperature reading.

NORMAL FINDINGS

■ 98.7°F to 100.5°F or 37.1°C to 38.1°C

ABNORMAL FINDINGS

■ Less than 98.7°F to greater than 100.5°F or less than 37.1°C to greater than 38.1°C

SENC Safety Alert Parents should be instructed to call their healthcare provider if their child has a fever, most often defined as a temperature above 38°C or 100.4°F.

TECHNIQUE 22-5: ASSESSING HEART RATE

Purpose: To assess the heart rate

Equipment: Watch or clock with second hand, stethoscope (age-appropriate)

TIP The best time to assess a child's heart rate and respiratory rate is when the child is quiet and not crying.

Assessing the heart rate of a child is similar to assessing it in adults.

■ Because the transmission of sound via the stethoscope relies on creating an airtight seal between the surface of the skin and the chest piece of the stethoscope, it is important to use the correct size stethoscope to obtain adequate surface contact on the smaller bodies of infants and children.

■ Appropriately sized stethoscopes allow the healthcare provider to focus on sounds in a specific area of the body (Fig. 22-5).

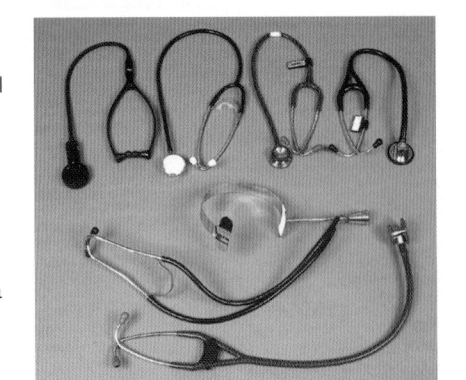

Fig. 22-5. Pediatric stethoscopes.

Technique 22-5A: **Auscultating an Apical Pulse**

Purpose: To assess the heart rate

Equipment: Stethoscope, watch with a second hand

ASSESSMENT STEPS

1. Explain the technique to the child (if age appropriate).
2. Wipe off the stethoscope with an alcohol swab to clean the diaphragm.
3. Warm the stethoscope.
4. Uncover the left side of the child's chest.
5. Gently place the diaphragm of the stethoscope directly over the left fourth or fifth intercostal space at the midclavicular line (apex of the heart) (Fig. 22-6).
6. Auscultate the heartbeat, assessing the rate and rhythm.
7. Count the beats per minute for 30 seconds, then multiply by two; if irregular, count the beats for 60 seconds.
8. Document the site and apical pulse rate.

NORMAL FINDINGS

■ Normal heart rates for infants and children are found in Table 22-4.

ABNORMAL FINDINGS

■ A heart rate that is abnormally fast or abnormally slow may indicate cardiac disease or arrhythmia.
■ **Tachycardia** is defined as a heart rate greater than 160 to 180 beats/min in the child over 5 years of age, although this can also be a normal response to stress.
■ **Bradycardia** is a heart rate less than 60 beats/min in a child.

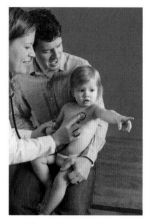

Fig. 22-6. Auscultating heart with pediatric stethoscope.

TABLE 22-4 Normal Heart Rates for Infants and Children (Beats/Min)			
Age	Normal Range	Average	Exercise or Fever
One to three years	80–120	100	Up to 200
Three to nine years	70–115	90	Up to 200
Nine to 14 years	65–109	80–85	Up to 200

Data from Hockenberry, 2011; Howlin, 2010.

Technique 22-5B: **Palpating the Radial Pulse**

Purpose: To assess the heartbeat through the wall of the radial peripheral artery at the wrist

ASSESSMENT STEPS

1. Explain the technique to the child (if age appropriate).

2. Gently place your second and third finger pads of your dominant hand on the radial artery at the flexor aspect of the wrist laterally along the radius bone.

> ▌ **TIP** Do not use your thumb because it has its own pulse that you may feel.

□ While palpating the pulsation, note the following characteristics of the pulse:
  • Rhythm of the pulse: regular versus irregular; missed or paused beats; or an abnormal pattern of beats
  • Amplitude (strength) of the pulse is the force of the blood in the arterial system. This is measured on a scale of 0 to 3 (see Chapter 6, Table 6-1).

3. Holding your watch in the opposite hand, start counting the pulsations (heartbeats) for 60 seconds starting the count with number 1.

4. Document both sites of the pulse, pulse rate, rhythm, and amplitude.

NORMAL FINDINGS

■ Normal heart rates for children are found in Table 22-4.

ABNORMAL FINDINGS

■ A heart rate that is abnormally fast or abnormally slow may indicate cardiac or arrhythmia.

> **SENC Safety Alert** When a child presents with tachycardia or bradycardia, be prepared to deliver pediatric life support and notify a physician healthcare provider immediately. Notify the healthcare provider if findings indicate an irregular heart rate or murmur.

Technique 22-5C: **Assessing Respiratory Rate**

Purpose: To assess the pulmonary ventilation

Equipment: Stethoscope, watch or clock with a second hand

Assessing the respiratory rate of a child is similar to assessing it in an adult.

ASSESSMENT STEPS

1. Position changes influence expansion of the lungs; sitting up or standing is the best position for improving respiratory depth; lying down (prone position) reduces respiratory depth.

2. Explain the technique to the child (if age appropriate).

3. Observe the child's rise (inspiration) and fall (expiration) of the chest area.

4. Observe the following characteristics of the respirations:
  □ **Depth:** even pattern, deep or shallow respirations
  □ **Rhythm:** regular or irregular
  □ **Effort:** amount of work required to take a breath

5. Count the number of respirations for 30 seconds and multiply by two; if irregular, count the number of respirations for 60 seconds.

6. Document the rate, depth, rhythm, and effort.

NORMAL FINDINGS

- Normal respiratory rates for children are listed in Table 22-5.

ABNORMAL FINDINGS

- Respiratory rate exceeding 60 breaths per minute or compromised breathing
- Retractions
- Nasal flaring
- Grunting or stridor
- Pale, mottled, or blue skin color
- Tachycardia
- Change in consciousness

SENC Safety Alert Never feed an infant or child orally if the respiratory rate exceeds 60 breaths/minute.

SENC Safety Alert Children have an uncanny ability to compensate for ineffective respiratory and cardiac function. Subtle changes will occur in the child's color, respirations, behavior, and heart rate before the child "crashes" and may then have a significantly diminished probability of recovery.

TIP Report even subtle changes in a child's overall appearance and trust your instincts when you sense something is going wrong.

TABLE 22-5 Normal Respiratory Rates for Children

Age (years)	Rate (breaths/min)
2	25
4	23
6	22
8	20
10	19
12	19
14	18
16	17
18	16–18

Data from Hockenberry, 2011.

Technique 22-5D: Assessing Blood Pressure

Purpose: To assess circulatory blood volume as the heart contracts and relaxes

Equipment: Noninvasive blood pressure (BP) device, size-appropriate BP cuff

- The most important factor in obtaining an accurate BP requires using a cuff that is appropriate for the size of the child's upper arm (Fig. 22-7).
- Having child cuffs of different sizes (Table 22-6) is necessary to measure BP in children, ages 3 through adolescence, and should include a standard adult cuff, a large adult cuff, and a thigh cuff. The latter two cuffs may be needed for use in adolescents.

  TIP When the correct size cuff is not available, use an oversized cuff rather than an undersized cuff. Do not choose a cuff based on the name of it (infant-sized, child-sized, etc.) because the cuff may be too small or too large for the child.

- BP values change with age and growth and are likely to vary when different sites are used for measurement, if the child is lying, sitting, or standing, or if the child is anxious.

TABLE 22-6 Recommended Dimensions for BP Cuff Bladders

Age Range	Width (cm)	Length (cm)	Maximum Arm Circumference (cm)*
Newborn	4	8	10
Infant	6	12	15
Child	9	18	22

From National Institutes of Health, National Heart, Lung, and Blood Institutes, 2006.

▇ **TIP** Always look in the child's record to compare BP readings.

ASSESSMENT STEPS

1. Explain the technique to the child.
2. Ask the child or adolescent if he or she has smoked or had any caffeine in the last 30 minutes; if no, proceed to take his or her BP; if yes, wait until 30 minutes has lapsed.
3. Ask the child not to move, talk, or cross the legs while taking the reading.
4. If sitting, seat the child comfortably with back supported, legs uncrossed, and palm facing up, the arm resting at the level of the fourth intercostal space (heart level) and not tensed; if the child is in supine position in the bed, place the arm flat with palm facing up on a pillow so that the arm is at heart's level.
5. Use a paper measuring tape, and measure the circumference of the midpoint of the upper arm between the shoulder and the elbow; choose the correct cuff size for the child.
6. Wrap the deflated cuff around the child's arm about 2.5 cm (1 inch) above the brachial artery and wrap evenly; make sure the artery marker is pointing to the brachial artery.
7. Have the child support the bare arm on the examination table or in your arm at the child's heart's level.
8. Turn the manual valve clockwise on the BP cuff to close it.
9. Palpate the brachial artery at the antecubical fossa or the radial artery at the wrist, and continue to feel for the pulsation of the brachial or radial artery.
10. Start squeezing the bulb at the end of the rubber tube attached to the BP cuff. When you no longer feel the pulsation of the brachial artery, make note of this number on the sphygmomanometer and continue to inflate the cuff pressure another 30 mm Hg. Slowly release the manual valve to deflate the BP cuff and note if the brachial pulse returns at the same point that it disappeared.
11. Place the bell or the diaphragm of the stethoscope on the brachial artery, and inflate the BP cuff 30 to 40 mm Hg above the palpable systolic BP number (Anderson, 2010). The numerical reading should be read to the nearest 2 mm Hg.

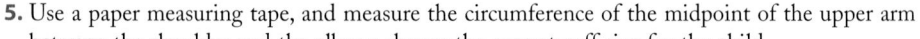

Fig. 22-7. Pediatric BP cuffs.

12. Slowly release the manual valve (2 to 3 mm/sec) to deflate the BP cuff, and listen for the first rhythmic Korotkoff sounds heard as blood begins to flow through the artery; this first sound is the systolic reading.
13. Continue to listen as the cuff pressure is released, for the last Korotkoff sound that you are able to hear; this last sound is the diastolic reading.
14. Document the location and BP reading.

NORMAL FINDINGS

■ See Table 22-7 for normal BP values in children.

ABNORMAL FINDINGS

■ BP that does not fall within normal ranges

TABLE 22-7 Normal BPs in Children		
Age	Systolic Pressure (mm Hg)	Diastolic Pressure (mm Hg)
Toddler (1–2 years)	86–106	42–63
Preschool (3–5 years)	89–112	46–72
School age (6–7 years)	97–115	57–76
Preadolescent (10–12 years)	102–120	61–80
Adolescent (12–15 years)	110–131	64–83

TECHNIQUE 22-6: **Assessing Pain**

Purpose: To assess actual or potential tissue damage

Special Considerations

■ Recognizing and treating pain in children can be challenging. They experience pain differently than do adults and even verbal children find it difficult to locate, describe, and quantify their pain.
■ Children in pain are not easily distracted and are often disinterested in activities that would ordinarily gain their attention.
■ More overt behaviors of children in pain include crying, guarding painful body parts, and exhibiting developmental regression.
■ Children in pain will say almost anything to avoid what they perceive as a negative consequence, such as an injection to relieve pain (Taddio, 2009).
■ A self-report is the preferred method for assessing pain. Because physiological measures such as oxygen saturation, BP, and respiratory rates cannot quantify a child's pain experience; they are most useful when used in conjunction with a pain assessment tool.
■ The verbal numerical rating scale is one of the most widely used scales for assessing pediatric pain intensity. This rating scale is a valid instrument for assessing pain intensity in children above 8 years of age (Castarlenas, Miró, & Sánchez-Rodríguez, 2013).
■ The best method for pain assessment in children includes selecting a tool that is validated and reliable and is age appropriate and accounts for the cognitive ability, language, and cultural background of the child. The selected tool should be used consistently over time and in combination with the nurse's objective measures and other assessments. Pain rating scales for children are as follows:

TABLE 22-8 FLACC Scale for Pain

Categories	Scoring			Date
	0	1	2	
Face	No particular expression or smile	Occasional grimace or frown; frequent to constant frown, clenched jaw, withdrawn, disinterested	Frequent to constant frown, clenched jaw, quivering chin	
Legs	Normal position or relaxed	Uneasy, restless, tense	Kicking or legs drawn up	
Activity	Lying quietly, normal position, moves easily	Squirming, shifting back and forth, tense	Arched, rigid, or jerking	
Cry	Arched, rigid, or jerking	Moans or whimpers, occasional complaint	Crying steadily, screams or sobs; frequent complaints	
Consolability	Crying steadily, screams or sobs; frequent complaints	Reassured by occasional touching, hugging, or being talked to; distractable	Difficult to console or comfort	

From Merkel, Voepel-Lewis, Shayevitz, & Malviya, 1997. The FLACC scale was developed by Sandra Merkel, MS, RN, Terri Voepel-Lewis, MS, RN, and Shobha Malviya, MD, at C. S. Mott Children's Hospital, University of Michigan Health System, Ann Arbor, MI.

- ☐ **Face, Legs, Activity, Cry, Consolability (FLACC) scale** (Table 22-8) is a measurement used to assess pain for children between the ages of 2 months and 7 years or individuals who are unable to communicate their pain.
  - The scale is scored between a range of 0 to 10, with 0 representing no pain.
  - The scale has five criteria (Face, Legs, Activity, Cry, Consolability) that are each assigned a score of 0, 1, or 2 (Merkel, 1997).
- ☐ **COMFORT-B (Comfort Behavior) Scale** (Table 22-9)
  - This is a tool to assess pain and sedation in infants and children.
  - Observe the child's face and body for a full 2 minutes.
  - Document pain intensity based on observations of alertness, calmness-agitation, respiratory response, crying, physical movement, muscle tone, and facial tension (van Dijik, Peters, van Deventer, & Tibboel, 2005).

SENC Evidence-Based Practice The COMFORT-B Scale requires nurses to do a 2-minute observation period of the infant. Some nurses consider this time to be too long. Boerlage, Ista, de Jong, Tibboel, & van Dijk (2012) performed an observational study to test the reliability of a 30-second observation period at a Level III intensive care unit at a university children's hospital. Sensitivity and positive predictive value for the 30-second observation were 0.44 and 0.80, respectively. A 30-second COMFORT behavior scale observation increases the risk of underscoring pain. Therefore, the 2-minute observation period should be adhered to in the best interest of the patients.

TABLE 22-9 COMFORT Behavior Scale

		Check
Alertness	Deeply asleep (eyes closed, no response to changes in the environment)	O 1
	Lightly asleep (eyes mostly closed, occasional responses)	O 2
	Drowsy (child closes his/her eyes frequently, less responsive to the environment)	O 3
	Awake and alert (child responsive to the environment)	O 4
	Awake and hyperalert (exaggerated responses to environmental stimuli)	O 5
Calmness/Agitation	Calm (child appears serene and tranquil)	O 1
	Slightly anxious (child shows slight anxiety)	O 2
	Anxious (child appears agitated but remains in control)	O 3
	Very anxious (child appears very agitated, just able to control)	O 4
	Panicky (severe distress with loss of control)	O 5
Respiratory Response (score only in mechanically ventilated children)	No spontaneous respiration	O 1
	Spontaneous and ventilator respiration	O 2
	Restlessness or resistance to ventilator	O 3
	Actively breathes against ventilator or coughs regularly	O 4
	Fights ventilator	O 5
Crying (score only in spontaneously breathing children)	Quiet breathing, no crying sounds	O 1
	Occasional sobbing or moaning	O 2
	Whining (monotonous sound)	O 3
	Crying	O 4
	Screaming or shrieking	O 5
Physical Movement	No movement	O 1
	Occasional, (three or fewer) slight movements	O 2
	Frequent (more than three) slight movements	O 3
	Vigorous movements limited to extremities	O 4
	Vigorous movements including torso and head	O 5

Continued

TABLE 22-9 COMFORT Behavior Scale—cont'd

		Check
Muscle Tone	Muscles totally relaxed; no muscle tone	O 1
	Reduced muscle tone; less resistance than normal	O 2
	Normal muscle tone	O 3
	Increased muscle tone and flexion of fingers and toes	O 4
	Extreme muscle rigidity and flexion of fingers and toes	O 5
Facial Tension	Facial muscles totally relaxed	O 1
	Normal facial tone	O 2
	Tension evident in some facial muscles (not sustained)	O 3
	Tension evident throughout facial muscles (sustained)	O 4
	Facial muscles contorted and grimacing	O 5
	Total Score	_____

© Copyright English version: B. Ambuel, K. Hamlett, & C. Marx, version 4, November 2003.

□ **OUCHER! Scale**
- The OUCHER! is a poster displaying two scales: a number scale for older children and a picture scale for younger children.
- The picture scale depicts children in varying degrees of pain (Fig. 22-8).
- The child selects the picture that best describes his or her pain. The picture is easily converted to a number value from 1 to 10, with 1 being no pain and 10 being the worst possible pain (Beyer, Denyes, & Villarruel, 1992).

■ **TIP** OUCHER! scale is available with African-American, Caucasian, Hispanic, and Asian versions.

SENC Evidence-Based Practice Multiple studies have been conducted to determine the reliability and validity of pain assessment tools. Developmentally appropriate pain assessment tools to obtain a self-report are available for children as young as 3 years old. Children who are able to count may be asked to rate their pain on a number scale from 0 (no pain) to 10 (worst possible pain imaginable). Children who are unable to count but are interactive may be asked to rate their pain on a continuum scale using colors, pictures of children, or drawings of faces. The FLACC (Face, Legs, Activity, Cry, Consolability) scale and the COMFORT-B scale are effective tools for identifying pain and no pain in nonverbal children (Bai, 2012; Baulch, 2010; Caple, 2012; Melby, 2011; Page, 2012; Raeside, 2011; Stapelkamp, 2011).

For more information on pain assessment, please see Chapter 7.

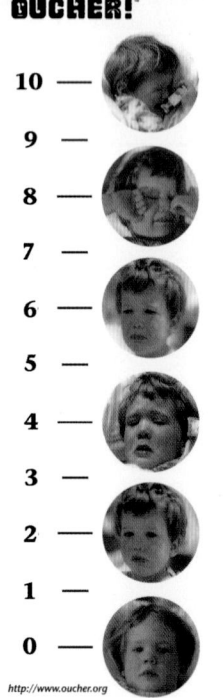

OUCHER!

10 —
9 —
8 —
7 —
6 —
5 —
4 —
3 —
2 —
1 —
0 —

http://www.oucher.org

Fig. 22-8. OUCHER! Scale (From www.oucher.org).

TECHNIQUE 22-7: **Assessing the Skin, Hair, and Nails**

Purpose: To assess for any abnormalities of the skin

Technique 22-7A: **Inspecting and Palpating the Skin**

Purpose: To identify changes in skin, including rashes, lesions, masses, and abnormal moles

Equipment: Penlight

> **SENC Safety Alert** If skin has an open area, always wear gloves to protect yourself from bacteria or germs.

ASSESSMENT STEPS

1. Inspect and palpate simultaneously to assess:

- Hygiene (including odors of the body or breath)
- Color
    - ☐ Assess for cyanosis in the lips, oral mucosa, and tongue.
    - ☐ Assess for pallor of the skin in the lips, fingernails, and mucus membranes.
    - ☐ Assess for jaundice of the skin in the sclera of the eyes, the overall skin, and lips.

CULTURAL CONSIDERATIONS

- Normal color in light-skinned children varies from milky white and rose to deeply hued pink.
- Dark-skinned children, such as Native American, or those of Hispanic or African descent, have inherited various brown, red, yellow, olive green, and bluish tones in their skin.

- **Vascularity:** presence of vascular lesions
- **Temperature:** use the dorsal surface of your hand to check temperature
- Thickness
    - ☐ Skin thickness varies; thin skin is on the eyelids, and the thickest areas are the soles of our feet, palms of our hands, and elbows.
- Skin turgor
    - ☐ The best location to assess skin turgor is the abdomen for toddler and younger child.
    - ☐ The best location to assess skin turgor is the clavicle area for the older child and adolescent.
- Moisture
- Rashes, lesions, tattoos, scars, and masses identifying
    - ☐ Location
    - ☐ Distribution

☐ Pattern and configuration of lesions (see Chapter 8)
☐ Color
☐ Size (use a ruler to measure in centimeters)

2. Document your findings.

NORMAL FINDINGS

- Good hygiene, no odors
- Skin warm, moist
- Uniform color
- Good skin turgor
- No abnormal lesions
- Nevi are uniform brown color, regular borders, less than 0.6 cm.

ABNORMAL FINDINGS

- Bruises
- Vascular lesions
- Changes in skin texture
- Poor skin turgor with tenting of skin
- Rash
- Bluish hue or yellowing of the skin

> **SENC Safety Alert** Suspect abuse in the event of unexplained bruising, red marks, cigarette burns or burns, or injury. Report findings to the appropriate authorities.

Technique 22-7B: Inspecting and Palpating the Hair and Scalp

Purpose: To assess for changes or abnormalities in the hair and scalp
Equipment: Gloves

> **TIP** Inspection of hair should include body hair, scalp, axillae, and pubic areas at 1-inch intervals.

ASSESSMENT STEPS

1. Inspect and palpate simultaneously to assess the following:
- General condition of hair (amount, distribution, cleanliness)
- Condition of scalp (lesions, color, and skin)
- Color
- Texture (thick, brittle, curly)

2. Document your findings.

- Hair clean, curly, or straight texture; uniform thickness and distribution
- Color brown, black, blonde, red
- Scalp clean and intact, no lesions

ABNORMAL FINDINGS

- **Hair loss**
  - □ Anorexia nervosa is one of the most common psychiatric disorders in girls and young women; it is a life-threatening eating disorder; symptoms may include hair loss, dry hair, and dry skin (NEDA, 2014).
  - □ **Alopecia areata** of scalp (spot baldness) is a loss of hair in patches.
- **Tinea capitis** (scalp ringworm) is a fungal infection of the scalp causing round, patchy hair loss, pustules, and scale on the skin.

Technique 22-7C: Inspecting and Palpating the Fingernails and Toenails

Purpose: To assess for healthy nails or presence of vitamin deficiency, malnutrition, disease, or infection

ASSESSMENT STEPS

1. Inspect and palpate simultaneously to assess the following:

- General condition (cleanliness, thinness, thickness)
- Color and markings
- Adherence to nailbed
- Shape and contour
- Capillary refill test (also part of assessing peripheral vascular circulation; easy to perform at this time of the assessment; see Chapter 15, Technique 15-5)

2. Document your findings for the skin, hair, and nail assessment.

NORMAL FINDINGS

- Nails smooth, short, uniform thickness, well groomed
- Nail base angle 160 degrees
- Firmly adhere to the nailbed
- Nailbed pink
- Capillary refill less than 3 seconds
- Nontender to palpation
- No redness, exudates, or signs of infection or inflammation
- White spots in the nail may result from forms of mild trauma.

ABNORMAL FINDINGS

- Changes in color, shape, texture, or thickness

TECHNIQUE 22-8: **Inspecting and Palpating the Head, Face, Mouth, and Neck**

Purpose: To assess for any alterations in growth and development or abnormalities

Special Considerations
- Assess for the anterior fontanel (usually closes between 12 and 18 months)
- Measure head circumference for children up to 3 years old (Fig. 22-9). (See also Chapter 20, Technique 2D.) Plot on growth chart.

  SENC Safety Alert Opisthotonos, hyperextension of the head, with pain on flexion is a serious indication of meningeal irritation. Immediate referral for further examination is required.

- Anxious children can find examination of the mouth frightening and will clench their teeth and purse their lips to prevent a glimpse into their mouths. Assistance from the parent in restraining the child may be needed; in this case, consider performing this examination last.
- Turn examining the child's mouth into a game. Ask, "Let's see what is in your mouth" or "Can you stick out your whole tongue?" or "Let me see your teeth."

  TIP Do not show the tongue depressor unless it is necessary, and praise the child enthusiastically for cooperating.

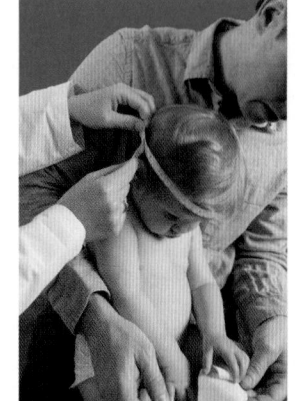

Fig. 22-9. Measuring head circumference for a child younger than 3 years old.

Technique 22-8A: **Inspecting and Palpating the Head**
Purpose: To assess for normal size and shape of the head
Equipment: Gloves (optional)
Inspecting and palpating may be done simultaneously.
ASSESSMENT STEPS
1. Put on gloves.
2. Inspect the child's head for:
  ☐ size
  ☐ shape
  ☐ configuration
  ☐ movement.
3. Palpate the head and assess for masses or depressions.

4. Remove and discard gloves.

5. Document your findings.

NORMAL FINDINGS

- Head growth slows to 1 inch per year by the end of age 2 years and then one-half inch per year until age 5 years.
- Head is symmetric, midline, round.
- Head is erect and still; no involuntary movements.
- No pain, tenderness, masses, or depressions during palpation are reported.

ABNORMAL FINDINGS

SENC Safety Alert Significant head lag after 6 months of age strongly indicates cerebral injury. The child should be referred for further evaluation.

- **Plagiocephaly** is a general term for cranial asymmetry, which basically refers to misshapen heads. The *Back to Sleep* campaign has been effective in reducing Sudden Infant Death Syndrome (SIDS), but concurrently, there is a marked increase in the diagnosis of positional head deformities in American newborns. Cases of positional plagiocephaly can range drastically. Very mild cases may correct themselves with preventative measures and through repositioning exercises, while severe cases can require corrective surgery and/or the use of helmet therapy.

Technique 22-8B: Inspecting and Palpating the Face

Purpose: To assess facial appearance, symmetry, tenderness, swelling, and inflammation

ASSESSMENT STEPS

Stand in front of the child and assess for the following:

1. Assess shape:
- ☐ Round
- ☐ Square
- ☐ Oval

2. Assess for symmetry of the face (cranial nerve VII):
- ☐ Nasal labial folds (the distance from the corner of each nostril to the corner of the lip bilaterally) should have equal measurements.
- ☐ Palpebral fissures (measure the distance between the upper and lower eyelids) should have equal measurements.

3. Assess for facial expression:
- ☐ Does the child make eye contact?
- ☐ Flat affect
- ☐ Sad or happy affect

4. Assess for involuntary movements (muscles).

5. Assess the condition and texture of the skin.

6. Assess for edema.

7. Using the finger pads of both hands, gently palpate the face for tenderness and swelling.

8. Place your fingers in front of the earlobes and corner of the eyes and palpate the temporal arteries simultaneously in front of each ear to assess for tenderness or inflammation.

9. Place your fingertips in front of each ear at the zygomatic arch and ask the child to open and close his or her mouth. Assess for any clicking sounds or decreased range of motion (ROM) of the jaw, including temporomandibular joint (TMJ) disorder.

10. Document your findings.

NORMAL FINDINGS

- Face (round, oval, or square)
- Bilaterally symmetrical facial structures
- Nasolabial folds and palpebral fissures equal
- Expression relaxed
- No involuntary muscle movement; no visible pulsations
- Skin smooth and clear
- No edema
- No tenderness
- Temporal artery nontender
- TMJ disorder has no clicking sounds or limited ROM.
- Mouth opens on the average 3 to 6 cm and moves laterally 1 to 2 cm.

ABNORMAL FINDINGS

- Asymmetry of the face may be related to abscess, infection, enlargement of parotid gland, neurological disorders.
- Flat affect may indicate depression or chronic pain.
- Temporal arteritis is an inflammation of the temporal arteries and blood vessels that supply blood to the head.
- TMJ disorder causes a clicking, popping, or grating sound; limited movement of the mouth; headaches, jaw, tooth, or ear pain.

Technique 22-8C: **Inspecting and Palpating the Nose**

Purpose: To assess for tenderness, inflammation, or deviation

CULTURAL CONSIDERATIONS The bridge of the nose is sometimes flat in Asian- and African-American children.

ASSESSMENT STEPS

1. Stand in front of the child and inspect the nose for the following:
   ☐ Symmetry
   ☐ Alignment of septum

☐ Color

☐ Swelling

2. Gently palpate the nose for tenderness or swelling.

3. Document your findings.

NORMAL FINDINGS

- Nose symmetrical
- Septum straight and midline
- Skin color same as face
- No lesions, swelling, or deformity

ABNORMAL FINDINGS

- Asymmetry
- Deviated septum
- Swelling or inflammation
- Redness, bruising, lesions
- Tenderness or swelling while palpating
- Boggy, bluish-purple or gray turbinates may indicate **chronic rhinorrhea** or **allergic rhinorrhea.**
- Nose: nasal flaring

SENC Safety Alert Nasal flaring indicates respiratory difficulty.

- Foreign object is lodged in nose

SENC Safety Alert Children are curious and will sometimes put an object up their nostril. If there is any question of the type of foreign object in the nose and the appropriate method to remove it, refer the child to the appropriate practitioner.

Technique 22-8D: Assessing the Patency of the Nose

Purpose: To assess for nasal passageway occlusion

ASSESSMENT STEPS

1. Ask the child to press on the right naris to occlude the passageway.

2. Ask the child to inhale through the left naris with his or her mouth closed.

3. Ask the child to press on the left naris to occlude the passageway.

4. Ask the child to inhale through the right naris with his or her mouth closed.

5. Document your findings.

NORMAL FINDINGS

- Each nasal passageway is patent.

ABNORMAL FINDINGS

- Absence of sniff may be an indication of nasal congestion or obstruction; obstruction may be related to a foreign object.
- Rhinitis may be related to a viral or bacterial infection.

Technique 22-8E: **Palpating the Maxillary and Frontal Sinuses**

Purpose: To assess for allergies or sinus infection

ASSESSMENT STEPS

Stand in front of the child and assess the following:

1. Place your thumbs slightly below the eyebrows.
2. Press up and under the eyebrows, palpating the frontal sinuses.
3. Assess for tenderness or pain.
4. Now, place your thumbs below the cheekbones, palpating the maxillary sinuses.
5. Assess for tenderness or pain.
6. Document your findings.

NORMAL FINDINGS

- No tenderness or pain is felt.

ABNORMAL FINDINGS

- Tenderness or pain that may indicate allergies or a sinus infection

Technique 22-8F: **Inspecting and Palpating the Mouth**

Purpose: To assess the structures of the mouth for redness, inflammation, lesions, or abnormalities
Equipment: Penlight, gloves

> **SENC Safety Alert** Always wear clean, nonsterile gloves for this part of the assessment because you will be coming in contact with the child's saliva.

> **SENC Safety Alert** A major difference in the upper tracheobronchial tree between the child and the adult is the tongue. The tongue is larger in the amount of space it takes up in the oropharynx increasing a child's risk for airway occlusion.

Technique 22-8G: **Inspecting the Lips**

Purpose: To assess shape and integrity of the lips
ASSESSMENT STEPS

1. Put on gloves.

2. Stand in front of the child and inspect the lips for the following:
- ☐ Symmetry
- ☐ Color
- ☐ Moisture
- ☐ Lesions
- ☐ Swelling

- ■ Lips are symmetric.
- ■ Upper lip is everted.
- ■ Lips are pink and moist.
- ■ There are no lesions, swelling, or cracking of skin.

- ■ Lips are inverted.
- ■ There is swelling, erythema, lesions, or cracking of skin.
  - ☐ **Angioedema** is edema of the lips; usually related to an allergic reaction.
- ■ Pallor of lips may indicate decreased perfusion related to respiratory or cardiovascular problems.
- ■ Mouth: A narrow, flat, or high arched palate affects the placement of the tongue and can interfere with feeding/eating and may cause speech problems.

Technique 22-8H: Inspecting the Teeth

Purpose: To assess for position, number, and integrity of teeth

1. Inspect the teeth for:
- ☐ missing teeth
- ☐ color.

2. Ask the child to clench teeth and assess for malocclusion, malposition of the teeth (Fig. 22-10).

- ■ Color of teeth white to an ivory color
- ■ Clean, free of debris
- ■ Smooth edges
- ■ 20 baby teeth by age 3; baby teeth begin to fall out by age 6
- ■ 32 adult teeth by age 14
- ■ Upper incisors should overlap the lower incisors; back teeth should meet

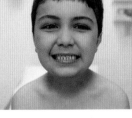

Fig. 22-10. Assessing an older child's teeth.

ABNORMAL FINDINGS
- Teeth are brown stained or dental caries are seen.
- Loose, broken, painful teeth
- Malocclusion of the teeth

Technique 22-8I: **Inspecting the Pharynx and Tonsils**

Purpose: To assess for redness and inflammation
Equipment: Tongue blade and penlight
ASSESSMENT STEPS
1. Explain the technique to the child (age appropriate).
2. Moisten a tongue blade with warm water.
3. Ask the child to open his or her mouth wide, tilt his or her head back, and say "aah." Using a penlight, inspect the rising of the soft palate and uvula.
4. Using the tongue depressor to hold the tongue down, ask the child to say "aah" again and assess the throat and tonsillar pillars.
   □ Note mouth odors.
5. Using the tongue depressor, gently touch the back of the pharynx to elicit a gag reflex.
6. Discard the tongue blade.
7. Remove and discard gloves.
8. Document your findings.
NORMAL FINDINGS
- Uvula rises midline symmetrically; glossopharyngeal (cranial nerve IX) and vagus (cranial nerve X) intact
- Throat pink
- Tonsils pink; may partially protrude or be absent
- Presence of a gag reflex
ABNORMAL FINDINGS
- Asymmetrical rise of the uvula
- Throat deep red, inflamed, with drainage
- Throat pain, dysphagia
- Tonsils protruding with or without drainage
- **Tonsillitis** is a viral or bacterial infection of the tonsils; tonsils become enlarged, swollen, may have white or yellow drainage. Enlargement of tonsils is graded on a 1 to 4 scale.
- **Pharyngitis** is a sore throat caused by inflammation of the mucous membranes of the back of the throat; may be related to viral or bacterial infection.

Technique 22-8J: **Assessing the Lymph Nodes in the Head and Neck Region**

Purpose: To assess for signs of inflammation or disease

Normally, lymph nodes are not palpated, but there are times that lymph nodes can be palpated.

ASSESSMENT STEPS

1. Explain the technique to the child.
2. Ask the child to sit up on the edge of the examination table.
3. Ask the child to slightly flex his or her neck forward to relax the muscles.
4. Warm your hands by rubbing them together.
5. Using the finger pads of your index and middle fingers, gently palpate using circular motions, the 10 facial and neck lymph nodes region, using both hands to examine corresponding sides.
   - ☐ Preauricular (in front of the ears)
   - ☐ Postauricular (behind the ears)
   - ☐ Suboccipital (area between the back of the neck and head)
   - ☐ Tonsilar (below the jaw bone)
   - ☐ Submandibular (under the jaw on both sides)
   - ☐ Submental (just below the chin)
   - ☐ Superficial cervical (upper neck)
   - ☐ Posterior cervical (on the side of the neck toward the back)
   - ☐ Deep cervical chain (near the internal jugular vein)

   TIP Use soft touch when palpating lymph nodes. If you palpate too deeply, you can move them.
6. Ask the child to slightly flex her or his neck to the right and shrug the shoulders, palpate the left supraclavicular lymph nodes in the hollow area just above the clavicle.
7. Ask the child to slightly flex his or her neck to the left and shrug the shoulders, palpate the right supraclavicular lymph nodes.
8. Document your findings.

NORMAL FINDINGS

- No lymph nodes are palpated.
- If palpated, the lymph node should be less than 1 cm, discrete, moveable, and nontender.
- "Shotty nodes" are small, enlarged, firm, nontender lymph nodes that may be related to past infection and are of no clinical significance.

ABNORMAL FINDINGS

- Nodes that are enlarged, greater than 1 cm, matted, hard, and tender may be signs of inflammation or a malignancy.

Technique 22-8K: **Inspecting the Neck**

Purpose: To assess symmetry, movement, and swelling of the neck

ASSESSMENT STEPS

1. Ask the child to sit up straight with neck in the normal position and then slightly hyperextended.
2. Assess the neck for symmetry and swelling.
3. Have the child turn his or her head to assess ROM:
   □ Turn neck side to side.
   □ Bend neck forward.
   □ Extend neck backward.
   □ Bend neck toward each shoulder.

■ **TIP** Sometimes you can make the steps of this assessment to be the "Simon says" game commands.

NORMAL FINDINGS
■ Neck is symmetrical; no swelling
■ No pain with ROM
■ Full ROM of neck

ABNORMAL FINDINGS
■ Symmetrical
■ Pain with movement
■ Unable to turn neck
■ **Torticollis** is a stiff neck or limited range of motion with muscle spasm of the sternocleidomastoid muscle on one side of the body causing a lateral flexion contracture of the cervical spine musculature; may be congenital or acquired (Venes, 2013).

Technique 22-8L: **Inspecting and Palpating the Trachea**

Purpose: To assess for tracheal shift or deviation

ASSESSMENT STEPS

1. Ask the child to sit up straight and bend her or his head slightly forward to relax the sternomastoid muscles.
2. Inspect the trachea below the thyroid isthmus.
3. Gently place your right index finger in the sternal notch.
4. Slip your finger off to each side noting distance from the sternomastoid muscle.
5. Assess the symmetrical spacing on each side and note any deviation from midline.
6. Document your findings.

- Trachea is midline.
- Space is symmetric on each side.

ABNORMAL FINDINGS
- Trachea is deviated to the right or left side and away from the midline.

Technique 22-8M: **Inspecting the Thyroid**

Purpose: To assess size, mobility, and enlargement

ASSESSMENT STEPS

1. Seat the child with his or her head in a neutral or slightly extended position.

2. Stand in front of the child.

3. Inspect the neck for swelling or enlargement of the thyroid gland below the cricoid cartilage.

4. Have the child take a sip of water and observe the upward motion of the thyroid gland.

NORMAL FINDINGS
- Neck area at the site of the thyroid gland should have a smooth, straight appearance.
- Thyroid gland as well as cricoid and thyroid cartilage move up with swallowing.

ABNORMAL FINDINGS
- Neck is enlarged, asymmetrical.
- Gland does not move during swallowing.

Technique 22-8N: **Palpating the Thyroid**

Purpose: To assess the thyroid gland for smoothness, enlargement, nodules, or tenderness

TIP The thyroid gland may be assessed using an anterior or posterior approach. Assessment is easier if you are able to find your landmarks first, the isthmus of the thyroid gland, cricoid cartilage, and suprasternal notch. Always explain what you are going to do so the child will not be afraid.

ASSESSMENT STEPS—POSTERIOR APPROACH

1. Stand behind the child.

2. Ask the child to sit up straight with his or her neck slightly flexed to the right to relax the neck muscles.

3. Place your finger pads between the sternomastoid muscle and trachea on the child's neck slightly below the cricoid cartilage.

4. Have the child take a sip of water or swallow and feel the rise of the thyroid gland.

 TIP The younger child may swallow using sippy cup or bottle.

5. Using your left-hand finger pads, gently push the trachea to the right side.

6. Using your right-hand finger pads, ask the child to take a sip of water or swallow and gently palpate laterally the right lobe of the thyroid for smoothness, enlargement, nodules, or tenderness.

7. Ask the child to slightly flex his or her neck to the left to relax the neck muscles.

8. Using your right-hand finger pads, gently push the trachea to the left side.
9. Using your left-hand finger pads, ask the child to take a sip of water or swallow and gently palpate laterally the left lobe of the thyroid for smoothness, enlargement, nodules, or tenderness.
10. Document your findings. Specifically, document the size, shape, and location of any nodule.

NORMAL FINDINGS

- Lateral lobes may or may not be palpable.
- If palpable, the lobes are smooth, firm, and nontender.

ABNORMAL FINDINGS

- Enlargement of one or both lobes
- Tenderness, presence of lumps or nodules
- Texture has variations of firmness

ASSESSMENT STEPS—ANTERIOR APPROACH

1. Stand in front of the child.
2. Ask the child to sit up straight with his or her neck slightly flexed to the right to relax the neck muscles.
3. Place your finger pads between the sternomastoid muscle and trachea on the child's neck slightly below the cricoid cartilage.
4. Have the child take a sip of water or swallow and feel the rise of the thyroid gland.
   - **TIP** The younger child may swallow using sippy cup or bottle.
5. Using the thumb of your right hand on the child's neck slightly below the cricoid cartilage, gently push the trachea to the right.
6. Position the finger pads of your left hand between the sternomastoid muscle and trachea, have the child take a sip of water or swallow and gently palpate the right lobe of the thyroid for smoothness, enlargement, nodules, or tenderness.
7. Ask the child to slightly flex his or her neck to the left to relax the neck muscles.
8. Using the thumb of your left hand on the child's neck slightly below the cricoid cartilage, gently push the trachea to the left.
9. Position the finger pads of your right hand between the sternomastoid muscle and trachea, have the child take a sip of water or swallow and gently palpate the left lobe of the thyroid for smoothness, enlargement, nodules, or tenderness.
10. Document your findings. Specifically, document the size, shape, and location of any nodule.

NORMAL FINDINGS

- Lateral lobes may or may not be palpable.
- If palpable, the lobes are smooth, firm, and nontender.

ABNORMAL FINDINGS

- Enlargement of one or both lobes
- Tenderness, presence of lumps or nodules
- Texture has variations of firmness

TECHNIQUE 22-9: **Inspecting the Ears**

Purpose: To assess for ear deformities

ASSESSMENT STEPS

1. Stand in front of the child and assess both ears for:
- □ size
- □ shape
- □ color
- □ symmetry
- □ landmarks.
  - • **Darwin's tubercle** (congenital deviation that is a small cartilaginous protuberance on the helix of the ear)

2. Assess the angle of attachment by doing the following:
- □ Draw an imaginary line from the external canthus of the eye to the top of the helix.
- □ Draw an imaginary line perpendicular to the ear (Fig. 22-11).
- □ Assess the angle of attachment.

3. Document your findings.

NORMAL FINDINGS

- ■ Equal size and shape bilaterally; normal size (4 to 10 cm) (Fig. 22-11A)
- ■ Firm consistency
- ■ Color same as facial skin
- ■ Symmetrical
- ■ Angle of attachment less than 10 degrees (Fig. 22-11B)
- ■ No deformities, inflammation, nodules, or drainage
- ■ Nontender to palpate external ear

ABNORMAL FINDINGS

- ■ Asymmetrical
- ■ Color is blue, red, white, or pale
- ■ Lesions

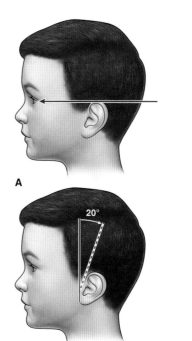
A

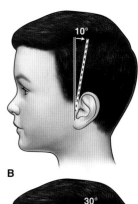
B

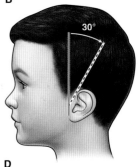
C

D

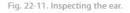
Fig. 22-11. Inspecting the ear.

- Cysts
- Drainage
- Angle of attachment is greater than 10 degrees (Fig. 22-11C, Fig. 22-11D)
- Abnormally large or small ears

SENC **Safety Alert** Bloody or clear drainage may be related to a perforated eardrum or head injury.

Technique 22-9A: **Palpating the Ears**

Purpose: To assess for tenderness

ASSESSMENT STEPS

1. Stand on the right side of the child.
2. Gently palpate the right ear:
   ☐ Auricles (Pinna)
   ☐ Tragus
   ☐ Ear lobes
   ☐ Mastoid process
3. Stand on the left side of the child and palpate the left ear.
4. Document your findings.

NORMAL FINDINGS

- No tenderness

ABNORMAL FINDINGS

- Tenderness may indicate inflammation.

TIP A child may tug or pull at an ear that has an otitis media (ear infection).

Technique 22-9B: **Assessing Hearing (CN VIII) using the Whispered Voice Test**

Purpose: To assess for impaired or loss of hearing

TIP Tests to assess hearing are subjective because you are relying on the individual's response to what the child says he or she hears. The tests will only screen for hearing loss.

ASSESSMENT STEPS

1. Place child in the sitting position.
2. Stand behind the child to his or her right side about 2 feet away so you cannot be seen.
3. Ask the child to cover the left ear that you are not testing.
4. Whisper three random letters or numbers.
5. Have the child repeat what you whispered.

6. Repeat steps 2 through 5 on the left side.

7. Document your findings.

NORMAL FINDINGS

■ Child repeats the letters or numbers correctly.

ABNORMAL FINDINGS

■ Tilting of head in awkward position to hear

■ Need to repeat requests

■ Loud or altered speech

■ Inattentive behavior

■ Foreign bodies

■ Child repeats fewer than half of the three letters or numbers correctly or did not hear what you whispered.

■ Audiometric testing is in order when there are abnormal findings (Sanders & Gillig, 2010, p. 19).

Technique 22-9C: **Assessing the Ears With an Otoscope**

Purpose: To assess the external auditory canal, middle ear, and eardrum

Equipment: Otoscope with disposable speculum

Special Considerations

■ **TIP** It may be helpful to demonstrate examining the parent's ear first.

■ Examining the internal structure of the ear of a young child can be challenging because the child cannot observe the procedure.

■ Position the child in one of two ways: (1) place the child in the supine position and, if needed, have the parent restrain the arms (Fig. 22-12A) or (2) have the child sit in the parent's lap facing front or sideways so the nurse can assess the inner ear (Fig. 22-12B).

■ Older children are likely to cooperate and should not need restraint.

■ In children less than 3 years of age, the external auditory canal is directed upward. Therefore, pull the pinna down and back to straighten the canal for the best view (Fig. 22-13A).

■ In children older than 3 years of age, the canal is curved downward and forward. Therefore, pull the pinna upward and backward to straighten the canal for the best view (Fig. 22-13B).

■ If examining a painful ear, examine the unaffected ear first.

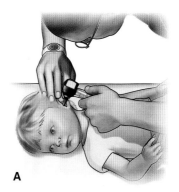 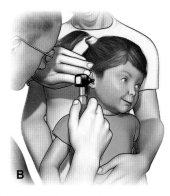

A   **B**

Fig. 22-12. Positions for ear assessment. (A) Supine. (B) Child on parent's lap.

CULTURAL CONSIDERATIONS The walls of the external auditory canal are pink although they may be more pigmented in dark-skinned children.

ASSESSMENT STEPS

1. Turn the light on for the otoscope and choose the largest and shortest speculum that fits comfortably in the individual's ear canal.
2. Ask the child (age appropriate) to sit up straight with the head tilted to the left side.
3. Hold the otoscope in your dominant hand with the handle either up or down.
4. With your other hand, use your fingers to grasp the right auricle and gently lift the auricle up and back (for a child older than 3 years of age) to clearly visualize the external auditory canal.
5. Gently insert the speculum into the outer third (about a half inch) of the ear canal (Fig. 22-14A, B).
6. Look through the magnifying lens to assess the:
   ☐ external ear canal
   ☐ tympanic membrane
   ☐ portions of the malleus (dense, whitish streak) assessed through the translucent tympanic membrane
   ☐ umbo (the central depressed portion of the concavity on the lateral surface of the tympanic membrane)
   ☐ cone of light (a triangular reflection when the light is focused on the malleus).
7. Gently move the light to get a full assessment of the tympanic membrane.
8. Repeat steps 4, 5, and 6 on the child's left ear.
9. Document your findings.

NORMAL FINDINGS

■ External ear canal patent
■ No inflammation or drainage

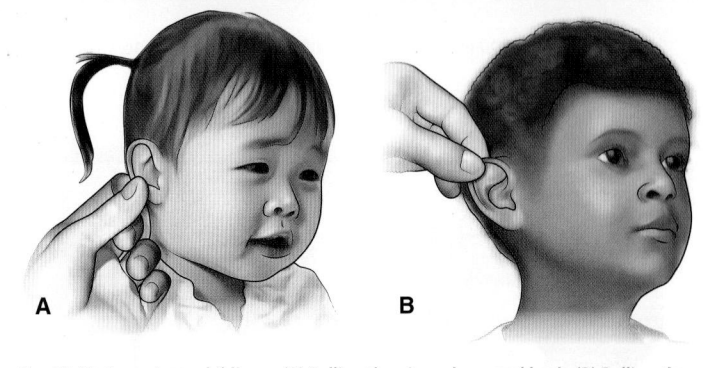

Fig. 22-13. Assessing a child's ear. (A) Pulling the pinna down and back. (B) Pulling the pinna up and back.

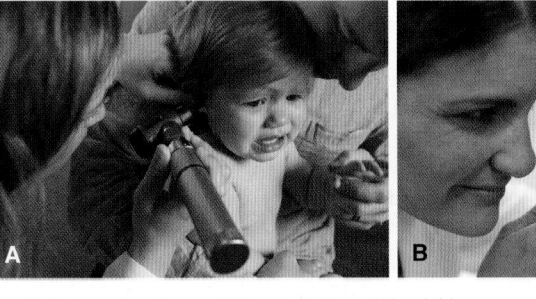

Fig. 22-14. Assessing the ear. (A) Young child. (B) Older child.

- Small amount of pale yellow, moist wax
- Tympanic membrane intact, pearly gray color; translucent; contour slightly conical
- Bony landmarks visible
- Cone of light present
- Ear tubes are intact (if present).

ABNORMAL FINDINGS
- Large amounts of earwax (**cerumen**).
- Sinuses or small openings around the ear may represent a fistula that drains into an area of the neck or ear.
- **Otitis externa** is inflammation of the outer ear causing redness, inflammation, discharge, and pain; may be related to infection or swimmer's ear.
- **Otitis media** is inflammation of the inner ear causing pain, inflammation, pressure, and a build-up of fluid; bright, red bulging eardrum with diminished or no cone of light visible.
- **Serous otitis media** is an accumulation of fluid in the middle ear caused by an obstruction of the eustachian tube; tympanic membrane will appear to be a yellowish color, air bubbles, and bulging.
- **Scarred tympanic membrane** has less blood supply and appears to have white, dense, streaks, and spotting; the individual may have had many ear infections during childhood.
- **Perforated tympanic membrane** is a ruptured tympanic membrane; a dark oval hole will be present in the membrane.

SENC Safety Alert If there is any question of the type of foreign object in the ear and the appropriate method to remove it, refer the child to the appropriate healthcare provider.

TECHNIQUE 22-10: **Inspecting the Eyes**

Purpose: To assess any abnormalities of the eye
Equipment: Penlight, ophthalmoscope

Special Considerations
- Prepare the child for the examination by showing the child the ophthalmoscope, demonstrating the light source, how it shines in the eye, and the need for darkening the room.
- For young children, it is best to use distraction to encourage them to keep their eyes open.

CULTURAL CONSIDERATIONS Epicanthal folds are often found in Asian children (Fig. 22-15).

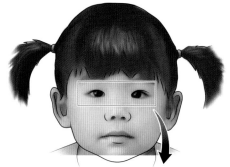
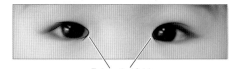

Epicanthal folds

Fig. 22-15. Epicanthal folds.

Technique 22-10A: **Inspecting the Structure of the Eyes**

Purpose: To assess the anterior eye structures

Equipment: Light source, gloves

▇ **TIP** Forcibly parting the lids results in a frightened, watery-eyed child and a frustrated nurse.

ASSESSMENT STEPS

1. Stand in front of the child.
2. Inspect the eyelids.
   - ☐ Observe that the eyelids open and close completely.
   - ☐ Assess for any drainage.
3. Inspect the eyelashes for:
   - ☐ distribution
   - ☐ drainage.
4. Inspect the eyebrows.
   - ☐ Assess symmetry.
   - ☐ Assess distribution of hair and any scaly, flaky, skin.
5. Inspect the cornea.
   - ☐ Use a light source to inspect side to side the cornea for smoothness and clarity.
6. Inspect the lens.
   - ☐ Use a light source to inspect side to side the lens of the eye for clarity.
   - ☐ Use light source to inspect the color and round shape.
7. Assess the sclera for color.
8. Inspect the conjunctiva.
   - ☐ Use your thumbs to slide the bottom eyelids down to assess the mucosa of the lower conjunctiva.
   - ☐ Ask the child to look up.
   - ☐ Inspect the color of the mucosa.
9. Inspect the lacrimal duct.
   - ☐ Wearing gloves, inspect and palpate the lacrimal duct for any swelling or excessive tearing.
10. Assess palpebral fissures.
    - ☐ Assess the distance of the upper lid to the lower lid for symmetry.
    - ☐ Compare the palpebral fissures on each side of the face.
11. Inspect for abnormal involuntary eye movements.
12. Document your findings.

NORMAL FINDINGS

- Eyes symmetrical; no protrusion
- Upper and lower eyelids close completely; no redness or drainage; no drooping of an eyelid (ptosis); upper eyelid covers half of the iris
- Eyelashes equally distributed; no drainage
- Eyebrows evenly distributed; no scaly or flaky skin; symmetrical
- Cornea clear with no opacities
- Lens transparent with no opacities
- Pupils equal in size
- Iris blue, green, brown, or hazel in color, smooth; controls diameter and size of pupil
- Sclera white
- Conjunctiva pink and moist
- Lacrimal duct clear with no swelling
- Palpebral fissures equal bilaterally
- No abnormal involuntary movement

ABNORMAL FINDINGS

- **Ptosis**, drooping of the eyelid caused by muscle or nerve dysfunction, injury, or disease.
- **Blocked lacrimal duct** causing excessive tearing because tears cannot drain properly
- **Conjunctivitis (pink eye)** is a bacterial or viral infection causing erythema of the sclera and yellow-green drainage of the conjunctiva.
- **Hordeolum** is an inflammation of a follicle of an eyelash that causes redness, inflammation, and a lump at the site.

  TIP Ocular **strabismus** ("cross-eyed" or "lazy-eye") can result in amblyopia, or reduced vision in an otherwise normal eye. If strabismus is left uncorrected it can lead to reduced visual acuity.

Technique 22-10B: **Assessing for Visual Acuity**

Purpose: To measure a child's vision to see details at near and far distances.

Equipment: Snellen chart, Tumbling E, HOTV, Kindergarten Eye Chart (Fig. 22-16A)

Special Considerations

- Test visual acuity beginning between ages 3 and 4 years.

  TIP U.S. Preventive Services Task Force (USPSTF) recommends vision screening of all children aged 3 to 5 years.

  ☐ Because children under 3 years of age have difficulty following the directions for testing and sometimes cannot identify the pictures on a chart, it is often not possible to test their visual acuity.

  ☐ For children unable to read letters (Snellen chart), the tumbling E or HOTV test is useful (Coats & Jenkins, 1997).

  • The tumbling E uses the capital letter E pointing in four different directions. The child, 3 to 5 years old, is standing 10 feet from the chart and is asked to point in the direction the E is facing.

- The HOTV test consists of a wall chart with the letters H, O, T, and V. The child, 3 to 5 years old, stands 10 feet from the chart and is given a board to hold containing the same letters. The examiner points to a letter on the wall chart and the child matches the letter on the board he or she is holding.
- The Snellen chart is used for children 6 years and older.
- The Kindergarten Eye Chart has easily recognizable symbols that a young child can identify.
■ In all tests of visual acuity, it is important that both eyes show the same results; otherwise, refer to an ophthalmologist for further testing.
■ For young children, turn the assessment into a game.
■ Visual fields can be assessed with the young child sitting in the parent's lap.

TIP If the child wears glasses, the glasses should be worn during the vision assessment. Reading glasses should not be worn. Document if the child has worn his or her glasses during the assessment.

ASSESSMENT STEPS
1. Place the chart at a comfortable height for the child's height.
2. Depending on the age of the child, have the child stand 10 or 20 feet from the chart (Fig. 22-16B).
3. Cover the left eye and have the child start reading the lines out loud starting from the top and working down the chart. The child reads the row from left to right.
4. Ask the child to read each line until he or she cannot identify all the letters in the line correctly.
5. Repeat steps 3 and 4 by covering the right eye.
6. Repeat steps 3 and 4 with both eyes uncovered.
7. Document the last line that was correctly read for each assessment.

NORMAL FINDINGS
■ Visual acuity for the toddler is 20/40.
■ For older children, the normal distant visual acuity is 20/20; this means that the child can read what a person with normal eyesight can read at 20 feet.

ABNORMAL FINDINGS
■ A higher denominator means poorer distant visual acuity.
■ **Nearsightedness,** known as **myopia,** is poor visual acuity; distant objects appear blurred because the images are focused in front of the retina rather than on it. The denominator is greater than 20.
■ **Farsightedness,** known as **hyperopia,** is the ability to see distant objects clearly, but objects nearby may be blurry.

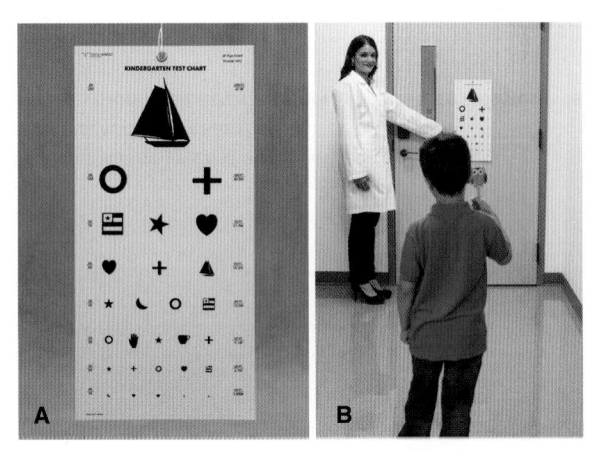

Fig. 22-16. (A) HOTV/Kindergarten chart. (B) Using the HOTV chart to assess the eyes.

Technique 22-10C: **Assessing for Color Blindness**

Purpose: To assess the ability to distinguish colors

Equipment: Ishihara plates

■ **TIP** Children with color blindness may have a poor sense of color coordinating of clothing and poor performance in academic skill that requires the use of color as a visual aid.

ASSESSMENT STEPS

1. Explain the technique to the child.

2. Ask the child to identify the embedded colored figures or numbers on each of the Ishihara plates within 3 to 5 seconds.

3. Document the child's results.

NORMAL FINDINGS

■ The child is able to correctly identify the colored embedded figures or numbers.

ABNORMAL FINDINGS

■ The child is unable to identify the colored embedded figure/numbers. This may indicate color blindness.

   SENC Safety Alert Adolescents who are color blind and learning to drive will have a lack of recognition of amber or red traffic lights, and brake lights.

TECHNIQUE 22-11: **Assessing the Respiratory System**

Purpose: To assess for any abnormalities of the respiratory system

Equipment: Appropriate-sized stethoscope

Assessing the respiratory assessment is similar to assessing it in the adult, but only an experienced healthcare provider should percuss the lungs.

■ **TIP** Younger children may be fearful of the stethoscope. Before you begin, let the child hold and touch the stethoscope. The best time to assess the respiratory system in a younger child is when the child is quiet or distracted.

■ **TIP** Children have thin chest walls that radiate sound making it essential to have the appropriate-sized stethoscope.

Technique 22-11A: **Inspecting the Thoracic Cage**

Purpose: To inspect the size and shape of the thoracic cage

ASSESSMENT STEPS

1. Put the child in the sitting position.

2. Inspect the anterior, posterior, and lateral thoracic cage for:
   □ size
   □ shape

☐ symmetry
☐ color
☐ respiratory rate and rhythm.
3. Document your findings.

NORMAL FINDINGS

- Less than age 6, anteroposterior (AP) diameter is 1:1; age 6 and older AP-to-lateral ratio is approximately 1:2 and the costal angle less than 90 degrees
- **Conical shape:** smaller at the top and widens at the bottom
- **Symmetry:** sternum is symmetrical; clavicles and scapula are the same height; chest movement is symmetrical.
- Skin color is uniform and intact.
- Even and smooth respirations
- No accessory muscle retractions

ABNORMAL FINDINGS

- Asymmetrical chest movement
- Bluish hue to skin color
- Uneven and irregular or fast respirations
- Accessory muscle retractions

SENC Safety Alert Use of accessory muscles indicates that the child is working harder to breathe; this is a sign of respiratory distress.

Technique 22-11B: **Palpating the Thorax**

Purpose: To assess surface characteristics or tenderness of the thoracic cage

ASSESSMENT STEPS

1. Place the child in the sitting position.
2. Using your finger pads, gently palpate the anterior, posterior, and lateral thoracic cage and assess the following:
   ☐ Surface characteristics
   ☐ Temperature
   ☐ Moisture
   ☐ Tenderness

NORMAL FINDINGS

- Surface is smooth and uniform
- Warm skin
- Skin dry
- No tenderness

ABNORMAL FINDINGS

- Irregular surface (lumps or masses)
- Temperature cool, clammy
- Tenderness
- **Crepitus** (a light crackling or popping feeling under the skin caused by leakage of air into the subcutaneous tissue); sounds like Rice Krispies popping under the skin.

Technique 22-11C: **Auscultating the Lungs**

Purpose: To assess airflow throughout all lobes of the lungs

Equipment: Age-appropriate stethoscope

ASSESSMENT STEPS

1. Place the child in the sitting position.
2. Warm the diaphragm of the stethoscope between your hands.
3. Ask the child to breathe in and out of the mouth.
4. **Assess anterior lung fields.** Auscultate at the intercostal spaces moving from the apex to the base on each side of the anterior lung fields noting breath sounds. Complete this assessment in its entirety.
5. **Assess posterior lung fields.** Auscultate at the intercostal spaces moving from the apex to the base on each side of the anterior lung fields and note breath sounds. Complete this assessment in its entirety.
6. **Assess lateral lung fields.** Auscultate at the intercostal spaces moving from the apex to the base on right and left lateral lung fields noting breath sounds.
7. Document your findings.

NORMAL FINDINGS

- Bronchial breath sounds are heard over the trachea and larger bronchi; expiratory sounds are louder and last longer than inspiratory sounds and have a pause between them; high-pitched, hollow, tubular breath sounds.
- Bronchovesicular sounds are heard anteriorly over the mid-chest anterior intercostal spaces and between the scapula posteriorly; these are medium-pitched sounds with the I:E ratio 1:1.
- Vesicular sounds are heard throughout the periphery of the lungs; inspiration sound is longer and louder than expiration; soft, low-pitched, rustling sounds.

ABNORMAL FINDINGS

- It is abnormal to hear bronchial breath sounds when they are not in the normal locations.
- Breath sounds are diminished.
- Adventitious breath sounds are sounds not normally heard in a chest (see Chapter 12, Table 12-3).

TECHNIQUE 22-12: **Assessing the Cardiac System**

Purpose: To assess for any abnormalities in cardiac system
Equipment: Age-appropriate stethoscope
■ **TIP** Children have thin chest walls that radiate sound making it essential to have the appropriate-sized stethoscope.

Technique 22-12A: **Palpating the Precordium and Apical Pulse**

Purpose: To assess for vibrations and the apical pulse
For infants and children up to age 7, the mitral area is located at or near the fourth intercostal space, slightly to the left of the midclavicular line; age 7 and older, the mitral area is located at or near the fifth intercostal space, at the midclavicular line.

ASSESSMENT STEPS
1. Explain the technique to the child (age appropriate).
2. Using the palmar surface of your right hand, gently palpate the five landmarks feeling for pulsations or vibrations.
   □ Right Sternal Border (RSB), Second Intercostal Space (Aortic Valve)
   □ Left Sternal Border (LSB), Second Intercostal Space (Pulmonic Valve)
   □ Left Sternal Border (LSB), Third Intercostal Space (Erb Point)
   □ Left Sternal Border (LSB) Fourth Intercostal Space (Tricuspid Valve)
   □ Left Sternal Border (LSB), Fifth Intercostal Space (Mitral Valve)
3. Using the palmar surface of your right hand, palpate the apical pulse.
   □ Location
   □ Amplitude
4. Document your findings.

NORMAL FINDINGS
■ No pulsations are felt at the five landmarks; apical pulse is palpated and auscultated at the fourth or fifth left intercostal space at the midclavicular line
   □ Amplitude: regular rhythmic tap

ABNORMAL FINDINGS
■ Visible pulsations may indicate increased cardiac output.
   □ **Heaves or lifts** are forceful *cardiac* contractions that cause a slight to vigorous movement of sternum and ribs.
   □ **Thrill** is a palpable vibration caused by very turbulent blood flow; usually correlates with a loud cardiac murmur.

Technique 22-12B: **Auscultating Heart Sounds**

Purpose: To assess heart sounds

Equipment: Age-appropriate stethoscope

ASSESSMENT STEPS

1. Explain the technique to the child (age appropriate).

2. Place the child in the supine position or sitting in the parent's lap.

3. Warm the stethoscope before placing on the precordium.

4. Using your second and third finger pads of your right or left hand, landmark each auscultatory site prior to placing the stethoscope on the skin.

5. Using the diaphragm of the stethoscope, auscultate the heart sounds ($S_{1\{lub\}}$ and $S_{2\{dub\}}$) at the five landmark sites, listening for:

☐ S_1 and S_2 heart sounds

☐ rhythm of the heart sounds

☐ abnormal or extra heart sounds.

6. With the child in the supine or sitting position, auscultate heart sounds at the five landmark sites.

7. Ask the child to lean forward; using the diaphragm of the stethoscope, auscultate the aortic and pulmonic valve areas listening for:

☐ murmurs

☐ extra heart sounds.

8. Using the bell of the stethoscope, auscultate for low-pitched heart sounds at the five landmark sites.

9. Document your findings.

NORMAL FINDINGS

- S_1 and S_2 sounds heard; regular pattern
- Children often have a sinus arrhythmia and a split second heart sound that may change with respiration.
- Systolic innocent murmurs and venous hum are common findings as well.

   TIP A venous hum in a child is heard in the supraclavicular area with the child in a sitting position; this murmur is caused by turbulent blood flow in the jugular veins and is considered to be normal in children (Laird, 2014).

ABNORMAL FINDINGS

- Extra or abnormal heart sounds are heard.
- Fixed splitting, in which the split in S_2 does not change during inspiration, is an important finding and may be a sign of atrial septal defect.
- Pericardial friction rubs result from inflammation of the pericardial sac surrounding the heart.

   SENC Safety Alert If you hear a murmur refer the child for follow-up.

TECHNIQUE 22-13: **Assessing the Abdomen**

Purpose: To assess for any abnormalities of the abdomen
Equipment: Age-appropriate stethoscope
■ **TIP** Except for the liver, successful identification of other organs, spleen, kidney, and part of the colon, requires considerable practice with tutorial supervision.

Technique 22-13A: **Inspecting the Abdomen**

Purpose: To assess abnormalities in shape, skin, or movement of the abdomen
Inspection of the abdomen should be done in two positions: at the child's side and standing at the child's feet.

ASSESSMENT STEPS

1. Assist child to supine position.
2. Standing at the child's right side, inspect the abdomen for:
   ☐ contour, size, and symmetry
   ☐ size and position and of the umbilicus
   ☐ condition of skin: color, lesions, hernias
   ☐ movements, pulsations, and peristalsis.
3. Document your findings.

NORMAL FINDINGS

■ Young children have prominent, cylindric abdomens, pot-bellied, because of the physiological lordosis of the spine that disappears as abdominal muscles strengthen.
■ Older children: contour (flat or rounded)
■ Bilaterally symmetrical
■ Umbilicus midline
■ Skin smooth and intact without pulsations or visible peristalsis
■ Peristalsis and aortic pulsations may be visible in very thin children
■ Visible peristaltic waves
■ Umbilical hernias are common in infants, especially African-American children.
■ A diastasis recti is a midline protrusion from the xiphoid to the umbilicus, or symphysis pubis, where the rectus abdominis muscles failed to join in utero; it is usually a variation of normal musculature development in the young child.

ABNORMAL FINDINGS

- Increased peristaltic waves (ripple-like movement from LUQ to RLQ) are seen with intestinal obstruction.
- Abdominal distention is caused by fluid, fat, feces, or flatulence.
- Inguinal hernia is a weakness in the muscles of the abdomen; a soft bulge is assessed in the groin area; a loop of intestine protrudes through the abdominal wall.

   TIP Acute intestinal obstruction occurs when there is an interruption in the forward movement of food or fluids through the small or large intestine. The classic physical examination findings are abdominal distension, tympany to percussion, and high-pitched bowel sounds (Jackson and Raihi, 2011).

Technique 22-13B: **Auscultating Bowel Sounds**

Purpose: To assess a normal pattern of bowel sounds

Equipment: Age-appropriate stethoscope

ASSESSMENT STEPS

1. Auscultate bowel sounds by placing the diaphragm of the stethoscope on the abdomen at the ileocecal valve (RLQ) where bowel sounds are usually present.

   TIP Listen for 3 to 5 minutes before documenting that there are no bowel sounds.

2. Note the intensity, pitch, and frequency of the bowel sounds (see Chapter 14, Table 14-2).

3. Document your findings.

NORMAL FINDINGS

- Five to 34 clicks or gurgles per minute

ABNORMAL FINDINGS

- Hyperactive, high-pitched bowel sounds may indicate early bowel obstruction or increased peristalsis.
- No bowel sounds could indicate a paralytic ileus, no peristalsis movement.

Technique 22-13C: **Percussing the Abdomen**

Purpose: To assist with identifying gas and solid or fluid-filled masses in the abdomen.

1. Using indirect percussion, percuss over each quadrant and note the quality of sounds heard.

2. Follow one of the two patterns for percussion. (See Chapter 14, Fig. 14-17.)

3. Document your findings.

NORMAL FINDINGS

- Tympany in all four quadrants; dullness over organs

ABNORMAL FINDINGS
- Excessive high-pitched tympanic sounds may indicate distention.
- Dullness may indicate increased tissue density such as organ enlargement or an underlying mass.
- Pain during percussion may indicate peritoneal inflammation.

Technique 22-13D: **Palpating the Abdomen**

Purpose: To assess surface characteristics, tenderness, enlarged organs, or fluid in the abdominal cavity

Special Considerations
- Have the child "help" with palpation by placing a hand over the palpating hand (Fig. 22-17). This can minimize the tickling sensation during the examination and provide comfort for the wary child.
- Always ask the child or parent if the child has any tenderness, abdominal discomfort, or pain. These areas should be assessed last.

Light Palpation
Purpose: To feel for surface characteristics and assess for tenderness

ASSESSMENT STEPS
1. Using the finger pads of one hand, press down about one-half inch.
2. Lightly palpate in a clockwise direction the entire abdomen.
3. Lift your fingers gently as you move to a different area.
4. Watch child's facial expression for signs of pain or abdominal guarding.
5. Document your findings.

NORMAL FINDINGS
- No tenderness, smooth surface characteristics

ABNORMAL FINDINGS
- Tenderness is present; nodular or mass felt.

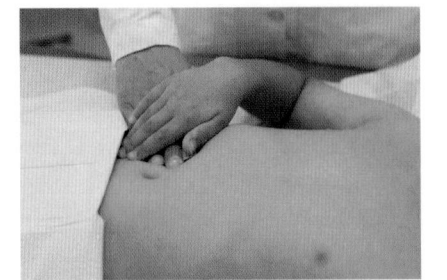

Fig. 22-17. Palpating the abdomen with the child's help.

Deep Palpation
Purpose: To assess for enlarged organs, masses, or tenderness

ASSESSMENT STEPS
1. Place your nondominant hand on top of your dominant hand (also known as bimanual palpation)
2. Gently press down about 1.5 inches using a circular or a dipping motion in a clockwise direction.
3. Lift your hands gently as you move to different areas.
4. Document your findings.

NORMAL FINDINGS
- No masses, enlarged organs, or tenderness

- An enlarged liver is palpable 3 centimeters (1.5 inch) below the right costal margin and requires further evaluation.
- An enlarged spleen is palpable more than 2 centimeters (0.8 inch) below the left costal margin and requires further evaluation.

Technique 22-13E: Palpating Femoral Pulses and Inguinal Nodes

Purpose: To assess arterial circulation and for enlarged lymph nodes

Equipment: Gloves

ASSESSMENT STEPS

1. Position the child in the supine position.
2. Expose the lower legs from the groin to the feet making sure to keep the genitalia covered for privacy.
3. Put on gloves.
4. Using your second, third, and fourth finger pads of your dominant hand, gently palpate the right and left inguinal groin areas near the saphenous vein to assess the inguinal lymph nodes.
5. Assess the pulses in the right and left lower extremities by gently placing your second and third finger pads of your dominant hand. Assess the rhythm, amplitude, and symmetry of the following:
   - ☐ **Femoral pulse** is located in the groin area below the inguinal ligament, halfway between the symphysis pubis and the anterior-superior iliac spine.
6. Remove and discard gloves.
7. Document your findings.

NORMAL FINDINGS

- Inguinal lymph nodes nonpalpable
- 2+ symmetrical, regular femoral pulses

ABNORMAL FINDINGS

- Enlarged inguinal lymph node(s)
- Absence of femoral pulses is a sign of narrowing of the aorta (coarctation of the aorta) and requires further medical evaluation.

TECHNIQUE 22-14: Assessing the Musculoskeletal System

Purpose: To assess for any abnormalities of the bones and muscles

TIP Playing a game with the younger child such as "Simon Says" may help to assess the range of motion of both the upper and lower extremities. If necessary, demonstrate the technique to the child.

Equipment Needed: Gloves

Sequence of Assessment

1. Inspecting
2. Palpating
3. Assessing ROM
4. Assessing strength
▤ **TIP** Always compare sides for all musculoskeletal assessments.

Technique 22-14A: **Inspecting Gait and Posture**

Purpose: To assess the ability of the child to ambulate
▤ **TIP** The child should not be wearing any shoes during this assessment.

ASSESSMENT STEPS

1. Explain the technique to the child (age appropriate).
2. Have the child walk away from you first and then back toward you. This allows for both anterior and posterior observation of gait.
3. Inspect any differences in leg swing and arm swing.
4. Assess the child's ability or inability to control any joints. Are they limping, unable to move a lower extremity joint through the functional ROM?
5. Inspect the child's posture while the child is walking (Fig. 22-18), assessing the following:
  □ Are the shoulders level and even?
  □ Is the head sitting centered on the axial skeleton?
  □ Inspect the location of the head in relation to the trunk.
  □ Is the head sitting forward?
  □ Is the head tipped to one side?
  □ Is the neck fixed in a flexed or extended position?
6. Document your findings.

NORMAL FINDINGS

■ Steady gait and straight posture
■ Extremities: toddlers can usually walk alone by 12 to 13 months. Their balance is unsteady, and they use a wide base of support for walking.
■ Toddlers are usually bowlegged, genu varum (Fig. 22-19), after beginning to walk until their back and leg muscles are well developed.

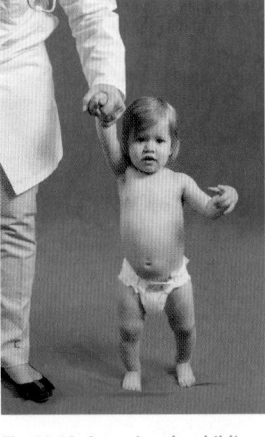

Fig. 22-18. Assessing the child's posture while the child is walking.

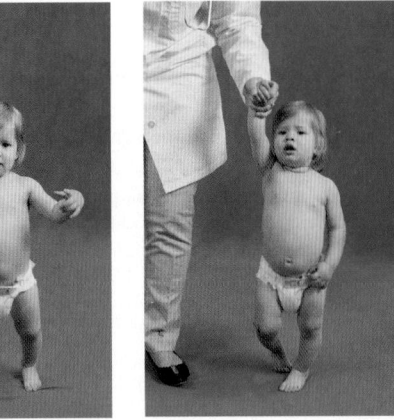

Fig. 22-19. Genu varum (bowleggedness).

- A child should be walking, jumping, and climbing by age 3.
- The preschooler's gait is more balanced as a smaller base of support is used to walk.
- Children from ages 2 to 7 years may be normally knock-kneed, genu valgum (Fig. 22-20).

ABNORMAL FINDINGS

- **Pigeon toe:** most common gait problem in children which usually results from an abnormal rotation or bowing of the tibia (Fig. 22-21).
- One leg shorter than the other leg may indicate a hip abnormality.

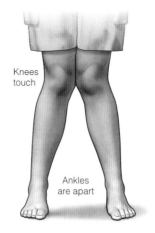
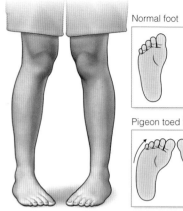
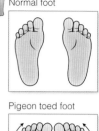

Knees touch

Ankles are apart

Normal foot

Pigeon toed foot

Fig. 22-20. Genu valgum (knock-knees).   Fig. 22-21. Pigeon-toe.

Technique 22-14B: Inspecting and Palpating the Vertebral Column

Purpose: To assess for abnormalities in the structure of the vertebral column

ASSESSMENT STEPS

1. Explain the technique to the child (age appropriate).
2. Ask the child to stand.
3. Facing the child's back, inspect the alignment of the vertebral column and assess for (Fig. 22-22):
   ☐ How straight is the vertebral column when the child is standing?
   ☐ Is there any noted deviation in the anterior-posterior plane?
4. Ask the child to bend at the waist. Assess whether the vertebral column is straight.
5. Facing the child's back, using two or three finger pads, starting at the top of the vertebral column, palpate the vertebral column assessing for:
   ☐ Areas of tenderness
   ☐ Noted deviations in the lateral plane. This would be noted as a deviation from a straight line that the vertebral column should maintain.
   ☐ Protrusions, something being more prominent along the vertebral column, or depressions, like a pit or hole, may indicate dysfunction within the vertebral column.
6. Document your findings.

NORMAL FINDINGS
- Vertebral column straight when child is standing and flexed forward
- No deviation noted in anterior-posterior plane and in the lateral plane
- No areas of tenderness
- No deviation in the lateral plane
- No protrusions or drop-offs within the vertebral column

Special Considerations
- **Spine:** newborns present with a rounded or *C*-shaped curve to the spine. The development of the cervical and lumbar curves approximates the development of various motor skills giving the older child the typical double *S* curve.

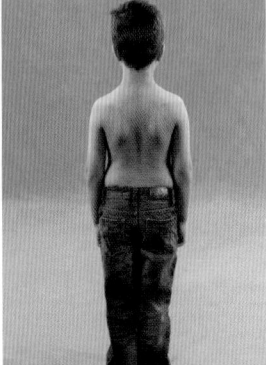
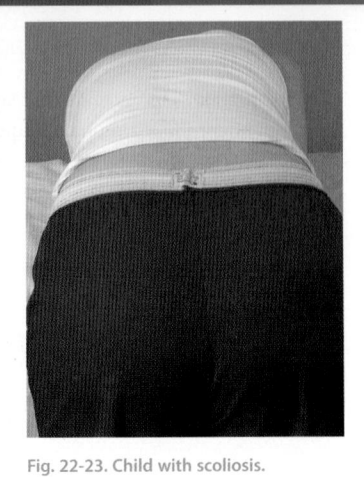

Fig. 22-22. Assessing alignment of child's back.

Fig. 22-23. Child with scoliosis.

ABNORMAL FINDINGS
- **Scoliosis** is an abnormal curvature of the spine that occurs in a lateral manner; it may look like a *C* or an *S* on visualization and may be palpable (Fig. 22-23).
  - □ When bending over at the waist, there is asymmetry of the shoulders.
  - □ A normal spine has no curvature; a child is diagnosed with scoliosis if the curvature of the spine is greater than 10 degrees (AAP, 2015).
  - □ Children are screened for scoliosis during annual physical examinations and by the school nurse.
- Areas of tenderness may indicate a problem with the bony structure or the ligaments within the vertebral column.
- Protrusions or depressions may indicate a displacement of one vertebral body on another vertebral body.

Technique 22-14C: Inspecting and Palpating the Upper Extremities
Purpose: To determine if there are any abnormalities within the upper extremity.
ASSESSMENT STEPS
1. Explain the technique to the child (age-appropriate).
2. Inspect the upper extremity on the right side then the left side; compare the right to the left side.
3. Using two or three finger pads, gently palpate the upper extremity on the right side:
  - □ Shoulder
  - □ Elbow
  - □ Wrist
  - □ Hand/fingers and joints

4. Assess for:
- ☐ tenderness
- ☐ depressions
- ☐ bulges
- ☐ changes in temperature.

5. Repeat steps 3 and 4 on the left side.

6. Document your findings.

NORMAL FINDINGS

With the child standing, inspection of the upper extremity should find the following:

- Symmetry between left and right upper extremity
- No forward rounding of the shoulder
- Straight upper arms
- Slight bending in the elbows
- Wrists in line with the lower arm and palms facing the upper leg
- Some slight flexion of the fingers
- No findings of tenderness/pain, depression or protrusions, increased warmth, increased joint size, or missing fingers

ABNORMAL FINDINGS

- Forward rounding of the shoulders may indicate tightness of muscles across the anterior thorax and a weakness of the muscles of the posterior thorax.
- Nonstraight upper arm may indicate a fracture (old or new) or a significant muscle tear.
- A straight or hyperextended elbow may indicate lack of bony structure or muscle tone to hold it in a slightly flexed position.
- A flexed elbow that is unable to be straightened may indicate a serious problem with the joint.
- If the wrist is out of line with the lower arm, there may be a new or old bony injury causing limitations to the motion.
- Areas of tenderness or pain may indicate an injury to bone, muscle, tendon, or ligament.
- Depressions may indicate a dislocated joint, significant muscle injury, or joint subluxation.
- Increased warmth in the joints may be an indication of infection or disease process within that joint.

Technique 22-14D: Assessing Range of Motion and Muscle Strength of the Upper Extremities

Purpose: To assess strength and limitations in ROM in the upper extremities

ASSESSMENT STEPS

1. Explain the technique to the child (age-appropriate). You will ask the child to perform specific motions independently first and then against resistance.

2. Ask the child to perform the following ROM activities of the right and left upper extremities:

☐ Shoulder motion

- **Flexion:** movement of the upper extremity as a whole, forward, with thumb facing forward when starting. Have the child lift both arms toward the ear.
- **Flexion against resistance:** movement of the upper extremity as a whole, forward, with thumb forward, to the ear. Place your palm on the anterior aspect of the elbow and provide resistance as the child attempts this motion.
- **Extension:** movement of the upper extremity as a whole, backward. The thumb should be facing forward when starting.
- **Extension against resistance:** movement of the upper extremity as a whole, backward. The thumb should be facing forward when starting. Place your palm on the posterior aspect of the elbow and provide resistance as the child attempts this motion.
- **Abduction:** movement of the upper extremity as a whole away from anatomic neutral position (0°) toward the ear (180°); ask the child to move the right arm away from the body up to 180°; repeat on the left side.
- **Abduction against resistance:** movement of the upper extremity as a whole away from anatomic neutral position toward the ear. Place your palm on the lateral aspect of the child's elbow and provide resistance as the child attempts the motion.
- **Adduction:** movement of the upper extremity as a whole away from the ear toward the waist and then across midline in front of the navel.
- **Adduction against resistance:** movement of the upper extremity as a whole away from the ear toward the waist and then across midline in front of the naval. Place your palm on the medial aspect of the child's elbow and provide resistance as the child attempts the motion.
- **Internal rotation:** ask the child to pretend to tuck a shirt into the waistband in the front and in the back. This is a functional assessment of the child's ability to perform internal rotation.
- **Internal rotation against resistance:** as the child holds the upper arms at the side with the elbow flexed to 90 degrees, place your palm against the child's palm and provide resistance as the child moves his or her hand toward the opposite hip or naval.
- **External rotation:** ask the child to rub the back of his or her head with the right hand and then the left hand.
- **External rotation against resistance:** as the child holds the right upper arm at the side with the elbow flexed to 90 degrees, place your palm on the back of the child's hand and provide resistance as the child moves his or her hand toward the starting point for internal rotation.

☐ Elbow motion

- **Flexion:** move the right hand to the shoulder from the anatomic neutral position; repeat using the left hand.
- **Flexion against resistance:** movement of the hand to the shoulder from anatomic neutral. Place your palm on the child's right forearm and resist as the child performs the above motion; repeat using the left elbow motion.
- **Extension movement:** move the hand from the shoulder to anatomic neutral position.
- **Extension against resistance:** move the hand from the shoulder to anatomic neutral. Place your palm on the posterior aspect of the child's forearm and resist as the child performs the motion.
- **Pronation:** with the elbow flexed to 90 degrees, move the hand from palm facing up to palm facing down.

- **Pronation against resistance:** with the elbow flexed to 90 degrees, move the hand from palm facing up to palm facing down. Hold the child's hand and resist the motion to determine the strength.
  - **Supination:** with the elbow flexed to 90 degrees, move the hand from palm facing down to palm facing up.
  - **Supination against resistance:** with the elbow flexed to 90 degrees, move the hand from palm facing down to palm facing up. Hold the child's hand and resist the motion to determine strength.
- ☐ Wrist motion
  - **Flexion:** move the palm toward the forearm.
  - **Flexion against resistance:** place your palm on the child's palm and resist the child's motion to determine strength.
  - **Extension:** move the palm from the forearm.
  - **Extension against resistance:** place your palm on the posterior aspect of the child's hand and resist the movement of the palm from the forearm.
  - **Radial deviation:** move the hand toward the radial head.
  - **Radial deviation against resistance:** place your palm over the thumb of the hand and resist movement of the hand toward the radial head.
  - **Ulnar deviation:** move the hand toward the ulnar head.
  - **Ulnar deviation against resistance:** place your palm over the medial aspect of the hand and resist movement of the hand toward the ulnar head.
- ☐ Finger motion
  - **Flexion:** move the fingers toward the palm into a fist-like position.
  - **Flexion against resistance:** have the child attempt to squeeze two of your fingers.
  - **Extension:** move the fingers out of the fist-like position into a straight and slightly flared position.
  - **Extension against resistance:** move the fingers out of the fist-like position into a straight and slightly flared position. Have the child try to open his or her fist against your palm that is over the child's fingers.

3. Document the motion and the strength grade.

NORMAL FINDINGS

- All motions should be symmetrical when compared to the same motion of the right and left upper extremities. (See Chapter 16, Tables 16-1, 16-2, 16-3.)
- The fingers should be able to flex fully, as demonstrated by making a closed fist, and extend as demonstrated by having the fingers flare out in a straight manner.
- Strength of extremities: strength is graded on a scale of 0 to 5 (see Chapter 16, Table 16-4). It is the measurement of the muscles' ability to contract and work against a load.

ABNORMAL FINDINGS

- Anything less than expected full ROM can be considered to be an abnormal finding. It may be due to a new injury, old injury, surgical procedure, or neurological problem.

- Strength of less than 4 of 5. This indicates muscular weakness. The weakness may be due to injury or deconditioning.
- Pain when meeting resistance: this may indicate injury to the muscle.

Technique 22-14E: **Inspecting and Palpating the Lower Extremities**

Purpose: To assess for any abnormalities within the lower extremities

TIP When assessing the lower extremities, it is recommended that each extremity be fully exposed for this assessment.

ASSESSMENT STEPS

1. Explain the technique to the child (age-appropriate). You will ask the child to perform specific motions independently first and then against resistance.

2. Ask the child to perform the following ROM activities of the right and left lower extremities.

3. Inspect the lower extremity on the right side then the left side; compare the right to the left side.

4. Using your finger pads, gently palpate the right and left lower extremities:
- ☐ Hip
- ☐ Knee
- ☐ Ankle
- ☐ Foot
- ☐ Toes

5. Assess the presence of:
- ☐ tenderness
- ☐ depressions
- ☐ bulges
- ☐ change in temperature.

TIP Palpation of the lower extremities may be done with the child on the examination table in a sitting or supine position.

6. Document your findings.

NORMAL FINDINGS

- No pain/tenderness, depressions or protrusions, swelling, increased joint size, or missing digits
- When the child is standing, he or she should be bearing weight on both lower extremities equally. There should be no forward flexing at the hip, and the upper leg should be straight.
- The knees should be slightly flexed and pointed forward.
- The ankle should be perpendicular to the straight lower leg.
- The foot should be straight forward, in line with the knee, and a slight arch should be noted on the medial aspect of the foot.

ABNORMAL FINDINGS

- The inability to bear weight equally on both lower extremities may indicate the presence of pain in one of the extremities.
- A shortened extremity may indicate a bony injury, hip disease, or be resultant from a disease or surgical procedure.
- Forward flexion at the hip may indicate problems within the hip joint, tightness of the muscular structure around the hip, or a problem with the lower back.
- Nonstraight upper leg may indicate a significant bony or muscular injury in the past. If the child is able to bear weight, the injury is most likely old.
- Knees that are straight may indicate a laxity in the ligaments supporting the knee or a problem with the bony structure of the knee.
- Knees that are more than slightly flexed may indicate increased bony buildup within the joint; a disease process; a loose body that locks the joint in this position; or an old injury.
- Lower legs that are not straight may indicate an injury to the bones or muscles.
- Ankles that are not perpendicular to the lower leg indicate a lack of ROM within the ankle joint.
- A foot without a slight arch may be indicative of problems with the following: plantar fascia injuries, fallen arches, and old bony injuries.

Technique 22-14F: Assessing Range of Motion and Strength of the Lower Extremities

Purpose: To assess strength and limitations in ROM in the lower extremities

■ **TIP** Always remember to compare one side with the other side.

ASSESSMENT STEPS

1. Explain the technique to the child (age appropriate) and tell the child you will be assessing each lower extremity separately and the child will have to perform specific motions without assistance.
2. Ask the child to perform the following ROM activities without and with resistance of each lower extremity; assess any differences in symmetry of motion and the fluid nature of the motion.
   □ Hip motion
     - **Flexion:** move the hip forward and toward the anterior aspect of the body.
     - **Flexion against resistance:** move the hip forward, toward the anterior aspect of the body. Place your palm on the anterior aspect of the upper thigh and resist the motion.
     - **Extension:** move the hip backward, away from the anterior aspect of the body.
     - **Extension against resistance:** move the hip backward, away from the anterior aspect of the body. Place your palm on the posterior aspect of the upper thigh and resist the motion.
     - **Abduction:** move the lower extremity away from the midline of the body.
     - **Abduction against resistance:** move the lower extremity away from the midline of the body. Place your palm on the lateral aspect of the thigh and resist the motion.
     - **Adduction:** move the lower extremity toward the midline of the body.

- **Adduction against resistance:** move the lower extremity toward the midline of the body. Place your palm on the distal one third of the medial aspect of the upper thigh and resist the motion.
- ☐ Knee motion
  - **Flexion:** move the heel toward the buttocks.
  - **Flexion against resistance:** move the heel toward the buttocks. Place your palm on the anterior aspect of the distal one third of the lower leg and resist the motion.
  - **Extension:** move the lower extremity toward the anterior aspect of the body.
  - **Extension against resistance:** move the lower extremity toward the anterior aspect of the body. Place your palm on the anterior aspect of the distal one third of the lower leg and resist the motion.
- ☐ Ankle motion
  - **Dorsiflexion:** move the sole of the foot away from the floor, toward the knee.
  - **Dorsiflexion against resistance:** move the sole of the foot away from the floor, toward the knee. Place your palm on the top of the foot and resist the motion.
  - **Plantarflexion:** move the sole of the foot toward the floor, away from the knee.
  - **Plantarflexion against resistance:** move the sole of the foot toward the floor, away from the knee. Place your palm on the sole of the foot and resist the motion.
  - **Inversion:** move the great toe/foot toward the midline of the body.
  - **Inversion against resistance:** move the great toe/foot toward the midline of the body. Place your palm on the medial aspect of the foot and resist the motion.
  - **Eversion:** move the great toe/foot away from the midline of the body.
  - **Eversion against resistance:** move the great toe/foot away from the midline of the body. Place your palm on the lateral aspect of the foot and resist the motion.

3. Document the motion and strength.

NORMAL FINDINGS

- The ROM of each joint is symmetric when compared with the opposite limb. Motion is fluid and without restrictions. Motion is without pain.
- The child should demonstrate strength of at least 4/5 in all of the motions in the lower extremities. Muscle strength is graded on a scale of 0 to 5 (see Chapter 16, Tables 16-5, 16-6, 16-7). It is the measurement of the muscles' ability to contract and work against resistance.
  - ☐ Strength of extremities: strength is graded on a scale of 0 to 5.

ABNORMAL FINDINGS

- The ROM of each joint is not symmetric to the opposite limb.
- Motion is not fluid. This may indicate a muscular strain.
- Limitation in ROM may indicate a problem in the joint or with the muscular strength.

- Pain is present with ROM activities. This may indicate injury to the muscle or joint.
- Alteration in strength with findings of 3/5 or less in one or more of the motions may indicate an injury to the muscle.
- Limitations in ROM against resistance may indicate a problem in the joint.
- Ability to resist at 4/5 or 5/5 for part of the ROM, but at a level of 3/5 or less for another part of the ROM may indicate that one of the muscles that performs the movement may be injured.

TECHNIQUE 22-15: Assessing the Neurological System

Purpose: To assess any gross abnormalities of the neurological system
Equipment: Easily identifiable scents, cotton wisp, flashlight, gloves, object with soft and sharp areas, ophthalmoscope, other scents, pupil scale chart, reflex hammer, Snellen or pediatric eye chart, teaspoon, tongue blade, tuning fork, water

Sequence of Assessment

1. Inspection/observation
2. Neurological assessments (major categories)
   □ Level of consciousness and mental status
   □ Cranial nerve function
   □ Motor system
   □ Reflexes
   □ Sensory system

Technique 22-15A: Assessing Cranial Nerve Function

Purpose: To assess the function of the 12 pairs of cranial nerves.
Cranial nerve assessment evaluates the motor and sensory systems combined. The 12 cranial nerves are

1. Olfactory (CN I)
2. Optic nerve (CN II)
3. Oculomotor nerve (CN III)
4. Trochlear (CN IV)
5. Trigeminal (CN V)
6. Abducent (CN VI)
7. Facial (CN VII)
8. Vestibulocochlear (CN VIII)

9. Glossopharyngeal (CN VIX)

10. Vagus (CN VX)

11. Spinal accessory nerve (CN VXI)

12. Hypoglossal nerve (CN VXII)

Each cranial nerve has a right and left side, and each child's side is assessed separately. Nurses should always compare the responses of each side.

Technique 22-15B: Assessing Sense of Smell (CN I)

Purpose: To assess the sense of smell

Equipment: Easily identifiable scents

> **TIP Make sure the child's nostrils are patent and not clogged or congested.**

ASSESSMENT STEPS

1. Explain the technique to the child (age appropriate).

2. Ask the child to close her or his eyes and occlude the right nostril.

3. Hold one of the available scents under the unoccluded left nostril and ask the child to sniff the scent.

4. Ask the child to identify the scent.

5. Ask the child to occlude the left nostril.

6. Hold a different available scent under the unoccluded right nostril.

7. Ask the child to identify the scent.

8. Document your findings.

NORMAL FINDINGS

■ Able to state the correct scent on each side

ABNORMAL FINDINGS

■ **Anosmia:** inability to smell or identify the correct scent, indicating loss of function to olfactory nerve

Technique 22-15C: Inspecting Pupil Size and Consensual Pupil Response (CN II and CN III)

Purpose: To assess the pupillary light reflex that controls the diameter of the pupil, and to assess the integrity of the optic pathways (consensual pupil response)

Equipment: Penlight, pupil measurement chart

ASSESSMENT STEPS

1. Explain the technique to the child (age appropriate).

2. Stand in front of the child.

3. Use the penlight to inspect the pupils.

4. Assess color.

5. Assess shape of each pupil.

6. Assess symmetry.

7. Assess direct reaction. Shine light into the right eye pupil and then left eye pupil.

8. Assess consensual reaction. Shine light into the left eye pupil and assess the right eye; right eye should constrict and have a consensual response. Repeat on the right eye.

9. Measure the size of each pupil in millimeters.

10. Document your findings.

NORMAL FINDINGS

- Pupil is round and black.
- Both pupils are equal size.
- Diameter is 2 to 8 mm.
- Both eyes have a consensual response to direct light.

ABNORMAL FINDINGS

- Pupils are unequal in size or both dilated or constricted and fixed.
- **Anisocoria** is unequal size of the pupils; may be genetics, medications, or related to a neurological disorder (see Chapter 11, Fig. 11-18).

   SENC Safety Alert Any change in a patient's pupil size, reaction, and shape can indicate an increase in intracranial pressure (Hickey, 2014).

- **Mydriasis** is bilateral dilated and fixed pupils; may be caused by eye drops, stimulation of sympathetic nerves, anesthesia, botulism, and central nervous system injury.
- **Miosis** is an abnormal constriction of the pupils; may be caused by a stroke, medications, brain damage.

Technique 22-15D: Assessing Sensation (CN V)

Purpose: To assess sensation of the skin; to assess facial sensation

Equipment: Cotton wisp, object with a sharp and dull side

TIP Make sure the object will not scare or hurt the child.

The trigeminal nerve is a motor and sensory nerve.

ASSESSMENT STEPS

1. Explain the technique to the child (age appropriate).

2. Tell the child that every time he or she feels the light wisp of cotton to say "now." Have the child feel the wisp of cotton.

3. Ask the child to close his or her eyes.

4. Standing in front of the child, touch the child lightly with the wisp of cotton on the following areas of the face:

   ☐ Forehead

   ☐ Right cheek

☐ Left cheek

☐ Jaw

5. Now, touch the child lightly with the wisp of cotton on the following areas of the upper and lower extremities:

☐ Upper arm bilaterally

☐ Forearm bilaterally

☐ Thigh bilaterally

☐ Lower shin bilaterally

6. Ask the child to open his or her eyes.

7. Explain the next assessment for identifying sharp and dull sensations.

8. Take an object with a sharp and dull side. Demonstrate on the child's skin what "sharp and dull" will feel like.

9. Advise child to close his or her eyes.

10. Use the object and follow steps 4 and 5, alternate patterns between sharp and dull.

11. Document the findings.

NORMAL FINDINGS

■ Light, sharp, and dull sensations are felt in all sites.

ABNORMAL FINDINGS

■ Light, sharp, or dull sensations are not felt at a site; this may indicate a peripheral nerve disorder.

Technique 22-15E: **Assessing Jaw Movement (CN V)**

Purpose: To assess the motor portion of this cranial nerve.

ASSESSMENT STEPS

1. Explain the technique to the child (age appropriate).

2. Advise child to open his or her eyes.

3. Ask the child to clench his or her teeth (to test motor component).

4. Palpate the temporal and masseter muscles, just above the mandibular angle; ask the child to open and close his or her jaw and move the jaw side to side.

5. Document your findings.

NORMAL FINDINGS

■ Child can clench teeth tightly.

■ Masseter muscles bulge when teeth are clenched.

■ On palpation, both masseter muscles feel equal in size and strength.

ABNORMAL FINDINGS

■ **Trigeminal neuralgia** is indicated when the child cannot clench jaw and move jaw side to side.

Technique 22-15F: Assessing Cranial Nerve VII (Facial Nerve)

Purpose: To assess facial movements

The facial nerve is a motor and sensory nerve.

ASSESSMENT STEPS

1. Explain the technique to the child (age appropriate).

2. Stand in front of the child.

3. Assess child's ability to perform the following facial movements. Ask the child to:

□ smile

□ frown

□ puff out his or her cheeks

□ close eyes and try to open eyes against resistance.

4. Document your findings.

NORMAL FINDINGS

■ Child is able to smile, frown, and puff out cheeks.

■ Muscles are symmetrical.

■ Eyes do not open against resistance.

ABNORMAL FINDINGS

■ Asymmetrical muscles while smiling, frowning, or puffing out cheeks

■ Eyes open against resistance

Technique 22-15G: Assessing Cranial Nerve IX (Glossopharyngeal Nerve) and Cranial Nerve X (Vagus Nerve)

Purpose: To assess pharyngeal sensation and function, and the presence or absence of a gag reflex

Equipment: Gloves, tongue blade, cup of water

The glossopharyngeal and the vagus nerves are sensory and motor nerves innervating the pharynx.

ASSESSMENT STEPS

1. Explain the technique to the child (age appropriate).

2. Put on gloves.

3. Ask the child to open his or her mouth.

4. Gently touch the posterior aspect of tongue or pharynx with the tip of the tongue blade to initiate a gag reflex.

5. Assess vocal quality by asking the child to say "ah, ah, ah."

6. Assess the bilateral symmetry of the elevation of the soft palate and central location of uvula.

7. Ask child to take a sip of water.

8. Assess the movement of the throat.

9. Document your findings.

NORMAL FINDINGS

- Positive gag reflex
- Positive pharyngeal sensation bilaterally
- Clear voice
- Able to swallow

ABNORMAL FINDINGS

- Absent gag reflex
- Absent or unilateral pharyngeal sensation indicates dysphagia
- Difficulty with swallowing indicates dysphagia
- Coarse raspy voice indicates poor pharyngeal function.

Technique 22-15H: **Assessing Cranial Nerve XI (Spinal Accessory Muscle)**

Purpose: To assess shoulder and head movement

The spinal accessory nerve is a motor nerve.

ASSESSMENT STEPS

1. Explain the technique to the child (age appropriate).

2. Have the child sit on the end of the bed or examining table.

3. Stand in front of the child.

4. Ask child to shrug shoulders against resistance of examiner pushing down on shoulders.

5. Ask child to turn head his or her head to the right side against the resistance of your hand.

6. Ask child to turn his or her head to the left side against the resistance of your hand.

7. Document your findings.

NORMAL FINDINGS

- Ability to shrug both shoulders against resistance and turn head both ways against resistance

ABNORMAL FINDINGS

- Inability to shrug shoulders or turn head against resistance may indicate paralysis or lesion to accessory nerve (Hickey, 2014).

Technique 22-15I: **Assessing Cranial Nerve XII (Hypoglossal Nerve)**

Purpose: To assess movement of tongue

The hypoglossal nerve is a motor nerve.

ASSESSMENT STEPS

1. Explain the technique to the child (age appropriate).

2. Ask the child to stick out tongue and inspect tongue for:
- ☐ symmetry
- ☐ alignment.

3. Ask the child to move the tongue from side to side.

4. Document your findings.

NORMAL FINDINGS

■ Tongue midline without tremor

■ Tongue moves smoothly from side to side.

ABNORMAL FINDINGS

■ Tongue is not midline or has tremors; this can indicate paralysis or stroke, or a lesion of cranial nerve XII (Hickey, 2014).

Technique 22-15J: **Assessing Gait and Position Sense**

Purpose: To assess balance, coordination, muscle strength, and tone

ASSESSMENT STEPS

1. Explain the technique to the child (age appropriate).

2. Identify a specific distance that you want the child to walk to in the room.

3. Ask the child walk from you first and then back toward you. This allows for both anterior and posterior observation of gait, balance, and posture.

4. Ask the child to walk on his or her toes and return walking toward you on his or her heels; this allows you to assess balance.

5. Instruct the child to walk heel-to-toe away from you and back toward you; this is called tandem walking. Tandem walking assesses for muscular weakness.

6. Ask the child to hop on the right foot and then alternate to the left foot; this assesses position sense and cerebellar function.

7. Ask the child to do a shallow knee bend; this assesses muscular weakness.

8. Document your findings.

NORMAL FINDINGS

■ Gaits, hopping, and knee bends are stable, smooth, and coordinated.

ABNORMAL FINDINGS

■ Gaits lack stability, smoothness, and coordination.
■ **Ataxia** is defective muscle coordination that may be related to loss of position sense, drugs, alcohol, or cerebellar disease.
■ Inability to walk on toes may indicate plantar flexion weakness. Inability to walk on heels may indicate dorsiflexion foot weakness. Inability to walk on both heels and toes may indicate muscular weakness, poor position sense, or vertigo.

Technique 22-15K: Heel-to-Shin Test

Purpose: To assess coordination of movement and position sense

SENC Safety Alert Child should be in the supine position to prevent a fall.

ASSESSMENT STEPS

1. Explain the technique to the child (age appropriate).
2. With the child in the supine position, ask the child to place the heel of his or her right leg on the left knee and slide it down the shin to the left ankle; assess smoothness and coordination.
3. Repeat step 2 using the left leg.
4. Have the child close his or her eyes and repeat steps 2 and 3 on the opposite leg; this assesses position sense.
5. Document your findings.

NORMAL FINDINGS

■ Movement of leg is smooth and coordinated

ABNORMAL FINDINGS

■ Heel does not stay on the shin or moves from side to side while running down the shin may indicate cerebellar disease or loss of motor coordination.

Technique 22-15L: Finger-to-Nose Test

Purpose: To assess cerebellar function, coordination, and point-to-point movements

ASSESSMENT STEPS

1. Explain the technique to the child (age appropriate).
2. Hold your index finger in front of the child at eye level.
3. Ask the child to touch the tip of your index finger and then touch the tip of his or her nose with his or her right index finger.
4. Repeat several times while you are moving your finger a few inches in each direction up, down, right, and left, each time the child attempts to touch your finger by extending his or her arm.
5. Repeat steps 2, 3, and 4 with the child's left index finger.
6. Hold your finger in one place and have the child touch it several times.

7. Ask the child to now close his or her eyes, and using his or her right index finger, have the child touch your finger several times; repeat using the left index finger with eyes closed.

8. Document your findings.

NORMAL FINDINGS

- Child touches the nurse's finger and nose accurately and smoothly in all locations.
- Child touches the nurse's finger accurately and smoothly in one location with eyes closed.

ABNORMAL FINDINGS

- Child is unsteady and unable to touch the stationary finger with the eyes closed; may indicate cerebellar disease.
- **Dysmetria** is the inability to perform point-to-point movements due to over- or underprojecting the finger to touch an object.

Technique 22-15M: **Assessing Rapid Alternating Movements**

Purpose: To assess coordination

TIP It may be helpful to demonstrate the technique to the child.

ASSESSMENT STEPS

1. Explain the technique to the child (age appropriate).
2. Upper extremities: ask the child to place both hands palm down on his or her thighs.
3. Lift both hands and place both hands palms up on his or her thighs.
4. Ask the child to repeat these alternating movements for 10 seconds.
5. Observe the alternating movements for speed and smoothness.
6. Lower extremities: Ask the child to rapidly pat your hand using the ball of the right foot for 10 seconds; observe speed and smoothness.
7. Repeat step 6 on the left foot.
8. Document the findings.

NORMAL FINDINGS

- Coordinated and smooth movements of both hands
- Coordinated and smooth movement of both feet

ABNORMAL FINDINGS

- **Dysdiadochokinesis** is uncoordinated, slow, and clumsy movements; may be a sign of cerebellar disease.

Technique 22-15N: **Pronator Drift**

Purpose: To assess motor function and proprioception

This assessment can be performed standing or sitting.

ASSESSMENT STEPS

1. Explain the technique to the child (age appropriate).

2. Ask the child to extend both arms out with palms up.

3. Ask the child to close his or her eyes and observe the child's arms for change in position for 20 to 30 seconds.

4. Document your findings.

■ **TIP** When the child closes his or her eyes, proprioception (sense of relative position) alone maintains the position of the arms.

NORMAL FINDINGS

■ Arms should remain in the extended position without drifting.

ABNORMAL FINDINGS

■ An arm does not remain raised, the palm may pronate or drop slightly; may indicate an abnormality in the corticospinal tract, the upper motor neurons in the brain and spinal cord that mediate voluntary muscle movement.

Technique 22-15O: **Romberg's Test**

Purpose: To assess position sense and cerebellar function, balance and coordination.

ASSESSMENT STEPS

1. Explain the technique to the child (age appropriate).

2. Ask the child to stand with feet together and arms at sides and look straight ahead for 30 seconds without any support.

3. Assess for any swaying to either side or loss of balance.

4. Now, with the child in this position, stand on the side of the child and extend your hands in the front and back of the child for child safety.

5. Ask the child to close her or his eyes and continue to stand in this position for 30 seconds; observe for swaying and balance.

6. Document your findings.

SENC Safety Alert Keep your hands in front and back of the child in case the child starts to sway or fall.

NORMAL FINDINGS

■ Negative Romberg's test: maintains position without swaying or falling to one side, with and without opening eyes

ABNORMAL FINDINGS

■ Positive Romberg's test: swaying or falling to one side may indicate cerebellar dysfunction, or lesions in the cerebellum or spinal cord.

Technique 22-15P: **Assessing Sensory Function**

Purpose: To assess for any loss in function to sensory nerves. The following techniques will be used when the examiner has detected sensory function or it is known that the child has spinal cord disease.

Technique 22-15Q: **Assessing Graphesthesia**

Purpose: To assess the sensation of touch or tactile stimulation

1. Explain the technique to the child (age appropriate).

2. Have child extend right arm and turn palm face up toward ceiling.

3. Ask child to close eyes.

4. Write a letter or number on the right palm and ask child to state which letter or number was written.

5. Repeat steps 2, 3, and 4 on the left palm.

6. Document your findings.

NORMAL FINDINGS

■ Child is able to state letter or number correctly on each side.

ABNORMAL FINDINGS

■ Child is unable to feel and state the letter or number.

Technique 22-15R: **Assessing Stereognosis**

Purpose: To assess the perception of a shape of an object

1. Explain the technique to the child (age appropriate).

2. Ask child to close eyes.

3. Put a small, familiar object in the palm of the child's right hand.

4. Ask the child to identify the object.

5. Using a different object, repeat steps 2, 3 and 4 using the left hand.

6. Document your findings.

NORMAL FINDINGS

■ Patient is able to perceive and identify the shape of the object.

ABNORMAL FINDINGS

■ **Tactile agnosia** is the inability to process sensory information and to perceive and recognize an object by touch.

TECHNIQUE 22-16: **Assessing the Genitalia and Rectum**

Purpose: To assess for any abnormalities of the genitalia or rectum

Equipment: Gloves

Examination of the female genitalia is limited to inspection and palpation of external structures. An appropriate referral is necessary if a vaginal examination is required.

■ **TIP** Same as adult with consideration to the Tanner scale.

SENC Patient-Centered Care This is a sensitive assessment for the older girl depending on the developmental stage. Be thoughtful in your approach and offer age-appropriate explanations. Make sure the child or adolescent is given time to voice any concerns or fears.

■ **Hymen:** a thin crescent-shaped or circular membrane that covers part of the vaginal opening in virgins

■ **TIP** Although an imperforated hymen denotes lack of penile intercourse, a perforated hymen does not always indicate sexual activity.

■ **Female circumcision:** the female genitalia appear different. The nurse should not display surprise or disgust but document the appearance and discuss the appearance with the female adolescent.

Technique 22-16A: Inspecting the External Female Genitalia

Purpose: To assess for inflammation, lumps, lesions, or abnormalities

Equipment: Light source, gloves

■ **TIP** The younger child may feel more comfortable sitting on her mother's lap.

ASSESSMENT STEPS

1. Explain the technique to the child (age appropriate).
2. Perform hand hygiene and put on gloves.
3. Talk to the child as you are performing the steps of the assessment.
4. Inspect the skin color of the labia majora and minora.
5. Inspect the following external genitalia for redness, swelling, or lesions:
   □ Mons pubis
   □ Labia majora
   □ Labia minora
   □ Perineum for hair distribution
6. Using your dominant gloved hand, gently separate the labia majora to inspect the urethral meatus for developmental abnormalities or discharge.
7. Inspect the clitoris and vestibule for size, color, presence of lesions, and discoloration or masses.
8. Inspect the perineum for swelling, ulcers, condylomata (warts), or changes in colors.
9. Inspect urethral meatus for position.
10. Inspect the vaginal orifice for discharge, protrusion of the walls, and condition of the hymen.
11. Inspect the perineum and anus for color and shape.
12. Remove and discard gloves.
13. Document your findings.

SENC Safety Alert Be alert to signs of infection for patients who have external genitalia piercings.

- Labia majora and labia minora are uniform color, symmetrical.
- Skin over mons pubis is smooth with even hair distribution (age appropriate).
- Pubic hair is evenly distributed and shaped like an inverse triangle (see Tanner's Staging, Table 22-1); no lice or nits.
- Clitoris does not have redness or swelling.
- Urethra is a slit-like opening; midline; no swelling, redness, or discharge.
- Bartholin glands are at 4 and 8 o'clock; no redness or inflammation.
- Skene's glands are at 1 and 11 o'clock; no redness or inflammation.
- Perineum is smooth and skin color is uniform.
- No vaginal discharge or bleeding is noted.
- Anus is dark brown; puckering of skin; no swelling, inflammation, or signs of trauma.

ABNORMAL FINDINGS

- Rashes, swelling, erythema, or vaginal discharge or bleeding
- Signs of trauma: When children have been sexually assaulted (raped), they may show medical signs of their attack including sexually transmitted infection, urinary tract infection, and other hard-to-explain injuries. These conditions could also occur in cases of children's voluntary sexual activity, but parents should not assume that case.

Technique 22-16B: Inspecting the External Male Genitalia

Purpose: To assess the external male genitalia for lesions, edema, and masses

Equipment: Gloves, tangential lighting

> **SENC Patient-Centered Care** Inspecting the genitalia may be embarrassing for the child; male patients are sensitive and very aware of nonverbal body language; always be professional and objective throughout the assessment.

ASSESSMENT STEPS

1. Explain the technique to the child (age appropriate).
2. Ask the child to lie on the examination table in the supine position.
3. Put on gloves.
4. Drape the child so that only the genital area being examined is exposed.
5. Inspect the skin of the male genitalia assessing for:
   - ☐ color
   - ☐ lesions
   - ☐ drainage
   - ☐ edema
   - ☐ hair distribution.

6. Assess the following structures:
   - ☐ Penis: assess the ventral, lateral, and dorsal sides.
   - ☐ Prepuce: note whether the patient is circumcised or not; if uncircumcised ask patient to retract the foreskin.
   - ☐ Urethral meatus: note location of the urethral opening.
   - ☐ Pubic hair: assess pattern of hair distribution. (See Tanner's staging, Table 22-1.)
7. Skin: assess for irritation or public lice.
8. Gently lift up the scrotum to assess the posterior side.
9. Assess the groin area for inguinal bulging; if suspected, ask the child to cough for better visualization of any suspected bulging.
10. Maintaining the child's dignity, ask the patient to turn on his side with his upper leg slightly bent, and gently spread the buttocks apart to inspect the anus.
11. Remove and discard gloves.
12. Document your findings.

NORMAL FINDINGS

- Penis: Caucasians, pink to light brown; dark-skinned or African Americans, light to dark brown; smooth, no hair; dorsal vein is visible; no lesions; no discharge; no nits or lice
  - ☐ Prepuce: circumcised foreskin is smooth and pink; uncircumcised foreskin easily retracts.

- ☐ Urethra meatus: pink, smooth, is located at the center of the glans.
- ☐ Pubic hair: at the base of the penis the hair distribution is in a triangular pattern consistent with age; coarse hair; no nits or lice.
- ☐ Anus: darker-colored skin, wrinkled around the orifice, no hemorrhoids, no signs of trauma.
- ☐ Scrotum: skin is a darker pigmentation; wrinkled surface, thin skin; left testis hangs lower than the right testis.
- ☐ Inguinal area: skin is smooth, free from lumps or bumps, no signs of a hernia.

ABNORMAL FINDINGS

- **Phimosis:** a narrowing or stenosis of the preputial opening of the foreskin in uncircumcised males (see Chapter 19, Figure 19-19)
- **Balanitis:** an inflammation or infection of the phimotic foreskin
- **Hydrocele:** a fluid-filled sack in the scrotum which usually resolves spontaneously by 1 year of age
- **Cryptorchidism:** failure of one or both testes to descend. In most cases, the testes will descend by 1 year of age.
- **Hypospadias:** the urethral opening of the penis is below the glans penis.

CHILD OR ADOLESCENT TEACHING

- Anticipatory guidance is child teaching that focuses on the issues specific to the developmental stage of the child that will promote health and prevent disease.
- Foundational to providing meaningful anticipatory guidance is gathering information (review of systems and health assessment)

from the child and the parent and establishing a therapeutic relationship.
- See Table 22-10 for specific anticipatory guidance topics for infants and young children, Table 22-11 for children aged 5 to 10 years, and Table 22-12 for preadolescent and adolescent youth.

Age	1–2 years	2 years Same as previous age group. Add:	3 years Same as previous age group. Add:	4 years Same as previous age group. Add:
Healthy Habits	Keep home and car smoke free Wash hands often Clean toys Avoid TV viewing	Teach child to wash hands Wipe nose with tissue Clean potty chairs after each use Limit screen time to 2 hours, watch programs together Reinforce bedtime routine	Teach child to wipe nose with tissue Reinforce bedtime routine	Remind child to wash hands
Injury Prevention	Use safety seat in back seat of car Never place child in front seat with a passenger air bag Childproof home (dangling cords, sockets, poisons, medicines, guns) Supervise near water: empty tub, buckets, pools, wells Supervise near pets, mowers, driveways, streets		Switch to belt-positioning booster seat in back seat when child weighs 40 lbs. Ensure playground safety Teach stranger safety Teach pedestrian safety skills	Keep cigarettes, matches, poisons, alcohol, electrical tools locked up and/or out of reach Use helmet for biking Be sure child learns how to swim Keep poison center number handy Keep guns unloaded and locked up, or remove from home

TABLE 22-10 Anticipatory Guidance: Early Childhood

Continued

TABLE 22-10 Anticipatory Guidance: Early Childhood—cont'd

Age	1–2 years	2 years Same as previous age group. Add:	3 years Same as previous age group. Add:	4 years Same as previous age group. Add:
Nutrition	Provide three nutritious meals Provide two to three healthy snacks daily Allow child to feed self, use cup If breastfeeding: Discuss weaning If bottlefeeding: Change to whole milk, begin weaning Let child experiment with food, do not force eating Avoid choke foods (grapes and raisins; nuts; hot dogs; chunks of meat or cheese; hard, gooey, or sticky candy and chewing gum; gobs of peanut butter, especially chunky peanut butter; popcorn; raw vegetables) Limit sugar Eat meals as a family	Offer variety of healthy foods, let child decide Avoid struggles Do not force eating Provide child-size utensils	Serve low-fat dairy products	Limit candy, chips, soft drinks Model good eating habits
Oral Health	Do not put child to bed with bottle Brush child's teeth with soft toothbrush, water only Discuss fluoride Schedule first dental examination Practice good family oral health habits (brushing, flossing)	Begin brushing child's teeth with fluoridated toothpaste Schedule dental appointment		Be sure child brushes teeth

TABLE 22-10 **Anticipatory Guidance: Early Childhood—cont'd**

Age	1–2 years	2 years Same as previous age group. Add:	3 years Same as previous age group. Add:	4 years Same as previous age group. Add:
Social Competence	Set limits (e.g., use distraction) Do not allow hitting, biting, aggressive behavior Limit rules Set routines Be consistent	Begin toilet training when child is ready	Encourage talking, reading Encourage safe exploration, socialization, physical activity Provide choices Reinforce limits, use "time out" Help child cope with fears	Encourage child to talk about feelings, experiences, school Set appropriate limits Provide structured learning (preschool, Sunday school)
Family Relationships	Hold, cuddle child Show affection in family Help child express emotions Limit caregivers, choose carefully	Help child express emotions Help siblings resolve conflicts Do not expect child to share all toys	Handle anger constructively Help siblings resolve conflicts	Create family time together Handle anger constructively Help siblings resolve conflicts
Sexuality Education		Expect curiosity about genitals Use correct terms	Expect normal curiosity Use correct terms, answer questions Explain that certain body parts are private	

From Bright Futures/American Academy of Pediatrics, 2008, with permission.

TABLE 22-11 Anticipatory Guidance: Childhood and Middle Childhood

Age	5 Years	6 Years Same as Previous Age Group. Add:	8 Years Same as Previous Age group. Add:	10 Years Same as Previous Age Group. Add:
Healthy Habits	Promote physical activity Limit screen time (TV, video, computer) to 2 hours. No TV or Internet in bedroom Teach hygiene, handwashing after toileting and before meals	Reinforce personal care/hygiene	Supervise activities with peers Counsel about avoiding alcohol, tobacco, drugs, inhalants	Set reasonable standards for TV, music, video, computer time
Injury Prevention	Use belt-positioning booster seat Never place child in front seat with a passenger air bag Emphasize pedestrian, neighborhood, stranger, playground safety Teach child how to swim; reinforce water safety rules Limit sun; use sunscreen Keep guns unloaded and locked up, or remove from home Teach child emergency phone numbers, home safety rules Provide safe after-school care	Teach stranger safety Keep firm, consistent rules	Reinforce water, bike, neighborhood, and sports safety	Ensure use of lap/shoulder safety belts in back seat of car Anticipate some errors in judgment and increased risk taking
Nutrition		Teach healthy food choices including fruits and vegetables Limit high-fat, low-nutrient foods		
Oral Health	Schedule dental appointment	Learn dental emergency care		Teach dangers of smoking and smokeless tobacco

TABLE 22-11 Anticipatory Guidance: Childhood and Middle Childhood—cont'd

Age	5 Years	6 Years Same as Previous Age Group. Add:	8 Years Same as Previous Age group. Add:	10 Years Same as Previous Age Group. Add:
Social Competence	Read interactively with child	Praise child and encourage talking about activities and feelings Read interactively with child, listen as the child reads aloud	Encourage reading and hobbies Spend time together as family Set limits and establish consequences	Encourage pursuit of talents Promote interaction/friendships through team or group activities Encourage positive interactions with teachers and other adults Reinforce limits, family rules for bedtimes, homework, chores
Family Relationships	Spend time playing together	Know child's friends and their families	Set reasonable but challenging expectations	Contribute to self-esteem with affection and praise Handle anger constructively in family Do not allow violence
Sexuality Education	Explain that certain body parts are private	Answer questions Use age-appropriate books	Discuss information given at school	Prepare child for sexual development, menstruation, wet dreams Discuss information given at school, provide more information as needed Teach importance of delaying sexual behavior
School	Meet with teachers Prepare child for school Become involved with school			

From Bright Futures/American Academy of Pediatrics, 2008, with permission.

TABLE 22-12 Anticipatory Guidance: Early to Late Adolescence

Age	11 Years	11 to 14 Years Same as Previous Age Group. Add:	15 to 17 Years Same as Previous Age Group. Add:	18–22 Years Same as Previous Age Group. Add:
Healthy Habits	Keep home and car smoke free Try to get 8 hours of sleep a night Engage in physical activity (30–60 minutes, three or more times a week) Discuss athletic conditioning, weight training, fluids, weight gain/loss, supplements Limit TV, computer time Learn to manage time, activities		Practice time management skills	Follow speed limits, drive responsibly, avoid distractions, use of cell phone Ride with designated driver or call for a ride if drinking
Injury Prevention	Use lap and shoulder belts in car Do not drink alcohol, especially when biking, swimming, operating machinery Limit sun, use sunscreen Do not use tanning beds Use bike helmet, mouth guards, protective gear Discuss home safety rules with parents (visitors, parties, emergencies) Do not carry or use weapons Learn to swim Avoid loud music Learn to protect self from abuse			Use protective gear at work, follow job safety rules Avoid high noise levels, especially with earphones Do not carry or use weapons Learn how to resolve conflicts

TABLE 22-12 Anticipatory Guidance: Early to Late Adolescence—cont'd

Age	11 Years	11 to 14 Years Same as Previous Age Group. Add:	15 to 17 Years Same as Previous Age Group. Add:	18–22 Years Same as Previous Age Group. Add:
Mental Health	Talk with health provider or trusted adult if feeling sad or if things are not going right Recognize and learn how to deal with stress			Take on new challenges to build confidence Continue to develop sense of identity and clarify values, beliefs Trust own feelings, listen to good friends and valued adults Seek help if often feeling angry, depressed, or hopeless Set reasonable, challenging goals Meet spiritual needs
Nutrition	Choose fruits, vegetables; breads, cereals, other grains; lean meats, chicken, fish; low-fat dairy products Maintain healthy weight with good eating habits, physical activity			Purchase/prepare a variety of healthy foods (fruits, vegetables; breads, cereals, other grains; lean meats, chicken, fish; low-fat dairy products) Limit high-fat, high-sugar foods Eat in pleasant environment with companions Maintain healthy weight with good eating habits, physical activity
Oral Health	Do not smoke or chew tobacco			
Social Competence		Participate in social activities, community groups, or sports Understand parental limits and consequences for unacceptable behavior	Discuss handling negative peer pressure Continue building decision-making skills, understand consequences of your behavior	Continue to maintain strong family relationships Develop good peer relationships, social support systems Use peer refusal skills to handle negative peer pressure Continue progress in independence, decision making, anticipating consequences of behavior

Continued

Age	11 Years	11 to 14 Years Same as Previous Age Group. Add:	15 to 17 Years Same as Previous Age Group. Add:	18–22 Years Same as Previous Age Group. Add:
Responsibility		Model respect, family values, safe driving practices, and healthy behaviors Respect adolescent's need for privacy Establish realistic expectations, clear limits and consequences Anticipate challenges to parental authority Minimize criticism; avoid nagging, negative messages Emphasize importance of school Show interest in school activities Ask for resources/referrals if needed Keep guns unloaded and locked up, or remove from home	Respect rights and needs of others Follow family rules (curfew, car) Share household chores Take on new responsibility Learn new skills (lifesaving, mentoring) Discuss taking responsibility for own health, becoming informed	Serve as positive role model Learn new responsibilities, skills Become an informed healthcare consumer Ask for help entering adult healthcare system Discuss future reproductive plans with health provider **If Thinking of Having a Baby...** Discuss responsibilities involved (physical, emotional, financial) Eat a variety of healthy foods, be physically active Take a folic acid supplement daily before and during pregnancy Avoid tobacco, alcohol, drugs before and during pregnancy Seek genetic counseling if needed

TABLE 22-12 Anticipatory Guidance: Early to Late Adolescence—cont'd

TABLE 22-12 **Anticipatory Guidance: Early to Late Adolescence—cont'd**

Age	11 Years	11 to 14 Years Same as Previous Age Group. Add:	15 to 17 Years Same as Previous Age Group. Add:	18–22 Years Same as Previous Age Group. Add:
Sexuality Education	Ask health provider about puberty, sexual development, contraception, STDs			Discuss LGBTQ issues; celibacy; questions/concerns Delay having sex until older; having sex should be a well-considered decision Abstinence is safest way to prevent pregnancy and STDs Learn to resist sexual pressures If sexually active, discuss contraception, STD prevention; practice safer sex Limit partners, use latex condoms and other barriers correctly
Prevention of Substance Use/Abuse	Do not use tobacco, alcohol, drugs, diet pills, inhalants Discuss how to resist peer pressure to smoke, drink, use drugs If smoking or using drugs or alcohol, discuss help and seek assistance Avoid situations where drugs or alcohol are present			Do not sell drugs Support friends who choose not to smoke, drink, use drugs
School Achievement	Discuss school transitions Become responsible for attendance, homework, course selection Discuss frustrations with school Participate in school activities Identify/pursue talents, interests	Discuss thoughts of dropping out	Make plans for after high school	Identify/pursue talents and interests Plan for the future

From Bright Futures/American Academy of Pediatrics, 2008, with permission.

CHAPTER 23

Assessment of the Pregnant Woman

Leslie White

INTRODUCTION

Assessment of the pregnant woman at regular intervals contributes to overall maternal and fetal health and well-being. All body systems are affected by pregnancy; thus, strong physical assessment skills are required for nurses who care for these patients. Pregnancy is divided into three trimesters, with a total average pregnancy length of 40 weeks. A robust knowledge base about normal anatomical changes in each trimester of pregnancy helps the nurse to determine which changes are expected and which are outside the norm.

The pregnant woman experiences profound anatomical and physiological changes in nearly every organ system of the body. These adaptations to pregnancy begin just after conception and continue through delivery. After delivery, the adaptations almost completely revert back to the nonpregnant state over a period of weeks.

REVIEW OF ANATOMY AND PHYSIOLOGY

The purpose of anatomical and physiological changes during pregnancy is to accommodate the changing needs of the mother and the fetus who work in concert throughout the pregnancy. Many normal alterations occur during this 9-month period.

Skin

- **Melasma or cholasma** ("mask of pregnancy") is a hyperpigmented area of skin that often occurs on the face. Melasma occurs in up to 75 percent of pregnant women (Pomerantz, 2012) (Fig. 23-1). Hyperpigmentation can also occur along the midsection of the abdomen as a thin vertical line called "linea nigra" (Fig. 23-2).
- **Spider angiomas,** palmar erythema, spider veins, and varicosities occur due to an increase in estrogen as well as increased blood volume and are common and benign conditions during pregnancy (Fig. 23-3).
- **Striae gravidarum** ("stretch marks") develop due to the mechanical stretching of the skin (Fig. 23-4). Hormonal effects on skin contribute to the development of stretch marks.

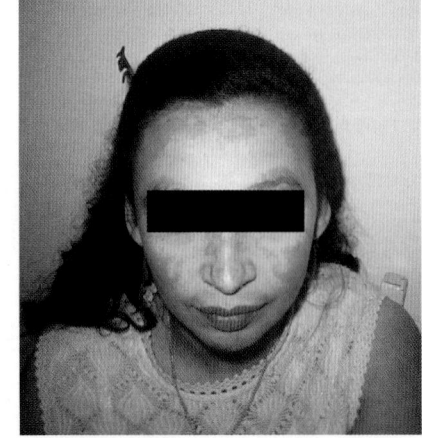

Fig. 23-1. Melasma.

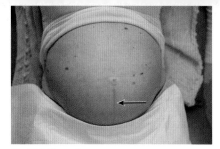
Fig. 23-2. Linea nigra.

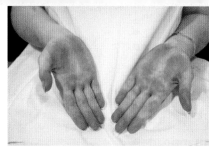
Fig. 23-3. Palmar erythema.

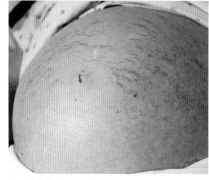
Fig. 23-4. Striae gravidarum.

- **Pruritus:** There are many causes for pruritus during pregnancy. The most common cause is pruritic urticarial papules and plaques of pregnancy (PUPPP).
  - □ PUPPP manifests as highly pruritic urticarial plaques and papules that may or may not have erythematous patches.
  - □ The PUPPP rash typically occurs first on the abdomen, often along striae.
  - □ The extremities are sometimes involved, but the face is usually spared.
  - □ PUPPP commonly occurs in the third trimester, often toward the end of pregnancy.

TIP If pruritus becomes generalized and is not associated with PUPPP, this must be evaluated because it can be a sign of intrahepatic cholestasis, an interruption with the excretion of bile. Typically, this form of pruritus is associated with excoriations from scratching and is generalized throughout the skin, although there are no specific lesions (Afshar & Esakoff, 2014).

- **Hirsutism,** a pattern of male pattern hair growth of the face in particular, but also occurring on the abdomen and extremities, is a normative change (Pomerantz, 2012).

Musculoskeletal System

Strain is placed on the axial skeleton and pelvis due to normal weight gain as well as hormonal changes. Common musculoskeletal changes include:

- **Lordosis:** the expanding uterus causes a shift in the center of gravity and progressive lumbar lordosis, or concave curvature of the spine. Lumbar lordosis leads to low back pain for many pregnant women (Fig. 23-5).
- **Low back pain, joint pain, and pubic symphysis separation** can occur as a result of the hormonal effects of relaxin. Relaxin is a hormone produced by the corpus luteum, decidua, and placenta (Cunningham, Leveno, Bloom, Spong, & Dashe, 2014).

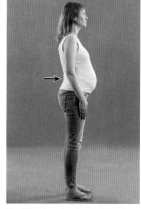
Fig. 23-5. Lumbar lordosis.

- **Pain in the round ligaments of the uterus** is very common. The round ligament of the uterus comes from the pelvis, passes through the internal abdominal ring, and then runs along the inguinal canal to the labia majora. The round ligaments hold the uterus suspended inside the abdominal cavity (Fig. 23-6).

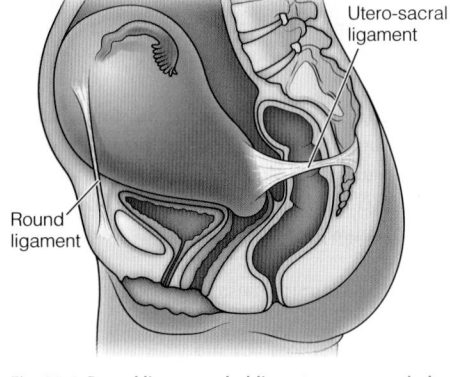

Fig. 23-6. Round ligaments holding uterus suspended.

- **Hip pain, knee pain, and foot pain** are common due to increased uterine size and weight, as well as normative changes in posture.
- **Cramping in the legs** is another expected change that many women experience in the second and third trimesters. Leg cramps may be caused by increases in body weight, circulatory changes, or electrolyte imbalances (Lowdermilk, Perry, & Cashion, 2013).

Breasts

Breast enlargement, increased vascularity, and hyperplasia of glandular tissue are normal and expected as a result of increased levels of estrogen and progesterone. The breasts can be different in appearance (Fig. 23-7). Common changes include:

- blood vessels are more visible
- nipples and areolae become darker, larger, and more erectile
- the sebaceous glands (Montgomery's glands) that help to lubricate the areolae are more pronounced

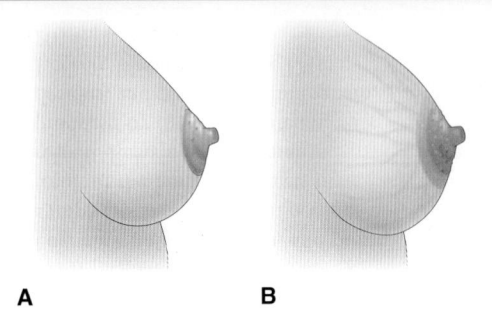

A   **B**

Fig. 23-7. Changes in breast appearance. (A) Early pregnancy. (B) Late pregnancy.

- colostrum, the yellow premilk, may be expressed as early as the 16th week of pregnancy (Lowdermilk et al, 2013).

SENC Patient-Centered Care The breasts may be integral to women's self-esteem and sexuality. Changes in physical appearance can be either distressing or pleasing. It is important for the nurse to validate the pregnant woman's emotions about her changing body and to remind her that changes to her appearance are indicative of the healthy process of pregnancy. Empathetic listening and support is critical.

Reproductive System

Uterus

The uterus makes several changes in shape and size as pregnancy progresses. The nonpregnant upside-down pear shape changes to spherical in the second trimester, and finally becomes ovoid in the third (Lowdermilk et al, 2013).

- At 12 to 14 weeks, the uterus is usually palpable at the symphysis pubis.
- The uterus typically enlarges by 1 cm per week rising to the umbilicus at 23 to 24 weeks.

- After reaching the umbilicus, the uterus continues to grow by 1 cm per week until approximately 38 weeks.
- At 38 weeks, the crest of the uterus is at the xiphoid process.
- The uterus often dips below the xiphoid in a process called "lightening" between the 38th and 40th weeks of gestation.
- Measurements of uterine growth are called "fundal height."
- **Braxton Hicks contractions** can be felt through the abdominal wall by 4 months of gestation and are painless and irregularly occurring. The etiology of Braxton Hicks contractions is unknown; however, it is thought that these contractions promote blood flow through the uterus (Lowdermilk et al, 2013).

Cervix

- Goodell's sign is a softening of the cervix.
- Chadwick's sign is a bluish appearance of the cervix (Fig. 23-8).
- Hegar's sign refers to a softening of the cervix and uterine isthmus.

Vagina and Vulva

- Increased vascularity, thickening, and lengthening of the vagina and vulva are normal and expected.
- **Chadwick's sign:** In the sixth to eighth weeks of pregnancy, a violet/bluish hue can be visualized that indicates increased vascularity of the vagina and vulva.

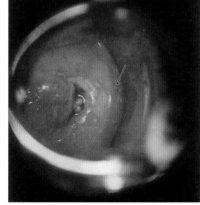

Fig. 23-8. Chadwick's sign.

- **Leukorrhea:** a noninfectious, odorless, white or slightly greyish vaginal discharge, is normal during pregnancy.
- **Vaginal pH is elevated** which protects against vaginal bacterial infections. Pregnant women are more likely to develop yeast infections due to increases in glycogen (Bickley & Szilagi, 2009).

Ovaries

- **Corpus luteum** is the follicle that was released from the ovum and was fertilized. The corpus luteum may be palpable on the affected side early in pregnancy.
- Follicle-stimulating hormone (FSH) levels decrease due to increased levels of estrogen and progesterone secreted by the ovaries and corpus luteum. FSH prevents ovulation and menstruation during pregnancy.

Cardiovascular System

- **Heart size** increases due to increases in diastolic filling and hypertrophy. Increased heart size causes a shift in the point of maximal impulse.
- **Blood volume** is increased 40 to 45 percent above pre-pregnancy levels.
- **Fibrinolytic (clotting) activity** is suppressed providing protection against hemorrhage during delivery and postpartum. Pregnant women are more at risk of thrombosis due to changes in coagulation activity (Lowdermilk et al, 2013).

SENC Safety Alert Pregnant women with leg pain, warmth, or edema should be immediately evaluated by the healthcare provider, as this may be a sign of thrombosis.

- Peripheral vascular resistance declines in the first and second trimesters, resulting in decreased diastolic blood pressures (BPs). BP returns to pre-pregnancy levels in the third trimester (Foley, 2012).

SENC Safety Alert Remind patients in the third trimester to avoid supine positions for long periods of time. Supine positions can result in compression of the inferior vena cava and lower aorta. Obstruction of the inferior vena cava reduces venous return to the heart leading to a fall in cardiac output, resulting in dizziness or weakness, as well as impaired blood flow to the uterus and reduced oxygenation to the fetus.

Respiratory System

■ In response to **estrogenic effect** on the respiratory tract, increased **chest expansion** is possible. This ability to expand the chest further allows for adequate oxygenation.
■ **Estrogenic effects** are also responsible for **capillary enlargement** that results in nasal congestion and possible epistaxis (nosebleed).
■ **Tidal volume** rises as a result of progesterone that enables increased depth of breathing.

SENC Safety Alert Pregnant women with epistaxis (nosebleed) that does not respond to typical techniques of suppression such as nose blowing and/or tamponade should be evaluated by the healthcare provider, as it may be associated with clotting disorders or postpartum hemorrhage (Dugan-Kim, Connell, Stika, Wong, & Gossett, 2009).

Gastrointestinal System

■ Increasing levels of human chorionic gonadotropin (hCG) or estrogen result in **nausea and vomiting in the first trimester,** commonly referred to as "morning sickness." This nausea and vomiting usually subsides by the 12th week of pregnancy.

TIP Nausea associated with pregnancy can often be relieved by a few basic techniques. Pregnant women should be advised to eat small, frequent meals. A dry simple food, such as a cracker, immediately upon arising can often help to stem nausea for the day. The addition of vitamin B_6 in the form of supplements can reduce nausea, although vitamin B_6 does not seem to help with vomiting (Matthews, Haas, O'Mathúna, Dowswell, & Doyle, 2014).

SENC Safety Alert Pregnant women who have excessive vomiting need prompt evaluation. This condition is called hyperemesis gravidarum. Women with hyperemesis may vomit multiple times each day, and develop orthostatic hypotension, laboratory abnormalities, and physical signs of dehydration. Hospitalization may be necessary (Temming et al, 2014).

■ Changes to taste may result in cravings.

SENC Safety Alert Pica is the habit of craving substances of no nutritional value such as ice, dirt, or chalk. The etiology of pica is unknown. Pregnant women who develop pica should be evaluated as the substances that are ingested may contain toxins or parasites.

■ Increased progesterone results in decreased motility and slower emptying times, which can cause acid reflux.
■ Progesterone is also responsible for increased water absorption from the colon, resulting in constipation. Gut motility slows down.
■ Iron is readily absorbed from the small intestine in response to increased nutritional needs.

TIP Despite increased absorption of iron, pregnant women are at risk for iron deficiency anemia. The developing fetus depletes the mother's stores of iron, and a fall in maternal hemoglobin levels results in anemia (Bauer, 2012). Supplementation with iron provides a simple solution. It is suggested that all pregnant women take a daily prenatal vitamin that includes extra calcium, folic acid, and iron. If iron deficiency anemia is present, additional iron supplements may be required.

Renal System

■ Ureters dilate resulting in increased retention of urine and slower rates of urine emptying. This dilation can result in increases in urinary tract infection, as urine remains in the ureters and renal pelvis for longer periods of time.

- Increased bladder sensitivity can result in frequent urination of small volumes of urine; as pregnancy progresses, the bladder becomes compressed by the expanding uterus, resulting in urinary urgency (Lowdermilk et al, 2013).
- The glomerular filtration rate (GFR) increases to allow for increased metabolic and circulatory demand (Lowdermilk et al, 2013).

Psychosocial Changes

- Emotional changes are normal as women adjust and adapt to life changes around childbearing. Psychological concerns during pregnancy such as anxiety, depression, or mood changes are very common (Lowdermilk et al, 2013).
- Women who have underlying mental illness may have improvement or worsening of symptoms and should continue receiving care from their mental health providers.
- "Postpartum blues," or feelings of sadness, are common in the days following delivery. These feelings usually rapidly resolve without treatment. While postpartum blues are transient, persistent feelings of depression or anxiety may indicate a more serious problem and should be evaluated promptly.

SENC **Safety Alert** Postpartum depression occurs in 10 to 20 percent of all childbearing women and is considerably underdiagnosed (Caple & Schub, 2012). Postpartum depression is treatable if found early but can persist if not addressed. If not treated, postpartum depression can result in significant risk to mother and baby. Screening instruments such as the Edinburgh Postnatal Depression Scale or EPDS (Cox, Holden, & Sagovsky, 1987) or the Postpartum Depression Screening Scale are very useful in determining which women need follow-up. The postpartum visit with obstetrical providers at 6 weeks after delivery is an optimal time to evaluate depression (Caple & Schub, 2012). Postpartum depression can accelerate to postpartum psychosis if untreated (Doucet, Dennis, Letourneau, & Blackmore, 2009). See the website (http://www2.aap.org/sections/scan/practicingsafety/toolkit_resources/module2/epds.pdf) for access to the EPDS.

Signs and Symptoms of Early Pregnancy

- **Presumptive symptoms** (symptoms that a woman experiences that are suggestive, but not conclusive of pregnancy) include:
  - ☐ amenorrhea (no menses)
  - ☐ breast tenderness
  - ☐ fatigue
  - ☐ nausea/vomiting
  - ☐ frequent urination.
- **Probable signs/symptoms** (signs or symptoms that indicate that pregnancy is likely, though not definite)
  - ☐ Abdominal enlargement
  - ☐ Piskacek's sign (asymmetry to the uterus)
  - ☐ Hegar's sign (softening of the lower uterine segment)
  - ☐ Goodell's sign (softening of the cervix)
  - ☐ Chadwick's sign (blue coloration of the vulva, vagina, and/or cervix)
  - ☐ Braxton Hicks contractions (painless, irregular, intermittent uterine contractions)
- **Positive signs:** signs that indicate that there is definitely a pregnancy occurring.
  - ☐ Fetal heart sounds detected by Doppler
  - ☐ Quickening (fetal movement usually felt by 19 to 20 weeks)
  - ☐ Visualization of fetus by ultrasound

TERMINOLOGY OF PREGNANCY

Assessing the pregnant woman requires specific considerations. This specialty has specific terminology that every nurse needs to know (Box 23-1).

Naegele's rule is the standard calculation to determine the expected date of delivery (Box 23-2).

BOX 23-1 Terminology of Pregnancy

- **GTPAL:** Gravida, Term, Preterm, Abortion, Living. A system used to summarize pregnancy history.
- **Gravida:** The absolute total number of times that a woman has been pregnant, regardless of the outcome of the pregnancy or the number of fetuses per pregnancy.
- **Parity:** The number of pregnancies in which the fetus (or fetuses) have reached 20 weeks of gestation when they are born. Whether the fetuses are born alive or not does not affect parity.
- **Viability:** The capacity of a fetus to live outside of the uterus; there is no absolute definition in terms of weeks, but 23 weeks is an accepted limit at this time (American Academy of Pediatrics, American Heart Association, & Kattwinkel, 2011).
- **Preterm:** A pregnancy that is between 20 and 37 weeks of gestation.
- **Term:** A pregnancy that is between 38 and 40 completed weeks of gestation.
- **Post-term or Post-dates:** A pregnancy that is between 41 and 42 completed weeks of gestation.

- **First trimester:** 0 to 12 completed weeks of pregnancy
- **Second trimester:** 13 to 28 completed weeks of pregnancy
- **Third trimester:** 29 weeks until delivery
- **Estimated Date of Confinement (EDC)**, also known as Estimated Date of Delivery (EDD), is based on last menstrual period (LMP) because conception usually occurs 2 weeks after the LMP based on a 28-day menstrual cycle.
- **Ballottement** is assessed during abdominal palpation and during cervical examination. Ballottement refers to the period of time when the fetus's head has not yet descended fully into the pelvis and is freely movable.
- **Braxton Hicks contractions,** also known as false labor, are irregular, typically mild intensity contractions. Braxton Hicks contractions will typically occur during the last trimester of pregnancy. These contractions may also occur more frequently if the woman is standing or sitting for long periods and will resolve with activity.
- **Abortions:** Both miscarriages and abortions
- **Living:** Living children

BOX 23-2 Calculating Naegele's Rule

Take the first day of the last menstrual period, count back 3 months, then add 7 days.

Example LMP: December 1
Month 12 – 3 months = 9 (September)
+ Day 1 + 7 (8th)
= EDC September 8th

DIAGNOSTICS

Confirmation of pregnancy must be determined. There are a number of methods used to determine that conception has occurred:

- **Urine pregnancy test** identifies the presence of human chorionic gonadotropin (hCG) in the urine. It is an inexpensive and reliable test that can be done at home or in the medical setting; hCG is detectable at 5 to 7 days after implantation (Carcio & Secor, 2010).

- **Serum qualitative test** (test of the presence of hCG in the serum) is a blood test. In a qualitative test, results are stated as "positive" or "negative" (Carcio & Secor, 2010).
- **Serum quantitative test** is the same as with qualitative, but given in numerical form (i.e., number above 25 mIU/mL).
- **Serum hCG levels** double every 2 days during the first 3 to 4 weeks after implantation; levels peak at 60 to 70 days after fertilization (Carcio & Secor, 2010).
- **Ultrasound** is an electronic technology that has become routine in developed countries. It uses the reflection of pulses of high-frequency sound to produce an image. During pregnancy, ultrasound is used diagnostically as well as for screening of a variety of conditions. It is done at various points during pregnancy, as well as to evaluate female reproductive organs (Whitworth, Bricker, Neilson James, & Dowswell, 2010).
  - ☐ Ultrasound is commonly performed in the first trimester at 7 to 9 weeks of gestation to confirm a pregnancy and to evaluate the size of the gestation as compared with the dates that are determined by a woman's last menstrual period (LMP).
  - ☐ Ultrasound during the first trimester is a reliable indicator of gestational age for women who are unsure of LMP or who have very irregular menstrual cycles.
  - ☐ Ultrasound is a part of "first trimester screening." This screening evaluates the risk of Down's syndrome (Trisomy 21) as well as Edward's syndrome (Trisomy 18) and Trisomy 13. First trimester screening is optional for pregnant women. The test involves collecting a maternal blood sample for specific biologic marker levels in combination with the results of a specialized ultrasound to generate a risk assessment. This screening test is considered to be 94 to 96 percent sensitive for the above trisomies (American College of Obstetricians and Gynecologists [ACOG], 2011).
  - ☐ Ultrasound is used at 18 to 20 weeks to evaluate the fetal anatomy and to determine gender if desired by the mother.

- ☐ Ultrasound is used to evaluate fetal position.
- ☐ Ultrasound is used to measure volume of amniotic fluid.
- ☐ Ultrasound is used to assess the placenta and placental blood flow.
- ☐ Specialized ultrasounds are also performed by highly trained personnel for in-depth views of suspected abnormalities and for guidance during surgical procedures.

TIP Standard and limited ultrasounds that look at viability, malformations, and presentation of a fetus, placental evaluation, and amniotic fluid volume can be performed by trained nurses.

Routine testing done during pregnancy includes:
- Complete blood count
  - ☐ Blood type (including Rh) and antibodies
  - ☐ Sexually transmitted infections (STIs)
    - Syphilis, hepatitis, and HIV
    - Chlamydia and gonorrhea

SENC Safety Alert Chlamydial and gonorrheal infections are associated with ophthalmia neonatorum, neonatal conjunctivitis, and pneumonia in newborns (Centers for Disease Control and Prevention [CDC], 2010).

- Thyroid screening
- Rubella and varicella titers
- Cystic fibrosis screening (if genetically appropriate/desired)
- Hemoglobinopathy (an inherited blood disorder) screening (if genetically appropriate/desired)
- Other genetic screening tests are performed based on specific ethnicities and patient preference.
- Urine culture and urinalysis
- Pap smear assesses cervical cellular changes. A Pap smear is only needed if it was not done prior to pregnancy. Pap smears should be done during pregnancy based on current guidelines at the same interval as with nonpregnant women (Splete, 2012).

- Vaginal/perianal cultures for Group B streptococcus (GBS) are performed at 35 to 37 weeks. Group B streptococcus can colonize the gastrointestinal and genital tract of pregnant women without causing symptoms. Maternal colonization can cause respiratory infection in neonates and young infants via vertical (mother-to-child) transmission from the vagina to the amniotic fluid (Baker, 2012).
- Gestational diabetes tests are performed at 28 weeks, and earlier if there are specific risk factors.
  - ☐ The screening test (**glucose challenge test**) involves a 50-g oral glucose solution followed by a single plasma glucose screen 1 hour later.
  - ☐ Fasting is not required for this test. If the result is elevated, a second test, called a **glucose tolerance test** is performed. A fasting blood glucose level is drawn, followed by the consumption of a 100-g oral glucose solution. Blood samples are then collected 1, 2, and 3 hours later (four samples are collected).
  - ☐ A woman is considered to have gestational diabetes if two or more of the four samples collected are elevated (Berghella, 2012).

SENC Evidence-Based Practice Analysis of risk reduction of perinatal complications following treatment for gestational diabetes mellitus was done during a trial conducted by Landon et al (2009). In this randomized controlled trial, 958 women with gestational diabetes mellitus were assigned either to prenatal dietary advice, blood glucose monitoring and insulin therapy (treatment group), or to routine care (control group). The incidences of pre-eclampsia, large for gestational age (LGA) births, shoulder dystocia, cesarean section, and gestational hypertension were significantly reduced in the treatment group (Landon et al, 2009).

SENC Patient-Centered Care United States Preventative Services Task Force (USPSTF) along with the American Congress of Obstetricians and Gynecologists (ACOG), and the CDC recommend the above screenings for all pregnant women. Genetic carrier screening for certain conditions is recommended (CDC, 2010; Lockwood & Magriples, 2012; USPSTF, 2011; ACOG, 2017).

HEALTH HISTORY

Review of Systems

Pregnancy affects all bodily systems and is a normal, healthy process. The challenge of a review of systems for a pregnant woman is to differentiate normal and expected changes from abnormal or concerning problems. It is important to remember that changes in any body system of the pregnant woman can relate to a health problem that may affect the health of the developing fetus.

Use the OLDCARTS mnemonic (**O**nset, **L**ocation, **D**uration, **C**haracteristics, **A**ggravating/Alleviating factors, **R**elieving factors, **T**reatment, **S**everity) to identify attributes of a symptom.

SENC Patient-Centered Care Using open-ended questions and querying about normal and expected changes helps to promote trust between the nurse and patient, in addition to providing needed support and education.

Ask the patient the following questions.

Physical Concerns

- Do you have headaches, changes in your vision, swelling in your legs?
  - ☐ This cluster of symptoms is associated with pre-eclampsia and/or pregnancy-induced hypertension (PIH).

- Have you noticed any rashes and/or changes in hair, skin, or nails?
- Do you have any pain with urination or urinary frequency?
- Do you have any vaginal discharge, odor, burning, or itching?
- Do you have any of the following?
  - ☐ Nausea/Vomiting/Food aversions
  - ☐ Heartburn
  - ☐ Constipation
  - ☐ Fatigue
  - ☐ Heart racing or skipping a beat
  - ☐ Shortness of breath
  - ☐ Breast tenderness/enlargement
  - ☐ Difficulty sleeping
  - ☐ Changes in mood
  - ☐ Changes in libido

Psychosocial History

Health Promotion and Lifestyle of the Pregnant Woman
- How have you been eating? Have you been nauseous or vomited?
- Tell me about your typical diet. Do you eat fresh fruits and vegetables? Are you getting enough protein? Taking prenatal vitamins?
- Tell me about what you typically drink in a day. Are you staying well hydrated?
- What medications or substances have you used since your last visit?
  - ☐ All prescription medications should be assessed for safety during pregnancy. Illegal drugs can cause fetal and maternal harm.
- Have you been exposed to sick children or adults?
  - ☐ Infectious diseases such as cytomegalovirus, Fifth disease (parvovirus B19), and Rubella can cause fetal harm including stillbirth (de Jong, Vossen, Walther, & Lopriore, 2013).
- Have you had any falls or accidents or been hurt in any other way?

- Do you feel safe at home and outside the home? Has anyone threatened or hurt you?
- Do you have any animals in the house? Who provides care for these animals?

SENC Safety Alert Exposure to cat feces that contains the parasite toxoplasma can cause birth defects. Pregnant women should avoid contact with cat litter and should wear gloves when gardening.

Health of the Fetus
- Has your baby been moving normally for your experience?
- Have you had any signs of labor including frequent, painful contractions, pelvic pain, or low back pain?
- Have you had any vaginal bleeding or leaking of fluid from the vagina?

CULTURAL CONSIDERATIONS Prenatal care in the United States follows a prescribed plan with interval visits starting in the first trimester. This model of care may seem foreign to women of other cultures where prenatal care may be delivered in the home, infrequently, or not at all.
- Due to cultural differences and expectations about pregnancy and medical care, women from some cultures may not keep appointments for prenatal care; this should not be interpreted as a lack of concern about the pregnancy (Lowdermilk et al, 2013).
- Avoidance of prenatal visits may also be the result of concerns about modesty, particularly where male caregivers are present.
- Exploration of these issues with the patient in a gentle but honest way provides the best outcomes.
- Nurses must be aware of cultural variations among the populations with which they work. Ideas about nutrition, self-care, sexuality, clothing, and hygiene during pregnancy vary widely.

Healthy People 2020
Goal: Increasing the proportion of women who receive prenatal care in the first trimester (HHS, 2010).

SENC Evidence-Based Practice In a retrospective study of approximately 29 million births over an 8-year period between 1995 and 2002, the risk of prematurity, stillbirth, neonatal death, and infant death increased when prenatal care was not available or inadequate. The authors concluded that public health focus should be on high-quality and available prenatal care programs specifically targeting adolescents, Black and Hispanic women, and women with less than a high school education (Partridge, Balayla, Holcroft, & Abenhaim, 2012).

PREPARATION FOR ASSESSMENT

Equipment Needed

Gloves
Measuring tape
Stethoscope
Blood pressure cuff
Thermometer
Doppler ultrasound
Conducting gel
Fetoscope (optional, if Doppler is not available)

Sequence of Assessment

1. Inspection
2. Auscultation
3. Palpation

Preliminary Steps

- Maintain privacy throughout the assessment.
- Drape parts of the body for minimal exposure of the area you are examining.
- Explain all steps of the assessment to the patient.
- Ask permission to assess private areas.
- Answer patient questions.
- Keep room warm, well lit, and comfortable for the patient.
- Wash and warm hands.
- **TIP** Warm hands by washing in warm water, drying well, and then rubbing hands together.
- Gather equipment.

TECHNIQUE 23-1: **Measuring Vital Signs**

Purpose: To monitor for normal values of blood pressure, pulse, respiratory rate, and temperature. Vital signs are assessed at each prenatal visit.
Equipment: Sphygmomanometer, stethoscope, thermometer
See Chapter 6, General Survey and Assessing Vital Signs for techniques of measuring vital signs.

> **SENC Safety Alert** Measurement of BP is one of the most important aspects of prenatal care. Pregnant women may develop pregnancy-induced hypertension (PIH). Elevated BPs may also indicate the presence of pre-eclampsia, a potentially life-threatening illness. The cause of pre-eclampsia is poorly understood, but signs usually include elevations in blood pressure, proteinuria (presence of protein in the urine), and edema (Lowdermilk et al, 2013). Pre-eclampsia has no cure but can be managed so that the risk to the mother and fetus are minimized.

TECHNIQUE 23-2: **Measuring Height and Weight**

Purpose: To provide baseline information. To ensure adequate caloric intake required for healthy maintenance of pregnancy.
See Chapter 5, Assessment Techniques for techniques of measuring height and weight.
- Height is assessed at the first prenatal visit.
- Weight is assessed at each visit.

NORMAL FINDINGS
- Weight gain of 25 to 35 lb throughout the pregnancy for women with normal BMI at start of pregnancy
- Expected weight gain is 1 to 5 lb during the first trimester and 1 lb for each week of pregnancy after 12 weeks (Cunningham et al, 2014).

ABNORMAL FINDINGS
- Weight gain less than 15 lb or greater than 35 lb during the course of the pregnancy

> **SENC Safety Alert** Large, abrupt weight gains in addition to elevations in blood pressure, edema, and/or proteinuria may indicate the presence of pre-eclampsia and should be promptly reported to the healthcare provider for further assessment.

> **TIP** Inadequate or excessive weight gain that is not associated with pre-eclampsia may point to the need for dietary counselling or a referral to a nutritionist.

TECHNIQUE 23-3: **General Assessment**

Purpose: To assess for normal and abnormal signs and symptoms of pregnancy. The general assessment of pregnant women does not greatly vary from the adult examination (Box 23-3).

SENC Patient-Centered Care A key task during the health assessment of the pregnant woman is to emphasize the normality of changes associated with pregnancy. Encouraging a woman to view her pregnant body as functional and normal allows for higher self-esteem, allows for fewer complications during delivery, and promotes effective parenting (Lowdermilk et al, 2013). Active listening and providing adequate time during prenatal visits are very important parts of assessment. As pregnancy is a normative process, much of the assessment time is focused on anticipatory guidance and supportive listening.

> **BOX 23-3 Variations of General Assessment**
>
> - Skin may be oily with increased acne.
> - Texture and distribution of hair may change.
> - Striae on abdomen are normal.
> - Pigmentation of skin such as cholasma (mask of pregnancy) and linea nigra (darkly pigmented abdominal line) are normal.
> - Nasal congestion and epistaxis are common during pregnancy.
> - Diaphragmatic elevation is expected as the uterus enlarges.
> - Normal cardiac variations include venous hum, a continuous diastolic sound, and S_3, an extra heart sound, which is also known as a ventricular gallop.

TECHNIQUE 23-4: **Inspecting and Palpating the Breasts**

Purpose: To assess for tissue changes and abnormal masses
Equipment: Gloves
ASSESSMENT STEPS

1. Explain the technique to the patient.
2. Put on clean gloves.
3. Inspect the nipples for the ability to evert (turn inside out or outward); ask the woman to gently roll the areolae between her fingers one side at a time.
   TIP If a woman has inverted nipples, ask if she has been able to evert them easily. Women with inverted nipples can often breastfeed with the use of an electronic breast pump.
4. Gently squeeze each areola and nipple to inspect for the presence of colostrum.
5. Palpate the breasts for masses, nodes, and tenderness.

6. Discard gloves.

7. Document your findings.

See Chapter 18, Assessing the Female Breasts, Axillae, and Reproductive System for more detail on the breast assessment.

NORMAL FINDINGS

- More visible veins throughout the breast
- Darkening of nipples and areolae
- Enlargement of Montgomery's tubercles
- Mild tenderness
- Expression of colostrum from one or both nipples

ABNORMAL FINDINGS

- Lumps or masses
- Moderate to severe pain or tenderness
- Nipple excoriation, cracking, or bleeding

TECHNIQUE 23-5: **Inspecting and Palpating the Abdomen**

Purpose: To assess for pregnancy-related changes and fetal well-being

Equipment: Paper tape or measuring tape, Doppler ultrasound or fetoscope

ASSESSMENT STEPS

1. Explain the technique to the patient.

2. Position the pregnant woman in a semi-sitting position with knees slightly bent (Fig. 23-9).

■ **TIP** The semi-sitting position allows for uterine palpation, allows for fetal heart rate assessment, and provides for comfort by reducing the weight of the uterus on the abdominal organs and vessels (Bickley & Szilagyi, 2009).

3. Inspect the abdomen for surgical scars, striae, hair, and linea nigra (Fig. 23-10).

4. Palpate for position and changes to the abdominal organs, and assess for abdominal masses, pain, and tenderness.

■ **TIP** As pregnancy progresses and the uterus enlarges, it may not be possible to palpate abdominal organs such as the spleen, kidneys, and liver.

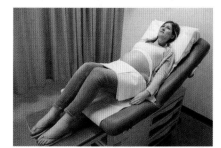

Fig. 23-9. Position of pregnant woman for abdominal exam.

SENC Safety Alert Abdominal pain in the upper abdomen that is severe, sudden, and constant is indicative of a disease process. The presence of peritoneal signs (rebound tenderness, abdominal guarding) is never normal in pregnancy (Kilpatrick & Orejuela, 2012).

5. Palpate for uterine contractions using the palmar surface of your fingers (Fig. 23-11A) or using the finger pads of both hands (bimanual palpation) (Fig. 23-11B).

6. Tightening and firming of the uterus can be felt by the examiner during uterine contractions. If the examiner's hand remains on the uterine fundus, relaxation can be palpated when the contraction ceases. Contractions are described as:
   □ mild (like the feeling of the cheek)
   □ moderate (like the feeling of the tip of the nose)
   □ strong (like the feeling of the forehead) (Murray, Huelsmann, & Koperski, 2011)

7. Palpate for fetal movement by placing the palmar surface of the hands over the abdomen. Fetal movement can usually be felt abdominally by the examiner after 24 weeks' gestation.

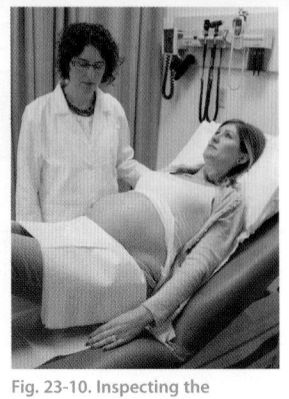

Fig. 23-10. Inspecting the pregnant abdomen.

SENC Safety Alert Pregnant women can usually feel internal fetal movement from around 16 to 20 weeks of gestation. Fetal movement in a healthy fetus can vary from 12 movements in 24 hours to 10 movements in 2 hours. When the fetus is not well, movements may be decreased, and may not be felt for one or more days. A sudden decrease in the number of fetal movements is suggestive of fetal compromise (Higgins, Johnstone, & Heazell, 2013). It is the obligation of the nurse to inform the healthcare provider about decreased or absent fetal movement.

SENC Patient-Centered Care In the case of decreased fetal movement, speak calmly and slowly to explain the concern to the pregnant woman. Position changes that increase patient comfort and fetal oxygenation are advised.

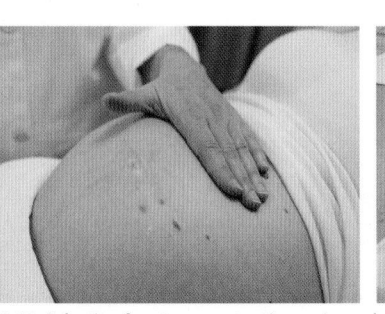

Fig. 23-11. Palpating for uterus contractions using palmar surface of fingers. (A) Manual. (B) Bimanual.

8. Palpate for fetal position using Leopold's maneuvers, illustrated and explained in Fig. 23-12 and Box 23-4.

NORMAL FINDINGS
- Striae and/or linea nigra
- Mild contractions after 38 weeks' gestation
- Fetal movement after 24 weeks' gestation
- Vertex (head down) position after 32 weeks' gestation

ABNORMAL FINDINGS
- Pain or tenderness to palpation
- Enlargement of any of the abdominal organs
- Peritoneal signs: abdominal pain, abdominal guarding and rebound tenderness
- Moderate to strong contractions that occur in a regular pattern with decreasing time between contractions prior to full term (38 weeks of gestation)
- Lack of fetal movement after 24 weeks of gestation
- Breech or transverse positions after 32 weeks of gestation

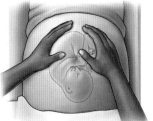

First maneuver

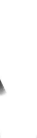

Second maneuver

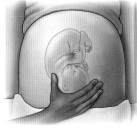

Third maneuver

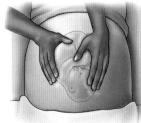

Fourth maneuver

Fig. 23-12. Leopold's maneuvers.

Technique 23–5A: **Measuring Fundal Height**

Purpose: To assess for fetal growth and volume of amniotic fluid

Equipment: Paper measuring tape

ASSESSMENT STEPS

1. Explain the technique to the patient.
2. Position the pregnant woman in a semi-sitting position with knees slightly bent (see Fig. 23-9).
3. Place the measuring tap at the top of the symphysis pubis and measure up to the top of the uterine fundus (Fig. 23-13).

   ■ **TIP** Fundal height at the level of the umbilicus roughly corresponds to 20 weeks of gestation. As an estimate, the uterus should grow 1 centimeter per week of pregnancy (±2 centimeters) through 36 weeks.
4. Record the length in centimeters.
5. Document your findings.

NORMAL FINDINGS

■ Fundal height is equal to weeks of gestation.

ABNORMAL FINDINGS

■ Fundal height that is greater than 2 centimeters above or below the weeks of gestation after 20 weeks of gestation

SENC Safety Alert Fundal heights below expected levels can indicate a small for gestational age fetus and need to be promptly reported to the healthcare provider for further assessment as they can result in fetal compromise (Lowdermilk et al, 2013). Fundal heights that are above expected heights may indicate an excess of amniotic fluid (hydramnios), uterine fibroids, multiple pregnancy, or fetal macrosomia and should also be promptly evaluated.

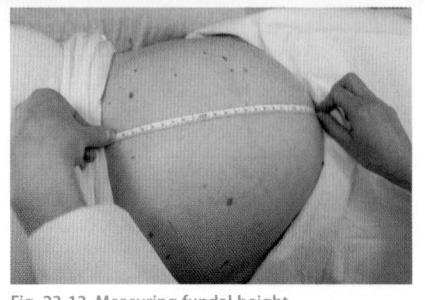

Fig. 23-13. Measuring fundal height.

Technique 23-5B: **Auscultating Fetal Heart Rate**

Purpose: To auscultate the fetal heart rate and assess for fetal viability (Box 23-5)

Equipment: Doppler stethoscope, fetoscope

ASSESSMENT STEPS

1. Explain the technique to the patient.
2. Position the pregnant woman in a semi-sitting position with knees slightly bent (see Fig. 23-9).
3. Place the Doppler ultrasound in the midline of the abdomen below the umbilicus.

   ■ **TIP** Fetal position affects where fetal heart sounds are heard. Performing Leopold's maneuvers before fetal auscultation guides the nurse where to place the Doppler to listen for the fetal heart rate.

4. Auscultate the fetal heart using a Doppler (beginning at around 10 weeks of gestation), or with a fetoscope (beginning at 18 weeks) (Durham & Chapman, 2013) (Fig. 23-14).
5. Document your findings (Box 23-5).

NORMAL FINDINGS

■ Fetal heart rate between 120 and 160 bpm

ABNORMAL FINDINGS

■ Fetal heart rate outside of the normal range of 120 to 160 bpm
■ Decelerations: slowing of the heart rate
■ Accelerations: elevated fetal heart rate above 160 bpm
■ Arrhythmia: irregular heart rate
■ Absent heart rate

BOX 23-5 **Definitions for Fetal Monitoring**

- **Baseline fetal heart rate (FHR):** a mean (average) FHR rounded to increments of five beats per minute (bpm) during a 10-minute segment of tracing expressed as a single number (for example, "135")
- **Variability:** fluctuations in the FHR baseline that are two cycles per minute or more and that are irregular in amplitude and frequency
- **Accelerations:** a visually apparent increase in the FHR (onset to peak in less than 30 sec)
- **Early decelerations:** in association with a uterine contraction, a visually apparent, gradual (onset to nadir 30 sec or more) decrease in FHR
- **Late decelerations:** a visually apparent gradual decrease (onset to nadir is ≥30 sec) of FHR below baseline
- **Variable decelerations:** a visually apparent abrupt decrease in the FHR (onset to nadir less than 30 sec)
- **Reassuring (normal) FHR pattern:** presence of fetal heart rate accelerations, usually indicating that there is no academia; generally indicative of fetal well-being

Adapted from the 2008 National Institute of Child Health and Human Development workshop report on electronic fetal monitoring (Macones, Hankins, Spong, Hauth, & Moore, 2008).

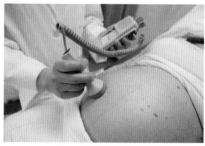

Fig. 23-14. Auscultating fetal heart with Doppler.

PATIENT EDUCATION

Healthy People 2020

Goals: Healthy People 2020 goals include the following:

- Increase the proportion of women delivering a live birth who received preconception care services and practiced key recommended preconception health behaviors.
- Improve pregnancy planning and spacing, and prevent unintended pregnancy.
- Reduce cesarean births among low-risk (full-term, singleton, vertex presentation) women.
- Reduce preterm births.
- Increase abstinence from alcohol, cigarettes, and illicit drugs among pregnant women.

Maternal and Fetal Health Promotion

Teaching about pregnancy begins prior to conception and continues through pregnancy and into the postpartum period. The focus of pregnancy teaching is to optimize maternal and fetal health and well-being. Some topics of focus include:

- contraception, family planning, and birth spacing
- nutrition, including vitamin intake and weight gain
- exercise
- safety, including seat belts
- travel
- warning signs
- when and how to call a provider
- vaccinations
- medications
- substance use and abuse
- work and environmental concerns
- sexual activity
- birth choices and options
- breastfeeding.

Assessment of the pregnant woman at regular intervals contributes to overall maternal and fetal health and well-being. Thorough assessments are critical to ensuring the welfare of pregnant women. Nurses directly impact the health and safety of mother and fetus by providing education and support; the effect of nursing interventions throughout pregnancy is lifelong.

CHAPTER 24

Assessing the Older Adult

INTRODUCTION

Aging is a universal, normal, inevitable biological phenomenon (Velhal, 2012). In the United States, life expectancy for women is 81 years and for men it is 76 years (Arias, 2016). For the first time since 1993, the CDC (2016) reported that life expectancy in the United States declined to 78.8 years, with women continuing to have a longer life expectancy than men. Most developed world countries have accepted the chronological age of 65 years as a definition of "elderly" or older person; however, there is no general agreement on the age at which a person becomes old (World Health Organization [WHO], 2016a). In 2011, the first baby boomers (adults born between 1946 and 1964) turned 65. In 2050, the number of people age 65 and older is expected to grow from 83.7 million (U.S. Census Bureau, 2014). Many people are able to age in good health and remain active participants in society throughout their lives. But others experience physical and cognitive limitations and may lose the ability to live independently (WHO, 2013a). Older adults want to maintain their quality of life for as long as they are physically and mentally able to care for themselves. The geriatric assessment is a multifaceted approach that focuses on understanding the physical, cognitive, psychological, and social domains of an older adult (Carlson, Merel, & Yukawa, 2015).

REVIEW OF ANATOMY AND PHYSIOLOGY

Nurses need the knowledge about common physiological changes that occur as an individual ages. The following are common physical changes and assessment findings.

Skin

Skin changes are the most visible signs of aging that are influenced by environmental, genetic, and lifestyle behaviors.
- The epidermal layer of skin becomes thinner and more fragile.
- Blood vessels in the dermal layer become more fragile and have a tendency to rupture and pool throughout the dermal layer.
- The number of nerve endings in the skin decreases, causing decreased sensation and sensitivity to pain.
- There is decreased function of the sweat glands; decreased perspiration and sweating.
- Sebaceous glands produce less oil; skin becomes dry and pale.
- The subcutaneous fat layer thins providing less insulation.
- Wrinkling of the skin is seen, especially in the chin and neck area.
  TIP Smoking causes increased wrinkling and premature aging of the skin.
- Skin pores become large and plugged with dead skin.

- Aging pigmented spots or lesions may appear on the skin.
- Narrowing of the arteries causes reduced peripheral circulation.

SENC Safety Alert Assess patients with decreased cognition and chronic illness for alterations in skin integrity; these patients may be more likely to be at risk for skin breakdown (See Box 24-2 for Risk Factors for Skin Breakdown).

Hair

- Less melanin is being produced causing hair to turn gray or white.
- Men's eyebrows and hair in their ears and nose become bushier, longer, and coarser.
- Women may begin to lose hair or develop facial hair due to hormonal changes.
- A decrease in hormones causes thinning of hair or hair loss of the scalp, axillary, and pubic areas.
- Senescent alopecia occurs when hair follicles produce thinner, smaller hairs or none at all.

Mouth

- Decreased sense of taste
- Less saliva is produced causing a dry mouth.
- Teeth wear down or fall out; gums recede increasing risk for periodontal disease.

Ears

Hearing loss affects approximately one third of adults 61 to 70 years of age and more than 80 percent of those older than 85 years. Men usually experience greater hearing loss and have earlier onset compared with women (Walling & Dickson, 2012).

- Hearing begins to decline because the cells within the organ of Corti are not replaced; therefore, there is a gradual loss of hearing as the person ages; decreased ability to discriminate sounds.
- Tympanic membrane in the ear becomes dull gray and less flexible.
- There is an increased accumulation of ear cerumen.
- Increased hair growth occurs in the outer ear canal.

Eyes

SENC Safety Alert Older adults have difficulty adapting to darkness; there is an increased risk of stumbling or falling when moving from dark to light environments and vice versa (Watson, 2009).

- Cornea curvature decreases and sight begins to decline.
- Slower pupillary reflex
- Pupils are smaller but equal in size; may react more sluggishly to light
- Loss of color discrimination
- Decreased production of lacrimal (tear) secretions; eyes become drier
- Decreased orbital and ciliary muscle strength
- Increased opacity and clouding of the lens; lens loses its elasticity

SENC Safety Alert The older adult has a need for brighter light; as people age, seeing in dim light becomes more difficult because the lens tends to become less transparent (Besdine, 2013).

TIP Visual changes among aging adults include problems with reading speed, seeing in dim light, reading small print, and locating objects (American Psychological Association, 2013).

Nose

- Reduction in the surface area of the olfactory epithelium
- Sense of smell decreases with a decreased ability to discriminate between smells (Blair, 2012)
- **Anosmia** is the inability to smell

Respiratory System

- Bone structure and density decrease in the thorax and vertebrae decreasing lung expansion.
- Vital capacity of the lung decreases.
- The number of alveoli decrease resulting in decreased perfusion and exchange of oxygen and carbon dioxide at the alveolar level.
- Lungs have less recoil and elasticity; causes increased demands to breathe and increased risk for shortness of breath.
- Cough reflex is decreased.
- Overall body changes in muscular strength, skeletal structure, and mobility, in addition to cardiovascular function, result in changes in pulmonary function.
- Decreased thirst response, and less moisture within the mucous membranes of the upper and lower respiratory tracts contribute to thickened mucus (Frederick, 2014).
- Lungs have less ability to fight off infection because the cells that sweep debris containing microorganisms out of the airways are less able to do so.

TIP Older adults are particularly susceptible to respiratory diseases. Signs of infection many not be as obvious (Mauk, 2013).

Cardiovascular System

TIP Nearly 40 percent of all deaths among those 65 and older can be attributed to heart problems. By age 80, men are nine times more likely to die of chronic heart failure than they were at age 50 (National Institute on Aging, 2016).

- Vasculature and valves within the heart become more rigid.
- The heart muscle becomes thinner, decreases in strength, and becomes less compliant; however, a thickening (hypertrophy) in the left ventricle is common.
- Decrease in elasticity and increased stiffness of the arterial system
- Loss of atrial pacemaker cells and bundle of HIS fibers can decrease the electrical activity in the heart; heart rate slows down.

- The heart's pumping mechanism declines and arterial resistance increases causing an increase in blood pressure (BP).
- The ability to meet cardiac output demands with increased workload is decreased.
- A S_3 or S_4 heart sound may be a sign of heart failure (HF) or cardiomyopathy, and weakening of the heart muscle.
- Jugular vein distention, swollen legs/feet, and/or shortness of breath may be signs of HF
- The S_4 heart sound is commonly heard due to decreased ventricular compliance and impaired ventricular filling; related to the stiffness of the ventricle as one ages.
- A widened pulse pressure (difference between systolic and diastolic pressures) may occur which is related to vascular vessel stiffness.
- More commonly, heart murmurs are auscultated related to changes in the structure and stiffness of heart valves.
- Chest pain may indicate angina (tissue ischemia).
- Atrial fibrillation (AF) is the most common arrhythmia in older adults (Tang, Ma, Dong, Yu, & Long, 2014). It is a fast irregular heartbeat. Older adults may experience symptoms of heart palpitations, dizziness, and shortness of breath. These patients are prescribed an anticoagulant to prevent blood clots from developing in the arterial system.

SENC Safety Alert Older adults may take medications that have the side effect of orthostatic hypotension. Reinforce to patients to change positions slowly to prevent dizziness and falls.

- Plaque accumulation in the arteries causes atherosclerosis and coronary artery disease (CAD) (Fig. 24-1).

TIP Older adults have a higher risk for developing CAD and peripheral arterial disease (PAD) due to an accumulation of plaque in the arteries throughout their body.

Peripheral Vascular System and Regional Lymphatics

- Elastic arteries show two major physical changes with age; they dilate and stiffen.

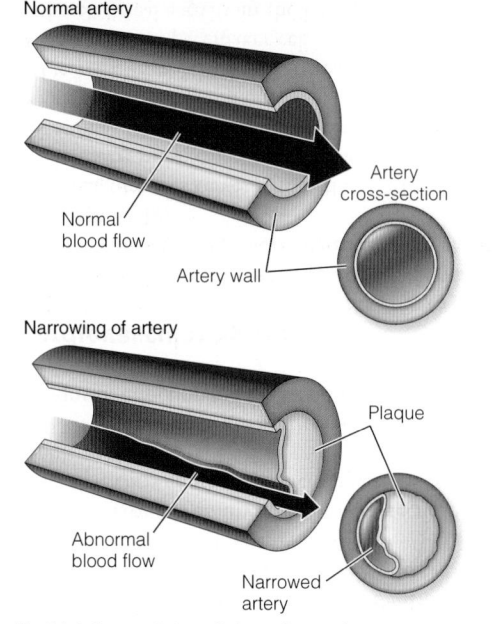

Normal artery

Artery
cross-section

Normal
blood flow

Artery wall

Narrowing of artery

Plaque

Abnormal
blood flow

Narrowed
artery

Fig. 24-1. Accumulation of plaque in arteries.

■ Less arterial compliance and increased risk for calcification of the arterial walls (Lionkis, Mendrinos, Sanidas, Favatas, & Georgopoulou, 2012).
■ Vein valves weaken causing increased risk of varicosities especially in the lower legs.
■ Veins bulge on the upper arm extremities with thin, frail, older adults.
■ Lymph nodes may decrease in numbers with aging influencing the immune system to lose its ability to fight off infections.

■ Immune system is less tolerant of its own cells; there is an increased risk for autoimmune diseases to develop (Dugdale, 2012).

Abdomen

■ Fatty tissue increases in the abdominal area and abdominal muscles weaken; older individuals have a tendency to have a "pot belly" appearance.
■ Gastric acidity is reduced in the elderly and may alter absorption of medications (Lehne, 2013); less lactase is produced causing an increased risk for lactose intolerance.
■ Pernicious anemia is a vitamin B_{12} deficiency caused by a decreased number of red blood cells.
■ Liver cells (hepatocytes) decrease; decreased blood circulation through the liver.

SENC Safety Alert The liver is the major organ to metabolize medications; if liver function declines, drug metabolism declines, causing increased risk for elderly to have accumulation of drugs and place them at risk for drug toxicity.

■ Liver mass and blood supply in the liver decrease with age; the liver's metabolic and detoxification ability is reduced.
■ Gall bladder has decreased function with slower emptying time which causes increased accumulation of biliary sludge and risk for gallstones.
■ Pancreatic enzymes, amylase and lipase, decrease in production causing malabsorption of essential nutrients.
■ Intestines have decreased peristalsis related to weakening in the smooth muscle wall.

TIP Older adults may suffer from chronic constipation; it is not uncommon to hear patients tell you that they use several laxatives; many times patients are embarrassed to report constipation; ask the patient about diet, exercise, and current medications and remedies to relieve constipation.

Kidneys and Bladder

SENC Safety Alert The older adult may have a decline in kidney functioning; it is important to assess the amount of medications an older adult takes because drug excretion may be reduced causing drugs to accumulate in the system.

- The number of nephrons and the overall amount of kidney tissue decreases, affecting the kidneys' ability to function properly.
- Blood vessels supplying the kidney can become hardened, and the kidneys filter blood more slowly.
- The muscles of the bladder weaken, and patients may experience incontinence or prolapse of the bladder; the bladder may not empty completely when urinating, and patients may have problems with urinary retention.

SENC Safety Alert Decreased renal output and glomerular filtration impair the kidney's ability to excrete sodium; this places the older adult at higher risk for hypertension; advise older adults to limit their salt intake.

- Older adults have an increased risk for urinary incontinence and urinary tract symptoms due to the aging of the bladder muscle that leads to a decrease in the bladder's capacity to store urine. Urinary incontinence is involuntary urination. There are four types of incontinence:
  1. **Stress** incontinence is leaking small amounts of urine with intra-abdominal pressure such as with coughing, sneezing, and exercising; may be related to the weakening of the pelvic floor muscles.
  2. **Urge** incontinence is the sudden urge to urinate.
  3. **Overflow** incontinence is caused by weakened bladder muscle or urethral blockage, causing an overflow of urine; individuals cannot completely empty their bladder.
  4. **Functional** incontinence occurs more often with older individuals with chronic arthritis, Parkinson's disease or Alzheimer's disease;

these individuals are unable to control their bladder before reaching the bathroom due to limitations in moving related to a physical or cognitive disability.

TIP Mixed incontinence shares the causes and symptoms of both stress and urge incontinence.

Musculoskeletal System

- Bones becomes less dense, and individuals are at risk for osteoporosis; bones that are weakened more than others are:
  - □ femur at the hip
  - □ the radius and ulna at the wrist
  - □ the vertebrae of the spine

    TIP Bone changes may be influenced by decreased intake of calcium and vitamin D, medications (i.e., steroids), smoking, and lack of weight-bearing exercises (Blair, 2012).

- Atrophy, skeletal muscle loss, or muscle wasting may occur.
- Joint surfaces lose cartilage and connective tissue.
- Muscles begin to lose fibers and degenerate.
- Tendons and ligaments stiffen.
- Height loss is related to aging changes in the bones, muscles, and joints (Fig. 24-2).

DIAGNOSTICS

Dual-energy x-ray absorptiometry (DEXA) is a form of x-ray technology that is used to measure bone loss. DEXA is the gold standard method for the evaluation of diagnosis and fracture risk in elderly (Naharci, Kocak, & Doruk, 2012) and to measure bone density.

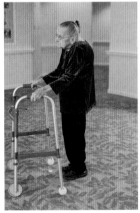

Fig. 24-2. Height loss related to aging.

Neurological System

- Brain and spinal cord begin to lose nerve cells and neural impulses begin to slow down causing a decrease in sensations and reflexes.
- Brain loses weight as the nerve cells die; these nerve cells are not usually replaced.
- Decline in balance

Breasts and Female Reproductive System

- Breast loses alveolar, glandular, and lobular tissue.
- Breasts begin to sag due to relaxation of the suspensory ligaments.
- Nipples become softer, smaller, and less erect.
- Vulva and genitalia shrink; vaginal secretions diminish causing the vagina to become dry.
- The vagina thins and loses elasticity due to decreased estrogen levels; uterine prolapse may occur.
- Women may begin to have a decreased interest in sexual activity.
- Atrophic changes occur in the external genitalia.
- Pubic hair thins and starts to turn gray.

Male Genitalia and Reproductive System

- Scrotum thins and testes drop lower in the scrotal sac.
- Penis shrinks and becomes smaller.
- There is increased incidence of problems with erectile dysfunction.
- Benign prostatic hypertrophy (BPH) is an enlargement of the prostate gland, may cause hesitancy, urine retention, and difficulty starting the stream in older men.

DIAGNOSTICS

- There are no significant changes in laboratory data in the older adult; however, some changes are affected by the physiology of aging (Blair, 2012). The following bloodwork is routinely ordered:

- Complete metabolic panel to assess electrolytes and kidney functioning
- Albumin and protein levels to assess nutritional stores
- Fasting blood sugars and hemoglobin A1C to assess diabetes
- Lipid panels to measure cholesterol and triglyceride levels
- Blood urea nitrogen (BUN) and creatinine levels to assess kidney functioning and for dehydration
- International normalized ratio (INR) is a test to measure blood clotting; used to monitor patients who are on warfarin (Coumadin), an oral anticoagulant to prevent blood clots.
- Because anemia is common in older adults, some levels that you may assess are:
  - ☐ Vitamin B_{12} levels are frequently monitored in the older adult; this vitamin is essential in DNA synthesis, hematopoiesis (creating new blood cells in the body), and central nervous system integrity (Van Leeuwen, Poelhuis-Leth, & Vroomen-Durning, 2013); lack of vitamin B_{12} may cause neurological damage and a diagnosis of pernicious anemia.
  - ☐ Serum iron levels assess red blood cell function; a low iron level is indicative of iron deficiency anemia.

CULTURAL CONSIDERATIONS Older adults may be part of a cultural group that values specific healthcare beliefs and practices (Wallace, 2008); a cultural assessment will help to identify specific healthcare practices.

- English may be a second language for older adults and the patient may have difficulty understanding (Jimenez, Cook, Bartels, & Alegria, 2012). If English is a patient's second language, an interpreter may be needed to obtain a health history.
- Some cultures designate a specific family member to make all the decisions; some cultures believe that the older adult should not be told his or her diagnosis and that it should only be shared with family members (Wallace, 2008); this needs to be respected.
- The American Psychological Association (2013) reports:

- older Americans are predominantly Caucasian, but the demographics of older America will undergo a dramatic transformation in the next few decades.
- the number of older African Americans will triple by the middle of the next century, moving them from 8 to 10 percent of Americans over age 65.
- the older Hispanic population will increase 11-fold, going from representing fewer than 4 percent of today's older adults to representing nearly 16 percent of older adults.
- the onset of chronic illness in minorities is usually earlier than in Caucasians.

HEALTH HISTORY

Collecting the health history of an older adult can be challenging for the patient and the nurse. The older adult may not have textbook presentations but may have atypical presentations and present differently. The term "geriatric syndrome" is used to capture those clinical conditions in older persons that do not fit into discrete disease categories (Strandberg et al., 2013). Symptoms of the geriatric syndrome may be found in Box 24-1.

■ During the interview, older adults will often share lifetime stories and reminisce or recall information about past experiences.
■ To obtain a good history, pay attention to detail, both verbal and nonverbal body language (Galvin, 2009).

SENC Patient-Centered Care Older adults often have cognitive and affective problems that make history taking difficult (Cress & Barber, 2007). You must have patience and understanding while collecting data. Do not rush the patient during the interview.

■ Assess the reliability of the patient.
    TIP The best way to assess reliability is to ask the patient questions to which you can confirm the answers. For instance, asking the patient's name, date of birth, place of residence, date and time, or names of his or her children or significant other; use secondary resources to validate the information is correct.
■ Explain what you are going to do in simple terms.
■ Ask short, simple, clear, open-ended, and focused questions.
■ Secondary sources (e.g., significant others, caregivers) may be needed to provide information on any concerns or symptoms the patient may be demonstrating if the individual cannot give a reliable health history.
■ Obtaining a family health history for familial risk factors and psychosocial history is necessary in a comprehensive assessment. However, it may be difficult for the older adult to recall specific information.

The review of systems (ROS) and physical assessment for the older adult are the same as for any adult. (See Chapter 3.) Use the OLDCARTS

BOX 24-1 **Signs and Symptoms of the Geriatric Syndrome**	
Anorexia	Impaired hearing
Dementia	Impaired vision
Dizziness	Malnutrition
Falls	Parkinson disease
Frailty	Pressure ulcers
Gait instability	Sleep complaints
Impaired cognition	Vertigo

mnemonic (**O**nset, **L**ocation, **D**uration, **C**haracteristics, **A**ggravating/ **A**lleviating factors, **R**elieving factors, **T**reatment, **S**everity) to identify attributes of a symptom.

TIP Sometimes patients do not know that their hearing aid battery is dead or do not know how to change their hearing aid batteries. Patients who have difficulty hearing speak loudly. You may also have to adjust your voice to be of low-pitched tone and speak loudly.

- Introduce yourself and tell the patient the purpose of your encounter.
- Respect every patient. Most older adults grew up in a time when one would not think of addressing an older adult by his or her first name (Nicklin, 2006). All patients should be addressed by their last name out of respect, unless they specifically say to call them by their first name.
- Do not use medical jargon.
- Working with older adults takes time; be patient and allow for extra time.
- Communicate with the patient in a compassionate and caring manner; make sure the patient hears and understands you.
- Reduce background noise so the patient is able to hear your questions clearly.
- Older adults experience feeling cold more often than the middle-aged adult. Provide a warm, comfortable environment.
- Be observant to whether the patient becomes short of breath during the interview; this may be a sign of respiratory disease.
- Minimize position changes; assist the patient as needed with position changes.
- Older individuals may be cognitively impaired making it difficult to assess the patient. (See Chapter 2.)
- Communicate directly with the older adult; if cognitively impaired, the patient's significant other, family member, or caregiver may help

to provide information. However, you still should ask the patient's permission.

- Patients with dementia or Alzheimer's disease may be uncooperative or restless during the assessment; be calm, reassuring and use clear, simple, one-step directions.
- The older adult may need assistance getting undressed and dressed as well as changing positions.

Psychosocial Assessment

Each population has special needs and considerations. The physical assessment is the same as for any adult except there are some special gerontological considerations. Particular attention should be given to the following assessment areas: living arrangements, functional assessment, falls, health promotion, driving, alcohol use, elder abuse, and sexuality.

Residential Living

There are many available living arrangements for the older adult such as single family home in retirement communities, senior housing apartment communities, assisted living facilities, rest homes or boarding houses, and skilled nursing care.

Ask the patient:
- Where do you live?
- Do you live alone? If not, with whom do you live?
- Are you comfortable where you are living now?
- Do you feel safe where you are living now?
- If you had a medical emergency, who and how would you call for help?

SENC Safety Alert Older adults who live independently should know how and whom to call in case of a medical or environmental emergency. Patients may wear a medical alert device to call for help when needed. Nurses should assess and recommend such a device if the patient lives alone.

Health Promotion

Today, the older adult is more informed about health promotion and caring for self. The Internet has become a resource for many aging individuals to increase their knowledge about health promotion activities, medications, diseases, and treatments. Many older adults are motivated to become more health conscious about diet, exercise, the need to stay active, and the need to maintain relationships and connections. However, all adults may not be aware of the importance of staying involved. As one ages, his or her social network may diminish. The National Institute on Aging (2015) recommends provisions for social support and involvement in social activities to foster positive effects on the health and longevity in older adults. Information related to social interactions should be assessed.

Ask the patient:

■ Do you have a spouse or significant other?
■ Whom do you consider to be your family?
■ Do you have friends who you socialize with?
■ Are you involved in any community activities or belong to a senior center?

Sleep

A common report of insomnia and changes in sleep patterns are part of the normal aging process. Some commonly reported changes in sleep patterns are as follows (National Sleep Foundation, 2009):

■ Stages 3 and 4 (deep sleep) decrease, and stage 1 (light sleep) increases.
■ Difficulty falling asleep
■ Nap more often during the daytime hours
■ Have frequent awakenings during the night
■ Insomnia related to pain or chronic health problems

Ask the patient:

■ What time do you usually go to bed, and what time do you wake up?
■ Do you feel rested when you wake up in the morning?
■ Do you nap during the day? If so, how many times during the day and for what period of time?

TIP Adults with progressive dementia or Alzheimer's disease will sleep throughout the day and night.

■ Do you take any medication to help you fall asleep?
■ Do you have sleep apnea? If so, do you use a continuous positive airway pressure (CPAP) machine?

SENC Safety Alert Sleep apnea is cessation of breathing for 10 or more seconds which causes oxygen saturation levels to drop. As the individual ages, muscle tone decreases within the muscles of the upper airway resulting in a more relaxed airway and airway occlusion. This places the older adult at risk for stroke or sudden death (Peters, 2013).

Medications

As one ages, organ systems begin to decline, and the intake of prescribed and over-the-counter (OTC) medications increases. Nurses must perform a thorough medication assessment. The elderly constitute 12 percent of the U.S. population and consume 31 percent of the nation's prescribed drugs (Lehne, 2013).

Polypharmacy continues to be an ongoing problem among older adults. Polypharmacy is frequently identified by the use of:

■ multiple medications
■ multiple prescribers
■ several filling pharmacies
■ too many forms of medication
■ medications taken when there is no clinical indication
■ multiple dosing schedules

Perform a thorough medication assessment. (See Chapter 3.)

TIP It is recommended that the older adult bring with her or him all the medications taken on a regular basis or bring a written list for your review.

SENC Patient-Centered Care Patients need to be educated on adherence to a medication regimen. Between 25 and 59 percent of older adult patients do not take their medications as prescribed. Most cases (75 percent) of nonadherence among older adults are intentional due to cost or side effects of the drugs (Lehne, 2013).

SENC Safety Alert The older adult may not review the expiration date of medications in the medication cabinet. Ask patients if they check the medication cabinet for expired medications at least once a year. Encourage patients to check their medication cabinets at the same time that they change their clocks for daylight savings time or when their smoke detector batteries are changed annually.

Pain Assessment

Older adults are able to give reliable self-reports of levels of pain using different measures. (See Pain Assessment Chapter 7.)

- When assessing pain in the older adult, be alert to the cognitive status of the patient (Malstrom & Tait, 2010).
- Older adults may not be able to report their pain accurately; some may be unwilling to report pain (Tsai, 2011).
- Close observation of the patient's nonverbal body language and behavior is essential when assessing this type of patient. Examples of nonverbal body language are restlessness, facial grimacing, frequent change in positions, and incomprehensible sounds.

Functional Assessment

Functional status is the patient's ability to care for him- or herself and meet essential tasks for daily life. Screening older adults for functional limitations has been identified as a "vital sign" (Studenski et al., 2003). The Barthel index of basic activities of daily living (ADLs) is considered a "core" to functional assessment (Appendix 24-1). The focus of the assessment must be on the patient and how he or she perceives his or her current level of functioning.

Nutritional Assessment

Older persons are vulnerable to malnutrition (WHO, 2016b), and inadequate micronutrient intake is common in older persons (Elsawy & Higgins, 2011). When assessing the older adult's nutrition, a nutritional assessment tool should be as ethnically specific as possible to account for cultural and anthropometric differences across populations (Tsai, Chang, Chen, & Yang, 2009). Modifiable risk factors such as weight, exercise, and diet influence health and the risk for developing chronic diseases. Older adults who are underweight (body mass index [BMI] less than 19) or overweight (BMI greater than 25) often have loss of muscle mass, a compromised immune system, and risk of health complications.

Ask the patient:

- How would you describe your appetite?
- Do you have your own teeth or dentures?
- Do you have any difficulty with chewing solid foods?
- Do you have any difficulty swallowing fluids?
- Do you notice any changes in your sense of taste?
- Tell me what you ate yesterday starting from the time you woke up.

SENC Safety Alert Unintentional weight loss may be influenced by decreased cognition, chronic or acute disease, or psychosocial factors. You must compare the patient's current weight with previous known weights and assess for weight loss.

Mini Nutritional Assessment (MNA)

The Mini Nutritional Assessment (MNA) is the most validated nutritional screening and assessment tool that can identify geriatric patients age 65 and above who are malnourished or at risk of malnutrition. It consists of six questions, streamlines the screening process, and is available in several languages (Nestle Nutrition Institute, n.d.) (Appendix 24-2).

This essential assessment tool is used in any type of setting. The user guide for the MNA tool is found at http://www.mna-elderly.com/forms/mna_guide_english.pdf and the free phone app can be downloaded from http://www.mna-elderly.com/mna_forms.html.

Assess for signs of poor nutrition:

- Anorexia (decreased appetite)
- Bleeding and inflamed gums
- Brittle hair and nails
- Pale conjunctiva
- Decreased urinary output
- Dry skin with decreased skin turgor
- Dry cracked or chapped lips
- Eyes appear sunken
- Fatigue and weakness
- Wounds that do not heal

Driving With Advancing Age

Motor vehicle injuries are the leading cause of injury-related deaths among 65- to 74-year-olds and are the second leading cause (after falls) among 75- to 84-year-olds. While traffic safety programs have reduced the fatality rate for drivers under age 65, the fatality rate for older drivers has consistently remained high (AARP, 2013). When you take the patient's history, be alert to "red flags"—that is, any medical condition, medications, or a symptom that can affect driving skills, either through acute effects or chronic functional deficits. Some symptoms to be alert to are:

- impaired personal care such as poor hygiene and grooming
- impaired ambulation such as difficulty walking or getting into and out of chairs
- difficulty with visual tasks
- impaired attention, memory, language expression, or comprehension

Ask the patient:

- Are you able to read signs easily?
- Can you recognize someone you know from across the street?
- Are you able to see street markings, other cars, people walking, especially at dawn, dusk, and at night?
- How do you handle headlight glare at night? (National Highway Traffic Association, n.d.)

The American Association of Retired Persons (AARP) (2010) has identified warning signs for when to stop driving. These are as follows:

- Almost crashing, with frequent "close calls"
- Finding dents and scrapes on the car, on fences, mailboxes, garage doors, curbs, etc.
- Getting lost, especially in familiar locations
- Having trouble seeing or following traffic signals, road signs, and pavement markings
- Responding more slowly to unexpected situations, or having trouble moving their foot from the gas to the brake pedal; confusing the two pedals
- Misjudging gaps in traffic at intersections and on highway entrance and exit ramps
- Experiencing road rage or causing other drivers to honk or complain
- Easily becoming distracted or having difficulty concentrating while driving
- Having a hard time turning around to check the rear view while backing up or changing lanes
- Receiving multiple traffic tickets or warnings from law enforcement

Alcohol Use

In the United States, 17.6 million people, about 1 in every 12 adults, abuse alcohol or are alcohol dependent (NIAAA, 2011). In general, more men than women are alcohol dependent or have alcohol problems. In this population, alcoholism is more challenging to assess and diagnose due to chronic illness, polypharmacy, and cognitive disorders. Older adults are more sensitive to the effects of alcohol. Women are more sensitive to the effects of alcohol than men. As people age, there is a decrease in the amount of water in the body, so when older adults drink, there is less water in their bodies to dilute the alcohol that is consumed. This causes older adults to have a higher blood alcohol concentration (BAC) than younger people after consuming an equal amount of alcohol (NIH Senior Health, 2015). Medications can have adverse interactions with alcohol. The older adult alcoholic usually:

- is male
- is grieving due to loss of spouse, family, or friends
- is socially isolated and lonely
- has comorbid psychiatric illness such as depression or anxiety
- has family history of alcohol dependence
- precipitated by losses, loneliness, social isolation, medical or psychiatric comorbidities
- has poor personal hygiene (Mahgoub, 2009).

The National Institute of Alcohol Abuse and Alcoholism (2011) makes the following recommendations:

- Adults over age 65 who are healthy and do not take medications should not have more than:
  - □ three drinks on a given day
  - □ seven drinks in a week.

Assess older adults for alcoholism using the CAGE questionnaire. (See Chapter 3, Psychosocial Assessment.)

Elder Abuse

SENC Safety Alert One out of 10 older adults experiences some form of abuse or neglect by a caregiver each year, and the incidence is expected to increase (Hoover & Polson, 2014).

During the assessment, it is essential that nurses assess for signs of elder abuse. Elder abuse is a growing, underreported problem. This type of abuse can affect people of all ethnic backgrounds and social status and can affect both men and women (National Center on Elder Abuse [NCEA], n.d.). The older adult is particularly vulnerable to elder abuse because they are more likely to suffer acute or chronic conditions resulting in physical or mental impairments.

■ **TIP** Most elder abuse is committed by relatives, spouses, significant others, and caregivers. The responsibilities and demands of elder caregiving, which escalate as the elder's condition deteriorates, can be very stressful to the caregiver.

According to the National Center for Elder Abuse (NCEA), there are seven types of elder abuse (Table 24-1).

■ **TIP** Many older adults do not report the abuse because they fear retaliation from the abuser; others believe that if they turn in their abusers, no one else will take care of them. Parents who are being abused by their children do not report because they do not want their children to get in trouble with the law.

It is essential for nurses to be alert to signs of elder abuse by:

- listening to seniors and their caregivers
- intervening when you suspect elder abuse
- educating others about how to recognize and report elder abuse.

  ■ **TIP** The laws in most states require helping professions in the front-line health-care providers to report suspected abuse or neglect. These professionals are called *mandated reporters* (NCEA, n.d.).

Sexuality

Humans are sexual beings from birth until death. Sexuality does not end when one reaches a certain age, nor does it end with the diagnosis of a chronic illness (Wilmoth, 2014). Sexual health has long been considered within the functional health patterns of nursing assessment and management (Wallace, 2013). Sexuality is not widely covered in nursing education programs, especially in relation to the care of older adults, so nurses are often uncomfortable assessing sexual issues (Wallace, 2008). Sexual

TABLE 24-1 Types of Elder Abuse

Physical abuse	The use of physical force that can result in bodily injury, physical pain, or impairment
Sexual abuse	Nonconsensual sexual contact of any kind with an elderly adult
Abandonment	The desertion of an older person by an individual who has assumed responsibility for providing care for the older adult or by a person with physical custody
Emotional or psychological abuse	The infliction of anguish, pain, or distress through verbal or nonverbal acts
Financial or material exploitation	The illegal or improper use of an older adult's funds, property, or assets
Neglect	The refusal or failure to fulfill any part of a person's obligations or duties to an older adult; refusal or failure to provide an elderly person with such life necessities
Self-neglect	A person's refusal or failure to provide himself/herself with adequate food, water, clothing, shelter, personal hygiene, medication, and safety precautions

National Center on Elder Abuse. *Major types of elder abuse*. Available at http://ncea.aoa.gov/FAQ/Type_Abuse/

interest and function is a very sensitive topic to discuss with the older patient. Older adults may not be as active as in their younger years but continue to have sexual relationships and sexual desire. Provide privacy and be sensitive to any discussion.

Ask the patient:

■ Are you involved in an intimate or sexual relationship with a partner?
  □ Intimacy involves a physical communion with another person but also involves intellectual or emotional closeness; each component

may be experienced separately with another person or two or three of the components may be shared with another person (Brown, 2012, p. 206).

■ Can you tell me how you express your sexuality?
■ What concerns or questions do you have about fulfilling your continuing sexual needs?
■ In what ways has your sexual relationship with your partner changed as you have aged? (Wallace, 2000)

FOCUSED ASSESSMENT

TECHNIQUE 24-1: **Surveying the Whole Person**

Purpose: To assess the general well-being and behavior of the patient

The assessment begins with a general observation of the patient when you first meet and greet the patient and continues throughout the entire assessment. During the general survey, use your senses of sight, hearing, and smell. As you progress through the comprehensive focused, or follow-up assessment, you will collect more specific subjective and objective data.

CULTURAL CONSIDERATIONS Always take the age and cultural considerations of the patient into account when completing a general survey.

ASSESSMENT STEPS

1. Greet the patient and introduce yourself to the patient (Fig. 24-3).
2. Explain your role and the sequencing of the assessment.
3. As you begin interviewing the patient, make the following general observations about the patient:

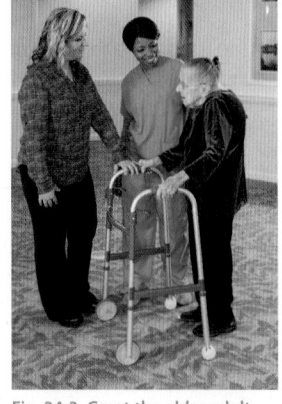

☐ **Physical appearance**
  • Health: does the patient look healthy or ill?
  • Age: does the patient look his or her stated age?
  • Patient hygiene, grooming, appropriate dress for climate or season; note body odors and breath
  • Body structure: tall, short, muscular, thin, or overweight; symmetry of body structures
  • Posture: is the patient able to stand up straight?
  • Mobility: is the patient able to walk or in need of assistive devices?
☐ **Behavior and mental status**
  • Level of consciousness: alertness and orientation
  • Reliable or unreliable when answering questions
  • Behavior: calm, cooperative, eye contact, clarity of speech
☐ **Facial expression:** relaxed, stressed, frowning, facial grimacing, symmetrical
☐ **Mood:** happy, depressed, flat affect, agitated
☐ **Speech:** clear, difficulty articulating words, slurring speech
4. Document your findings.

Fig. 24-3. Greet the older adult and inspect general appearance.

NORMAL FINDINGS
■ **Health:** Appears healthy with no signs of illness or debilitation
■ **Physical appearance:** Age: patient looks stated age; hygiene: well groomed, appropriately dressed for climate, no odors; body structure: well built, symmetrical body structures

- **Mobility:** gait steady and symmetrical, no difficulty walking; posture: stands straight, sits up straight without support; range of motion: ability to move all joints and extremities, actively participates in the assessment
- **Posture:** able to stand up straight (Fig. 24-4)
- **Level of consciousness:** alert and oriented × 4 (person, place, time, situation); calm and cooperative; may or may not have direct eye contact (depends on culture), speech clear, facial expression relaxed and symmetrical; mood calm; reports understanding reason for assessment
- **Reliability:** understands questions and is able to answer
- **Facial expression:** relaxed with no signs of discomfort
- **Speech:** clear
- **Distress:** no signs of general discomfort or pain; no signs of cardiac or respiratory distress

ABNORMAL FINDINGS

- **Physical appearance**
  - ☐ Frailty, cachectic (wasting syndrome), tired, may be a sign of acute or chronic illness
  - ☐ Age: patient looks much older than stated age; may indicate chronic stress or illness
  - ☐ Patient hygiene: unkempt grooming, inappropriate dress for climate, clothing that is too tight or too loose, odors of the body or breath, weight gain or weight loss; may indicate mental status or cognitive dysfunction
  - ☐ Body structure: tall, short, muscular, thin, or overweight (Chapter 6, Nutritional Assessment); symmetry of body structures (Chapter 17, Neurological Assessment)
- **Mobility**
  - ☐ Gait and posture: Unsteady difficulty walking, limping, poor posture, use of assistive devices (walker, cane, wheelchair) (Chapter 16, Musculoskeletal System)
  - ☐ Range of motion: inability to move all joints and extremities; unable to participate in the examination (Chapter 16, Musculoskeletal System)
- **Behavior and mental status**
  - ☐ Level of consciousness: disoriented, decreased mentation (Chapter 3, Psychosocial Assessment; Chapter 17, Neurological Assessment)
  - ☐ Behavior: inappropriate (Chapter 3, Psychosocial Assessment; Chapter 17 Neurological Assessment)
  - ☐ Mood: depressed, flat affect (Chapter 3, Psychosocial Assessment)
  - ☐ Speech: difficulty articulating words, slurring speech (Chapter 17, Neurological Assessment)
  - ☐ Unreliable when giving answers
- **Distress:** signs of respiratory distress (Chapter 12, Respiratory System), signs of cardiac distress (Chapter 13, Cardiovascular System), signs of pain (Chapter 7, Pain Assessment).

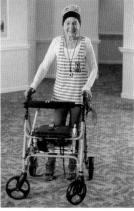

Fig. 24-4. Posture.

TECHNIQUE 24-2: **Assessing Height, Weight, and Body Mass Index**

Body mass index (BMI) is a measure of body fat based on height and weight that applies to adult men and women.

Purpose: To assess for body fat

Equipment: Scale, stadiometer, BMI chart

■ **TIP** Always compare the current weight with previous weight measurements.

ASSESSMENT STEPS

1. Ask patient to remove shoes and place feet together before measuring height.

■ **TIP** If shoes are left on for safety reasons, document that patient was weighed with shoes on.

2. Measure the patient's height by standing upright under a stadiometer.

3. Carefully lower the horizontal bar until it touches the top of the patient's head.

4. Record the measurement.

5. Weigh the patient on a scale (Fig. 24-5).

■ **TIP** Scales need to be calibrated to zero prior to taking the patient's weight; when using a calibrated balance-beam scale, balance the scale by sliding both weight bars to zero.

6. Look at a BMI chart to identify where on the chart the height and weight intersect for the BMI.

7. Record and interpret the BMI number.

8. Document height, weight, and BMI.

■ **TIP** Be aware that BMI numbers decrease in the older adult patient.

NORMAL FINDINGS

■ BMI is between 18.5 and 24.9.

ABNORMAL FINDINGS

■ BMI less than or equal to 18.5: underweight

■ BMI greater than or equal to 25 to 29.9: overweight

■ BMI 30 or higher: obese (CDC, 2016)

SENC **Safety Alert** For the older adult, monitor for a 5 percent weight loss in 1 month and a 10 percent weight loss in 6 months.

SENC **Evidence-Based Practice** Evidence links malnutrition to worse clinical outcomes, increased hospital stays, a longer duration of convalescence, a reduced quality of life, increased morbidity, and increased mortality in the general patient population (Freeman, 2012).

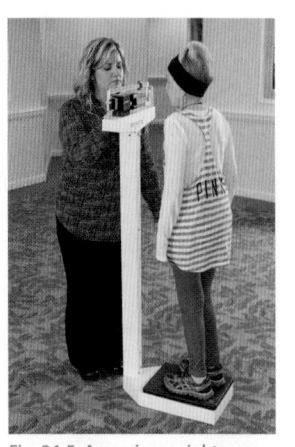

Fig. 24-5. Assessing weight.

TECHNIQUE 24-3: **Assessing Oral Temperature**

Purpose: To assess the core body temperature
Equipment: Electronic thermometer

▇ **TIP** Always make sure your thermometer is fully charged and calibrated.
The oral sublingual site has a rich blood supply from the carotid arteries that quickly responds to changes in inner core temperature.

▇ **TIP** The oral temperature should not be used on a patient who cannot follow directions to keep her or his mouth closed, has decreased mentation, or breathes through his or her mouth.

ASSESSMENT STEPS

1. Take the thermometer off the charger prior to assessing the patient.
2. Explain the procedure to the patient.
3. Ask the patient if he or she has smoked or consumed any hot or cold foods or beverages in the last 30 minutes, if so, wait until 30 minutes has passed to maintain the accuracy of the reading.
4. Take the thermometer probe out of the holder and attach a plastic disposable probe cover.
5. Ask the patient to open his or her mouth and lift up the tongue.
6. Gently place the thermometer probe underneath the tongue (sublingually).
7. Ask the patient to gently but firmly close her or his mouth.
8. Observe the calculation of the thermometer; a sound or blinking will occur as the temperature reading registers.
9. Dispose of the dispensable thermometer probe cover.
10. Return the thermometer to the charger.
11. Document the site and temperature reading.

NORMAL FINDINGS

■ 97.7°F to 99.5°F or 36°C to 38°C

ABNORMAL FINDINGS

■ Less than 97.7°F to greater than 100°F or less than 36.5°C to greater than 37.8°C

TECHNIQUE 24-4: **Assessing Tympanic Temperature**

Purpose: To assess the core body temperature
Equipment: Tympanic thermometer

ASSESSMENT STEPS

1. Explain the procedure to the patient.
2. Take the tympanic thermometer off the charging stand.
3. Attach a clear dispensable plastic ear probe.
4. Gently pull the upper earlobe up and back.
5. Insert the ear probe snugly pointing it toward the tympanic membrane.
6. Push the button to register the temperature reading.
7. Once the temperature reading registers, dispose of the dispensable thermometer probe cover.
8. Return the thermometer to the charger.
9. Document the site and temperature reading.

NORMAL FINDINGS

■ 98.2°F to 100°F or 36.8°C to 37.8°C

ABNORMAL FINDINGS

■ Less than 98.2°F to greater than 100°F or less than 36.8°C to greater than 37.8°C

TECHNIQUE 24-5: **Palpating the Radial Pulse**

Purpose: To assess the heartbeat through the wall of the radial peripheral artery at the wrist

ASSESSMENT STEPS

1. Explain the technique to the patient.

2. Gently place your second and third finger pads of your dominant hand on the radial artery at the flexor aspect of the wrist laterally along the radius bone. While palpating the pulsation, note the following characteristics of the pulse:

□ Rhythm of the pulse: regular versus irregular; missed or paused beats; or an abnormal pattern of beats

□ Amplitude (strength) of the pulse is the force of the blood in the arterial system. This is measured on a scale of 0 to 3. (See Chapter 6, Table 6-2.)

■ **TIP** Compare pulses on both sides to make sure they have the same rate, rhythm, and amplitude.

3. Holding your watch in the opposite hand, start counting the pulsations (heartbeats) for 30 seconds starting the count with number 1.

4. If the heartbeat is regular, multiply this number by 2; if the heart rate is irregular, take a radial pulse for 60 seconds.

5. Now, take the pulse on the opposite wrist and compare the numbers.

6. Document both sites of the pulse, pulse rate, rhythm, and amplitude.

NORMAL FINDINGS

■ Rate: resting pulse: 60 to 100 bpm

■ Rhythm: regular

■ Amplitude: 2+

ABNORMAL FINDINGS

■ Pulse rate less than 60 and greater than 100

■ Rhythm: irregular with pauses may be indicative of an irregular heart rate (arrhythmia).

■ Amplitude: absent (no heart rate), weak (decreased stroke volume), or bounding (increased stroke volume) may be indicative of changes in the circulatory system.

■ **TIP** Review the patient's medication list. Older adults commonly take cardiac medications that slow down the heart rate.

TECHNIQUE 24-6: **Auscultating an Apical Pulse**

Purpose: To assess the heart rate
Equipment: Stethoscope, watch with a second hand
ASSESSMENT STEPS
1. Explain the technique to the patient.
2. Warm the stethoscope.
3. Uncover the left side of the patient's chest.
4. Gently place the diaphragm of the stethoscope directly over the left fifth intercostal space at the midclavicular line (apex of the heart).
5. Auscultate the heartbeat, assessing the rate and rhythm.
6. Count the beats per minute for 30 seconds, then multiple by 2; if irregular, count the beats for 60 seconds.
7. Wipe off the stethoscope with an alcohol swab to clean the diaphragm.
8. Document the site and apical pulse rate.
NORMAL FINDINGS
■ Rate: resting pulse: 60 to 100 bpm
■ Rhythm: regular
ABNORMAL FINDINGS
■ Pulse rate less than 60 and greater than 100
■ Rhythm: irregular with pauses may be indicative of an irregular heart rate (arrhythmia).

TECHNIQUE 24-7: **Assessing the Respiratory Rate**

Purpose: To assess the pulmonary ventilation
Equipment: Watch with a second hand
TIP The best time to take a respiratory rate is after taking the pulse without the patient knowing that you are counting his or her respirations.

1. Observe the patient's rise (inspiration) and fall (expiration) of the chest area.
2. Observe the following characteristics of the respirations:
   ☐ Depth: even pattern, deep or shallow respirations
   ☐ Rhythm: regular or irregular
   ☐ Effort: amount of work required to take a breath
3. Count the number of respirations for 30 seconds and multiply by 2; if irregular, count the number of respirations for 60 seconds.
4. Document the rate, depth, rhythm, and effort.

NORMAL FINDINGS
■ 12 to 18 breaths per minute; pattern is even; rhythm is regular.

ABNORMAL FINDINGS
■ Less than 12 breaths and greater than 18 breaths per minute
■ Depth: deep or shallow respirations
■ Rhythm: irregular
■ Effort: using accessory muscles to breathe
   ☐ Specific abnormalities of respiratory rates (see Chapter 12, Table 12-1)

TECHNIQUE 24-8: **Assessing Blood Pressure in the Upper Arm**

Purpose: To assess circulatory blood volume as the heart contracts and relaxes
Equipment: Manual sphygmomanometer, stethoscope, Electronic BP automated device (optional)
ASSESSMENT STEPS

1. Explain the technique to your patient.
2. Ask the patient if she or he has smoked or had any caffeine in the last 30 minutes; if no, proceed to take the BP; if yes, wait until 30 minutes has lapsed.
3. If the patient is ambulatory, have patient sit in a chair with his or her feet flat on the floor for 5 minutes.
4. Ask the patient not to move, talk, or cross the legs while taking the reading (Hyatt, 2011).
5. If sitting, seat the patient comfortably with back supported, legs uncrossed, and palm facing up, the arm resting at the level of the fourth intercostal space (heart level) and not tensed; if the patient is in supine position in the bed, place the arm flat with palm facing up on a pillow so that the arm is at heart's level.

6. Use a paper measuring tape, and measure the circumference of the midpoint of the upper arm between the shoulder and the elbow; choose the correct cuff size for your patient. (See Chapter 6, Table 6-4.)

7. Wrap the deflated cuff around the patient's arm about 2.5 cm (1 inch) above the brachial artery and wrap evenly; make sure the artery marker is pointing to the brachial artery.

8. Have the patient support the bare arm on the examination table or in your arm at the patient's heart level.

9. Turn the manual valve clockwise on the BP cuff to close it.

10. Palpate the brachial artery at the antecubital fossa or the radial artery at the wrist, and continue to feel for the pulsation of the brachial or radial artery.

11. Start squeezing the bulb at the end of the rubber tube attached to the BP cuff, inflating the BP cuff until you no longer feel the pulsation of the brachial artery; make note of this number on the sphygmomanometer. Release the manual valve to deflate the BP cuff.

12. Place the bell or diaphragm of the stethoscope on the brachial artery, and inflate the BP cuff 30 to 40 mm Hg above the palpable systolic BP number (Anderson, 2009).

13. Slowly release the manual valve (2 to 3 mm/s) to deflate the BP cuff, and listen for the first rhythmic Korotkoff sounds heard as blood begins to flow through the artery; this first sound is the systolic reading.

14. Continue to listen as the BP cuff pressure is released, for the last Korotkoff sound that you are able to hear; this last sound is the diastolic reading.

15. Document your findings.

NORMAL FINDINGS

- Normotensive (normal BP); aged 60 years or older less than 140/90 mm Hg
- Systolic hypertension (systolic blood pressure is >140 and diastolic is <90) is a common assessment finding for the older adult.

    TIP Increased arterial stiffness is the reason for developing systolic hypertension, especially of the large arteries. Elevated systolic BP is even more associated with cardiovascular morbidity and mortality than diastolic BP (Duprez, 2012).

ABNORMAL FINDINGS

- Hypotension is BP below 90/60.
- Hypertension is BP greater than 150 systolic or greater than 90 diastolic.

SENC Safety Alert Older adults often complain of dizziness, placing them at risk for falls; take orthostatic BPs to identify orthostatic hypotension. (See Chapter 6, Technique 6-6.)

TECHNIQUE 24-9: **Inspecting and Palpating the Skin**

Purpose: To identify changes in skin, including rashes, lesions, masses, and abnormal moles

SENC **Safety Alert** Always wear gloves if skin has an open area to protect yourself from bacteria or germs.

ASSESSMENT STEPS

1. Inspect the patient's hygiene, including odors of the body or breath.
2. Inspect the patient's color.
  ☐ Assess for cyanosis in the lips, oral mucosa, and tongue.
  ☐ Assess for pallor of skin in the lips, fingernails, and mucus membranes.
  ☐ Assess for jaundice of skin in the lips, sclera of the eyes, and across the rest of the body.
3. Palpate for temperature, comparing side to side using the dorsal surface of your hand.
4. Palpate skin thickness. Remember that skin thickness varies. The thinnest skin is found on the eyelids, and the thickest areas of skin are found on the soles of the feet, palms of the hands, and elbows. Assess the hands and feet for calluses caused by pressure areas and rubbing (Fig. 24-6).
5. Palpate skin turgor.
6. Palpate skin moisture.
7. Assess rashes, lesions, scars, and masses, making sure to identify location, distribution, pattern and configuration, color, and size, making sure to use a ruler to measure in centimeters.
8. Document your findings.

NORMAL FINDINGS
■ Good hygiene, no odors
■ Uniform color
■ Skin warm, moist
■ No abnormal lesions (see Abnormal Findings)
■ **Nevi** are uniform brown color, regular borders, less than 0.6 cm.

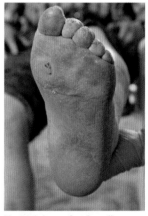

Fig. 24-6. Assess feet for calluses or pressure areas.

- **Acrochordon** (skin tag) is composed of skin and subcutaneous tissue; soft hanging skin commonly occurring on the trunk, armpits, and under the arms (Fig. 24-7).
- **Solar lentigo** (liver spots) are hyperpigmented macular lesions commonly seen on the exposed body surface areas (Fig. 24-8).
- **Cherry hemangiomas** are small, bright cherry red spots seen on the trunk and extremities; usually are the size of a pinhead or one-quarter-inch diameter (Bermin, 2012) (Fig. 24-9).
- **Seborrheic keratosis** are noncancerous pigmented waxy lesions; color ranges from light tan, brown, to black (Fig. 24-10).
- **Cutaneous horn** is caused by an overgrowth of keratin that resembles a miniature horn; may be normal or malignant; vary in color from yellow to brown or black; referral to a dermatologist is recommended (Stoppard, 2014) (Fig. 24-11).
- **Senile purpura** are areas of ruptured fragile capillaries and bruising of the skin; caused by loss of subcutaneous fat (Fig. 24-12).

SENC Safety Alert As a person ages, the skin becomes thin and fragile increasing the risk for skin tears. Immobility, decreased nutrition, dehydration, and incontinence place the older adult at higher risk for skin breakdown and pressure ulcers (Box 24-2); wounds take longer to heal. Nurses have to be cautious when handling older adults because of their thin skin; nurses need to check the skin more often for potential areas of breakdown.

ABNORMAL FINDINGS

- **Changes in a pre-existing lesion.** Use the ABCDE mnemonic to note changes (Box 24-3) in lesions that may indicate signs of a malignancy.

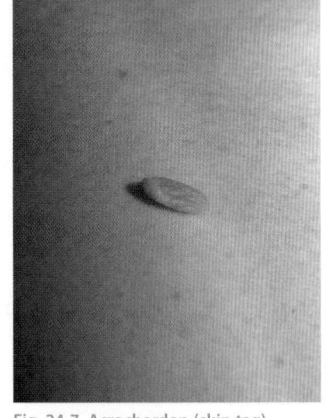

Fig. 24-7. Acrochordon (skin tag).

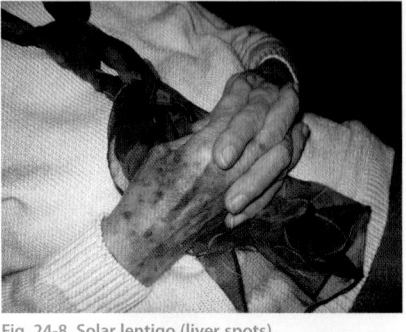

Fig. 24-8. Solar lentigo (liver spots).

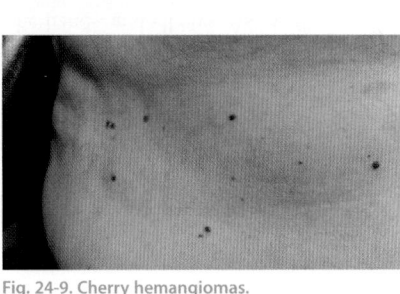

Fig. 24-9. Cherry hemangiomas.

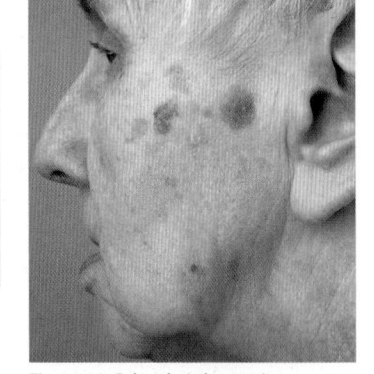

Fig. 24-10. Seborrheic keratosis.

BOX 24-2 Risk Factors for Skin Breakdown

Aging	Frailty
Bony prominences	Immobility
Diabetes	Incontinence
Cognitive impairment	Malnutrition
Chronic disabilities	Obesity
Dehydration	Polypharmacy
Depression	Reduced mobility
Diabetes	Reduced peripheral sensation
Dry skin	Weight loss

BOX 24-3 ABCDE Mnemonic for Changes in a Lesion

Asymmetry   **D**iameter greater than 6 mm
Border irregularity   **E**volution or **e**volving
Change in color

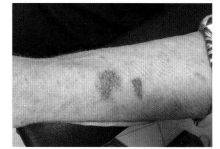

Fig. 24-12. Senile purpura.

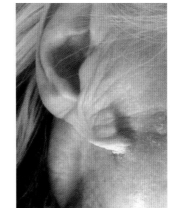

Fig. 24-11. Cutaneous horn.

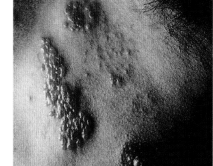

Fig. 24-13. Shingles.

- **Actinic keratosis** is a rough, scaly patch that most often develops on chronically sun-exposed areas such as the face, the dorsum of the hands and forearms, the upper chest, and the scalp of bald men (Sarnoff, 2014); often described as "stuck-on cornflakes" (Wheeler, 2009); commonly seen in Caucasian older adults.
  ▨ **TIP** Basal cell carcinomas are the most common cancerous lesions seen in the older population.
- **Shingles** (herpes zoster) is caused by the varicella-zoster virus, the same virus that causes chicken pox. The vesicular lesion develops into a rash that presents on one side of the body where the dormant virus reactivates; the rash is painful and forms blisters and may take weeks to resolve. Older individuals are at greater risk because their immune response decreases with age (Fig. 24-13).
  ▨ **TIP** The vaccine for shingles (Zostavax) is recommended for use in people 60 years old and older to prevent shingles. The older a person is, the more severe the effects of shingles typically are, so all adults 60 years old or older are encouraged to get the shingles vaccine (CDC, 2016).
- **Petechiae** or **purpura** may indicate a clotting or liver disorder.

- **Erythema** may indicate inflammation or excoriation or open wounds of the skin
- **Tenting of skin** commonly seen in the abdomen in older adults may indicate dehydration or weight loss.

    SENC Safety Alert Older adults may be at increased risk for fungal infections due to decreased immune system and increased use of medications altering the normal healthy bacteria. Assess the skin for rashes and the mouth for thrush; thrush is oral candidiasis, a fungus infection characterized by raised white patches on the tongue and/or buccal mucosa.

HEAD, HAIR, SCALP

TECHNIQUE 24-10: **Inspecting and Palpating the Head, Hair, and Scalp**

Purpose: To assess for changes or abnormalities in the head, hair, and scalp
Equipment: Gloves
ASSESSMENT STEPS
1. Put on gloves
2. Inspect the patient's head for:
   ☐ size
   ☐ shape
   ☐ configuration
   ☐ movement.
3. Palpate the head and assess for masses or depressions.
4. Assess general condition of the hair, including amount, distribution, and cleanliness.
5. Assess the condition of the scalp; inspect scalp skin and color, and inspect for lesions.
6. Assess hair color.
7. Assess hair texture (thick, brittle, curly).
8. Document your findings.
NORMAL FINDINGS
- Head is symmetric, midline, round.
- Normocephalic; a person's head and all major organs of the head are in normal condition and without significant abnormalities.
- Head erect and still; no involuntary movements
- No pain, tenderness, masses, or depressions during palpation
- Hair clean, curly, or straight texture; uniform thickness and distribution

- Color brown, black, blonde, red, white, or gray
- Scalp clean and intact, no lesions

ABNORMAL FINDINGS

- Pain
- Tenderness
- A mass
- Involuntary movements
- Depression of the skull
- **Alopecia,** defined as hair loss, may be due to nutritional deficiencies, medications, illness, endocrine disorders, radiation, or the physiological changes of aging.
- **Alopecia areata** of scalp, or spot baldness, is a loss of hair in patches involving the scalp or beard; thought to be related to an autoimmune disorder.
- **Folliculitis** is inflammation of a hair follicle developing on the face, arms, legs, or buttocks; white pustules appear around the hair follicle; may be related to *Staphylococcus aureus* infection.
- **Seborrheic dermatitis** is a chronic, greasy scale that accumulates and thickens on the scalp with or without redness; may extend to the forehead, eyebrows, and face.

FINGERNAILS AND TOENAILS

TECHNIQUE 24-11: **Inspecting and Palpating the Fingernails and Toenails**

Purpose: To assess for healthy nails or presence of vitamin deficiency, malnutrition, disease, or infection

ASSESSMENT STEPS

1. Inspect general condition of the nails, including cleanliness, thinness, and thickness.
2. Inspect color and markings.
3. Inspect adherence to nailbed.
4. Inspect shape and contour.
5. Perform the capillary refill test. (See Chapter 15, Technique 15-5.)
6. Document your findings.

NORMAL FINDINGS
- Nails smooth, short, uniform thickness, well groomed
- Nail base angle 160 degrees
- Firmly adhere to the nailbed
- Nailbeds pink
- Capillary refill less than 3 seconds
- Nontender to palpation
- No redness, exudates, or signs of infection or inflammation
- Dark-skinned individuals have pigmented bands in their nails.
- Nails may become brittle or hard and thick, especially the toenails.
- Color of the nails may change from clear to dull or opaque color.
- Longitudinal ridges may form; tips of fingernails may become brittle and split.

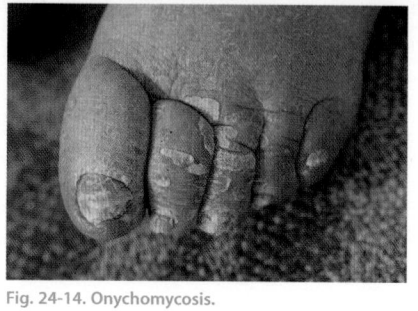

Fig. 24-14. Onychomycosis.

ABNORMAL FINDINGS
- Changes in color, shape, texture, or thickness indicate an abnormal finding.
- **Beau's line** is a white, horizontal groove across the nailbed; usually caused by disease, toxic reaction, or trauma.
- **Onychomycosis** is thickening, yellow discoloration, and scaling of the nailbed due to a fungal infection; more common in diabetics and older adults (Fig. 24-14).

SENC Patient-Centered Care Older adults may not be able to wash their feet or cut their toenails; a referral to a podiatrist may be recommended. Older adults who are diabetics should see a podiatrist regularly.

FACE

TECHNIQUE 24-12: **Inspecting the Face**

Purpose: To assess facial appearance and symmetry

ASSESSMENT STEPS
1. Stand in front of the patient and assess for the shape of the face:
   - ☐ Round
   - ☐ Square
   - ☐ Oval

2. Assess for symmetry of the face (CN VII).
   □ Nasolabial folds (the distance from the corner of each nostril to the corner of the lip bilaterally); should be equal measurements
   □ Palpebral fissures; measure the distance between the upper and lower eyelids; should be equal measurement
3. Assess for facial expression.
   □ Does the patient make eye contact?
   □ Flat affect
   □ Sad or happy affect
4. Assess for involuntary movements.
5. Assess the condition and texture of the skin.
6. Assess for edema.
7. Document your findings.

NORMAL FINDINGS
- Face (round, oval, or square)
- Bilaterally symmetrical facial structures
- Nasolabial folds and palpebral fissures equal
- Expression relaxed
- No involuntary muscle movement; no visible pulsations
- Skin smooth and clear
- No edema

ABNORMAL FINDINGS
- Asymmetry of the face may be related to abscess, infection, enlargement of parotid gland, neurological disorders.
- Flat affect may indicate depression.
- Parkinson's disease causes a "masklike" facial appearance.
- Kidney diseases may cause swelling of the face or around the eyes (periorbital edema).
- Cardiac, respiratory, and autoimmune disorders may present with different facial changes.

TECHNIQUE 24-13: **Palpating the Face**

Purpose: To assess tenderness, swelling, and inflammation
ASSESSMENT STEPS
Stand in front of the patient and assess for the following:
1. Using the finger pads of both hands, gently palpate the face for tenderness and swelling.

2. Place your fingers anterior to the tragus palpate to the corner of the eyes and palpate the temporal arteries simultaneously anterior to each ear to assess for tenderness or inflammation.

3. Place your fingertips anterior to each ear at the zygomatic arch and ask the patient to open and close his or her mouth. Assess for any clicking sounds or decreased range of motion (ROM) of the jaw, including TMJ disease.

4. Document your findings.

NORMAL FINDINGS

■ No tenderness

■ Temporal arteries nontender

■ TMJ has no clicking sounds or limited ROM. Mouth opens on the average 3 to 6 cm and moves laterally 1 to 2 cm.

ABNORMAL FINDINGS

■ Temporal arteritis is an inflammation of the temporal arteries and blood vessels that supply blood to the head; cause is unknown; patients may complain of a throbbing headache on one side of the head, fever, jaw pain, and tenderness of the face and temporal area.

■ TMJ syndrome causes a clicking, popping, or grating sound; limited movement of the mouth; headaches, jaw, tooth, or ear pain.

TECHNIQUE 24-14: **Inspecting and Palpating the Nose**

Purpose: To assess for tenderness, inflammation, or deviation.

ASSESSMENT STEPS

1. Stand in front of the person and inspect the nose for the following:
  □ Symmetry
  □ Alignment of septum
  □ Color
  □ Swelling

2. Gently palpate the nose for tenderness or swelling.

3. Document your findings.

NORMAL FINDINGS

■ Nose symmetrical

■ Septum straight and midline

■ Skin color same as face

■ No lesions, swelling, or deformity

ABNORMAL FINDINGS

■ Asymmetry

■ Deviated septum

- Swelling or inflammation
- Redness, bruising, lesions
- Tenderness or swelling while palpating

TECHNIQUE 24-15: **Assessing the Patency of the Nose**

Purpose: To assess for nasal passageway occlusion

ASSESSMENT STEPS

1. Ask the patient to press on the right naris to occlude the passageway.

2. Ask the patient to inhale through the left naris with his mouth closed.

3. Ask the patient to press on the left naris to occlude the passageway.

4. Ask the patient to inhale through the right naris with his mouth closed.

5. Document your findings.

NORMAL FINDINGS

- Each nasal passageway is patent.
- Decreased sense of smell

ABNORMAL FINDINGS

- Absence of sniff may be an indication of nasal congestion or obstruction; obstruction may be related to a foreign object.
- Rhinitis may be related to a viral or bacterial infection.
- Nasal polyp is a soft, painless, noncancerous growth on the lining of the nasal passages or sinuses.

TECHNIQUE 24-16: **Palpating the Maxillary and Frontal Sinuses**

TIP Percussion may be done instead of palpating the sinuses. Tap over the maxillary and frontal sinuses instead of palpating.

Purpose: To assess for allergies or infection.

ASSESSMENT STEPS

Stand in front of the patient and assess the following:

1. Place your thumbs slightly below the eyebrows.

2. Press up and under the eyebrows, palpating the frontal sinuses.

3. Assess for tenderness or pain.

4. Now, place your thumbs below the cheekbones, palpating the maxillary sinuses.

5. Assess for tenderness or pain.

6. Document your findings.

NORMAL FINDINGS

■ No tenderness or pain is felt.

ABNORMAL FINDINGS

■ Tenderness or pain may indicate allergies or a sinus infection.

TECHNIQUE 24-17: **Inspecting and Palpating the Mouth**

Purpose: To assess the structures of the mouth for redness, inflammation, lesions, or abnormalities

Equipment: Penlight and gloves

> **SENC Safety Alert** Always wear clean, nonsterile gloves for this part of the assessment, because you will be coming in contact with the patient's saliva.

> **TIP** You need good lighting for visualization of all structures in the mouth and throat. Assess from the front of the mouth and work toward the back of the throat. Some older adults may not be able to follow directions or open their mouth wide.

> **SENC Patient-Centered Care** While assessing the mouth, the patient will have to keep his or her mouth wide open. It may take some time. If you observe that the patient is having difficulty doing that, have him or her close the mouth for a rest period.

TECHNIQUE 24-18: **Inspecting the Lips**

> **TIP** Women should remove lipstick prior to this assessment.

Purpose: To assess shape and integrity of the lips

ASSESSMENT STEPS

1. Put on gloves.

2. Stand in front of the patient and inspect the lips for:

☐ symmetry

☐ color

☐ moisture

☐ lesions

☐ swelling

- Lips are symmetric
- Upper lip is everted
- Pink, moist, no lesions, swelling, or cracking of skin

ABNORMAL FINDINGS
- Lips are inverted
- Swelling, erythema, lesions, cracking of skin
    - ■ **TIP** A sore that does not heal in the mouth requires further evaluation.
    - □ **Angular cheilitis** are sore, cracked corners of the lips; commonly caused by yeast infections, dry mouth, or vitamin deficiency.
    - □ **Angioedema** is edema of the lips; usually related to an allergic reaction.
- Pallor of lips may indicate decreased perfusion related to respiratory or cardiovascular problems.
    - □ **Herpes simplex virus** manifests with cold sores or blisters on the lips.

TECHNIQUE 24-19: **Inspecting the Teeth**

Purpose: To assess for position, number, and integrity of teeth
1. Inspect the teeth for:
- □ dentures, caps, or missing teeth
- □ color

2. Ask the patient to clench teeth and assess for malocclusion, malposition of the teeth.
- ■ **TIP** Adults have between 28 and 32 teeth. Ask people if they have dentures or implants.

NORMAL FINDINGS
- Color of teeth white to an ivory color (Fig. 24-15)
    - ■ **TIP** Teeth may be stained yellow from smoking or brown from drinking tea or coffee.
- Clean, free of debris
- Smooth edges
- 32 teeth or 28 teeth if wisdom teeth have been removed
    - □ The upper incisors should overlap the lower incisors; back teeth should meet.

ABNORMAL FINDINGS
- Loose, broken, painful teeth; surfaces of the teeth may be worn off and decaying (Fig. 24-16).
- Malocclusion of the teeth

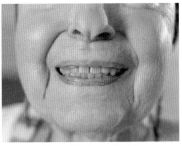

Fig. 24-15. Normal findings of teeth.

- Loss of teeth or rotting teeth
- Gums begin to recede trapping food and causing decay, increasing the risk for periodontal disease.
- Ill-fitting dentures cause difficulty eating.

SENC Safety Alert Poor fitting dentures, fewer or no teeth may attribute to unintentional weight loss.

- Missing teeth, discolored teeth, or no teeth
- Teeth appear longer, gums recede.
- Tooth decay and periodontal disease in the older adult can lead to loss of teeth and infection.

SENC Safety Alert Periodontal disease has also been linked to stroke and coronary artery disease (CAD); the more severe the periodontitis, the greater the risk for heart problems (University of Maryland Medical Center, 2009a).

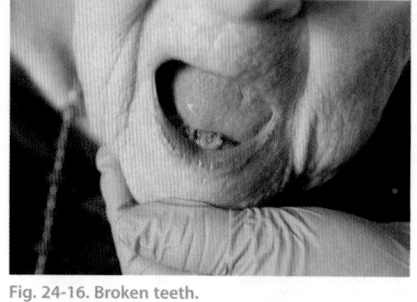
Fig. 24-16. Broken teeth.

- Taste buds decrease causing a decreased sensation of taste.

TIP One type of taste disorder (dysgeusia) is characterized by a persistent bad taste in the mouth, such as a bitter or salty taste. It occurs in older people, usually because of medications, poor nutrition, smoking, or oral health problems (Sorllitto, 2013).

TECHNIQUE 24-20: **Inspecting and Palpating the Buccal Mucosa**

Purpose: To assess for inflammation, lesions, or abnormalities

ASSESSMENT STEPS

1. If a patient has full or partial dentures, have her or him remove the dentures for inspection and palpation of gum area.

2. Inspect and palpate the buccal mucosa and gums.

3. Gently use a tongue blade to hold the tongue out of the way for full visualization of the gums and mucosa.

NORMAL FINDINGS

- Pink, smooth, moist, no lesions, swelling, or bleeding
- Tight margin around each tooth
- No tenderness with palpation
- Halitosis, or bad breath, may occur due to a dry mouth
- Xerostomia is dry mouth; less saliva is being produced

- Red, inflamed, or bleeding mucosa; lesions
- Tenderness with palpation
  - □ **Aphthous stomatitis** (canker sore) is the most common nontraumatic form of oral ulceration with 20 to 40 percent incidence in the population; ulcer formation is the main clinical presentation (Jefferson, 2011).
  - □ **Thrush** is a candidiasis fungal infection that creates thick, white to yellow patches on the tongue or buccal mucosa; occurs frequently with a weakened immune system and antibiotic therapy.
  - □ **Gingivitis** is the mildest type of periodontal disease; red, swollen, bleeding gums.
  - □ **Gingival hyperplasia** is an enlargement or overgrowth of the gum tissue; firm and nonpainful; may be related to systemic illness, side effects of medications such as phenytoin (Dilantin), and poor oral hygiene.
  - □ **Periodontal disease** is a chronic infection of the gums and is caused by bacteria in the plaque on teeth.

SENC Safety Alert A dry mouth can cause dysphagia, difficulty swallowing. The older adult may take several medications of which one of the side effects causes a dry mouth. This may lead to anorexia (decreased appetite) and weight loss. Monitor patients for unintentional weight loss. Calorie counts and or food diaries may be helpful assessment tools.

TECHNIQUE 24-21: **Inspecting and Palpating Hard and Soft Palates**

Purpose: To assess for color, tenderness, or abnormal deviations

ASSESSMENT STEPS

1. Using a penlight, inspect the anterior hard and posterior soft palates.
2. Inspect Stensen's ducts on each side of the soft palate.
3. Using your index finger, gently palpate the following structures:
  - □ Hard palate
  - □ Soft palate

NORMAL FINDINGS

- Transverse rugae, irregular ridges are firm, pink to light red; moist
- No tenderness
- Soft palate is pink, moist; no lesions or ulcerations
- Integrity of hard and soft palate intact
- Nodular bony ridge down the middle of the posterior hard palate

ABNORMAL FINDINGS
■ Deep red color, ulcerations, lesions, or growths
  ☐ Hard palate is a shade of yellow if jaundice is present.

TECHNIQUE 24-22: **Inspecting and Palpating the Tongue**

Purpose: To assess color, movement, and abnormalities

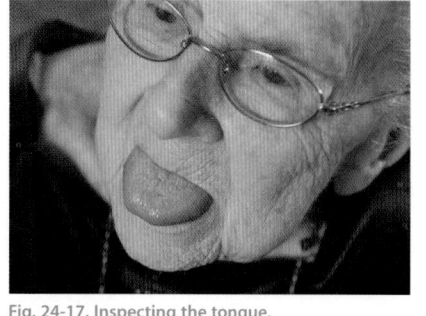

Fig. 24-17. Inspecting the tongue.

ASSESSMENT STEPS
1. Ask the patient to stick out his or her tongue (Fig. 24-17).
2. Inspect the dorsal surface of the tongue for color, lesions, or coating on the tongue.
3. Assess:
  ☐ lateral edges of the tongue
  ☐ voluntary movement of the tongue
  ☐ fine tremors (fasciculations) of the tongue
  ☐ position of the tongue.
4. Ask the patient to touch the roof of the mouth with the tongue; inspect the:
  ☐ floor of the mouth
  ☐ frenulum, which is a small fold of mucous membrane dividing the tongue in half; secures the tongue
  ☐ ventral surface of the tongue
  ☐ Wharton's ducts.
5. Using a sterile gauze, gently palpate the tongue for any lumps or nodules.

NORMAL FINDINGS
■ Color pink and saliva present
■ Papillae on dorsal surface
■ Tongue is in a midline position
■ Ventral surface smooth, pink, moist
■ No lumps or nodules with palpation
■ Wharton's and Stensen's ducts visible

ABNORMAL FINDINGS
■ Cracked, dry, red, presence of ulcers or lesions, bleeding, thick white or yellow coating on tongue
  ☐ **Atrophic glossitis** is a smooth red or pink tongue; may indicate nutritional deficiencies
  ☐ **Hairy tongue** is a white plaque to a dark, hairy surface that may indicate systemic immune suppression.

- **Leukoplakia** are patches on the tongue (usually white or gray); progress to cancer 19 percent of the time (Jefferson, 2011).
- **Squamous cell carcinoma** of the tongue is thickened white or red patch or plaque; may develop nodularity or ulceration; usually develops laterally on the tongue.
  - Tongue lesions require a biopsy to determine if the lesion is cancerous.

TECHNIQUE 24-23: **Inspecting the Pharynx and Tonsils**

Purpose: To assess for redness and inflammation
Equipment: Tongue blade

ASSESSMENT STEPS

1. Moisten a tongue blade with warm water.
   ■ **TIP** A moistened tongue blade may help to decrease the patient from gagging.
2. Ask the patient to open his or her mouth wide, tilt the head back, and say "aah." Inspect the rising of the soft palate and uvula.
3. Using the tongue depressor to hold the tongue down, ask the patient to say "aah" again and assess the throat and tonsillar pillars.
   - Note mouth odors.
4. Using the tongue depressor, gently touch the back of the pharynx to elicit a gag reflex.
5. Discard the tongue blade.
6. Remove and discard gloves.
7. Document your findings.

NORMAL FINDINGS

- Uvula rises midline symmetrically; glossopharyngeal (CN IX) and vagus (CN X) nerves intact
- Throat pink
- Tonsils pink; may partially protrude or be absent
- Presence of a gag reflex

ABNORMAL FINDINGS

- Asymmetrical rise of the uvula
- Throat deep red, inflamed, with drainage
- Throat pain, dysphagia
- Tonsils protruding with or without drainage

TECHNIQUE 24-24: **Assessing Swallowing**

Purpose: To assess for difficulty swallowing (dysphagia)
Equipment: Cup of water
ASSESSMENT STEPS
1. Explain to the patient that you are going to have him or her drink some fluid (i.e., water or juice)
2. Give the patient a cup, and ask the patient to drink.
3. Assess the patient's ability to swallow, observing for (Fig. 24-18):
   ☐ coughing
   ☐ drooling
   ☐ pocketing of fluid on side of the cheek
4. Document your findings.

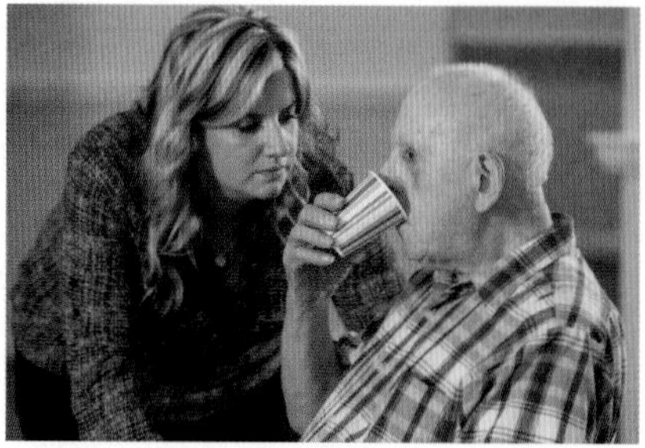

Fig. 24-18. Assess swallowing.

NORMAL FINDINGS
■ No difficulty swallowing liquids or food

ABNORMAL FINDINGS
■ Coughing, drooling, throat clearing, or pocketing fluids on the side of the mouth are signs of dysphagia.
   ■ **TIP** A speech therapist evaluates patients for dysphagia. Soft or pureed diets with thickened fluids may be ordered. The patient will be placed on aspiration precautions.

TECHNIQUE 24-25: **Assessing the Lymph Nodes in the Head and Neck Region**

Purpose: To assess for signs of inflammation or disease
Normally, lymph nodes are not palpated, but there are times that lymph nodes can be palpated. See Chapter 15, Table 15-1 for differences between normal and abnormal lymph node characteristics.
ASSESSMENT STEPS
1. Explain the technique to the patient.
2. Ask the patient to sit up on the edge of the examination table.
3. Ask the patient to slightly flex his or her neck forward to relax the muscles.
4. Warm your hands by rubbing them together.
5. Using the finger pads of your index and middle fingers; gently palpate using circular motions, the 10 facial and neck lymph nodes regions, using both hands to examine corresponding sides:

☐ Preauricular (anterior to the ears)
☐ Postauricular (posterior to the ears)
☐ Suboccipital (area between the back of the neck and head)
☐ Tonsillar (below the jaw bone)
☐ Submandibular (under the jaw on both sides)
☐ Submental (just below the chin)
☐ Superficial cervical (upper neck)
☐ Posterior cervical (on the side of the neck toward the back)
☐ Deep cervical chain (near the internal jugular vein)

6. Ask the patient to slightly flex her or his neck to the right and shrug the shoulders; palpate the left supraclavicular lymph nodes in the hollow area just above the clavicle.

7. Ask the patient to slightly flex his or her neck to the left and shrug the shoulders; palpate the right supraclavicular lymph nodes.

8. Document your findings.

NORMAL FINDINGS
■ No lymph nodes are palpated.
■ If palpated, the lymph node should be less than 1 cm, discrete, moveable, and nontender.

ABNORMAL FINDINGS
■ Enlarged, greater than 1 cm, matted, hard, and tender may be signs of inflammation or a malignancy.

CAROTID ARTERIES

TECHNIQUE 24-26: **Inspecting and Palpating the Carotid Arteries**

Purpose: To assess carotid artery circulation

■ **TIP** Palpating the carotid arteries may be more difficult in an obese patient; ask the patient to slightly turn his or her neck to the opposite side that you are trying to assess the pulse.

ASSESSMENT STEPS

1. Explain the technique to the patient.

2. Place the patient in a sitting or supine position.

3. Ask the patient to turn his or her head to the right side, inspect and palpate the left carotid artery for pulsations between the trachea and sternocleidomastoid muscle.

4. Ask the patient to turn his or her head to the left side, inspect and palpate the right carotid artery for pulsations between the trachea and sternocleidomastoid muscle.

5. Note the following characteristics of the carotid pulses:
- ☐ Rate
- ☐ Rhythm
- ☐ Amplitude

6. Document your findings.

NORMAL FINDINGS
- Visible symmetrical pulsations
- Pulse rate between 60 and 100
- Amplitude 2+

ABNORMAL FINDINGS
- No pulsations or asymmetrical pulsatile bulge may indicate decreased circulation or obstruction.
- Pulse rate less than 60 and greater than 100
- Rhythm: irregular with pauses; may be indicative of an irregular heart rate (arrhythmia)
- Amplitude: absent (no heart rate), weak (decreased stroke volume), or bounding (increased stroke volume); may be indicative of changes in the circulatory system.

TECHNIQUE 24-27: **Auscultating the Carotid Arteries**

Purpose: To assess carotid artery flow for signs of obstruction
Equipment: Stethoscope
A bruit is an abnormal "swooshing" sound that blood makes when it rushes past an obstruction in an artery.

ASSESSMENT STEPS

1. Explain the technique to the patient.

2. Ask the patient to take a breath and hold it.

■ **TIP** It is important that you listen for a carotid bruit while the patient is holding her or his breath so that you do not get confused by the patient's tracheal breath sounds.

3. Using either the bell or the diaphragm of the stethoscope, auscultate the left carotid artery for a bruit as the patient holds her or his breath.

4. Instruct the patient to take a breath and again hold the breath.

5. Using either the bell or the diaphragm of the stethoscope, auscultate the right carotid artery for a bruit.

6. Document your findings.

■ No bruit heard

■ A swooshing sound (bruit) indicates turbulent blood flow.

■ Bruit may indicate partial obstruction of the carotid artery due to plaque in the artery.

JUGULAR VEINS

TECHNIQUE 24-28: Inspecting for Jugular Venous Distention

Purpose: To assess for signs of increased central venous pressure (pressure in the right atrium of the heart)

The internal jugular veins are located deep beneath the sternocleidomastoid muscle, lateral to the carotid arteries. The veins are not normally visualized or protruding. Sometimes, the pulsations of the internal jugular veins are transmitted through the skin. The external jugular veins are lateral to the internal jugular veins and are superficial.

Equipment: Penlight

ASSESSMENT STEPS

1. Explain the technique to the patient.

2. Position patient in a sitting or semi-Fowler's (30 to 45 degree) position.

3. Ask the patient to turn his or her head to the left side.

4. Using a penlight, inspect the right side of the patient's neck for jugular vein distention.

5. Note any pulsations.

6. Repeat steps 3 through 5 on the left side.

7. Document your findings.

NORMAL FINDINGS

■ No visible pulsation or jugular vein distention

ABNORMAL FINDINGS

■ Visible distention is a sign of venous pressure elevation, commonly seen in congestive heart failure and fluid overload.

NECK

TECHNIQUE 24-29: **Inspecting the Neck**

Purpose: To assess symmetry, movement, and swelling of the neck

ASSESSMENT STEPS

1. Ask the patient to sit up straight with neck in the normal position and then slightly hyperextended.

2. Assess the neck for symmetry and swelling.

3. Have the patient turn his or her head to assess ROM:
- ☐ Turn neck side to side.
- ☐ Bend neck forward.
- ☐ Extend neck backward.
- ☐ Bend neck toward each shoulder.

   ▮ **TIP** Instruct the patient to try to keep the shoulders down, not up, when bending the neck to the shoulder to increase the full visibility of the neck.

NORMAL FINDINGS

- ▪ Neck is symmetrical; no swelling
- ▪ No pain with range of motion
- ▪ Full ROM of neck

ABNORMAL FINDINGS

- ▪ Asymmetrical
- ▪ Pain with movement
- ▪ Unable to turn neck

TECHNIQUE 24-30: **Inspecting and Palpating the Trachea**

Purpose: To assess for tracheal shift or deviation

▮ **TIP** A mass in the neck or pathology in the lung may cause the trachea to shift or deviate toward the affected or unaffected side.

ASSESSMENT STEPS

1. Ask the patient to sit up straight and bend her or his head slightly forward to relax the sternomastoid muscles.

2. Inspect the trachea below the thyroid isthmus.

3. Gently place your right index finger in the sternal notch.

4. Slip your finger off to each side noting distance from the sternomastoid muscle.

5. Assess the symmetrical spacing on each side, and note any deviation from midline.

6. Document your findings.

NORMAL FINDINGS

■ Trachea is midline.

■ Space is symmetric on each side.

ABNORMAL FINDINGS

■ Trachea is deviated to the right or left side and away from the midline.

TECHNIQUE 24-31: **Inspecting the Thyroid**

Purpose: To assess size, mobility, and enlargement

ASSESSMENT STEPS

1. Seat the patient with his or her head in a neutral or slightly extended position.

2. Stand in front of the patient.

3. Inspect the neck for swelling or enlargement of the thyroid gland below the cricoid cartilage.

4. Have the patient take a sip of water and observe the upward motion of the thyroid gland.

NORMAL FINDINGS

■ Neck area at the site of the thyroid gland should have a smooth, straight appearance.

■ Thyroid gland as well as cricoid and thyroid cartilage move up with swallowing.

ABNORMAL FINDINGS

■ Neck is enlarged, asymmetrical.

■ Gland does not move during swallowing.

TECHNIQUE 24-32: **Palpating the Thyroid**

Purpose: To assess the thyroid gland for smoothness, enlargement, nodules, or tenderness

■ **TIP** The thyroid gland may be assessed using an anterior or posterior approach. Assessment is easier if you are able to find your landmarks first: the isthmus of the thyroid gland, cricoid cartilage, and suprasternal notch.

Equipment: Cup of water (optional)

Posterior Approach
ASSESSMENT STEPS
1. Stand behind the patient.
2. Ask the patient to sit up straight with his or her neck slightly flexed to the right to relax the neck muscles.
3. Place your finger pads between the sternomastoid muscle and trachea on the patient's neck slightly below the cricoid cartilage.
4. Have the patient take a sip of water or swallow and feel the rise of the thyroid gland.
5. Using your left hand finger pads, gently push the trachea to the right side.
6. Using your right finger pads, ask the patient to take a sip of water or swallow and gently palpate laterally the right lobe of the thyroid for smoothness, enlargement, nodules, or tenderness.
7. Ask the patient to slightly flex his or her neck to the left to relax the neck muscles.
8. Using your right hand finger pads, gently push the trachea to the left side.
9. Using your left finger pads, ask the patient to take a sip of water or swallow and gently palpate laterally the left lobe of the thyroid for smoothness, enlargement, nodules or tenderness.
10. Document your findings. Specifically, document the size, shape, and location of any nodule.

NORMAL FINDINGS
- Lateral lobes may or may not be palpable.
- If palpable, the lobes are smooth, firm, and nontender.

ABNORMAL FINDINGS
- Enlargement of one or both lobes
- Tenderness, presence of lumps or nodules
- Texture has variations of firmness

Anterior Approach
ASSESSMENT STEPS
1. Stand in front of the patient.
2. Ask the patient to sit up straight with his or her neck slightly flexed to the right to relax the neck muscles.
3. Place your finger pads between the sternomastoid muscle and trachea on the patient's neck slightly below the cricoid cartilage.
4. Have the patient take a sip of water or swallow and feel the rise of the thyroid gland.
5. Using the thumb of your right hand on the patient's neck slightly below the cricoid cartilage, gently push the trachea to the right.
6. Position the finger pads of your left hand between the sternomastoid muscle and trachea, have the patient take a sip of water or swallow and gently palpate the right lobe of the thyroid for smoothness, enlargement, nodules, or tenderness.
7. Ask the patient to slightly flex his or her neck to the left to relax the neck muscles.
8. Using the thumb of your left hand on the patient's neck slightly below the cricoid cartilage, gently push the trachea to the left.

9. Position the finger pads of your right hand between the sternomastoid muscle and trachea, have the patient take a sip of water or swallow and gently palpate the left lobe of the thyroid for smoothness, enlargement, nodules, or tenderness.

10. Document your findings. Specifically, document the size, shape, and location of any nodule.

NORMAL FINDINGS
- Lateral lobes may or may not be palpable.
- If palpable, the lobes are smooth, firm, and nontender.

ABNORMAL FINDINGS
- Enlargement of one or both lobes
- Tenderness, presence of lumps or nodules
- Texture has variations of firmness.
- **Goiter** is an enlarged thyroid gland; may be related to hyperfunction or hypofunction of the thyroid gland.

EARS

TECHNIQUE 24-33: **Inspecting and Palpating the Ears**

Purpose: To assess for ear deformities and tenderness

ASSESSMENT STEPS

1. Stand in front of the patient and assess both ears for
- ☐ size
- ☐ shape
- ☐ color
- ☐ symmetry
- ☐ landmarks.

2. Gently palpate the right ear and assess for tenderness.
- ☐ Auricles (Pinna)
- ☐ Tragus
- ☐ Earlobes
- ☐ Mastoid process

3. Stand on the left side of the patient and palpate the left ear for tenderness.

4. Document your findings.

NORMAL FINDINGS
- Equal size and shape bilaterally; normal size (4 to 10 cm)
- Firm consistency
- Color same as facial skin
- Symmetrical
- Angle of attachment less than 10 degrees
- No deformities, inflammation, nodules, or drainage
- Nontender to palpate external ear

ABNORMAL FINDINGS
- Asymmetrical
- Lesions
- Cysts
- Drainage
- Color is blue, red, white, or pale.
- Tenderness
- **Tophi** are hard, whitish or cream colored, nontender deposits of uric acid crystals indicative of gout.

TECHNIQUE 24-34: **Assessing Hearing (CN VIII)**

Purpose: To assess for impaired or loss of hearing

▌**TIP** Tests to assess hearing are subjective because you are relying on the individual's response to what he or she says is heard. The tests will only screen for hearing loss.

Technique 24-34A: **Conducting the Whispered Voice Test**

Purpose: To assess for impaired or loss of hearing

ASSESSMENT STEPS
1. Place individual in the sitting position.
2. Stand behind the person to his or her right side about 2 feet away so you cannot be seen.
3. Ask the individual to cover the left ear that you are not testing.
4. Whisper three random words, letters, or numbers.
5. Have the individual repeat what you whispered.
6. Repeat steps 2 through 5 on the left side.
7. Document your findings.

- Individual repeats the words, letters, or numbers correctly.
- **Presbycusis** is normal progressive sensorineural hearing loss (CN VIII) that is more prevalent after 50 years of age; sensorineural hearing loss demonstrates with high-frequency hearing loss and difficulty discriminating spoken words.

  TIP Older people with hearing loss have difficulty hearing with background noise or when other people are all talking at once; these individuals usually talk louder than normal or turn their good ear toward the person talking.

  SENC Patient-Centered Care Presbycusis is the third most common disease of the elderly and can cause significant social isolation (Venes, 2013). Nurses need to assess patients for hearing loss and and notify the healthcare provider. A referral to an audiologist may be needed. Position yourself to face the patient when speaking to him or her and speak slowly, clearly, and in a lower frequency.

ABNORMAL FINDINGS

- Individual repeats fewer than half of the three words, letters, or numbers correctly or did not hear what you whispered.
- Audiometric testing is in order when there are abnormal findings (Sanders & Gillig, 2010, p. 19).

EYES

TECHNIQUE 24-35: **Inspecting the Eyes**

Purpose: To assess the anterior eye structures
Equipment: Light source
ASSESSMENT STEPS

1. Stand in front of the patient.
2. Inspect the eyelids.
   - ☐ Observe that the eyelids open and close completely.
   - ☐ Assess for any drainage.
3. Inspect the eyelashes for
   - ☐ distribution
   - ☐ drainage.
4. Inspect the eyebrows.
   - ☐ Assess symmetry.
   - ☐ Assess distribution of hair and any scaly, flaky, skin.

5. Inspect the cornea.

  ☐ Use a light source to inspect side to side the cornea for smoothness and clarity.

6. Inspect the lens.

  ☐ Use a light source to inspect side to side the lens of the eye for clarity.

  ☐ Use light source to inspect the color and round shape.

7. Assess the sclera for color.

8. Inspect the conjunctiva.

  ☐ Use your thumbs to slide the bottom eyelids down to assess the mucosa of the lower conjunctiva (Fig. 24-19).

  ☐ Ask the patient to look up.

  ☐ Inspect the color of the mucosa.

9. Inspect the lacrimal duct.

  ☐ Wearing gloves, inspect and palpate the lacrimal duct for any swelling or excessive tearing.

10. Assess palpebral fissures.

  ☐ Assess the distance of the upper lid to the lower lid for symmetry.

  ☐ Compare the palpebral fissures on each side of the face.

11. Inspect for abnormal involuntary eye movements.

12. Document your findings.

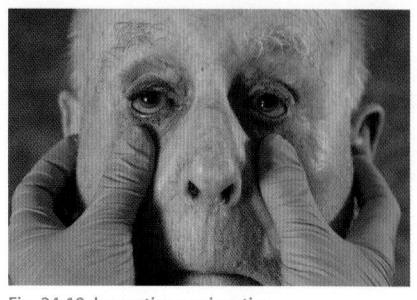

Fig. 24-19. Inspecting conjunctiva.

NORMAL FINDINGS

■ Eyes symmetrical; no protrusion

■ Upper and lower eyelids close completely; no redness or drainage; no drooping of an eyelid (ptosis); upper eyelid covers half of the iris

■ Eyelashes equally distributed; no drainage

■ Eyebrows evenly distributed; no scaly or flaky skin; symmetrical

■ Cornea clear with no opacities

■ Lens transparent with no opacities

■ Pupils equal in size

■ Iris blue, green, brown, or hazel in color, smooth

■ Sclera white

■ Conjunctiva pink and moist

■ Lacrimal duct clear with no swelling

■ Palpebral fissures equal bilaterally

■ No abnormal involuntary movement

- **Arcus senilis** is a thin gray-white line that encircles the cornea; may be a sign of increased cholesterol levels (Fig. 24-20).

ABNORMAL FINDINGS
- **Ptosis** is drooping of the eyelid caused by muscle or nerve dysfunction, injury, or disease.
- **Blepharitis** is an inflammation and infection of the eyelid margins. The eyelid margin becomes red, crusty, and greasy due to too much oil being produced by the eye glands.
- **Blocked lacrimal duct** causes excessive tearing because tears cannot drain properly.
- **Cataract** is an opacity of the lens caused by aging, long-term exposure to ultraviolet light, metabolic disorders, trauma, and medications.

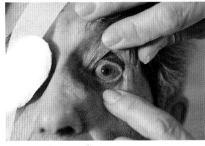
Fig. 24-20. Arcus senilis.

CULTURAL CONSIDERATION Cataracts are the leading cause of decreased vision in older adults; women are more likely to develop cataracts than men, and African Americans and Hispanic Americans are at particularly high risk (University of Maryland Medical Center, 2013b).

- **Conjunctivitis** is a bacterial or viral infection causing erythema of the sclera and yellow-green drainage of the conjunctiva.
- **Corneal abrasion** is a painful scratch to the clear surface of the eye, usually related to trauma to the eye.
- **Ectropion** is an everted eyelid.
- **Entropion** is an inverted eyelid.
- **Exophthalmos** is a protrusion of the anterior portion of the eyeball; common in hyperthyroidism; may cause patient to have dry eyes and difficulty closing the lids.
- **Hordeolum** is an inflammation of a follicle of an eyelash that causes redness, inflammation, and a lump at the site.
- **Scleral jaundice** (Icterus) is a sign of elevated bilirubin in the blood
- **Pterygium** is a gelatinous, abnormal growth of the conjunctiva; occurs more commonly on the nasal side.
- **Periorbital edema** is swelling around the tissues of the eye.
- **Glaucoma** is increased ocular pressure in the eye that damages the optic nerve; loss of peripheral vision.
- **Macular degeneration** is loss of central vision.

TECHNIQUE 24-36: **Assessing for Visual Acuity**

Purpose: To measure a patient's vision to see details at near and far distances
Equipment: Snellen chart

■ **TIP** If the patient wears glasses or contact lenses, the glasses or contact lenses should be worn during the vision assessment. Reading glasses should not be worn. Document if the patient has worn his or her glasses or contact lenses during the assessment.

ASSESSMENT STEPS

1. Explain the technique to the patient.
2. Place the chart at a comfortable height for the patient's height.
3. Have the patient stand 20 feet from the chart.
4. Cover the left eye and have the patient start reading the lines out loud starting from the top and working down the chart. The patient reads the row from left to right.
5. Ask the patient to read each line. The patient can miss one or two letters and be considered to have vision equal to that line.
6. Repeat steps 4 and 5 by covering the right eye.
7. Repeat steps 4 and 5 with both eyes uncovered.
8. Document the last line that was correctly read for each assessment.

NORMAL FINDINGS

■ Normal distant visual acuity is 20/20; this means that the patient can read what a person with normal eyesight can read at 20 feet.

ABNORMAL FINDINGS

■ A higher denominator means poorer distant visual acuity.
■ **Nearsightedness,** known as **myopia,** is poor visual acuity; distant objects appear blurred because the images are focused in front of the retina rather than on it. The denominator is greater than 20.
■ **Farsightedness,** known as **hyperopia,** is the ability to see distant objects clearly, but objects nearby may be blurry.
■ **Presbyopia** is the inability to focus clearly on near objects; the patient holds the print farther away to focus; magnifying glasses are used to read.
■ **Legal blindness** is visual acuity of 20/200 or more; this means that the patient standing at 20 feet can see what a normal patient can see at 200 feet. A patient can be legally blind if he or she only has central vision and 20/200 visual acuity; these patients can only see straight in front of them.

TECHNIQUE 24-37: **Using the Amsler Grid for Assessing Central Vision**

Purpose: To assess central vision
Equipment: Amsler grid
Reading glasses should be worn during this assessment. Instruct the patient to hold the Amsler grid the same distance from his or her eyes as if reading any type of reading material.

1. Explain the technique to the patient.
2. Have the patient cover the left eye.
3. Instruct the patient to focus on the dark dot in the center of the grid with the exposed right eye.
4. Ask if any of the lines are distorted, broken, or blurred.
5. Ask if there are any missing areas or dark areas in the grid.
6. Ask if he or she can see all the corners and sides in the grid.
7. Have the patient cover the right eye and repeat the test.
8. Mark the areas on the Amsler grid that the patient is not seeing correctly.
9. Document your findings.

NORMAL FINDINGS

■ No lines look distorted, broken, or blurred

ABNORMAL FINDINGS

■ Lines look distorted, broken, or blurred
■ **Macular degeneration,** which is a breakdown of cells in the macula of the retina, causes loss of central vision.

TECHNIQUE 24-38: **Using Confrontation Test for Visual Field Testing (CN III, IV, and VI)**

Purpose: To assess peripheral vision, overall field of vision, and for blind spots

ASSESSMENT STEPS

1. Face the patient.
2. Cover your right eye; the patient covers his or her left eye with a hand.
3. Instruct the patient to look directly into your uncovered eye.
4. Move the fingers of your left hand into your field of vision from four different angles:
    ☐ Temporal (90 degrees)
    ☐ Nasal (angle 60 degrees)
    ☐ Superiorly (50 degrees)
    ☐ Inferiorly (70 degrees)

5. Ask the patient to say "now" when he or she can see your fingers and state how many fingers he or she can see.

6. Assess whether the patient's peripheral vision corresponds with your visual fields.

7. Cover the opposite eye and repeat steps 2 through 6.

8. Document your findings.

NORMAL FINDINGS

■ The patient sees your fingers at the same time as you do and correctly states the number of fingers he or she sees.

ABNORMAL FINDINGS

■ This test is considered to be significant when the patient does not see your fingers; may be related to blind spots in the eye. The patient will need a referral to an ophthalmologist.

TECHNIQUE 24-39: **Testing for Ocular Motility: Six Cardinal Positions of Gaze (CN III, CN IV, CN VI)**

Purpose: To assess for weakness or problems with the ocular muscles

Equipment: Pencil (optional)

ASSESSMENT STEPS

1. Use your finger or hold an object in your hand (e.g., pencil) about 12 to 14 inches from the patient's face.

2. Instruct the patient not to move his or her head but to follow your finger or the object with just the eyes.

3. If the patient is unable to follow without moving his head, gently hold his or her head in place.

4. Move the object in six different positions using a wide "H" or "star" pattern to assess the six cardinal positions; pause between lateral and upward movements.

5. Document your findings.

NORMAL FINDINGS

■ The eyes have a normal pattern of movement in each of the six cardinal directions. Mild nystagmus in the lateral angles is normal.

ABNORMAL FINDINGS

■ Patient is not able to follow the pattern of movement in each of the six cardinal directions; patient may experience double vision (diplopia) or uncontrolled eye movements.

☐ **Diplopia** is a subjective complaint that may be related to a muscular dysfunction of the eye or neurologic problem.

☐ **Nystagmus** is an involuntary, cyclical movement of the eyes; occurs when the patient gazes or follows an object; may also occur if the patient has a fixed gaze in the peripheral field; may indicate a neurological disorder.

TECHNIQUE 24-40: **Testing for Convergence and Accommodation (CN II and CN III)**

Purpose: To assess the accommodation reflex of the eye
Equipment: Pencil (optional)

ASSESSMENT STEPS

1. Explain the technique to the patient.
2. Hold a pencil or your finger in front of the patient's eyes about 14 inches in front of his or her nose.
3. Instruct the patient to focus on your finger or object for 30 seconds.
4. Instruct the patient to follow your finger or object as you move it toward his or her nose.
5. Document your findings.

NORMAL FINDINGS

■ Both eyes converge and both pupils constrict (accommodation) simultaneously to focus on a near object.

ABNORMAL FINDINGS

■ Pupils do not converge or constrict.

RESPIRATORY

TECHNIQUE 24-41: **Inspecting the Thoracic Cage**

Purpose: To inspect the size and shape of the thoracic cage

ASSESSMENT STEPS

1. Position patient in the sitting position.
2. Inspect the anterior and posterior thoracic cage for:
   □ size
   □ shape
   □ symmetry
   □ color
   □ respiratory rate and rhythm.
3. Document your findings.

NORMAL FINDINGS

- Transverse diameter is approximately twice the anteroposterior (AP) diameter; AP-to-lateral ratio is approximately 1:2, and the costal angle is less than 90 degrees.
- Conical shape: smaller at the top and widens at the bottom
- Symmetrical; sternum is symmetrical; clavicles and scapula are the same height; chest movement is symmetrical.
- Skin color is uniform and intact; hair distribution consistent with gender and ethnicity.
- Normal adult respiratory rate (eupnea) is 12 to 20 breaths per minute; even and smooth respirations; normal inspiratory to expiratory ratio (I:E) is 1:2; the expiratory phase is longer than the inspiratory phase.

  TIP Do not tell the patient that you are taking the respiratory rate because this may change the breathing pattern.

ABNORMAL FINDINGS

- **Barrel chest:** Anterior posterior-to-lateral ratio is 1:1 and the costal angle greater than 90 degrees; increase in the costal angle may be a sign of chronic obstructive pulmonary disease (COPD).
- **Intercostal and accessory muscle retractions** may indicate problems with air movement; prolonged inspiratory phase may indicate upper airway obstruction; prolonged expiratory phase may indicate lower airway obstruction.
- **Abnormal respirations** (See Chapter 12, Table 12-1.)
- **Abnormal skin** color (See Chapter 12, Table 12-2.)
- **Pursed lip breathing** is breathing through the nose and exhaling through pursed lips; lips look like the patient is whistling; commonly seen in patients with chronic obstructive pulmonary disease.
- **Clubbing of nail plates** occurs with chronic lack of oxygen or hypoxia. The tips of the fingers and nails change in shape and size.

TECHNIQUE 24-42: **Palpating the Thorax**

Purpose: To assess surface characteristics or tenderness of the thoracic cage

  SENC Patient-Centered Care Tell the patient to let you know if she or he feels any tenderness, discomfort, or shortness of breath.

ASSESSMENT STEPS

1. Position the patient in the sitting position.

2. Using your finger pads, gently palpate the anterior, posterior, and lateral thoracic cage and assess:

  □ Surface characteristics

  □ Temperature

    TIP Use the dorsal surface of your hand to assess temperature.

  □ Moisture

  □ Tenderness

- Smooth and uniform surface
- Warm skin
- Skin dry
- No tenderness

ABNORMAL FINDINGS
- Irregular surface (lumps or masses)
- Temperature cool, clammy
- Tenderness
- **Crepitus** (a light crackling or popping feeling under the skin caused by leakage of air into the subcutaneous tissue); sounds like Rice Krispies popping under the skin

TECHNIQUE 24-43: **Palpating Tactile Fremitus**

Purpose: To palpate voice sound vibrations through the bronchi

ASSESSMENT STEPS

1. Explain the technique to the patient and then position the patient in the sitting position.
2. Instruct the patient to repeat words such as "ninety-nine," "coin," "toy," or "boy" in a low-pitched voice.
3. Starting just below the clavicle, use palmar base (ball of your hand) or the ulnar side of your hand and palpate down the anterior lobes as the patient keeps repeating the same word.
4. Starting just below the scapula, use palmar base (ball of your hand) or the ulnar side of your hand and palpate down the posterior lobes as the patient keeps repeating the same word.
5. Document your findings.

NORMAL FINDINGS
- Palpable vibrations of sounds are felt equally on both sides of the lungs.

ABNORMAL FINDINGS
- The palpable vibration is not felt equally on both sides.
- **Increased fremitus** may indicate increased density of the lung tissue; may be related to fluid or pathology in the lung that is changing the density or compressing the lung tissue, such as pneumonia.
- **Decreased fremitus** may indicate the vibrations are obstructed, air is trapped, decreased air movement (emphysema), or the lung tissue is solid.

TECHNIQUE 24-44: **Percussing the Thorax**

Purpose: To assess presence of air in each lung and the density of underlying lung tissue

ASSESSMENT STEPS

1. Explain the technique to the patient and then position the patient in the sitting position.

2. Assess anterior lungs. Using the indirect percussion technique, percuss the intercostal spaces moving from the apex to the base on each side of the anterior lung fields noting the tones of the percussion sounds.

3. Assess posterior lungs. Using the indirect percussion technique, percuss each side of the posterior lung fields moving from the apex to the base, noting the tones of the percussion sounds.

4. Instruct patient to raise each arm, and percuss the lateral lung fields. Using the indirect percussion technique, percuss each side of the lateral lung fields moving from the apex to the base noting the tones of the percussion sounds.

5. Document your findings.

NORMAL FINDINGS

■ Resonance is the low-pitched, clear, hollow sound that is percussed over healthy, air-filled lung fields.

ABNORMAL FINDINGS

TIP Lung consolidation means that the lung tissue that is normally filled with air has now become filled with a dense, solid exudate or tissue; may occur in pneumonia.

■ **Dullness sounds** are soft and muffled and heard over areas of increased density; may be heard over solid mass or areas of increased consolidation such as pneumonia or pleural effusion (fluid between the layer of tissues that line the lungs) (Dugdale & Hadjiliadis, 2012).

■ **Hyperresonance** is a low-pitched accentuated percussion sound heard in the lungs when the bronchi and alveoli are overinflated.

SENC Safety Alert Older patients with poor functional status are at higher risk of developing community-acquired pneumonia (CAP), due to the frequent presence of underlying respiratory and cardiac diseases, alteration of mental status, renal impairment, or hepatic failure; this places the older adult at great risk for an infection-related death (Russo, Falcone, & Venditti, 2013).

TECHNIQUE 24-45: **Auscultating the Lungs**

Purpose: To assess airflow throughout all lobes of the lungs

Equipment: Stethoscope

1. Explain the technique to the patient and then position the patient in the sitting position.

TIP Never auscultate over the patient's clothing to ensure clarity of the sounds.

2. Warm the diaphragm of the stethoscope between your hands.

3. Instruct the patient to lean forward slightly.

4. Instruct the patient to inhale and exhale through the mouth.

SENC Safety Alert The patient should breathe more deeply than normally. If the patient begins to feel lightheaded or starts to hyperventilate, allow the patient to rest.

5. Assess anterior lung fields. Start at the apex of the lungs. Place your stethoscope above the clavicle, then go to the 2nd ICS, and continue to auscultate down to the bases noting what lobe of the lung that you are auscultating. Listen to one full inhalation and exhalation cycle.

6. Assess posterior lung fields. Start at the apex of the lungs. Place your stethoscope above the scapula, then go in-between the spine and the shoulder blades; continue to auscultate down to the bases noting what lobe of the lung that you are auscultating. Listen to one full inhalation and exhalation cycle.

7. Assess lateral lung fields. Auscultate at the intercostals spaces moving from the apex to the base on right and left lateral lung fields noting breath sounds.

8. Document your findings.

NORMAL FINDINGS

■ Bronchial breath sounds are heard over the trachea; expiratory sounds are louder and last longer than inspiratory sounds and have a pause between them; high-pitched, hollow, tubular breath sounds.

■ Bronchovesicular sounds are heard anteriorly over the mid-chest and between the scapula posteriorly; these are medium-pitched sounds with the I:E ratio 1:1.

■ Vesicular sounds are heard throughout the periphery of the lungs; inspiration sound is longer and louder than expiration; soft, low-pitched, rustling sounds.

ABNORMAL FINDINGS

■ It is abnormal to hear bronchial breath sounds when they are not in the normal locations.

■ Breath sounds are diminished.

■ Adventitious breath sounds are sounds not normally heard in a chest. (See Chapter 12, Table 12-3.)

□ Some adventitious sounds are cleared with coughing; ask the patient to cough and then reassess the breath sound.

CARDIAC SYSTEM

TECHNIQUE 24-46: **Inspecting Anterior Chest**

Purpose: To assess the anterior chest for pulsations, symmetry, and heaves
Equipment: Tangential lighting

ASSESSMENT STEPS

1. Explain the technique to the patient.
2. Adjust the head of the examination table so that the patient is lying supine with his or her head and chest elevated 30 degrees.
3. Inspect the symmetry of the chest.
4. Inspect for surgical scars of the chest.
5. Inspect the anterior chest at the five landmark locations of the precordium for
☐ Pulsations
☐ Lifts or heaves
• A **lift** or **heave** is a sustained, forceful, outward thrusting of the ventricle secondary to increased workload.
6. Document your findings.

NORMAL FINDINGS

■ An apical pulsation may or may not be visible at the left fifth midclavicular line (MCL); no heaves or lifts; chest symmetrical

ABNORMAL FINDINGS

■ A right ventricular lift or heave is visualized at the sternal border; a left ventricular heave is seen at the apex.

TECHNIQUE 24-47: **Palpating the Precordium and Apical Pulse**

Purpose: To assess for vibrations and the apical pulse

ASSESSMENT STEPS

1. Explain the technique to the patient.
2. Using the palmar surface of your right hand, gently palpate the five landmarks feeling for pulsations or vibrations.
☐ Right Sternal Border (RSB), Second Intercostal Space (Aortic Valve)
☐ Left Sternal Border (LSB), Second Intercostal Space (Pulmonic Valve)

- ☐ Left Sternal Border (LSB), Third Intercostal Space (Erb's Point)
- ☐ Left Sternal Border (LSB) Fourth Intercostal Space (Tricuspid Valve)
- ☐ Left Sternal Border(LSB), Fifth Intercostal Space (Mitral Valve)

3. Ask the patient to turn slightly to the left lateral recumbent position, using your second and third finger pads of your dominant hand, palpate the apical pulse at the fifth left intercostal space at the midclavicular line noting the:
- ☐ location
- ☐ amplitude.

4. While auscultating the apical pulse, use your other hand to palpate the carotid pulse or radial pulse; count and compare the beats per minute and note the:
- ☐ amplitude
- ☐ beats per minute.

5. Document your findings.

NORMAL FINDINGS

■ No pulsations are felt at the five landmarks; apical pulse is palpated and auscultated at the fifth left intercostal space at the midclavicular line:
- ☐ Amplitude: Regular rhythmic tap
- ☐ Carotid or radial pulse is synchronous with the apical pulse.

ABNORMAL FINDINGS

■ Visible pulsations may indicate increased cardiac output.
■ Pulse deficit is a difference in beats per minutes between an apical pulse and palpable pulse; may be indicative of atrial fibrillation.

TECHNIQUE 24-48: **Auscultating Heart Sounds**

Purpose: To assess heart sounds

Equipment: Stethoscope with a bell and diaphragm

> **SENC Safety Alert** Prior to auscultating heart sounds, follow standard precautions and make sure to clean off the stethoscope to prevent any cross-contamination.

ASSESSMENT STEPS

1. Explain the technique to the patient.
2. Place the patient in a comfortable position.

3. Warm the stethoscope before placing on the precordium.

4. Using the second and third finger pads of your right or left hand, landmark each auscultatory site prior to placing the stethoscope on the skin.

5. Using the diaphragm of the stethoscope, auscultate the heart sounds ($S_{1[lub]}$ and $S_{2[dub]}$) at the five landmark sites, listening for:
- ☐ S_1 and S_2 heart sounds
- ☐ rhythm of the heart sounds
- ☐ abnormal or extra heart sounds

6. With the patient in the sitting position, ask the patient to lean forward; using the diaphragm of the stethoscope, auscultate the aortic and pulmonic valve areas listening for:
- ☐ murmurs
- ☐ extra heart sounds.

7. Using the bell of the stethoscope, press gently on the skin and auscultate for low-pitched heart sounds at the five landmark sites.

8. Assist the patient to lie on his or her left lateral side. Using the bell of the stethoscope, auscultate the apical area listening for:
- ☐ heart murmurs
- ☐ extra heart sounds.

9. Document your findings.

NORMAL FINDINGS
- ■ S_1 and S_2 sounds heard; regular pattern
- ■ Split S_2 [dub] sound is a normal heart sound that is affected by respirations

ABNORMAL FINDINGS
- ■ Extra or abnormal heart sounds are heard.
  - ☐ S_3, the third heart sound, may indicate congestive heart failure, aortic valve regurgitation, and be present after a myocardial infarction.
  - ☐ S_4, the fourth heart sound, may indicate thickening (hypertrophy) of the left ventricle, hypertension, aortic stenosis, or be heard after a myocardial infarction.
  - ☐ Murmurs may indicate increased turbulent blood flow is regurgitation.
  - ☐ Opening snap may indicate mitral stenosis.
  - ☐ Ejection clicks may be heard at valves with defective leaflets such as in mitral valve prolapse.
  - ☐ Pericardial friction rubs result from inflammation of the pericardial sac surrounding the heart.

TECHNIQUE 24-49: **Inspecting the Abdomen**

Purpose: To assess abnormalities in shape, skin, or movement of the abdomen

Inspection of the abdomen should be done in two positions: at the patient's side and standing at the patient's feet.

ASSESSMENT STEPS

1. Assist patient to supine position.

2. Inspect the abdomen by standing at the patient's feet for:

☐ contour, size, and symmetry

☐ size and position of the umbilicus

☐ condition of skin: color, lesions, veins, hernias, hair distribution

☐ movements, pulsations, and peristalsis

3. Stoop by the patient's side so the abdomen is at eye level. Inspect the abdomen for:

☐ contour, size, and symmetry

☐ size and position of the umbilicus

☐ condition of skin: color, lesions, veins, hernias, hair distribution

☐ movements, pulsations, and peristalsis

4. Document your findings.

NORMAL FINDINGS

■ Contour (flat or rounded)

■ Bilaterally symmetrical

■ Umbilicus midline

■ Skin smooth and intact without pulsations or visible peristalsis

■ Peristalsis and aortic pulsations may be visible in very thin patients.

ABNORMAL FINDINGS

■ A scaphoid, distended, or protuberant abdomen is usually seen with an underlying pathology such as cancer, weight loss, hernia, or accumulation of fluid.

■ Increased peristaltic waves (ripple-like movement from LUQ to RLQ) are seen with intestinal obstruction.

- Pulsations are increased with the presence of aortic aneurysm.
- Abdominal distention is caused by fluid, fat, feces, flatulence, fibroids, and fetus.
- Ascites is an abnormal accumulation of fluid in the peritoneal cavity.
- Diastasis recti is a bulging area in the abdomen occurring with the separation of the two halves of the rectus abdominis muscles in the midline at the linea alba.
- Hernias
- Cullen's sign is superficial bleeding under the skin (ecchymosis) around the umbilicus and may indicate intra-abdominal bleeding.

TECHNIQUE 24-50: **Auscultating Bowel Sounds**

Purpose: To assess a normal pattern of bowel sounds
Equipment: Stethoscope
ASSESSMENT STEPS
1. Explain the technique to the patient.
2. Auscultate bowel sounds by placing the diaphragm of the stethoscope lightly on the abdomen at the ileocecal valve (RLQ) where bowel sounds are usually always present.
3. Note the intensity, pitch, and frequency of the bowel sounds (see Chapter 14, see Table 14-2).
4. Listen for 3 to 5 minutes before documenting no bowel sounds.
5. Document your findings.
NORMAL FINDINGS
- 5 to 34 clicks or gurgles per minute
- Hypoactive bowels sounds
ABNORMAL FINDINGS
- Hyperactive, high-pitched bowel sounds may indicate early bowel obstruction or increased peristalsis.
- No bowel sounds could indicate a paralytic ileus, no peristalsis movement.

   TIP Nurses should assess older adults for constipation or diarrhea to prevent complications. Patients with decreased cognition are unable to identify whether they have normal bowel patterns or tell you when was they had their last bowel movement.

TECHNIQUE 24-51: **Auscultating Vascular Sounds**

Purpose: To assess a normal pattern of blood flow in the abdominal vasculature
Equipment: Stethoscope

ASSESSMENT STEPS

1. With the bell of the stethoscope, press down firmly to listen over the aorta, renal, iliac, and femoral arteries.
2. Auscultate over the liver (bell) for a venous hum, turbulent blood flow in the jugular venous system that may indicate liver disease or portal hypertension.
3. Document your findings.

NORMAL FINDINGS

■ No bruits over arteries

ABNORMAL FINDINGS

■ Bruits are turbulent, blowing sounds heard over a partially or totally obstructed artery.
■ Venous hum is a continuous, medium-pitched sound caused by blood flow in a large vascular organ (Cox & Steggall, 2009).
■ Friction rub is a grating sound heard over inflamed organs with serous surfaces; most commonly heard in the RUQ (liver) or LUQ (spleen)

TECHNIQUE 24-52: **Percussing the Abdomen**

Purpose: To assist with identifying gas and solid or fluid-filled masses in the abdomen

ASSESSMENT STEPS

1. Percuss over each quadrant and note the quality of sounds heard.
2. Follow one of the two patterns for percussion (Fig. 24-21).
3. Document your findings.

NORMAL FINDINGS

■ Tympany in all four quadrants; dullness over organs

ABNORMAL FINDINGS

■ Excessive, high-pitched tympanic sounds may indicate distention.
■ Dullness may indicate increased tissue density such as organ enlargement or an underlying mass.
■ Pain during percussion may indicate peritoneal inflammation.

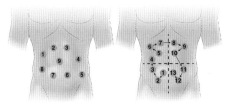

Fig. 24-21. Two patterns for percussion.

TECHNIQUE 24-53: **Palpating the Abdomen**

Purpose: To assess surface characteristics, tenderness, enlarged organs, or fluid in the abdominal cavity

■ **TIP** Warm your hands by rubbing them together prior to palpating the abdomen.

Technique 24-53A: **Light Palpation**

Purpose: To feel for surface characteristics and assess for tenderness

ASSESSMENT STEPS

1. Using the finger pads of one hand, press down about a half inch.
2. Lightly palpate in a clockwise direction the entire abdomen.
   ☐ Always palpate tender areas last.
3. Lift your fingers gently as you move to a different area.
4. Watch the patient's facial expression for signs of pain or abdominal guarding.
5. Document your findings.

NORMAL FINDINGS

■ No tenderness, smooth surface characteristics

ABNORMAL FINDINGS

■ Tenderness is present; nodule or mass felt

Technique 24-53B: **Deep Palpation**

Purpose: To assess for enlarged organs, masses, or tenderness

ASSESSMENT STEPS

1. Place your nondominant hand on top of your dominant hand (also known as bimanual palpation)
2. Deeply palpate; press down about 1.5 to 2 inches using a circular or a dipping motion in a clockwise direction.
3. Lift your hands gently as you move to different areas.
4. Document your findings.

NORMAL FINDINGS

■ No masses, enlarged organs, or tenderness

ABNORMAL FINDINGS

■ Masses are palpated.
■ Enlarged organs are noted.
■ Tenderness or pain is present.

Technique 24-53C: Palpating the Bladder

Purpose: To assess for a distended bladder

This assessment should be performed on an empty bladder.

ASSESSMENT STEPS

1. Ask the patient when she or he last emptied the bladder.

2. Watch for nonverbal body language; tenderness or pain may indicate bladder infection.

3. Lightly palpate for a distended bladder between symphysis pubis and umbilicus.

4. Note the size and location of the bladder.

5. Document your findings.

NORMAL FINDINGS

■ An empty bladder is not palpable.

■ A partially filled bladder will feel firm and smooth.

ABNORMAL FINDINGS

■ A distended bladder is palpated as a smooth, round, and firm mass extending as far up as the umbilicus.

TECHNIQUE 24-54: Palpating Inguinal Lymph Nodes and Femoral Pulses

▉ **TIP** You have to be flexible in the sequencing and clustering your assessments to minimize position changes. The femoral pulse assessment can be done while assessing the inguinal area or during the peripheral vascular assessment.

Purpose: To assess for enlarged or abnormal lymph nodes

Equipment: Gloves

ASSESSMENT STEPS

1. Put on gloves.

2. Place patient in the supine position.

3. Using the finger pads of the second, third, and fourth fingers, gently palpate the right inguinal lymph node using a rotary motion.

4. Using the finger pads of the second and third fingers, gently palpate the right femoral pulse. Assess rhythm and amplitude.

5. Repeat steps 3 and 4 on the left side.

6. Document your findings.

NORMAL FINDINGS

■ No lymph nodes are felt or are small (less than 1 cm), movable, and nontender nodes

■ Femoral pulses are regular, 2+ amplitude

ABNORMAL FINDINGS

■ Lymph nodes greater than 1 cm, firm, tender, and immobile could indicate lymphoma, cancer, or infection.

TECHNIQUE 24-55: **Percussing Costovertebral Tenderness**

Purpose: To assess tenderness or inflammation of the kidney

■ **TIP** You can do this assessment when the patient is already sitting up to minimize position changes.

You may use the indirect blunt percussion technique or the fist percussion technique to test for kidney inflammation.

SENC Safety Alert Do not percuss an organ transplant patient.

ASSESSMENT STEPS

1. Place patient in a sitting position; stand facing the patient's back.

2. To assess the kidney, place the palm of one hand over the 12th rib at the costovertebral angle on the back.

3. Thump that hand with the ulnar edge of your other fist.

4. Document your findings.

NORMAL FINDINGS

■ Elicits no pain

ABNORMAL FINDINGS

■ Tenderness or pain may indicate kidney infection or the presence of kidney stones.

SENC Safety Alert Urinary tract infection is the most common bacterial infection occurring in older populations. The older adult may not be able to report symptoms due to cognitive impairment. Symptoms may include a change in mental status, fatigue, lethargy, falls, incontinence, and foul smelling urine.

MUSCULOSKELETAL SYSTEM

SENC Safety Alert Older adults may have poor posture and problems with balance. Place your patient in a safe position to perform ROM techniques. Some older adults may not be able to perform the entire assessment due to physical limitations. Stop a musculoskeletal assessment if you observe a patient having difficulty performing a technique.

TECHNIQUE 24-56: **Inspecting and Palpating the Vertebral Column**

Purpose: To assess for abnormalities in the structure of the vertebral column.

ASSESSMENT STEPS

1. Explain the technique to the patient.

2. Ask the patient to stand.

3. Facing the patient's back, inspect the alignment of the vertebral column and assess the following:
- ☐ How straight is the vertebral column when the patient is standing?
- ☐ Is there any noted deviation in the anterior-posterior plane?

4. Ask the patient to bend at the waist and assess whether the vertebral column is straight.

5. Facing the patient's back, using two or three finger pads, starting at the top of the vertebral column, palpate the vertebral column assessing for:
- ☐ Areas of tenderness
- ☐ Noted deviations in the lateral plane
- ☐ Protrusions

6. Document your findings.

NORMAL FINDINGS

■ The vertebral column is straight when the patient is standing and flexed forward.
■ No deviation noted in anterior-posterior plane and in the lateral plane.
■ No areas of tenderness
■ No deviation in the lateral plane
■ No protrusions or drop-offs within the vertebral column

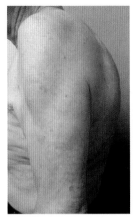

Fig. 24-22. Senile kyphosis.

ABNORMAL FINDINGS

■ **Scoliosis** is an abnormal curvature of the spine that occurs in a lateral manner; it may look like a *C* or an *S* on visualization and be palpable.
■ **Senile kyphosis** is a debilitating curvature of the thoracic spine which looks like a slouching, or hunchback, posture; this can lead to problems with posture, gait, and balance (Fig. 24-22).
■ **Lordosis** is a curvature of the spine that looks like an arched lower back: it is an increased inward curvature of the lumbar spine.
■ Areas of tenderness may indicate a problem with the bony structure or the ligaments within the vertebral column.
■ Protrusions or depressions may indicate a displacement of one vertebral body on another vertebral body.

> **SENC Safety Alert** Vertebral compression fractures are one of the most common fractures in patients with osteoporosis; the prevalence of this condition increase as people age. It is estimated that 40 percent of women age 80 and older are affected; it is also a major health concern for older men (American Association of Neurological Surgeons, 2017).

TECHNIQUE 24-57: **Inspecting and Palpating the Upper Extremities**

Purpose: To determine if there are any abnormalities within the upper extremity.

ASSESSMENT STEPS

1. Explain the technique to the patient.
2. Inspect the upper extremity on the right side and then the left side; compare the right to the left side.

3. Using two or three finger pads, gently palpate the upper extremity on the right side:
   ☐ Shoulder
   ☐ Elbow
   ☐ Wrist
   ☐ Hand/fingers and joints
4. Assess for:
   ☐ tenderness
   ☐ depressions
   ☐ bulges
   ☐ changes in temperature.
5. Repeat steps 3 and 4 on the left side.
6. Document your findings.

NORMAL FINDINGS

With the patient standing, inspection of the upper extremity should find:
- symmetry between left and right upper extremity
- no forward rounding of the shoulder
- straight upper arms
- slight bending in the elbows
- wrists in line with the lower arm and palms facing the upper leg
- some slight flexion of the fingers
- no findings of tenderness/pain; depression or protrusions; increased warmth; increased joint size or missing fingers

ABNORMAL FINDINGS

- Forward rounding of the shoulders may indicate tightness of muscles across the anterior thorax and a weakness of the muscles of the posterior thorax.
- Nonstraight upper arm may indicate a fracture (old or new) or a significant muscle tear.
- A straight or hyperextended elbow may indicate lack of bony structure or muscle tone to hold it in a slightly flexed position.
- A flexed elbow that is unable to be straightened may indicate a serious problem with the joint.
- If the wrist is out of line with the lower arm, there may be a new or old bony injury causing limitations to the motion.
- When the palms do not face the upper leg, there may be some bony limitation to ROM within the wrist joint.
- Fingers that are more than slightly flexed may indicate some sort of disease process that limits the ROM.
- Areas of tenderness or pain may indicate an injury to bone, muscle, tendon, or ligament.
- Depressions may indicate a dislocated joint, significant muscle injury, or joint subluxation.
- Protrusions may also indicate a dislocated or subluxated joint, a displaced fracture, the buildup of calcium within the muscle, a type of arthritis, or a tumor.
   ☐ **Bouchard's nodes** are bony enlargements on the proximal interphalangeal (PIP) joints; commonly seen in osteoarthritis or rheumatoid arthritis.
   ☐ **Heberden's nodes** are bony enlargements on the distal interphalangeal (DIP) joints; commonly seen in osteoarthritis.

- Increased warmth in the joints may be an indication of infection or disease process within that joint.
- Missing fingers may indicate old trauma, or disease process.

TECHNIQUE 24-58: **Assessing Range of Motion and Muscle Strength of the Upper Extremities**

Purpose: To assess strength and limitations in ROM in the upper extremities

ASSESSMENT STEPS

1. Explain the technique to the patient. You will ask them to perform specific motions independently first and then against resistance.
2. Ask the patient to perform the following ROM activities of the right and left upper extremities.
   - ☐ Shoulder motion
     - **Flexion:** movement of the upper extremity as a whole, forward, with thumb facing forward when starting. Have the patient lift both arms toward the ear.
     - **Flexion against resistance:** movement of the upper extremity as a whole, forward, with thumb forward, to the ear. Place your palm on the anterior aspect of the elbow and provide resistance as the patient attempts this motion.
     - **Extension:** movement of the upper extremity as a whole, backward. The thumb should be facing forward when starting.
     - **Extension against resistance:** movement of the upper extremity as a whole, backward. The thumb should be facing forward when starting. Place your palm on the posterior aspect of the elbow and provide resistance as the patient attempts this motion.
     - **Abduction:** movement of the upper extremity as a whole away from anatomic neutral position (0°) toward the ear (180°); ask the patient to move the right arm away from the body up to 180°; repeat on the left side.
     - **Abduction against resistance:** movement of the upper extremity as a whole away from anatomic neutral position toward the ear. Place your palm on the lateral aspect of the patient's elbow and provide resistance as the patient attempts the motion.
     - **Adduction:** movement of the upper extremity as a whole away from the ear toward the waist and then across midline in front of the naval (16-20A)
     - **Adduction against resistance:** movement of the upper extremity as a whole away from the ear toward the waist and then across midline in front of the naval. Place your palm on the medial aspect of the patient's elbow and provide resistance as the patient attempts the motion.
     - **Internal rotation:** ask the patient to pretend to tuck a shirt into his or her waistband in the front and in the back. This is a functional assessment of the patient's ability to perform internal rotation.
     - **Internal rotation against resistance:** as the patient holds the upper arms at the side with his or her elbow flexed to 90 degrees, place your palm against the patient's palm and provide resistance as the patient moves his or her hand toward the opposite hip or naval.
     - **External rotation:** ask the patient to rub the back of his or her head with the right hand and then the left hand.

- **External rotation against resistance:** as the patient holds his or her right upper arm at the side with the elbow flexed to 90 degrees, place your palm on the back of the patient's hand and provide resistance as the patient moves his or her hand toward the starting point for internal rotation.

☐ Elbow motion
  - **Flexion:** move the right hand to the shoulder from the anatomic neutral position; repeat using the left hand.
  - **Flexion against resistance:** movement of the hand to the shoulder from anatomic neutral. Place your palm on the patient's right forearm and resist as the patient performs the above motion; repeat using the left elbow motion.
  - **Extension movement:** move the hand from the shoulder to anatomic neutral position.
  - **Extension against resistance:** move the hand from the shoulder to anatomic neutral. Place your palm on the posterior aspect of the patient's forearm and resist as the patient performs the motion.
  - **Pronation:** with the elbow flexed to 90 degrees, move the hand from palm facing up to palm facing down.
  - **Pronation against resistance:** with the elbow flexed to 90 degrees, move the hand from palm facing up to palm facing down. Hold the patient's hand and resist the motion to determine the strength.
  - **Supination:** with the elbow flexed to 90 degrees, movement of the hand from palm facing down to palm facing up
  - **Supination against resistance:** with the elbow flexed to 90 degrees, movement of the hand from palm facing down to palm facing up. Hold the patient's hand and resist the motion to determine strength.

☐ Wrist motion
  - **Flexion:** move the palm toward the forearm.
  - **Flexion against resistance:** place your palm on the patient's palm and resist the patient's motion to determine strength.
  - **Extension:** movement of the palm from the forearm.
  - **tension against resistance:** place your palm on the posterior aspect of their hand and resist the movement of the palm from the forearm.
  - **Radial deviation:** movement of the hand toward the radial head.
  - **Radial deviation against resistance:** place your palm over the thumb of the hand and resist movement of the hand toward the radial head.
  - **Ulnar deviation:** movement of the hand toward the ulnar head.
  - **Ulnar deviation against resistance:** place your palm over the medial aspect of the hand and resist movement of the hand toward the ulnar head.
  - **Tinel's test** is performed to assess for carpal tunnel syndrome; with the patient's right palm facing up, tap on the median nerve (on the thumb side of the hand) (see Figure 16-31); if the patient complains of tingling or pain radiating to the thumb, index finger, or middle finger, perform the Phalen's test (Bostock, 2012). Repeat this assessment on the left hand.
  - Perform **Phalen's test:** Ask the patient to flex both wrists with the fingers extended and pointing downward and press them together for one full minute; ask the patient if he or she feels any tingling or numbness.

☐ **Finger motion**
- **Flexion:** movement of the fingers toward the palm into a fist-like position
- **Flexion against resistance:** have the patient attempt to squeeze two of your fingers.
- **Extension:** movement of the fingers out of the fist-like position into a straight and slightly flared position.
- **Extension against resistance:** movement of the fingers out of the fist-like position into a straight and slightly flared position. Have the patient try to open his or her fist against your palm that is over the patient's fingers.

3. Document your findings.

- All motions should be symmetric when compared to the same motion of the right and left upper extremities (see Chapter 16, Tables 16-1, 16-2, 16-3).
- The fingers should be able to flex fully, as demonstrated by making a closed fist, and extend as demonstrated by having the fingers flare out in a straight manner.
- Tinel's test: no pain, tingling, or numbness sensation felt in the wrist, hand, and fingers
- Strength of extremities: strength is graded on a scale of 0 to 5 (see Chapter 16, Table 16-4). It is the measurement of the muscles' ability to contract and work against a load.

ABNORMAL FINDINGS
- Anything less than expected full ROM can be considered to be an abnormal finding. It may be due to a new injury, old injury, a surgical procedure, or a neurological problem.
- Tinel's or Phelan's test produces pain or tingling sensations that may indicate carpal tunnel syndrome.
- Strength of less than 4 of 5. This indicates muscular weakness. The weakness may be due to injury or deconditioning.
- Pain when meeting resistance: this may indicate injury to the muscle. Document the motion and the strength grade. For example, elbow flexion 4/5 with pain.

TECHNIQUE 24-59: **Inspecting and Palpating the Lower Extremities**

Purpose: To assess for any abnormalities within the lower extremity

TIP When assessing the lower extremity, it is recommended that each extremity be fully exposed for this assessment.

ASSESSMENT STEPS
1. Explain the technique to the patient. You will ask the patient to perform specific motions independently first and then against resistance.
2. Ask the patient to perform the following ROM activities of the right and left lower extremities.
3. Inspect the lower extremity on the right side and then the left side; compare the right to the left side.

4. Using your finger pads, gently palpate the right and left lower extremities:

☐ Hip

☐ Knee

☐ Ankle

☐ Foot

☐ Toes

■ **TIP** Palpation of the lower extremities may be done with the patient on the examination table in a sitting or supine position.

5. Assess the presence of:

☐ tenderness

☐ depressions

☐ bulges

☐ change in temperature.

6. Document your findings.

SENC Safety Alert For the older patient, or patient who does not demonstrate good balance, the use of an examination table is preferred. The patient will need to sit and lay on the table to complete the assessment of the hips, knees, and ankles. For other patients, sitting on the table will allow for improved assessment of the knee, ankle, and foot.

NORMAL FINDINGS

■ No pain/tenderness, depressions or protrusions, swelling, increased joint size, or missing digits

■ When the patient is standing, the patient should be bearing weight on both lower extremities equally. There should be no forward flexing at the hip, and the upper leg should be straight.

■ The knees should be slightly flexed and pointed forward.

■ The ankle should be perpendicular to the straight lower leg.

■ The foot should be straight forward, in line with the knee, and a slight arch should be noted on the medial aspect of the foot.

ABNORMAL FINDINGS

■ The inability to bear weight equally on both lower extremities may indicate the presence of pain in one of the extremities.

■ A shortened extremity may indicate a bony injury, or be resultant from a disease or surgical procedure.

■ Forward flexion at the hip may indicate problems within the hip joint, tightness of the muscular structure around the hip, or a problem with the lower back.

■ Nonstraight upper leg may indicate a significant bony or muscular injury in the past. If the patient is able to bear weight, the injury is most likely old.

■ Knees that are straight may indicate a laxity in the ligaments supporting the knee or a problem with the bony structure of the knee.

- Knees that are more than slightly flexed may indicate increased bony buildup within the joint; a disease process; a loose body that locks the joint in this position; or an old injury. Sometimes the knee will appear rotated inward or outward. This is an indication of bony rotation above or below the knee.
- Lower legs that are not straight may indicate an injury to the bones or muscles. The ability to bear weight on this type of lower leg deformity indicates that it is not a new injury.
- **Generalized edema** in the lower extremity may indicate a circulatory problem. Note this in the documentation and inform the healthcare provider.
- Ankles that are not perpendicular to the lower leg indicate a lack of ROM within the ankle joint. This may be caused by tight tendons, bony deformity within the ankle joint or old injury, or surgery that caused a loss of normal joint function.
- A foot without a slight arch may be indicative of problems with the following: plantar fascia injuries, fallen arches, and old bony injuries.
- **Hallux valgus** (bunion) is a lateral deviation and an enlarged joint of the great toe.
- **Hammer toe** is a permanent contracted toe deformity; the proximal interphalangeal joint of the second, third, or fourth toe may be affected.

TECHNIQUE 24-60: **Assessing Range of Motion and Strength of the Lower Extremities**

Purpose: To assess strength and limitations in ROM in the lower extremities

TIP Always remember to compare one side with the other side.

ASSESSMENT STEPS

1. Explain the technique to the patient and tell the patient you will be assessing each lower extremity separately and the patient will have to perform specific motions without assistance.
2. Ask the patient to perform the following ROM activities without and with resistance of each lower extremity; assess any differences in symmetry of motion and the fluid nature of the motion.
   - ☐ Hip motion
     - **Flexion:** move the hip forward and toward the anterior aspect of the body.
     - **Flexion against resistance:** move the hip forward, toward the anterior aspect of the body. Place your palm on the anterior aspect of upper thigh and resist the motion.
     - **Extension:** move the hip backward, away from the anterior aspect of the body.
     - **Extension against resistance:** move the hip backward, away from the anterior aspect of the body. Place your palm on the posterior aspect of the upper thigh and resist the motion.
     - **Abduction:** move the lower extremity away from the midline of the body.
     - **Abduction against resistance:** move the lower extremity away from the midline of the body. Place your palm on the lateral aspect of the thigh, and resist the motion.

- **Adduction:** move the lower extremity toward the midline of the body.
- **Adduction against resistance:** move the lower extremity toward the midline of the body. Place your palm on the distal third of the medial aspect of the upper thigh, and resist the motion.

☐ Knee motion
- **Flexion:** movement of the heel toward the buttocks
- **Flexion against resistance:** movement of the heel toward the buttocks. Place your palm on the anterior aspect of the distal third of the lower leg, and resist the motion.
- **Extension:** movement of the lower extremity toward the anterior aspect of the body.
- **Extension against resistance:** movement of the lower extremity toward the anterior aspect of the body. Place your palm on the anterior aspect of the distal third of the lower leg, and resist the motion.

☐ Ankle motion
- **Dorsiflexion:** movement of the sole of the foot away from the floor, toward the knee.
- **Dorsiflexion against resistance:** movement of the sole of the foot away from the floor, toward the knee. Place your palm on the top of the foot, and resist the motion.
- **Plantar flexion:** movement of the sole of the foot toward the floor, away from the knee.
- **Plantar flexion against resistance:** movement of the sole of the foot toward the floor, away from the knee. Place your palm on the sole of the foot, and resist the motion.
- **Inversion:** movement of the great toe/foot toward the midline of the body.
- **Inversion against resistance:** movement of the great toe/foot toward the midline of the body. Place your palm on the medial aspect of the foot, and resist the motion.
- **Eversion:** movement of the great toe/foot away from the midline of the body.
- **Eversion against resistance:** movement of the great toe/foot away from the midline of the body. Place your palm on the lateral aspect of the foot, and resist the motion.

3. Document your findings.

NORMAL FINDINGS
- The ROM of each joint is symmetric when compared with the opposite limb. Motion is fluid and without restrictions. Motion is without pain.
- The patient should demonstrate strength of at least 4/5 in all of the motions in the lower extremities. Muscle strength is graded on a scale of 0 to 5 (see Chapter 16, Tables 16-5, 16-6, 16-7). It is the measurement of the muscles' ability to contract and work against resistance.
   ☐ Strength of extremities: strength is graded on a scale of 0 to 5. It is the measurement of the muscles' ability to contract and work against a load.

ABNORMAL FINDINGS
- The ROM of each joint is not symmetric to the opposite limb.
- Motion is not fluid. This may indicate a muscular strain.

- Limitation in ROM may indicate a problem in the joint or with the muscular strength.
- Pain is present with ROM activities. This may indicate injury to the muscle or joint.
- Alteration in strength with findings of 3/5 or less in one or more of the motions may indicate an injury to the muscle.
- Limitations in ROM against resistance may indicate a problem in the joint such as a loose body or a tendon getting caught when movement is attempted.
- Ability to resist at 4/5 or 5/5 for part of the ROM, but at a level of 3/5 or less for another part of the ROM. This may indicate that one of the muscles that performs the movement may be injured.

TECHNIQUE 24-61: **Get Up and Go Test**

Purpose: To assess patient's gait and balance and risk for falling

▧ **TIP** The test allows the patient to use any walking aids needed such as a cane or walker.

Equipment: Chair with arm rest, watch or clock with a second hand

ASSESSMENT STEPS

1. Explain to the patient that you will be giving him or her commands to follow and that this is a timed test. Give the patient one time to practice. The second attempt is timed.
2. Say "Go," to the patient, and start timing the test.
3. Give the command, "Stand up from the arm chair" (Fig. 24-23A).
4. Give the command, "Walk in a line for 3 meters or 10 feet."

   ▧ **TIP** Have a marking on the floor so that the patient knows where to stop walking.
5. Give the command "Turn around."
6. Give the command, "Walk back to the chair" (Fig. 24-23B).
7. Give the command, "Sit down" (Fig. 24-23C).
8. Time the second effort while assessing:
   ☐ postural stability
   ☐ steppage
   ☐ stride length
   ☐ sway

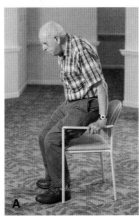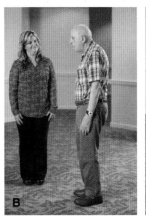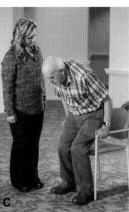

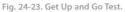
Fig. 24-23. Get Up and Go Test.

9. Document your findings.

NORMAL FINDINGS

- Completes task in 10 seconds or less
- Low scores correlate with good functional independence

ABNORMAL FINDINGS

- Completes task in greater than 10 seconds
- High scores correlate with poor functional independence and higher risk of falls (Mathias, Nayak, & Isaacs, 1986; Podsiadlo & Richardson, 1991).

PERIPHERAL VASCULAR SYSTEM

TECHNIQUE 24-62: **Inspecting and Palpating the Upper Extremities**

Purpose: To assess for peripheral circulation
Equipment: Gloves (only if there are open wounds or signs of bodily fluids), measuring tape
ASSESSMENT STEPS
1. Explain the technique to the patient.
2. Put on gloves.
3. Position the patient in a sitting or supine position.
4. Inspect each arm from the fingertips to the shoulder for:
   □ symmetry
   □ color
   □ texture
   □ edema.
5. Closely inspect the fingernail beds of both hands for:
   □ color
   □ nail thickness
   □ profile sign (clubbing of the nail plates is discussed in Chapter 12).
6. Using the dorsal surface of your hand, palpate the temperature of each arm; compare the temperatures of both arms.

7. Assess the epitrochlear lymph nodes by flexing the patient's elbow to about 90°. Hold the patient's left hand in your left hand and palpate with your left hand behind the patient's left elbow between biceps and triceps muscle; hold the patient's right hand in your right hand and palpate with your right hand behind the patient's right elbow between biceps and triceps muscle.
8. Assess the pulses in each arm by gently placing the second and third finger pads of your dominant hand on each of the following pulses (see Chapter 6, General Survey and Assessing Vital Signs).
   ☐ Radial pulse is palpated at the wrist on the radial artery.
   ☐ Brachial pulse is palpated at the medial side of the arm at the antecubital fossa space.
9. Document your findings.

NORMAL FINDINGS
- Arms are symmetrical.
- Color is uniform.
- No edema or ulcerations
- Fingernail beds pink
- Venous pattern normal
- Fingernails even thickness
- Fingernails 160° angle of attachment
- Temperature warm to touch
- Amplitude 2+ radial and brachial pulses

ABNORMAL FINDINGS
- Signs of altered peripheral circulation
- Discoloration, change in texture of skin, cool extremities, bilateral or unilateral edema
- Enlarged epitrochlear nodes (may indicate an infections of the hand or forearm or some types of blood cancer)

TECHNIQUE 24-63: Inspecting and Palpating the Lower Extremities

Purpose: To assess arterial or venous circulation
Equipment: Measuring tape, Doppler ultrasonic stethoscope (optional), Doppler gel, gloves
ASSESSMENT STEPS
1. Explain the technique to the patient.
2. Position the patient in the supine position.

3. Expose the lower legs from the groin to the feet making sure to keep the genitalia covered for privacy.

4. Inspect each leg from the groin to the toes for (Fig. 24-24):
- ☐ symmetry
- ☐ color
- ☐ texture
- ☐ edema
- ☐ venous pattern
- ☐ hair distribution
- ☐ ulcerations.

5. Closely inspect the toenail beds of both feet for:
- ☐ color
- ☐ nail thickness.

6. Using the dorsal surface of your hand, palpate the temperature of each leg; compare the temperatures of both legs.

7. Put on gloves.

8. Assess the pulses in the right and left lower extremities by gently placing your second and third finger pads of your dominant hand. Assess the rhythm, amplitude, and symmetry of each of the following pulses:
- ☐ Femoral pulse
- ☐ Popliteal pulses
- ☐ Dorsalis pedis pulse
- ☐ Posterior tibial pulse

9. Ask the patient to sit up on the side of the examining table, after approximately one minute, inspect the veins of the legs in the dependent position for distention.

10. Remove and discard gloves.

11. Document your findings.

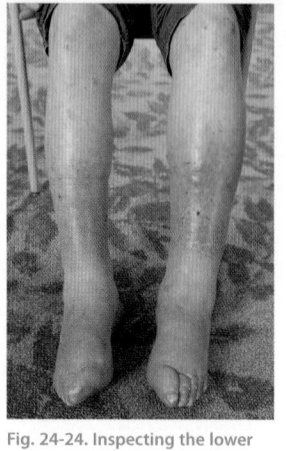

Fig. 24-24. Inspecting the lower legs.

NORMAL FINDINGS
- Legs are symmetrical.
- Color is uniform.
- No edema or ulceration is present.
- Toenails are pink with even thickness.
- Temperature is warm to touch bilaterally.

- Leg hair is evenly distributed; no ulcerations.
- Amplitude 2+ symmetrical, regular femoral, popliteal, dorsalis pedis, and posterior tibial pulses are noted.
- Venous pattern nondistended

ABNORMAL FINDINGS

- Color: discoloration (cyanosis, bright red, pale, or rubor) may indicate arterial or venous insufficiency; rubor color is a red/bluish color when the legs are in the dependent position (Fig. 24-25); indicates decreased circulation.
- Texture: decreased texture; thick leathery skin (venous insufficiency), dry and shiny skin (arterial insufficiency)
- Hair: loss of hair of one or both legs or feet (arterial insufficiency)
- Temperature: cool skin (arterial insufficiency)
- Toenails: thick (arterial insufficiency)

Pulses are diminished or absent (arterial insufficiency).

- Arterial or venous insufficiency wounds (see Chapter 15, Table 15-2)
- Presence of bilateral or unilateral edema
- Varicose veins (protruding veins of the lower extremities) resulting from incompetent valves; pooling of blood in the veins
- **Cellulitis** is a bacterial skin infection (Fig. 24-26).
- **Edema** is an accumulation of fluid seeping into the tissues; accumulation of fluid in the legs and feet is called peripheral edema (Fig. 24-27).
- **Ulcerations** (commonly occur with decreased circulation)
  □ Tissue ischemia is a risk factor for the development of foot ulcers; it also contributes to delayed wound healing. (See Chapter 15, Box 15-3.)

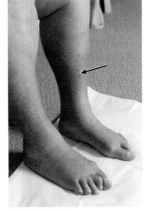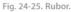

Fig. 24-25. Rubor.

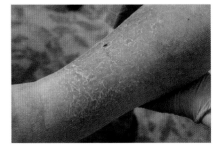

Fig. 24-26. Cellulitis.

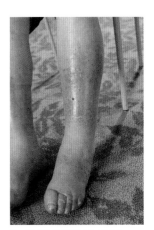

Fig. 24-27. Peripheral edema.

NEUROLOGICAL ASSESSMENT

Equipment Needed

Coffee beans
Cotton wisp
Flashlight
Gloves
Object with soft and sharp areas
Ophthalmoscope
Other scents
Pen with a cap
Pupil scale chart
Reflex hammer
Snellen chart
Teaspoon

Tongue blade
Tuning fork
Water

Sequence of Assessment

1. Inspection/observation
2. Neurological assessments (major categories):
    ☐ Level of consciousness and mental status
    ☐ Cranial nerve function
    ☐ Motor system
    ☐ Reflexes
    ☐ Sensory system

TECHNIQUE 24-64: **Assessing Cranial Nerve Function**

Purpose: To assess the function of the 12 pairs of cranial nerves

Technique 24-64A: **Assessing Sense of Smell (CN I)**

Purpose: To assess the sense of smell
Equipment: Coffee beans, other available scents.
■ **TIP** Make sure the patient's nostrils are patent and not clogged or congested.
ASSESSMENT STEPS
1. Explain the technique to the patient.
2. Ask the patient to close her or his eyes and occlude the right nostril.
3. Hold one of the available scents under the unoccluded left nostril, and ask the patient to sniff the scent.
4. Ask the patient to identify the scent.
5. Ask the patient to occlude the left nostril.

6. Hold a different available scent under the unoccluded right nostril
7. Ask the patient to identify the scent.
8. Document your findings.

NORMAL FINDINGS
- Able to state the correct scent on each side

ABNORMAL FINDINGS
- **Anosmia:** inability to smell or identify the correct scent, indicating loss of function to olfactory nerve

Technique 24-64B: **Inspecting Pupil Size and Consensual Pupil Response (CN II and CN III)**

Purpose: To assess the pupillary light reflex that controls the diameter of the pupil, and to assess the integrity of the optic pathways (consensual pupil response)

Equipment: Penlight, pupil measurement chart

TIP Prior to assessing the pupils, note any pre-existing abnormality such as cataracts, eye injury, and false eye. Note if patient is taking any medications that may cause pupillary dilation such as topical beta blockers and narcotics.

ASSESSMENT STEPS
1. Stand in front of the patient.
2. Use the penlight to inspect the pupils.
3. Assess color.
4. Assess shape of each pupil.
5. Assess symmetry.
6. Assess direct reaction. Shine light into the right eye pupil; right pupil should constrict.
7. Assess consensual reaction. Shine light into the right eye pupil and assess the left eye; left eye should constrict and have a consensual response.
8. Repeat steps 6 and 7 in the left eye.
9. Measure the size of each pupil in millimeters.
10. Document your findings.

NORMAL FINDINGS
- Pupil is round and black.
- Both pupils are equal size.
- Diameter is 2 to 8 mm.
- Both eyes have a direct and consensual response to direct light.

ABNORMAL FINDINGS
- Pupils are unequal in size or both dilated or constricted and fixed.
- Pupil does not have a direct and consensual response.

Technique 24-64C: **Assessing Sensation (CN V)**

Purpose: To assess sensation of the skin; to assess facial sensation

Equipment: Cotton wisp, paper clip

The trigeminal nerve is a motor and sensory nerve.

ASSESSMENT STEPS

1. Explain the technique to the patient.
2. Tell the patient that every time he or she feels the light wisp of cotton to say "now."
3. Ask the patient to close his or her eyes.
4. Standing in front of the patient, touch the patient lightly with the wisp of cotton on the following areas of the face:
   - ☐ Forehead
   - ☐ Right cheek
   - ☐ Left cheek
   - ☐ Jaw
5. Now, touch the patient lightly with the wisp of cotton on the following areas of the upper and lower extremities:
   - ☐ Upper arm bilaterally
   - ☐ Forearm bilaterally
   - ☐ Thigh bilaterally
   - ☐ Lower shin bilaterally
6. Ask the patient to open his or her eyes.
7. Explain the next assessment for identifying sharp and dull sensations.
8. Take an object with a sharp and dull side. Demonstrate on the patient's skin what "sharp and dull" will feel like.
9. Advise patient to close his or her eyes.
10. Use the object and follow steps 4 and 5, alternating patterns between sharp and dull.
11. Document the findings.

NORMAL FINDINGS

■ Light, sharp, and dull sensations are felt in all sites.

ABNORMAL FINDINGS

■ Light, sharp, or dull sensations are not felt at a site; this may indicate a peripheral nerve disorder.

Technique 24-64D: **Assessing Jaw Movement (CNV)**

Purpose: To assess the motor portion of this cranial nerve.

ASSESSMENT STEPS

1. Explain the technique to the patient.
2. Advise patient to open his or her eyes.

3. Ask the patient clench his or her teeth (to test motor component).

4. Palpate the temporal and masseter muscles, just above the mandibular angle; ask the patient to open and close his or her jaw and move the jaw side to side.

5. Document your findings.

NORMAL FINDINGS

- Patient can clench teeth tightly.
- Masseter muscles bulge when teeth are clenched.
- On palpation, both masseter muscles feel equal in size and strength.

ABNORMAL FINDINGS

- **Trigeminal neuralgia** is indicated when the patient cannot clench jaw and move jaw side to side.

Technique 24-64E: Assessing Cranial Nerve VII (Facial Nerve)

Purpose: To assess facial movements

The facial nerve is a motor and sensory nerve.

ASSESSMENT STEPS

1. Explain the technique to the patient.

2. Stand in front of the patient.

3. Assess patient's ability to perform the following facial movements. Ask the patient to:

    ☐ smile

    ☐ frown

    ☐ puff out his or her cheeks

    ☐ close eyes and try to open eyes against resistance.

4. Document your findings.

NORMAL FINDINGS

- Patient is able to smile, frown, and puff out cheeks.
- Muscles are symmetrical.
- Eyes do not open against resistance.

ABNORMAL FINDINGS

- Asymmetrical muscles while smiling, frowning, or puffing out cheeks
    ☐ **Drooping of one side of face and/or mouth** can indicate stroke.
- Eyes open against resistance.

Technique 24-64F: **Assessing Cranial Nerve IX (Glossopharyngeal Nerve) and Cranial Nerve X (Vagus Nerve)**

Purpose: To assess pharyngeal sensation and function, and the presence or absence of a gag reflex

Equipment: Gloves, tongue blade, teaspoon, water

■ **TIP** This may be a difficult assessment for older patients because they have to keep their mouth open. Wetting the tongue blade prior to assessing the gag reflex may provide less discomfort.

ASSESSMENT STEPS

1. Explain the technique to the patient.

2. Put on gloves.

3. Ask the patient to open his or her mouth.

4. Gently touch the posterior aspect of tongue or pharynx with the tip of the tongue blade to initiate a gag reflex.

5. If gag reflex is absent, assess for pharyngeal sensation by asking the patient to close his or her eyes.

6. Instruct the patient to lift the right or left hand to the side in which the patient feels the tip of the tongue blade. If the tip is felt on the correct side, this indicates positive pharyngeal sensation.

7. Touch the tongue blade to right side of pharynx.

8. Remind the patient to lift the arm on the side where the patient is feeling the sensation.

9. Touch the tongue blade to the left side of the pharynx.

10. Remind the patient to lift his or her arm on the side he or she is feeling the sensation.

11. Assess vocal quality by asking the patient to say "ah, ah, ah."

12. Assess the bilateral symmetry of the elevation of the soft palate and central location of uvula.

13. Ask patient to swallow a teaspoon of water.

14. Assess the movement of the throat.

15. Document your findings.

NORMAL FINDINGS

■ Positive gag reflex

■ Positive pharyngeal sensation bilaterally

■ Clear voice

■ Able to swallow

ABNORMAL FINDINGS

■ Absent gag reflex

■ Absent or unilateral pharyngeal sensation indicates dysphagia

■ Difficulty with swallowing indicates dysphagia

■ Coarse raspy voice indicates poor pharyngeal function.

Technique 24-64G: **Assessing Cranial Nerve XI (Spinal Accessory Muscle)**

Purpose: To assess the strength of the sternocleidomastoid and trapezius muscles

ASSESSMENT STEPS

1. Explain the technique to the patient.

2. Have the patient sit on the end of the bed or examining table.

3. Stand in front of the patient.

4. Ask the patient to shrug shoulders against resistance as you push down on the shoulders; assess the strength of both shoulders.

5. Ask the patient to turn his or her head to the right side against the resistance of your hand; assess the strength of the right side of the face.

6. Ask the patient to turn his or her head to the left side against the resistance of your hand; assess the strength of the left side of the face.

7. Document your findings.

NORMAL FINDINGS

■ Ability to shrug both shoulders against resistance using equal strength on both sides.

■ Turn head both ways against resistance with equal strength on each side.

ABNORMAL FINDINGS

■ Inability to shrug shoulders or turn head against resistance may indicate paralysis or lesion to the accessory nerve (Hickey, 2014).

Technique 24-64H: **Assessing Cranial Nerve XII (Hypoglossal Nerve)**

Purpose: To assess movement of tongue

ASSESSMENT STEPS

1. Explain the technique to the patient.

2. Ask the patient to stick out tongue and inspect the tongue for:

☐ symmetry

☐ alignment.

3. Ask the patient to move the tongue from side to side.

4. Document your findings.

NORMAL FINDINGS

■ Tongue is symmetrical and midline without tremor

■ Tongue moves smoothly from side to side

ABNORMAL FINDINGS

■ Tongue is not mid-line or has tremors; this can indicate paralysis or stroke, or a lesion of cranial nerve XII (Hickey, 2014).

Technique 24-64I: **Assessing Gait and Position Sense**

Purpose: To assess balance, coordination, muscle strength, and tone

■ **TIP** Older adults may not be able to perform some the steps in this assessment, do not push your patient if they cannot perform the assessment. Safety is always priority.

ASSESSMENT STEPS

1. Explain the technique to the patient.
2. Identify a specific distance that you want the patient to walk to in the room.
3. Ask the patient to walk from you first and then back toward you. This allows for both anterior and posterior observation of gait, balance, and posture.
4. Ask the patient to walk on his or her toes and return walking toward you on his or her heels; this allows you to assess balance.
5. Instruct the patient to walk heel-to-toe away from you and back toward you; this is called tandem walking. Tandem walking assesses for muscular weakness.
6. Ask the patient to hop on the right foot and then alternate to the left foot; this assesses position sense and cerebellar function.
7. Ask the patient to do a shallow knee bend; this assesses muscular weakness.
8. Document your findings.

NORMAL FINDINGS

■ Gaits, hopping, and knee bends are stable, smooth, and coordinated.

ABNORMAL FINDINGS

■ Gaits lack stability, smoothness, and coordination.
■ Ataxia

SENC Safety Alert As an individual ages, he or she may experience muscle weakness and an unstable gait placing the individual at risk for falls.

Technique 24-64J: **Heel-to-Shin Test**

Purpose: To assess coordination of movement and position sense

SENC Safety Alert Patient should be in the supine position to prevent a fall.

ASSESSMENT STEPS

1. Explain the technique to the patient.
2. With the patient in the supine position, ask the patient to place the heel of his or her right leg on the left knee and slowly run it down the shin to the left ankle; assess smoothness and coordination.
3. Repeat step 2 using the left leg.
4. Have the patient close his or her eyes, and repeat steps 2 and 3; this assesses position sense.
5. Document your findings.

■ Movement of leg is smooth and coordinated.

■ Heel that does not stay on the shin or moves from side to side while running down the shin may indicate cerebellar disease or loss of motor coordination.

Technique 24-64K: **Finger-to-Nose Test**

Purpose: To assess cerebellar function, coordination, and point-to-point movements

ASSESSMENT STEPS

1. Explain the technique to the patient.
2. Hold your index finger in front of the patient at eye level.
3. Ask the patient to touch the tip of your index finger and then touch the tip of his or her nose with his or her right index finger.
4. Repeat several times while you are moving your finger a few inches in each direction up, down, right, and left, each time the patient attempts to touch your finger by extending his or her arm.
5. Repeat steps 2, 3, and 4 with the patient's left index finger.
6. Hold your finger in one place, and have the patient touch it several times.
7. Ask the patient to now close his or her eyes, and using his or her right index finger, have the patient touch your finger several times; repeat using the left index finger with eyes closed.
8. Document your findings.

NORMAL FINDINGS

■ Patient touches the nurse's finger and nose accurately and smoothly in all locations.
■ Patient touches the nurse's finger accurately and smoothly in the one location with eyes closed.

ABNORMAL FINDINGS

■ Patient's finger is unsteady and unable to touch the moving target.
■ Patient is unsteady and unable to touch the stationary finger with the eyes closed
■ Dysmetria is the inability to perform point-to-point movements.

Technique 24-64L: **Assessing Rapid Alternating Movements**

Purpose: To assess coordination

ASSESSMENT STEPS

1. Explain the technique to the patient.

   ■ **TIP** If the older adult has difficulty understanding, demonstrate and ask them to follow what you are doing.

2. Upper extremities: Ask the patient to place both hands palm down on his or her thighs.

3. Lift both hands and place both hands palm up on his or her thighs.

4. Ask the patient to repeat these alternating movements for 10 seconds.

5. Observe the alternating movements for speed and smoothness.

6. Lower extremities: Ask the patient to rapidly pat your hand using the ball of the right foot for 10 seconds; observe speed and smoothness.

7. Repeat step 6 on the left foot.

8. Document the findings.

NORMAL FINDINGS

■ Coordinated and smooth movements of both hands

■ Coordinated and smooth movements of both feet

ABNORMAL FINDINGS

■ **Dysdiadochokinesis** is uncoordinated, slow, and clumsy movements; may be a sign of cerebellar disease, Parkinson's disease, or multiple sclerosis.

Technique 24-64M: **Pronator Drift**

Purpose: To assess motor function and proprioception

This assessment can be performed standing or sitting.

ASSESSMENT STEPS

1. Explain the technique to the patient.

2. Ask the patient to extend both arms out with palms up.

3. Ask the patient to close his or her eyes and observe the patient's arms for change in position for 20 to 30 seconds.

4. Document your findings.

NORMAL FINDINGS

■ Negative Pronator Drift: arms should remain in the extended position without drifting.

ABNORMAL FINDINGS

■ Positive Pronator Drift: an arm does not remain raised, the palm may pronate or drop slightly

Technique 24-64N: **Romberg's Test**

Purpose: To assess position sense and cerebellar function, balance, and coordination.

ASSESSMENT STEPS

1. Explain the technique to the patient.

2. Ask the patient to stand with feet together and arms at sides and look straight ahead for 30 seconds without any support.

3. Assess for any swaying to either side or loss of balance.

4. Now, with the patient in this position, stand on the side of the patient and extend your hands in the front and back of the patient for patient safety.

5. Ask the patient to close her or his eyes and continue to stand in this position for 30 seconds; observe for swaying and balance.

6. Document your findings.

SENC Safety Alert Keep your hands in front and back of the patient in case the patient starts to sway or fall.

NORMAL FINDINGS
- **Negative Romberg's test:** Maintains position without swaying or falling to one side, with and without opening eyes.

ABNORMAL FINDINGS
- **Positive Romberg's test:** swaying or falling to one side may indicate cerebellar dysfunction, or lesions in the cerebellum or spinal cord.

TECHNIQUE 24-65: **Assessing Sensory Function**

Purpose: To assess for any loss in function to sensory nerves. The following techniques will be used when the examiner has detected sensory function or it is known that the patient has spinal cord disease.

Technique 24-65A: **Assessing Graphesthesia**
Purpose: To assess the sensation of touch or tactile stimulation

ASSESSMENT STEPS
1. Explain the technique to the patient.
2. Have patient extend right arm and turn palm face up toward ceiling.
3. Ask patient to close eyes.
4. Write a letter or number on the right palm, and ask patient to state which letter or number was written.
5. Repeat steps 2, 3, and 4 on the left palm.
6. Document your findings.

NORMAL FINDINGS
- Patient is able to feel and state letter or number correctly on each side.

ABNORMAL FINDINGS
- Patient is unable to feel and state the letter or number on each side.

Technique 24-65B: **Assessing Stereognosis**
Purpose: To assess the perception of a shape of an object

ASSESSMENT STEPS
1. Explain the technique to the patient.
2. Ask patient to close his or her eyes.

3. Put a small object in the palm of the patient's right hand.

4. Ask the patient to identify the object.

5. Using a different object, repeat steps 2, 3, and 4 using the left hand.

6. Document your findings.

NORMAL FINDINGS

- Patient is able to perceive and identify the shape of the object.

ABNORMAL FINDINGS

- Tactile Agnosia is the inability to process sensory information and to perceive and recognize an object by touch; caused by lesions in the brain's parietal lobe.

Fall Risk Assessment

Falls are a public health problem that is largely preventable. One of three adults over the age of 65 falls each year but less than half tell their healthcare provider (CDC, 2016). Older adults are at greater risk for falls due to sensory, gait, and cognitive impairments. Patients who fall once continue to have the fear of falling again especially if they had a traumatic injury. This fear causes restrictions in activities and mobility, which can shorten the life span (Hendrich, Bender, & Nyhuis, 2003). Assess for risk factors:

- Advancing age
- Cognitive impairment
- Environmental factors
- Functional limitations
- Gait instability
- Incontinence
- Medications
- Muscle weakness
- More than one chronic illness
- Previous history of falls

 TIP Document whether the fall was witnessed or unwitnessed. If witnessed, ask the witness, "*What did you see? Did the person hit his or her head?*"

When assessing a patient directly after the fall occurred, the priority assessments are:

- assess airway
- assess breathing
- assess circulation
- assess whether the patient hit his head
- assess vital signs.

Many patients fracture a bone during a fall. Identifying information prior to, during, and after the fall is also important. A mnemonic for assessing an actual fall is:

S Symptoms experienced at the time of the fall (i.e., dizziness)
P Previous number of falls or near-falls
L Location of falls
A Activity engaged in or attempted at time of fall
T Time (hour) of fall
T Trauma (e.g., physical or psychological) associated with falls (Tideiksaar, 1998)

■ **TIP** The Medi Alert device is a simple push button device worn around the neck or on the wrist; the individual pushes the button that alerts a call center that help is needed (Fig. 24-28). Nurses should provide safety education about this device.

In acute care, a best practice approach incorporates use of the Hendrich II Fall Risk Model™ (Table 24-2) which is quick to administer and provides a determination of risk for falling based on:

■ gender
■ mental and emotional status
■ symptoms of dizziness
■ known categories of medications increasing risk (Hendrich et al., 2003). This assessment tool screens for primary prevention and is essential in a post-fall assessment for secondary prevention of falls (Hendrich et al., 2003).

Assessing Frailty

The most problematic expression of the population aging is the clinical condition of frailty. Frailty develops as a consequence

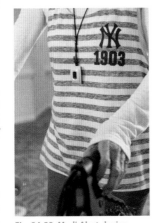

Fig. 24-28. Medi Alert device.

TABLE 24-2 Hendrich II Fall Risk Model

Risk Factor	Risk Points	Score
Confusion/Disorientation/Impulsivity	4	
Symptomatic Depression	2	
Altered Elimination	1	
Dizziness/Vertigo	1	
Gender (Male)	1	
Any Administered Antiepileptics (anticonvulsants) (Carbamazepine, Divalproex Sodium, Ethotoin, Ethosuximide, Felbamate, Fosphenytoin, Gabapentin, Lamotrigine, Mephenytoin, Methsuximide, Phenobarbital, Phenytoin, Primidone, Topiramate, Trimethadione, Valproic Acid)[1]	2	
Any Administered Benzodiazepines:[2] (alprazolam, Chlordiazepoxide, Clonazepam, Clorazepate Dipotassium, Diazepam, Flurazepam, Halazepam,[3] Lorazepam, Midazolam, Oxazepam, Temazepam, Triazolam)	1	
Get Up and Go Test: "Rising From a Chair" If unable to assess, monitor for change in activity level, assess other risk factors, document on patient chart with date and time.		
Ability to rise in single movement: no loss of balance with steps	0	
Pushes up, successful in one attempt	1	
Multiple attempts but successful	3	
Unable to rise without assistance during test If unable to assess, document this on the patient chart with the date and time	4	
(A score of 5 or greater = High Risk)	Total Score	

of age-related decline in many physiological systems, which collectively results in vulnerability to sudden health status changes and functional status (Clegg, Young, Iliffe, Rikkert, & Rockwood, 2013). Frail individuals are at high risk for falls, disability, hospitalization, and mortality (Fried et al., 2001).

- Adults at risk for becoming frail are individuals with the following impairments:
  - ☐ Medical
  - ☐ Emotional
  - ☐ Nutritional
  - ☐ Cognitive
  - ☐ Activity (Venes, 2013, p. 972)
- Symptoms and clinical presentation of frailty include:
  - ☐ weakness
  - ☐ fatigue
  - ☐ unexplained weight loss
  - ☐ muscle wasting
  - ☐ frequent infections
  - ☐ balance and gait impairments
  - ☐ acute confusion such as with delirium
  - ☐ fluctuating disability: day-to-day instability, resulting in a patient having "good" and "bad" days on which professional care is often needed (Clegg et al., 2013)

TIP Sarcopenia (loss of muscle mass with aging) is a key manifestation of frailty; frail patients are most vulnerable to safety issues (Fried, Walston, & Ferrucci, 2009).

Assess the patient for the presence of three of the eight components:

- Unintentional weight loss
- Decreased activity and engagement
- Self-reported exhaustion
- Low energy expenditure
- Weakness
- Balance and gait abnormalities
- Cognitive impairment
- Slow walking speed (Fried et al., 2001)

Cognitive Assessment

Psychological and cognitive impairment is correlated with decreased quality of life and functional deficits. Cognitive decline can cause changes in:

- short-term memory
- long-term memory
- mentation, such as confusion.

Some questions that you may want to ask the patient (if the patient is reliable) or with permission, ask family, caregivers, or significant others are:

- Do you have any family history of mental illness or dementia?
- Have you had any recent falls?
- Are you able to care for yourself?
- Has there been a change in your sleep patterns?
- Has there been a change in your daily activities or ability to care for yourself?
- Have you noticed a change in your mental function? If so, when did this change begin?

Mini-Cog Assessment is a simple screening tool to identify early mental decline and mild cognitive decline (Appendix 24-3).

- This tool uses a three-item recall test to assess memory and a simple scored clock-drawing test that takes about 3 minutes to administer.
- The Mini-Cog is less affected by the older adult's ethnicity, language, and education (Borson, Scanlan, Brush, Vitaliano, & Dokmak, 2000).

Assessing the Three "Ds"—Dementia, Delirium, and Depression

Cognitive disorders commonly seen in the older adult are

- **Dementia:** a progressive, irreversible, decline in mental function, marked by memory impairment and, often deficits in:
  - ☐ reasoning
  - ☐ judgment
  - ☐ abstract thought
  - ☐ registration
  - ☐ comprehension
  - ☐ learning
  - ☐ task execution

Instructions: Score 1 point for each bolded answer. A score of 5 or more suggests depression.

1. Are you basically satisfied with your life?	Yes	**No**
2. Have you dropped many of your activities and interests?	**Yes**	No
3. Do you feel that your life is empty?	**Yes**	No
4. Do you often get bored?	**Yes**	No
5. Are you in good spirits most of the time?	Yes	**No**
6. Are you afraid that something bad is going to happen to you?	**Yes**	No
7. Do you feel happy most of the time?	Yes	**No**
8. Do you often feel helpless?	**Yes**	No
9. Do you prefer to stay at home, rather than going out and doing new things?	**Yes**	No
10. Do you feel you have more problems with memory than most?	**Yes**	No
11. Do you think it is wonderful to be alive now?	Yes	**No**
12. Do you feel pretty worthless the way you are now?	**Yes**	No
13. Do you feel full of energy?	Yes	**No**
14. Do you feel that your situation is hopeless	**Yes**	No
15. Do you think that most people are better off than you?	**Yes**	No
Total score	___	/15

Fig. 24-29. Geriatric Depression Scale. From the Aging Clinical Research Center (ACRC), a joint project of Stanford University and the VA Palo Alto Health Care System.

☐ use of language (Venes, 2013).

☐ The **AD8** is an 8-item questionnaire that distinguishes between people who have dementia and people who do not have dementia. The AD8 has a yes or no format and takes only 3 minutes or so to complete (Rosenzweig, 2010). The questions may be given to the patient for self-administration or the patient's informant (usually a spouse, child, or nonfamily caregiver) who is asked to assess whether there have been changes in the past few years in certain areas of cognition and functioning, including:
  - Memory
  - Orientation
  - Executive functioning
  - Interest in activities

■ **Delirium:** an acute, reversible state of disorientation and confusion

☐ It is the the most acute condition of the three Ds and is a true medical emergency (Lang, 2012). The development of delirium is complex. Among elderly patients, dementia is the most prominent risk factor, being present in up to two-thirds of all cases of delirium (Fong, Tulebaev, & Inouye, 2009).

■ **Depression:** mood disorder marked by loss of interest or pleasure in living (Venes, 2013)

☐ Depression is a common problem among older adults, but it is not a normal part of aging. Depression in older adults may be difficult to recognize because the older adult has less obvious symptoms (NIH Senior Health, 2016).

☐ The USPSTF (2009) recommends screening older adults for depression when staff-assisted depression care supports are in place to assure accurate diagnosis, effective treatment, and follow-up.

☐ The **Geriatric Depression Scale** (short form) is a 15-question assessment survey for depression (Fig. 24-29). The short form is scored by the answers indicating depression are in bold and italicized; score one point for each one selected. A score of 0 to 5 is normal. A score greater than 5 suggests depression.

PATIENT TEACHING

Healthy People 2020

Goal: Improve the health, function, and quality of life of older adults (HHS, 2010). The 12 objectives related to the older adult may be found at https://www.healthypeople.gov/2020/topics-objectives/topic/older-adults/objectives

Preventive health services are valuable for maintaining the quality of life of older adults. Nurses need to take time to educate and carefully explain health promotion practices. Patient teaching includes verbal and written instructions.

■ Handouts given to older adults should be easy to read; font may need to be larger than 12 font.

- Due to poor eyesight or illiteracy, some older adults cannot read; ask the patient to read a portion of the handout to you to assess the patient's ability to read and follow directions. Family members and caregivers are critical to assist and care for these individuals.

Health Promotion and Preventive Services

Older adults need to have education related to maintaining their health and well-being. The Affordable Care Act, the health insurance reform legislation passed by Congress and signed into law by President Obama on March 23, 2010, provides for affordable and accessible health care for all Americans, including those enrolled in Medicare. People on Medicare no longer have to pay any out-of-pocket costs for most preventive services. Medicare covers the cost of an annual wellness visit; the following services are now available free of charge to the patient:

- Routine measurements such as your height, weight, BP, body-mass index (or waist circumference, if appropriate)
- Review of your medical and family history, including medications and current care by other healthcare providers
- A personal risk assessment (including any mental health conditions)
- A review of your functional ability and level of safety, including an assessment of any cognitive impairment and screening for depression
- The following preventive services that Medicare currently covers are provided free of charge to the patient:
  - ☐ Mammograms every 12 months for eligible beneficiaries age 40 and older
  - ☐ Colorectal cancer screening, including flexible sigmoidoscopy or colonoscopy
  - ☐ Cervical cancer screening, including a Pap smear test and pelvic examination
  - ☐ Cholesterol and other cardiovascular screenings
  - ☐ Diabetes screening
  - ☐ Medical nutrition therapy to help people manage diabetes or kidney disease
  - ☐ Prostate cancer screening
  - ☐ Bone mass measurement
  - ☐ Abdominal aortic aneurysm screening to check for a bulging blood vessel

Immunizations

Immunizations protect against vaccine preventable diseases. Immunizations recommended for older adults are:

- Tetanus/diphtheria/pertussis (Tdap) is recommended for adults 65 years and younger if they have not received this vaccine previously; also older adults who have contact with infants 12 months of age and younger.
- Influenza vaccine is recommended annually for all older adults; protects against the influenza virus.
- Pneumococcal vaccine is recommended for all adults ages 65 and older; protects against pneumonia.
- Zoster vaccine is recommended for all adults age 60 and older to protect against shingles, the same virus as the chicken pox.

Fall Prevention

- Encourage the patient to exercise regularly. It is important that the exercises focus on increasing leg strength and improving balance, and that they get more challenging over time. Tai Chi programs are especially good.
- Tell patients to ask their doctor or pharmacist to review their medicines (both prescription and over-the-counter) to identify medicines that may cause side effects or interactions such as dizziness or drowsiness.
- Discuss adequate calcium and vitamin D intake from food and supplements.

- Have eyes checked at least once a year; prescription lenses should be updated to maximize vision.
- Instruct patients how to make their homes safer by reducing tripping hazards, adding grab bars inside and outside the tub or shower and next to the toilet, adding railings on both sides of stairways, and improving the lighting (CDC, 2014b).

Advanced Directives

- An advanced directive is a legal document identifying the individual's types of decisions that might need to be made, considering those decisions ahead of time, and then letting others know about his or her preferences. This directive goes into effect only if the individual is incapacitated and unable to speak for him- or herself (National Institute on Aging, 2016).
- During the assessment, the patient should be asked about whether they have a living will or advanced directive document. More than one out of four older Americans face questions about medical treatment near the end of life but are not capable of making those decisions (National Institute on Aging, 2012).
- Discussing advance care directives is essential during an assessment. As one ages, older adults need to give some thoughts about their end-of-life wishes and decisions.

Barthel Activities of Daily Living (ADL) Index

Scoring: When assessment is complete, total the score.
Specify the informant when the Barthel Index is done in the community.

Patient ☐ Main support person ☐ Both ☐ Other ☐

If other, specify who _____

Mobility indoors: 0 Immobile 1 Wheelchair independent (including corners/doors) 2 Help of one untrained person, including supervision 3 Independent (may use aid)	☐
Transfers 0 Unable– no sitting balance, two to life 1 Major help: physical help, 1 strong/ skilled or 2 normal 2 Minor help: 1 person easily or supervision for safety 3 Independent	☐
Stairs 0 Unable 1 Needs help (verbal/physical, carrying aid) 2 Independent up and down, carrying walking aid	☐
Toilet Use 0 Dependent 1 Needs help but can do something (including wiping self) 2 Continent over 7 days	☐
Bladder 0 Incontinent or catheterized and unable to manage 1 Occasional accident (maximum once/ 24 hours) 2 Continent over 7 days	☐
Bowels 0 Incontinent (or needs to be given and enema) 1 Occasional accident (less than 1/week) 2 Continent over 7 days	☐
Bathing 0 Dependent 1 Independent Bath must be in and out unsupervised, wash self Shower: unsupervised/ unaided	☐
Grooming 0 Dependent 1 Independent: implemented can be provided by helper	☐
Dressing 0 Dependent 1 Needs help in cutting up food, spreading butter, etc, but feeds self 2 Independent (food cooked served and provided within reach but not cut up. Normal food (not only soft food)	☐

From Wade, D., Collins, C. (1988) The Barthel ADL index: a standard measure of physical disability. *International disability Studies*, 10, 64–67.

Appendix 24-1. Barthel Activities of Daily Living (ADL) Index. (From Wade, D., & Collin, C., [1988]. The Barthel ADL index: A standard measure of physical disability. *International Disability Studies, 10,* 64–67.)

Mini Nutritional Assessment
MNA®

Nestlé
NutritionInstitute

Last name:		First name:	
Sex:	Age:	Weight, Kg:	Height, cm:	Date:

Complete the screen by filling in the boxes with the appropriate numbers. Total the numbers for the final screening score.

Screening

A Has food intake declined over the past 3 months due to loss of appetite, digestive problems, chewing or swallowing difficulties?
0 = severe decrease in food intake
1 = moderate decrease in food intake
2 = no decrease in food intake ☐

B Weight loss during the last 3 months
0 = weight loss greater than 3 kg (6.6 lbs)
1 = does not know
2 = weight loss between 1 and 3 kg (2.2 and 6.6 lbs)
3 = no weight loss ☐

C Mobility
0 = bed or chair bound
1 = able to get out of bed / chair but does not go out
2 = goes out ☐

D Has suffered psychological stress or acute disease in the past 3 months?
0 = yes   2 = no ☐

E Neuropsychological problems
0 = severe dementia or depression
1 = mild dementia
2 = no psychological problems ☐

F1 Body Mass Index (BMI) (weight in kg) / (height in m)^2
0 = BMI less than 19
1 = BMI 19 to less than 21
2 = BMI 21 to less than 23
3 = BMI 23 or greater ☐

IF BMI IS NOT AVAILABLE, REPLACE QUESTION F1 WITH QUESTION F2.
DO NOT ANSWER QUESTION F2 IF QUESTION F1 IS ALREADY COMPLETED.

F2 Calf circumference (CC) in cm
0 = CC less than 31
3 = CC 31 or greater ☐

Screening score (max. 14 points) ☐☐

12 - 14 points: Normal nutritional status
8 - 11 points: At risk of malnutrition
0 - 7 points: Malnourished

References
1. Vellas B, Villars H, Abellan G, et al. Overview of the MNA® - Its History and Challenges. J Nutr Health Aging. 2006;**10**:456-465.
2. Rubenstein LZ, Harker JO, Salva A, Guigoz Y, Vellas B. Screening for Undernutrition in Geriatric Practice: Developing the Short-Form Mini Nutritional Assessment (MNA-SF). J. Geront. 2001;**56A**: M366-377.
3. Guigoz Y. The Mini-Nutritional Assessment (MNA®) Review of the Literature - What does it tell us? J Nutr Health Aging. 2006; **10**:466-487.
4. Kaiser MJ, Bauer JM, Ramsch C, et al. Validation of the Mini Nutritional Assessment Short-Form (MNA®-SF): A practical tool for identification of nutritional status. J Nutr Health Aging. 2009; **13**:782-788.
® Société des Produits Nestlé, S.A., Vevey, Switzerland, Trademark Owners © Nestle, 1994, Revision 2009. N67200 12/99 10M
For more information: www.mna-elderly.com

Appendix 24-2. Mini-Nutrition Assessment (MNA). (MNA is a registered trademark from the Société des Produits Nestlé S.A. MNA is also a registered trademark of Société des Produits Nestlé S.A.)

MINI-COG™

ADMINISTRATION	SPECIAL INSTRUCTIONS
1. Get patient's attention and ask him or her to remember three unrelated words. Ask patient to repeat the words to ensure the learning was correct.	• Allow patient three tries, then go to next item. • The following word lists have been validated in a clinical study.[1-3] **Version 1** • Banana • Sunrise • Chair **Version 2** • Daughter • Heaven • Mountain **Version 3** • Village • Kitchen • Baby **Version 4** • River • Nation • Finger **Version 5** • Captain • Garden • Picture **Version 6** • Leader • Season • Table
2. Ask patient to draw the face of a clock. After numbers are on the face, ask patient to draw hands to read 10 minutes after 11:00 (or 20 minutes after 8:00).	• Either a blank piece of paper or a preprinted circle (other side) may be used. • A correct response is all numbers placed in approximately the correct positions AND the hands pointing to the 11 and 2 (for the 4 and 8). • These two specific times are more sensitive than others. • A clock should not be visible to the patient during this task. • Refusal to draw a clock is scored abnormal. • Move to next step if clock not complete within three minutes.
3. Ask the patient to recall the three words from Step 1.	Ask the patient to recall the three words you stated in Step 1.

3 recalled words — Negative for cognitive impairment
1-2 recalled words + normal CDT — Negative for cognitive impairment
1-2 recalled words + abnormal CDT — Positive for cognitive impairment
0 recalled words — Positive for cognitive impairment

1. Borson S, Scanlan J, Brush M, Vitaliano P, Dokmak A. The mini-cog: a cognitive "vital signs" measure for dementia screening in multi-lingual elderly. Int J Geriatr Psychiatry. 2000;15(11):1021-1027.
2. Borson S, Scanlan JM, Chen P, Ganguli M. The Mini-Cog as a screen for dementia: validation in a population-based sample. J Am Geriatr Soc. 2003;51(10):1451-1454.
3. McCarten JR, Anderson P, Kuskowski MA et al. Finding dementia in primary care: the results of a clinical demonstration project. J Am Geriatr Soc. 2012;60(2):210-217.

Mini-Cog™ Copyright S Borson. Reprinted with permission of the author (soob@uw.edu). All rights reserved.

800.272.3900 | alz.org®

alzheimer's association®

Appendix 24-3. Mini-Cog Assessment.